CARDIAC HYPERTROPHY

CONTRIBUTORS

R. Albin
Norman R. Alpert
Ruth A. Altschuld
Ezra A. Amsterdam
V. Aschenbrenner
Anthony C. L. Barnard
William A. Baxley
M. Beznak
Oscar H. L. Bing
Sanford P. Bishop
John P. Boineau
F. Norman Briggs
Stanley A. Briller
Arnold L. Brown, Jr.
Robert A. Buccino
Henry Neal Coleman
Laval N. Cothran
A. Cutilletta
H. Davis Dear
Harold T. Dodge
Milton Draper
Paul Dreizen
Barry L. Fanburg
Donald A. Fischman
Vincent J. Fisher
L. W. Forney
Arthur C. Fox
John Gergely
Lewis C. Gershman
Edward W. Gertz
David B. Geselowitz
K. E. Giger
Alfred L. Goldberg
M. J. Goodkind
Richard J. Goss
N. J. Gross
D. Grove
Burt B. Hamrell
Edward D. Harris, Jr.
Edward W. Hawthorne
Paul F. Hoar
John H. Holt, Jr.
William P. Hood, Jr.
Paul H. Jewett
L. S. Jefferson
Horton A. Johnson
William B. Jones
Arnold M. Katz
Frederick Kavaler
Robert R. Kohn
B. Korecky
Frances Kraft-Hunter
John O. Kramer, Jr.
E. M. Kritcher
Allan M. Lefer
Michael Lesch
Herbert J. Levine
R. J. Luchi
Dean T. Mason
Satoru Matsushita
H. E. Morgan
E. Neil Moore
Eugene Morkin
A. A. Moscona
K. G. Nair
M. Oratz
Peter E. Pool
Barry I. Posner
Murray Rabinowitz
Charles E. Rackley
M. A. Rothschild
Harold Sandler
Sidney S. Schreiber
Arnold Schwartz
Kathleen T. Shiverick
R. John Solaro
Joachim R. Sommer
Edmund H. Sonnenblick
James F. Spann, Jr.
Natsu Taylor
P. T. Thyrum
Richard L. Verrier
M. Lucius Walker, Jr.
William V. Whitehorn
E. B. Wolpert
Radovan Zak
Robert Zelis

Cardiac Hypertrophy

Edited by NORMAN R. ALPERT

DEPARTMENT OF PHYSIOLOGY AND BIOPHYSICS
UNIVERSITY OF VERMONT
SCHOOL OF MEDICINE
BURLINGTON, VERMONT

ACADEMIC PRESS New York and London 1971

ACADEMIC PRESS, INC.
111 Fifth Avenue, New York, New York 10003

United Kingdom Edition published by
ACADEMIC PRESS, INC. (LONDON) LTD.
Berkeley Square House, London W1X 6BA

LIBRARY OF CONGRESS CATALOG CARD NUMBER: 71-137629

PRINTED IN THE UNITED STATES OF AMERICA

CONTENTS

Part V The Mechanical Characteristics of Hypertrophied Heart Muscle

Part VI Energetics of the Hypertrophied Heart

LIST OF CONTRIBUTORS

Numbers in parentheses indicate the pages on which the authors' contributions begin.

R. ALBIN, Departments of Medicine, Biochemistry, and Physiology of the Pritzker School of Medicine of the University of Chicago, and the Argonne Cancer Research Hospital, Chicago, Illinois (283)

NORMAN R. ALPERT, Department of Physiology, University of Vermont, College of Medicine, Burlington, Vermont (315, 333)

RUTH A. ALTSCHULD, Departments of Pathology and Medicine, The Ohio State University, Columbus, Ohio (567)

EZRA A. AMSTERDAM, The Section of Cardiopulmonary Medicine, University of California at Davis, School of Medicine, Davis, California (433)

V. ASCHENBRENNER, Departments of Medicine, Biochemistry, and Physiology of the Pritzker School of Medicine of the University of Chicago, and the Argonne Cancer Research Hospital, Chicago, Illinois (283)

ANTHONY C. L. BARNARD, Department of Biomathematics, University of Alabama School of Medicine, Birmingham, Alabama (589, 611)

WILLIAM A. BAXLEY, Department of Medicine, Division of Cardiology, University of New Mexico, Albuquerque, New Mexico (425, 453)

M. BEZNAK, Department of Physiology, University of Ottawa, Faculty of Medicine, Ottawa, Ontario, Canada (55)

OSCAR H. L. BING, Department of Medicine, Tufts University School of Medicine, Boston, Massachusetts (361)

SANFORD P. BISHOP, Department of Pathology, The Ohio State University, Columbus, Ohio (107, 567)

JOHN P. BOINEAU, Departments of Pediatrics and Medicine, Duke University Medical Center, Durham, North Carolina (595)

F. NORMAN BRIGGS, Department of Physiology, University of Pittsburgh School of Medicine, Pittsburgh, Pennsylvania (167)

STANLEY A. BRILLER, Department of Medicine, University of Pennsylvania School of Medicine, Philadelphia, Pennsylvania (623)

ARNOLD L. BROWN, JR., Department of Experimental and Anatomic Pathology, Mayo Clinic, Rochester, Minnesota (11)

ROBERT A. BUCCINO, Cardiology Section, Department of Medicine, Temple University, Health Sciences Center, Philadelphia, Pennsylvania (141)

HENRY NEAL COLEMAN, Sections of Physiology and Cardiology, Mayo Clinic, Rochester, Minnesota (485)

LAVAL N. COTHRAN, Department of Physiology, Howard University College of Medicine, Washington, D.C. (407)

A. CUTILLETTA, Cardiopulmonary Division, Hospital of the University of Pennsylvania, Philadelphia, Pennsylvania (157)

H. DAVIS DEAR, Division of Cardiology, Department of Medicine, University of Alabama Medical Center, South Birmingham, Alabama (453)

HAROLD T. DODGE, Department of Medicine, Division of Cardiology, University of New Mexico, Albuquerque, New Mexico (425, 453)

MILTON DRAPER, Department of Physiology, University of Vermont, College of Medicine, Burlington, Vermont (315)

PAUL DREIZEN, Department of Medicine and Program in Biophysics, Downstate Medical Center, State University of New York, Brooklyn, New York (177)

BARRY L. FANBURG, Cardiovascular Research Institute, University of California School of Medicine, San Francisco, California (273, 361)

DONALD A. FISCHMAN, Departments of Biology and Anatomy, University of Chicago, Chicago, Illinois (125, 247)

VINCENT J. FISHER, Department of Physiology, Downstate Medical Center, State University of New York, Brooklyn, New York (371)

L. W. FORNEY, Department of Physiology, College of Medicine, The Pennsylvania State University, Philadelphia, Pennsylvania (345)

ARTHUR C. FOX, Department of Medicine, New York University School of Medicine, New York, New York (203)

JOHN GERGELY, Department of Muscle Research, Boston Biomedical Research Institute, Boston, Massachusetts (355)

LEWIS C. GERSHMAN, Department of Medicine and Program in Biophysics,

Downstate Medical Center, State University of New York, Brooklyn, New York (177)

EDWARD W. GERTZ, Department of Physiology, University of Pittsburgh School of Medicine, Pittsburgh, Pennsylvania (167)

DAVID B. GESELOWITZ, Biochemical Engineering Department of the Moore School of Electrical Engineering, University of Pennsylvania, Philadelphia, Pennsylvania (623)

K. E. GIGER, Department of Physiology, The Pennsylvania State University, College of Medicine, Philadelphia, Pennsylvania (345)

ALFRED L. GOLDBERG, Department of Physiology, Harvard Medical School, Boston, Massachusetts (39, 301)

M. J. GOODKIND, Division of Cardiology, Philadelphia General Hospital, and Department of Internal Medicine, University of Pennsylvania, Philadelphia, Pennsylvania (65)

RICHARD J. GOSS, Division of Biological and Medical Sciences, Brown University, Providence, Rhode Island (1)

N. J. GROSS, Departments of Medicine, Biochemistry, and Physiology of the Pritzker School of Medicine of the University of Chicago, and the Argonne Cancer Research Hospital, Chicago, Illinois (283)

D. GROVE, Hospital of the University of Pennsylvania, Cardiopulmonary Division, Philadelphia, Pennsylvania (157)

BURT B. HAMRELL, Department of Physiology, University of Vermont, College of Medicine, Burlington, Vermont (333)

EDWARD D. HARRIS, JR., Cardiology Section, Department of Medicine, Temple University, Health Sciences Center, Philadelphia, Pennsylvania (141)

EDWARD W. HAWTHORNE, Department of Physiology, Howard University, Washington, D.C. (387, 407)

PAUL F. HOAR, Department of Physiology, University of Vermont, College of Medicine, Burlington, Vermont (333)

JOHN H. HOLT, JR., Department of Medicine, University of Alabama School of Medicine, and Veterans Administration Hospital, Birmingham, Alabama (611)

WILLIAM P. HOOD, JR., Department of Medicine, University of Alabama Medical Center, Birmingham, Alabama (445)

PAUL H. JEWETT, Departments of Pathology and Pediatrics, Duke University Medical Center, and Veterans Administration Hospital, Durham, North Carolina (89)

L. S. JEFFERSON, Department of Physiology, The Pennsylvania State University, College of Medicine, Philadelphia, Pennsylvania (345)

HORTON A. JOHNSON, Medical Department, Brookhaven National Laboratory, Upton, New York (21)

WILLIAM B. JONES, Division of Cardiology, Department of Medicine, University of Alabama Medical Center, South Birmingham, Alabama (453)

ARNOLD M. KATZ, Department of Medicine, Mount Sinai School of Medicine, New York, New York (85)

FREDERICK KAVALER, Cardiology Section and Cardiopulmonary Laboratory, New York Veterans Administration Hospital, New York, New York (371)

ROBERT R. KOHN, Department of Pathology, Case Western Reserve University, Cleveland, Ohio (19)

B. KORECKY, Department of Physiology, Faculty of Medicine, University of Ottawa, Ottawa, Canada (55)

FRANCES KRAFT-HUNTER, Department of Physiology, Howard University, College of Medicine, Washington, D.C. (407)

JOHN O. KRAMER, JR., Veterans Administration Hospital, Birmingham, Alabama (611)

E. M. KRITCHER, Department of Medical Research, Veterans Administration Hospital, Iowa City, Iowa (65)

ALLAN M. LEFER, Department of Physiology, University of Virginia School of Medicine, Charlottesville, Virginia (73)

MICHAEL LESCH, Department of Medicine, Peter Bent Brigham Hospital, Harvard Medical School, Boston, Massachusetts (147)

HERBERT J. LEVINE, Department of Medicine, Tufts University School of Medicine, Boston, Massachusetts (361)

R. J. LUCHI, Department of Medical Research, Veterans Administration Hospital, Iowa City, Iowa (65)

DEAN T. MASON, Cardiopulmonary Section, University of California at Davis, Davis, California (433)

Satoru Matsushita, Cardiovascular Research Institute, University of California, School of Medicine, San Francisco, California (273, 361)

H. E. Morgan, Department of Physiology, The Pennsylvania State University, College of Medicine, Philadelphia, Pennsylvania (345)

E. Neil Moore, The Comparative Cardiovascular Studies Unit, The University of Pennsylvania School of Veterinary Medicine, Philadelphia, Pennsylvania (595)

Eugene Morkin, Department of Medicine, Beth Israel Hospital, and Harvard Medical School, Boston, Massachusetts (259)

A. A. Moscona, Department of Biology, The University of Chicago, Chicago, Illinois (125)

K. G. Nair, Departments of Medicine, Biochemistry, and Physiology of the Pritzker School of Medicine of the University of Chicago, and the Argonne Cancer Research Hospital, Chicago, Illinois (157, 283)

M. Oratz, Radioisotope Service, New York, New York (215)

Peter E. Pool, University of California, Department of Medicine, San Diego, La Jolla, California (539)

Barry I. Posner, Cardiovascular Research Institute, University of California School of Medicine, San Francisco, California (273)

Murray Rabinowitz, Hospital of the University of Pennsylvania, Cardiopulmonary Division, Philadelphia, Pennsylvania (157, 283)

Charles E. Rackley, Division of Cardiology, Department of Medicine, University of Alabama Medical Center, South Birmingham, Alabama (153)

M. A. Rothschild, Radioisotope Service, New York, New York (215)

Harold Sandler, Biomedical Research Branch, NASA-Ames Research Center, Moffette Field, California (387)

Sidney S. Schreiber, Radioisotope Service, New York, New York (215)

Arnold Schwartz, Division of Myocardial Biology, Baylor University, College of Medicine, Houston, Texas (511, 549)

Kathleen T. Shiverick, Department of Physiology, University of Vermont, College of Medicine, Burlington, Vermont (333)

R. John Solaro, Department of Physiology, University of Pittsburgh School of Medicine, Pittsburgh, Pennsylvania (167)

JOACHIM R. SOMMER, Departments of Pathology and Pediatrics, Duke University Medical Center, and Veterans Administration Hospital, Durham, North Carolina (89)

EDMUND H. SONNENBLICK, Cardiology Section, Department of Medicine, Temple University, Health Sciences Center, Philadelphia, Pennsylvania (141)

JAMES F. SPANN, JR., Cardiology Section, Department of Medicine, Temple University, Health Sciences Center, Philadelphia, Pennsylvania (141, 433, 465)

NATSU TAYLOR, Department of Physiology, University of Vermont, College of Medicine, Burlington, Vermont (315)

P. T. THYRUM, Research Service, Veterans Administration Hospital, Houston, Texas (65)

RICHARD L. VERRIER, Department of Physiology, University of Michigan School of Medicine, Ann Arbor, Michigan (73)

M. LUCIUS WALKER, JR., Department of Mechanical Engineering, Howard University, Washington, D. C. (387)

WILLIAM V. WHITEHORN, Hulliken Hall, University of Delaware, Newark, Delaware (27)

E. B. WOLPERT, Department of Physiology, The Pennsylvania State University, College of Medicine, Philadelphia, Pennsylvania (345)

RADOVAN ZAK, Hospital of the University of Pennsylvania, Cardiopulmonary Division, Philadelphia, Pennsylvania (157, 247, 283)

ROBERT ZELIS, The Section of Cardiopulmonary Medicine, University of California at Davis, School of Medicine, Davis, California (433)

PREFACE

This book deals with the many problems involved in understanding the hypertrophied heart. Normal hearts pump an adequate quantity of blood through the lungs and tissues to meet the varying metabolic needs of the organism. A failing heart is incapable of meeting this demand. When a normal heart is subjected to a sustained stress, long-term compensation is accomplished by means of hypertrophy. Initially the hypertrophied myocardium is capable of meeting the substantially increased work demands. However, it has the seeds of deterioration incorporated into its structure. If the stress persists, the overgrown heart muscle progresses to the irreversible failing state. Thus, myocardial hypertrophy may be considered the interface between the normal and the failing condition. Understanding the circumstances which obligate adaptive cardiac growth to become pathological enlargement is the boundary where clinical medicine and basic science must meet.

The fundamental questions may be divided into three main categories. These are (a) the biological and biochemical correlates of myocardial growth, (b) the mechanical and energetic characteristics of the enlarged heart, and (c) the electrical correlates of increased myocardial mass.

How does heart muscle compare with other tissues in terms of its response to stress? Is the pattern of enlargement determined by the mitotic potential? Can maturation and stress-induced enlargement be considered the same phenomenon? Do all the stresses which induce compensatory growth work through the same final trigger? Once the hypertrophy is initiated what role is played by the hormonal environment? How do the alterations in ultrastructure and chemical composition relate to the initiation, maintenance, and characteristics of increased protein synthesis in cardiac hypertrophy? These questions are dealt with in Parts I, II, III, and IV of this book.

After the hypertrophy is established, are there alterations in the mechanical properties of the myocardium and energy transduction into work? These questions are considered in light of a number of experiments in animals and man in which isolated muscle strips as well as the intact heart have been studied. Parts V and VI are concerned with these problems.

Finally, it is necessary to know if there are better ways of evaluating the electrical activity of the enlarged myocardium. This problem is considered in Part VII.

Many questions have been raised. Some of them have been answered. It is my hope that this book will be useful to the scientist working in the area, the human and animal biologist, as well as to the clinician who must deal with the many problems associated with cardiac hypertrophy.

In a book of this sort the editor owes a great debt to many others. The extent of the debt and to whom it is owed will be obvious to the reader. In addition a special measure of gratitude must be offered to Doctors A. C. L. Barnard, H. Neal Coleman, Richard Goss, Edward Hawthorne, Arnold Katz, and William B. Whitehorn who were creatively involved in identifying the many important areas which are covered in the text. Indebtedness must also be expressed to Miss Kathleen Shiverick whose dedicated work on the index made it comprehensive and useful. Thanks are also due to the National Institutes of Health, the American Heart Association, and the Cardiac Muscle Society for their moral and financial support of this project. Harold Sandler deserves special recognition for having cajoled, prodded, and helped all of us bring this project to fruition. Finally, without competent and loyal secretarial help a book of this type would have been much more difficult to complete. It is with pleasure that I express my sincere appreciation to Chris Audette, Katharine Fenn, Sandra Marlowe, and Marie Luhr for help much beyond the call of duty and good sense.

CARDIAC HYPERTROPHY

Part I
Adaptive Growth and Heart Muscle

ADAPTIVE GROWTH OF THE HEART

Richard J. Goss

Introduction

There are two kinds of biological adaptation: One is genetic, the other physiological. The genetic kind provides that an animal shall be equipped not only with enough of each kind of organ required for survival, but with a generous margin for safety, regardless of whether the surplus tissues are ever needed. Physiological adaptations are called forth by temporary alterations in the demands for the services of various tissues and organs. Such adaptations as these can result in either growth or atrophy, depending on whether the physiological demands go up or down. Thus, in addition to the wherewithal for living under the normal conditions of our environment, nature provides us with the capacity to adjust to changes in that environment, should the need arise.

When an engineer designs a machine he must decide how many parts of a given kind should be installed, and what size of each part will best fulfill the functions to be performed. Automobiles, for example, are equipped with more than enough cylinders than are required for ordinary driving. The maximum attainable horsepower may be twice as much as is ever called into play, reflecting the engineer's estimation of the magnitude of various contingencies which should be provided for. At the present time a single spare tire is considered sufficient because the chances of two blowouts occurring at the same time are vanishingly small. Thus, the margin for safety built into inanimate machines represents a compromise between the probabilities of what might go wrong on the one hand, and the cost of providing surplus safety devices on the other.

Animate systems are likewise equipped with parts that are larger or more numerous than may ordinarily be required just for survival. There is a redundancy built into most organs of the body which may be severalfold greater than the minimal amount needed to sustain life. Living as we do in a competitive world, no organism could survive perpetually on the brink of extinction. All animals eventually die because sooner or later the vicissitudes of the environment overcome their innate capacities to react. Clearly, in the course of evolution the margin for safety has been dictated by the magnitude of these environmental fluctuations. Natural selection has favored the development of more than enough of each organ, but for reasons of economy, the production of tissue over and above this comfortable margin for safety has been selected against. Hence, like the efficient machine it is, the animal body has a built-in reserve which can be relied on in case of emergency. Provisions of this kind often keep man-made machines going until they can be repaired by some external agency. In a living system, the mechanism for repair resides within. It may take the form of wound healing, or it may be expressed as regeneration (Goss, 1969). In most internal organs, however, an insufficiency is coped with by a compensatory reaction in which the physiological overload triggers a growth response designed eventually to reestablish the original functional and morphological balance of the system (Goss, 1965).

Modes of Compensation

Compensatory hypertrophy can be caused in a variety of ways. In many organs a reduction in mass by surgical excision calls forth a growth response in what remains behind. It is possible to elicit the same response by creating a functional overload without reducing the amount of the organ. The nature of this functional overload varies from organ to organ depending upon what physiological activities are normally carried out. In those cases in which organs may have more than one function, there may be more than one way to elicit the growth response. All that is necessary, apparently, is to create an imbalance between the functional demands and the capacity of the organ in question to meet these demands.

The ways in which growth is achieved vary with the kind of organ—and the level of organization (Goss, 1966, 1967). Some organs can increase their mass by adding new units at the histological level of organization. New follicles, for example, can be added to the thyroid and ovary, and exocrine glands have varying capacities for augmenting their compliments of secretory acini. Other organs, unable to produce such complicated structures, enlarge solely by cellular proliferation. The kidney, for instance, cannot make new nephrons, but can enlarge the ones it has by multiplying their component cells. In like manner, the lungs, which cannot make new alveoli beyond infancy, increase their size by cell division. Other organs, including many endocrine glands, grow in the same way. Cell replication is also the mode of growth characteristic of such renewing tissues as blood, epidermis, intestinal mucosal epithelium, and the spermatogenic epithelium lining seminiferous tubules. Finally, there are some tissues and organs which are incapable of multiplying their functional units at the histological or cellular levels of organization. These mitotically static tissues must rely on molecular turnover in order to renew themselves. This subcelluar renewal is the basis for growth in the muscular and nervous systems. Here the capacity for compensatory growth is limited to cellular hypertrophy. Although such a mechanism provides the additional morphological substrate for doing extra work, the extent of compensatory growth in such organs is considerably restricted owing to the impossibility of mitotic proliferation, and the upper limit beyond which a cell cannot enlarge without increasing its DNA.

These several modes of growth represented by different organs and tissues of the body reflect certain relationships between growth and function. There is overwhelming evidence that increases in functional demand promote growth of specifically affected organs. Whether such growth is mitotic or not seems to depend on whether a given organ or tissue works part time or full time (Goss, 1970). Organs that work intermittently, such as most of the glands in the body, tend to grow by cell division. The rate at which their cells proliferate is controlled by, and is dependent upon, those physiological factors which promote functional activity. So it is that most glands adjust their size to the needs of the body, enlarging when the demands are high and undergoing atrophy when thrown out of work. Other parts of the body must function continuously. Should their cell division be subject to the stimulation of functional demands, they would then be in danger of serious overproduction. There are two ways to avoid this fate. One is to make new cells at top speed but to dispose of them at an equal rate. This is how renewing tissues have solved the problem of working, and therefore growing, continuously. The alternative is to abandon mitotic activity altogether. Nerves and muscles have adopted this solution to the problem. Being composed of potentially immortal cells, these tissues can function constantly in the absence of cell division without depleting themselves.

The heart fits into the above scheme of things in that it functions constantly but is composed of muscle fibers which do not normally undergo mitosis. Nevertheless, the heart is subject to the demands of functional overload, and will become hypertrophic in response to a variety of physiological stimuli. Exactly what stimuli affect the size of the heart, and how they do it, is central to the general problem of adaptive growth. Knowledge of comparable mechanisms in other organs and tissues of the body may be applied in principal to the special case of the heart; what we learn about the heart may in turn enhance our understanding of other systems, especially since the problem of cardiac growth is unique in a number of ways.

Half-Hearted Hypertrophy

Like many other parts of the body the heart is a paired organ. Yet it is one of the few in which the two parts perform different functions. The differences between the two halves are reflected in their divergent growth responses. There are many ways to stimulate the heart to enlarge, but they do not all affect both ventricles in the same way. Various forms of hypertension, for example, are well known to promote left ventricular hypertrophy. Whether the hypertension is caused by encapsulation of the kidney (Carney and Brown, 1964; McCallister and Brown, 1965; Matsumoto *et al.*, 1965), unilateral nephrectomy, DCA and saline drinking water (Beznak, 1967; Beznak *et al.*, 1969; Wannemacher and McCoy, 1969), constriction of the renal artery (Byrom and Dodson, 1949; Tobian *et al.*, 1960), or aortic stenosis (Beznak, 1952; Gluck *et al.*, 1964b; Spann *et al.*, 1964; Kleitke and Sydow, 1965; Wollenberger *et al.*, 1966; Moroz, 1967; Kaku, 1968; Beznak *et al.*, 1969), the results are always the same. The myocardium of the left ventricle is the tissue which grows to compensate for the heightened physiological demands. A similar response can be elicited by feeding a diet rich in cholesterol (Spraragen *et al.*, 1962), or in consequence of a lesion in the aortic valve (Tomita, 1966). None of the above procedures has more than a passive effect on the right ventricle.

The right side of the heart, however, is responsive to its own set of stimuli. Constrict the pulmonary artery, for example, and the right ventricle enlarges (Overy *et al.*, 1966; Spann *et al.*, 1967; Bishop and Cole, 1969; Fox and Reed, 1969). Exposure to high altitudes (or hypoxia) also brings about a greater hypertrophy of the right ventricle than of the left (Rotta, 1947; Barnard, 1958; Alexander and Jensen, 1959; Norman and Coers, 1960; Swigart, 1962; Hultgren and Miller, 1965; Van Liere *et al.*, 1965; Burton and Smith, 1967, 1969; Burton *et al.*, 1968; McGrath *et al.*, 1969), as does treatment with cobalt chloride (Swigart, 1962, 1965; Souhrada, 1968). Both of these procedures stimulate erythropoiesis, leading to polycythemia (Swigart, 1965; Burton and Smith, 1967). In fact, it has been shown that simply by making an animal polycythemic by means of hypertransfusion, the size of the right ventricle will increase (Swigart, 1965). In our search for the ultimate explanation of cardiac hypertrophy, we have a bewildering profusion of causes which are not easily unraveled. One possibility is that right ventricular hypertrophy is most directly attributable to pulmonary arterial hypertension (Burton *et al.*, 1968). This can be caused by ligation (Spann *et al.*, 1967; Bishop and Cole, 1969; Fox and Reed, 1969), or may be brought about by the increased viscosity of polycythemic blood in the lungs (Swigart, 1965; Burton and Smith, 1967). This could also explain the effects of cobalt chloride or exposure to the hypoxia of high altitude, both of which promote polycythemia in addition to cardiac hypertrophy.

It is noteworthy, however, that polycythemia is of necessity a systemic condition and whatever resistance it presents to the right ventricle should also be felt by the left. Such is evidently the case, for Barnard (1958), Van Liere *et al.* (1965), and Burton and Smith (1967) have all noted that although hypoxia predominately stimulates right ventricular hypertrophy, the left ventricle is also affected, albeit to a lesser degree.

Finally, it must be noted that still another category of stimuli exerts a bilateral effect on the cardiac ventricles, the presumption being that these factors overburden both sides of the heart at the same time. Probably the most common stimulation of general cardiac hypertrophy is chronic strenuous exercise (Steinhaus *et al.*, 1932; Tung *et al.*, 1934; Tepperman and Pearlman, 1961; Van Liere *et al.*, 1965; Crews and Aldinger, 1967), a condition that creates demands not only on the respiratory system, but also on the delivery of oxygen to the bodily tissues. Hence, the resources of both the left and right ventricles are called upon under these conditions. Another way to promote hypertrophy of both ventricles is to cause anemia (Norman and McBroom, 1958; Tepperman and Pearlman, 1961; Korecky and French, 1967). Whether this anemia is the result of hemolysis or iron deficiency, the resulting condition also calls into play both sides of the heart. The right ventricle must work harder to enhance the efficiency of the lungs in compensation for the reduced number of red blood cells. The left ventricle is overworked in delivering the blood more efficiently to the other tissues and organs of the body. Thus, both sides of the heart are important if the metabolic rate of the organism is to be elevated to compensate for the anemia. Perhaps this explains why the administration of thyroxine, which increases the rate of metabolism, also causes bilateral cardiac hypertrophy (Sandler and Wilson, 1959; Swynghedauw *et al.*, 1968). Administration of androgens (Burton and Smith, 1967) likewise stimulates growth of both ventricles. Exactly how these various factors are translated into a growth response we do not know. A clue to the problem may be found in the fact that isoproterenol, a sympathomimetic drug, will bring about enlargement of the entire heart (Stanton *et al.*, 1969). This could mean that various increases in physiological demand all may be funneled through the sympathetic nervous system as a common denominator. Unfortunately, such an explanation cannot account for the various instances of unilateral hypertrophy noted above, unless, of course, the release of sympathetic agents is itself controlled separately on either side of the heart.

The natural inequity in size between the left and right ventricles is itself a revealing curiosity. The preponderance of the left ventricle normally runs around twice the weight of the right—an exception is the giraffe in which it is said that the left side is inordinately large owing to the extremely high head of pressure against which it must pump. This lopsided shape is characteristic only of the postnatal mammalian heart. At or before birth the left and right human ventricles are nearly equal in weight (Scammon, 1927; Keen, 1955), or the right side may even outweigh the left (Emery and Mithal, 1961; Recavarren and Arias-Stella, 1964). A similar situation obtains in the newborn pig (Booth *et al.*, 1966), rabbit (Gluck *et al.*, 1964a), and dog (Latimer, 1965).

In view of the changes in the pattern of mammalian circulation at the time of birth, one cannot escape the conclusion that the differential growth of the two ventricles must reflect their altered functions consequent upon closure of the ductus arteriosus. The significance of these conclusions is that the left ventricle is not larger than the right by virtue of genetic expression, but that the difference in size is nothing more than a growth response to a regularly occurring physiological adaptation. This view is sustained by the finding that although the cardiac muscle fibers are larger in the left ventricle than in the right ventricle (Boellaard, 1952; Chanutin and Barksdale, 1933), the number of such fibers is approximately equal on the two sides (Linzbach, 1950, 1960).

The Limits of Hypertrophy

This state of affairs raises the interesting question of how hypertrophy differs from normal growth. During maturation of the individual, the fibers of the left ventricle clearly become hypertrophic in relation to those on the right. Yet if we call this hypertrophy, the enlargement of heart muscle fibers during normal ontogeny must fall into the same category. Now if one extrapolates from the normal adult dimensions to the hypertrophic heart proper, the only difference is one of degree. Herein lies the distinction between the normal and the pathological. Compensatory growth should be regarded as a normal reaction to the usual ups and downs of the physiological landscape. It is only when the adaptive capacity of the reacting tissues or organs is not equal to the functional stress confronting them that destructive changes occur leading to pathological consequences.

In the case of the heart, the transition from so-called normal dimensions to compensatory hypertrophy occurs when the average fiber diameter is about 14 μ or so (Harrison *et al.*, 1932; Roberts and Wearn, 1941; Ashley, 1945; Lowe and Bate, 1948a), and the transition from adaptive hypertrophy to pathological enlargement occurs when fiber widths measure in the twenties (Roberts and Wearn, 1941; Wearn, 1941; Lowe and Bate, 1948a,b). Thus, there seems to be an upper limit beyond which myocardial fibers cannot grow without risking untoward consequences.

Why this should be so is a difficult question to answer. For many years it has been assumed that beyond a critical upper size limit the growth of cardiac muscle fibers exceeded that of their accompanying blood vessels (Shipley *et al.*, 1937; Roberts and Wearn, 1941; Wearn, 1941). Such a situation, of course, would eventually lead to serious problems of metabolic exchange. Recent evidence, however, has indicated that vascularization does keep pace with hypertrophy of heart muscles (Tepperman and Pearlman, 1961; Kerr *et al.*, 1968; Arai *et al.*, 1968). If this is indeed so, then some other explanation must be sought for the inability of heart muscle fibers to grow larger than they normally do. The possibility suggests itself that nucleocytoplasmic relationships may be involved.

In this regard, a comparison between cardiac and skeletal muscle fibers may be instructive. Inasmuch as skeletal muscle fibers can become as large as 90 μ in diameter (Gutmann, 1948; Bosanquet *et al.*, 1960), it seems unlikely that cardiac muscle fibers should not be able to exceed widths of 20–30μ on the basis of diffusion problems alone. Skeletal muscle fibers, however, differ from cardiac fibers in that they are multinucleate, a condition which very probably accounts for such phenomenal expansion of their cytoplasm. On this basis, the compulsory mononucleate condition of cardiac muscle fibers may very well account for their limited growth potential, especially in view of their lack of anaerobic respiration (Lawrie, 1952). In addition to this, little or no cell division is possible among cardiac muscle fibers (Erokhina, 1968; Sasaki *et al.*, 1968; Shafiq *et al.*, 1968). There does not even seem to be a reserve population of myoblasts from which new muscle fibers could be recruited such as may be represented by the satellite cells of skeletal muscle. Hence, the mammalian heart is very vulnerable to insufficiency should the demands upon it exceed its built-in structural limitations.

By way of contrast, the cardiac ventricles of lower vertebrates may be endowed with far greater adaptive capacities than are those of birds and mammals. Among reptiles, amphibians, and especially fishes, there are species that seem to grow as long as they live, and to live as long as they grow. It follows that the hearts of such animals must also exhibit indeterminate growth if they are to keep pace with the enlargement of the body as a whole. They must do so either by hyperplasia or hypertrophy of cardiac muscle fibers. Assuming that the former possibility is at least partly involved, where do the new muscle cells come from? Perhaps preexisting myocardial fibers divide from time to time. Alternatively, myogenic stem cells may persist throughout life. Whatever the explanation, it is clear that such hearts should have certain attributes not enjoyed by those of warm-blooded vertebrates. Their fibers should never have to become hypertrophic; and in the event of infarction, they should be capable of regenerating more muscle to replace what was lost. One wonders why such obvious advantages were not perpetuated as higher vertebrates evolved.

Cardiac Atrophy

Insofar as heart muscle can adapt to increased functional demands by hypertrophy, it would not seem unreasonable to expect it to undergo disuse atrophy should the right circumstances come about. There is some evidence from studies of neonatal hearts that this may occur. Here it will be recalled that the two ventricles are of approximately equal size because they are both pumping blood through the same channels. When the ductus arterious closes after birth, the work load on the right ventricle is suddenly reduced from sharing half the burden of pumping blood through the systemic circulation to the responsibility for the pulmonary circulation only (Dawes, 1968). In keeping with these changes, some investigators have recorded an actual decrease in the absolute size of the right ventricle during early postnatal periods (Keen, 1955; Averill *et al.*, 1963; Recavarren and Arias-Stella, 1964); others record no change (Emery and Mithal, 1961). Aside from this, there have been occasional reports of various forms of congenital cardiac atrophy (Karsner *et al.*, 1925; Roberts and Wearn, 1941; Lumb and Dawkins, 1961; Dawes, 1968), but these may be the result of failure to grow in the first place, rather than a decrease in size previously attained. In any event, the explanation for such conditions eludes us.

An actual decrease in heart size can and does occur when a previously established hypertrophy is reversed following withdrawal of the original growth stimulus. This has been shown to be the case following hypoxia (Van Liere *et al.*, 1965), forced exercise (Leon and Bloor, 1968), and renal hypertension, thyroxine administration, aortic constriction, and nutritional anemia (Beznak *et al.*, 1969). Upon reversal of these conditions the formerly hypertrophic hearts promptly begin to lose weight until they reach normal dimensions.

An experimental approach to this facet of the problem may be feasible by taking advantage of recently developed techniques for transplanting extra hearts into rats (Abbott *et al.*, 1965; Ono and Lindsey, 1969). This can be done by suturing the aorta and pulmonary artery of the heart to the abdominal aorta and inferior vena cava of the host, respectively. Blood enters the transplant via the aorta, is shunted into the coronary arteries, perfuses the heart muscle, and returns through the coronary veins to the right atrium from which it passes to the right ventricle and back into the host by way of the pulmonary artery. Such transplanted hearts survive and continue to elicit electrical impulses even though they are actually pumping little or no blood. With such a reduced work load there is every reason to believe that their overall size might diminish and that the dimensions of their component muscle fibers might shrink proportionately.

How extensive this atrophy might be is hard to predict. Some tissues in the body have been known to disappear altogether when totally unemployed over a long period of time. Still others unaccountably persist in a permanent state of atrophy. Since cardiac muscle, with its intrinsic beat, is independent of innervation, it would seem reasonable that it might be self-perpetuating at some minimal dimension, a dimension representing the point at which genetic adaptations are abandoned and physiological ones take over.

References

Abbott, C. P., DeWitt, C. W., and Creech, O., Jr. (1965). *Transplantation* **3**, 432.

Alexander, A. F., and Jensen, R. (1959). *Amer. J. Vet. Res.* **20**, 680.

Arai, S., Machida, A., and Nakamura, T. (1968). *Tohoku J. Exp. Med.* **95**, 35.

Ashley, L. M. (1945). *Amer. J. Anat.* **77**, 325.

Averill, K. H., Wagner, W. W., Jr., and Vogel, J. H. K. (1963). *Amer. Heart J.* **66**, 632.

Barnard, P. J. (1958). *Lab. Invest.* **7**, 81.

Beznak, M. (1952). *J. Physiol.* **116**, 74.

Beznak, M. (1967). *Can. J. Physiol. Pharmacol.* **45**, 993.

Beznak, M., Korecky, B., and Thomas G. (1969). *Can. J. Physiol. Pharmacol.* **47**, 579.

Bishop, S. P., and Cole, C. R. (1969). *Lab. Invest.* **20**, 219.

Boellaard, J. W. (1952). *Z. Kreisforsch.* **41**, 101.

Booth, N. H., Hastings, S. G., Hopwood, M. L., and Maaske, C. A. (1966). *Proc. Soc. Exp. Biol. Med.* **122**, 186.

Bosanquet, F. D., Daniel, P. M., and Parry, H. B. (1960). *In* "The Structure and Function of Muscle" (G. H. Bourne, ed.), Vol. 3, pp. 321–358. Academic Press, New York.

Burton, R. R., and Smith, A. H. (1967). *J. Appl. Physiol.* **22**, 782.

Burton, R. R., and Smith, A. H. (1969). *Fed. Proc. Fed. Amer. Soc. Exp. Biol.* **28**, 1170.

Burton, R. R., Besch, E. L., and Smith, A. H. (1968). *Amer. J. Physiol.* **214**, 1438.

Byrom, F. B., and Dobson, L. F. (1949). *Clin. Sci.* **8**, 1.

Carney, J. A., and Brown, A. L., Jr. (1964). *Amer. J. Pathol.* **44**, 521.

Chanutin, A., and Barksdale, E. E. (1933). *Arch. Intern. Med.* **52**, 739.

Crews, J., and Aldinger, E. E. (1967). *Amer. Heart J.* **74**, 536.

Dawes, G. S. (1968). "Foetal and Neonatal Physiology. A Comparative Study of the Changes at Birth." Year Book Medical Publishers, Chicago, Illinois.

Emery, J. L., and Mithal, A. (1961). *Brit. Heart J.* **23**, 313.

Erokhina, I. L. (1968). *Tsitologiya.* **10**, 1391.

Fox, A. C., and Reed, G. E. (1969). *Amer. J. Physiol.* **216**, 1026.

Gluck, L., Talner, N. S., Gardner, T. H., and Kulovich, M. V. (1964a). *Nature (London)* **202**, 770.

Gluck, L., Talner, N. S., Stern, H., Gardner, T. H., and Kulovich, M. V. (1964b). *Science* **144**, 1244.

Goss, R. J. (1965). "Adaptive Growth." Academic Press, New York.

Goss, R. J. (1966). *Science* **153**, 1615.

Goss, R. J. (1967). *In* "Control of Cellular Growth in Adult Organisms" (H. Teir and T. Rytomäa, eds.), pp. 3–27. Academic Press, New York.

Goss, R. J. (1969). "Principles of Regeneration." Academic Press, New York.

Goss, R. J. (1970). *In* "Advances in Cell Biology" (D. M. Prescott, L. Goldstein, and E. McConkey, eds.), pp. 233–296, Appleton, New York.

Gutmann, E. (1948). *J. Neurophysiol.* **11**, 279.

Harrison, T. R., Ashman, R., and Larson, R. M. (1932). *Arch. Intern. Med.* **49**, 151.
Hultgren, H. N., and Miller, H. (1965). *Ann. N.Y. Acad. Sci.* **127**, 627.
Kaku, I. (1968). *Jap. Heart J.* **9**, 393.
Karsner, H. T., Saphir, O., and Todd, T. W. (1925). *Amer. J. Pathol.* **1**, 351.
Keen, E. N. (1955). *J. Anat.* **89**, 484.
Kerr, A., Jr., Bommer, W. J., and Pilato, S. (1968). *Amer. Heart J.* **75**, 144.
Kleitke, B., and Sydow, H. (1965). *Acta Biol. Med. German.* **14**, 447.
Korecky, B., and French, I. W. (1967). *Circ. Res.* **21**, 635.
Latimer, H. B. (1965). *Anat. Rec.* **152**, 225.
Lawrie, R. A. (1952). *Nature (London)* **170**, 122.
Leon, A. S., and Bloor, M. (1968). *J. Appl. Physiol.* **24**, 485.
Linzbach, A. J. (1950). *Virchow's Arch. Pathol. Anat.* **318**, 575.
Linzbach, A. J. (1960). *Amer. J. Cardiol.* **5**, 370.
Lowe, T. E., and Bate, E. W. (1948a). *Med. J. Austral.* **1**, 467.
Lowe, T. E., and Bate, E. W. (1948b). *Med. J. Austral.* **1**, 618.
Lumb, G., and Dawkins, W. A. (1961). *Amer. Heart J.* **60**, 378.
McCallister, B. D., and Brown, A. L., Jr. (1965). *Lab. Invest.* **14**, 692.
McGrath, J., Bullard, R. W., and Komives, G. K. (1969). *Fed. Proc. Fed. Amer. Soc. Exp. Biol.* **28**, 1307.
Matsumoto, S., Kishii, T., Ito, Y., and Kobayashi, T. (1965). *Jap. Heart J.* **6**, 443.
Moroz, L. A. (1967). *Circ. Res.* **21**, 449.
Norman, T. D., and McBroom, R. D. (1958). *Circ. Res.* **6**, 765.
Norman, T. D., and Coers, C. R. (1960). *Arch. Pathol.* **69**, 181.
Ono, K., and Lindsey, E. S. (1969). *J. Thorac. Cardiovasc. Surg.* **57**, 225.
Overy, H. R., Vogel, J. H. K., Grover, R. G., and Blount, S. G., Jr. (1966). *Circ. Res.* **18**, 634.
Recavarren, S., and Arias-Stella, J. (1964). *Brit. Heart J.* **26**, 187.
Roberts, J. T., and Wearn, J. T. (1941). *Amer. Heart J.* **21**, 617.
Rotta, A. (1947). *Amer. Heart J.* **33**, 669.
Sandler, G., and Wilson, M. (1959). *Quart. J. Exp. Physiol.* **44**, 282.
Sasaki, R., Morishita, T., and Yamagata, S. (1968). *Tohoku J. Exp. Med.* **96**, 405.
Scammon, R. E. (1927). *Radiology* **9**, 89.
Shafiq, S. A., Gorycki, M. A., and Mauro, A. (1968). *J. Anat.* **103**, 135.
Shipley, R. A., Shipley, L. J., and Wearn, J. T. (1937). *J. Exp. Med.* **65**, 29.
Souhrada, J. (1968). *Physiol. Bohemoslav.* **16**, 469.
Spann, J. F., Jr., Chidsey, C. A., and Braunwald, E. (1964). *Science* **145**, 1439.
Spann, J. F., Buccino, R. A., and Sonnenblick, E. H. (1967). *Proc. Soc. Exp. Biol. Med.* **125**, 522.
Stanton, H. C., Brenner, G., and Mayfield, E. D., Jr., (1969). *Amer. Heart J.* **77**, 72.
Spraragen, S. C., Bond, V. P., and Dahl, L. K. (1962). *Circ. Res.* **11**, 982.
Steinhaus, A. H., Hoyt, L. A., and Rice, H. A. (1932). *Amer. J. Physiol.* **99**, 512.
Swigart, R. H. (1962). *Anat. Rec.* **142**, 284.
Swigart, R. H. (1965). *Circ. Res.* **17**, 30.
Swynghedauw, B., Courtault, D., and Wanstok, F. (1968). *Pathol. Biol.* **16**, 691.
Tepperman, J., and Pearlman, D. (1961). *Circ. Res.* **9**, 576.
Tobian, L., Severseike, O., and Cich, J. (1960). *Proc. Soc. Exp. Biol. Med.* **103**, 774.
Tomita, K. (1966). *Jap. Heart J.* **7**, 566.
Tung, C. L., Hsieh, C. K., Bien, C. W., and Dieuaide, F. R. (1934). *Amer. Heart J.* **10**, 79.
Van Liere, E. J., Krames, B. B., and Northrup, D. W. (1965). *Circ. Res.* **16**, 244.
Wannemacher, R. W., Jr., and McCoy, J. R. (1969). *Amer. J. Physiol.* **216**, 781.
Wearn, J. T. (1941). *Bull. Johns Hopkins Hosp.* **68**, 363.
Wollenberger, A., Kleike, B., and Schulze, W. (1966). *Acta. Biol. Med. German.* **17**, 334.

MORPHOLOGIC FACTORS IN CARDIAC HYPERTROPHY

Arnold L. Brown, Jr.

The Myocardium as a Polycellular Tissue

The myocardium consists of more than just muscle cells—this obvious fact requires emphasis because of the preoccupation with the muscle cell that is apparent in the literature concerning cardiac growth and hypertrophy. Whereas it is most probably true that the hypertrophic process and cardiac failure can be completely understood only in terms of muscle cell structure and function, it would be well for the investigator studying this cell to remember that he must allow for the presence of connective tissue, endothelial, nerve, and smooth muscle cells in his isolated muscle preparations and, most importantly, in homogenates.

The Muscle Cell

The fine structure of the myocardial muscle cell has been recently reviewed in detail by Fawcett and McNutt (1969). The organelles of chief interest in the study of the hypertrophic heart have been the myofibril, mitochondria, and the sarcoplasmic reticulum, accounting for the contractile elements, the energetic supply, and the contraction–relaxation stimulating system. Each of these organelles can be isolated in relatively pure form—the myofibrils because they are unique to thc muscle cell, and mitochondria and the sarcotubular system because they far outnumber similar elements in nonmuscle cells. The nuclei of the muscle cells are generally larger than those of the other cells of the myocardium but their DNA content is presumably the same. No method has as yet been devised to isolate muscle nuclei free from nonmuscle nuclei. Muscle cells contain ribosomes and rarely seen Golgi systems, but there is no reason to believe that they are qualitatively different from those found in connective tissue and endothelial cells. Preparations of these organelles from myocardial homogenates must be assumed to be contaminated by those from nonmuscle cells.

Nonmuscle Cells

Any unified concept of cardiac hypertrophy and failure must take into account the cellular dynamics and function of at least the connective tissue, nerve, and endothelial cells. Little is known concerning either their proliferative ability in the enlarging heart or the restraints they may impose on the structural maturation or the functional integrity of the myocardium. But the least that can be said is that the nonmuscle cells are not simply passive elements in cardiac function, normal or abnormal.

Muscle Cell Hypertrophy or Hyperplasia as the Basis of Cardiac Growth and Hypertrophy

Growth in any organ can proceed by an enlargement of already existing cells (cell hypertrophy), by an increase in the number of cells (cellular hyperplasia), or by a combination of both. It is unlikely that different cell populations within an organ use the same mechanisms in contributing to the growth process. It is equally apparent that proliferation is the basis of organogenesis in the embryo. The question then arises: Does proliferation end at some point in organ development with subsequent growth proceeding by cell enlargement? In asking this question, however, care must be taken to specify the kind of cell. Functional cells, the neuron for example, can be expected to behave differently from so-called supportive elements, e.g., the endothelial cell.

Mitotic Activity of Myocardial Muscle Cells

There is little doubt that muscle cells in the heart continue to divide mitotically for some time after birth (Overy and Priest, 1966; Zhinkin and Andreeva, 1963). In the rat this activity appears to cease at about 28 days and in humans at 3 to 6 months. Mitotic division of mature muscle cell nuclei has been observed only following focal injury to the myocardium, as in experimentally induced infarction (Klinge, 1967; Robledo, 1956; Rumyantsev, 1968; Zhinkin and Andreeva, 1963). Amitotic division has been invoked to explain an apparent increase in the number of muscle cells during growth and hypertrophy, but this controversial concept of cytokinesis (Bloom and Fawcett, 1968) has not been convincingly demonstrated in the heart. The absence of mitotic activity in cardiac muscle cells in the postnatal growth period and hypertrophy have been reported by several workers (Enesco and Leblond, 1962; Klinge, 1967; Merkow and Leighton, 1967; Rumyantsev, 1963; Walker and Adrian, 1966).

Evidence for an Increase in Muscle Cells in Growth and Hypertrophy

Two lines of evidence have been cited in favor of muscle cell proliferation as the basis of cardiac growth and hypertrophy. One of these is the observation that the DNA content of the heart increases as the heart enlarges (Grimm *et al.*, 1966; Koplitz and Priest, 1962; Korecky and French, 1967; Meerson *et al.*, 1964; Norman and Carter, 1961; Nowy and Frings, 1960). Assuming that DNA content per nucleus remains constant, the only conclusion that can be reached is that the number of cells has also increased. However, as Norman and Carter (1961) suggested some years ago, this increase is due to proliferation of other than muscle cells; this has recently been confirmed by Grove and colleagues (1969b). The second line of evidence is morphological and is related to the observation that muscle fibers increase in the hypertrophic myocardium (King, 1940; Linzbach, 1960; Sandritter and Scomazzoni, 1964). Both of these studies were performed on human myocardium; confirmation by other techniques has not been possible.

Polyploidy in Cardiac Muscle Cells

Morphologists have recognized for many years that the nuclei of cardiac muscle cells in hypertrophic human hearts are not only enlarged, but are frequently hyperchromatic as well. Using cytophotometry, Kompmann and colleagues (1966) reported that relatively large numbers of muscle cell nuclei contained polyploid amounts of DNA, thus substantiating quantitatively the older qualitative observation. Grove and associates (1969a) also found polyploid muscle nuclei in hypertrophic rat hearts but to a considerably lesser proportion than in Sandritter's study on human hearts. The significance of polyploidy in cardiac cells is unknown, but there is general agreement that the process does not lead to cell mitosis.

Muscle Cell Organelle Dynamics in Cardiac Growth and Hypertrophy

Cells can enlarge just as organs can, by an increase in number and/or size of their constituent organelles. In the heart, muscle cells appear to grow as a result of an increase in number, rather than in size, of their organelles.

The Sarcomere

Measurements of sarcomere length in the hypertrophic heart have shown no change over the normal value (Grimm *et al.*, 1963; Linzbach, 1956). The constituent myofibrils, however, increase in diameter (Richter and Kellner, 1963), leading to an increase in fiber diameter (Karsner *et al.*, 1925; Lowe and Bate, 1948).

Myofilaments

The increase in size of the myofibrils is due to an increase in number of myofilaments, at least in the A band (Richter and Kellner, 1963). However, the diameter of the thick filaments does not enlarge (Carney and Brown, 1964).

Myosin

The molecular conformation of cardiac myosin has been studied in the hypertrophic canine heart. No increase in the length or diameter of the head or of the shaft portions of the molecule could be found (Carney and Brown, 1967). The same is probably true in the human heart (Carney and Brown, 1965).

Mitochondria

Differences of opinion have developed over the capacity of mitochondria to increase in number at the same rate as the myofilaments in the heart that is undergoing hypertrophy. Wollenberger and Schulze (1962) reported that myofibrils increase at a faster rate than do mitochondria, substantiating an earlier study by Tobian and associates (1960). A more recent report, however, (McCallister and Brown, 1965) stated that a parallel increase of mitochondria does occur, at least in the hypertrophic rat myocardium. Wollenberger and Schulze (1962) as well as McCallister and Brown (1965) agree that changes in the cristal structure of the mitochondria are present in the hypertrophic heart.

Cell Dynamics in the Hypertrophic Heart

Cardiac growth during the prenatal and early postnatal period is characterized by proliferation of both muscle and nonmuscle cells. But after this, the number of muscle cells does not increase, proliferation being confined to connective tissue, endothelial, and other nonmuscle cells. Hypertrophy is a continuation of the normal growth pattern: muscle cell enlargement and nonmuscle cell hyperplasia. Muscle cells enlarge during growth and hypertrophy by a proliferation of intracellular organelles; cell hypertrophy follows organelle hyperplasia.

The Human Heart

The above summary of events at the cell level occurring in growth and hypertrophy is based on animal experimentation. However, at least one important difference must be recognized between animal models and human cardiac hypertrophy: The former seldom, if ever, approach the degree of hypertrophy that the human heart often does. Regardless of the method used to produce hypertrophy in animals, the heart weight attained is usually between 50% and 70% more than the expected normal weight. In the human, heart weights of 100% and more over so-called normal weights occur, and considerably greater heart weights are not uncommon. That this may not be considered a trivial difference can be recognized in a paper by Linzbach (1960) in which he reported data that he interpreted as an indication that cell dynamics in human hearts above a critical weight (500 gm) are different from those in hearts below that weight. This might also explain the difference in ploidy values observed by Sandritter's group (Kompmann *et al.*, 1966; Sandritter and Scomazzoni, 1964) in human hearts, and by Grove and associates (1969a) in rat hearts.

Restraints on Cardiac Hypertrophy

The heart does not appear capable of unlimited hypertrophy in response to an increasing work load. Two restraints on the hypertrophic process have been studied and a third will be discussed.

Hormonal Milieu

Beznak (1963) has shown that the hypophysectomized rat does not develop cardiac hypertrophy following aortic constriction, but it occurs when growth hormone and thyroxine are given. She postulated (Beznak, 1964) that thyroxine restored the metabolic rate to normal but that growth hormone was required for the development of cardiac hypertrophy. The role of various hormones in limiting or inducing human cardiac hypertrophy has not been systematically established.

Capillary Blood Supply

An adequate supply of blood is obviously necessary for cardiac growth, normal and hypertrophic, as well as for optimal myocardial function. Wearn (1941) and Shipley and associates (1937) concluded from their studies of some years ago that the number of capillaries per enlarged fiber in hypertrophy markedly decreases. Linzbach (1956), however, found that capillaries increase in number in proportion to the increase in the number of fibers. Of perhaps more importance is the ability of active transport mechanisms of the sarcolemma and sarcotubular system to provide substrates and cofactors in adequate amounts at proper sites in the interior of an enlarging fiber.

Nuclear Sphere of Influence

Nuclear activity is a requirement for cell function and growth. Protein turnover and growth require continuous transcriptional activity by the operons of DNA. The transcriptional capacity of a given DNA charge within a nucleus has some upper limit. If the amount of DNA per nucleus remains constant, then this limit could act as a restraint on the ultimate volume to which the cytoplasm could grow. Other rate-limited functions within the nucleus could also have a similar effect on cell enlargement. The concept that a nucleus can "administer" only a limited amount of cytoplasm was first developed by Strasburger (1893), embellished by Hertwig (1908), and emphasized by Mazia (1961). In this view a cell approaches a critical size at which point it either ceases to grow or divides. If division is not possible, as appears to be the case with cardiac muscle cells, then the "nuclear sphere of influence" would establish an upper limit on cell size. Such a limitation on cell size in a non-dividing cell population would establish the extent to which an organ could grow normally or in response to an increased work load. If division of cardiac muscle cells does not occur after the postnatal period, then the upper limit of cardiac growth would be established at that early point in life. A possible means for extending the "nuclear sphere of influence" is suggested by the data of Sandritter and Scomazzoni (1964) and of Grove and associates (1969a,b), who found polyploid muscle cells in hypertrophic myocardia—one in humans, the other in rats. It is conceivable that DNA might be added in geometric ploidy increments and the transcriptional capacity of the nucleus thereby proportionally increased.

Summary

The structural aspects of cardiac hypertrophy and their functional implications can be understood only in terms of the myocardium as a polycellular tissue. The various populations of cells that make up the myocardium—muscle, connective tissue, endothelial, and nerve cells—contribute to cardiac growth and hypertrophy by different mechanisms. Muscle cells proliferate during embryonic and postnatal cardiac growth. After this, they contribute to growth by cell enlargement, apparently being no longer capable of division. Non-muscle cells, however, continue to divide. Muscle cells increase in size by a proliferation, not an enlargement, of their organelles. The hormonal milieu and capacity of the capillary system may act as restraints on the ultimate size to which muscle cells may grow. The "nuclear sphere of influence" may also act as such a restraint. Muscle cell polyploidy is suggested as a means of increasing the coding capacity of the nucleus and the ultimate size to which a muscle cell may grow. Much of the knowledge concerning the morphologic factors in the growing and hypertrophic heart is from experimental animals. Because such models seldom approach the degree of hypertrophy occurring in humans, present concepts must be regarded as tentative until definitive observations on hypertrophied human hearts can be made.

ACKNOWLEDGMENT

This investigation was supported in part by Research Grant HE-4856 from the National Institutes of Health, Public Health Service.

REFERENCES

Beznak, M. (1963). *Amer. J. Physiol.* **204**, 279.
Beznak, M. (1964). *Circ. Res.* **15**, Suppl. 2, 141.
Bloom, W., and Fawcett, D. W. (1968). "A Textbook of Histology," 9th Ed., p. 72. Saunders, Philadelphia, Pennsylvania.
Carney, J. A., and Brown, A. L. Jr. (1964). *Amer. J. Pathol.* **44**, 521.
Carney, J. A., and Brown, A. L., Jr. (1965). *Circ. Res.* **17**, 336.
Carney, J. A., and Brown, A. L., Jr. (1967). *Lab. Invest.* **16**, 36.
Enesco, M., and Leblond, C. P. (1962). *J. Embryol. Exp. Morphol.* **10**, 530.
Fawcett, D. W., and McNutt, N. S. (1969). *J. Cell Biol.* **42**, 1.
Grimm, A. F., Kubota, R., and Whitehorn, W. V. (1963). *Circ. Res.* **12**, 118.
Grimm, A. F. Kubota, R., and Whitehorn, W. V. (1966). *Circ. Res.* **19**, 552.
Grove, D., Nair, K. G., and Zak, R. (1969a). *Circ. Res.* **25**, 463.
Grove, D., Zak, R., Nair, K. G., and Aschenbrenner, V. (1969b). *Circ. Res.* **25**, 473.
Hertwig, R. (1908). *Arch. Zellforsch.* **1**, 1.
Karsner, H. T., Saphir, O., and Todd, T. W. (1925). *Amer. J. Pathol.* **1**, 351.
King, E. S. J. (1940). *Brit. Heart J.* **2**, 155.
Klinge, O. (1967). *Z. Zellforsch Mikrosk. Anat.* **80**, 488.
Kompmann, M., Paddags, I., and Sandritter, W. (1966). *Arch. Pathol.* **82**, 303.
Koplitz, R. M. and Priest, R. E. (1962). *Fed. Proc. Fed. Amer. Soc. Exp. Biol.* **21**, 199.
Korecky, B., and French, I. W. (1967). *Circ. Res.* **21**, 635.
Linzbach, A. J. (1956). *Arch. Pathol. Anat. Physiol.* **328**, 165.
Linzbach, A. J. (1960). *Amer. J. Cardiol.* **5**, 370.
Lowe, T. E., and Bate, E. W. (1948). *Med. J. Austral.* **1**, 467.
McCallister, B. D., and Brown, A. L., Jr. (1965). *Lab Invest.* **14**, 692.
Mazia, D. (1961). *In* "The Cell" (J. Brachet and A. E. Mirsky, eds.), Vol. III, p. 87. Academic Press, New York.
Meerson, F. Z., Beloshapkina, T. D., Lushnikov, E. F., Leikina, E. M., Markovskaya, G. N., and Chernyshova, G. V. (1963). *Vestn. Akad. Med. Nauk. SSSR* **18**, 27. (English translation in *Fed. Proc. Fed. Amer. Soc. Exp. Biol.* **23**, T667, 1964.)
Merkow, L., and Leighton, J. (1967). *Amer. J. Pathol.* **50**, 975.
Norman, T. D., and Carter, W. J. (1961). *Fed. Proc. Fed. Amer. Soc. Exp. Pathol.* **20**, 128.
Nowy, H., and Frings, H.-D. (1960). *Z. Ges. Exp. Med.* **132**, 538.
Overy, H. R., and Priest, R. E. (1966). *Lab. Invest.* **15**, 1100.
Richter, G. W., and Kellner, A. (1963). *J. Cell. Biol.* **18**, 195.
Robledo, M. (1956). *Amer. J. Pathol.* **32**, 1215.
Rumyantsev, P. P. (1963). *Folia Histochem. Cytochem.* **1**, 463.
Rumyantsev, P. P. (1968). *Experentia* **24**, 1234.
Sandritter, W., and Scomazzoni, G. (1964). *Nature* (*London*) **202**, 100.
Shipley, R. A., Shipley, Louise J., and Wearn, J. T. (1937). *J. Exp. Med.* **65**, 29.
Strasburger, E. (1893). "Histologische Beiträge," Vol. 5. Fischer, Jena.
Tobian, L., Severseike, O., and Cich, J. (1960). *Proc. Soc. Exp. Biol. Med.* **103**, 774.

Walker, B. E., and Adrian, E. K., Jr. (1966). *Cardiologia* **49**, 319.
Wearn, J. T. (1941). *Bull. Johns Hopkins Hosp.* **68**, 363.
Wollenberger, A., and Schulze, W. (1962). *Naturewissenschaften* **49**, 161.
Zhinkin, L. N., and Andreeva, L. F. (1963). *J. Embryol. Exp. Morphol.* **11**, 353.

SOME THOUGHTS ON ADAPTIVE GROWTH OF HEART MUSCLE

Robert R. Kohn

Tissues and organs throughout the body have the capacity to respond to functional demands by increasing or decreasing cell size or number. Cardiac and skeletal muscle are particularly reactive in this regard. Lack of function causes a rapid atrophy; 50% of the total skeletal muscle mass may be lost in 12 days following denervation in the rat. Hypertrophy as a result of increased functional demand is similarly rapid in cardiac and skeletal muscle.

Although the size of a muscle cell appears to be determined largely by the work it must do, intrinsic cellular mechanisms must also exert some control over growth, at least to a point. Muscle fibers have been grown in tissue culture in the absence of any function. On the other hand, if muscles that have been working are deprived of function by neurological disease or denervation, the myofibers undergo profound atrophy, and finally degenerate and disappear. It would appear that function is necessary to maintain myofibers after minimal growth has occurred.

It is tempting to postulate that atrophy and hypertrophy involve the same intracellular mechanisms, working in opposite directions in the two instances. The amounts of intracellular components present depend on the balance between rates of synthesis and rates of degradation. In various forms of muscle atrophy, rates of degradation are markedly increased. Rates of synthesis are also increased, but not sufficient to keep up with degradation, and the net effect is loss of muscle components. In hypertrophy of skeletal and cardiac muscle there is a rapid increase in RNA and protein synthesis. Very little is known about degradative mechanisms in hypertrophy. One might guess that degradation would also be accelerated, but to rates insufficient for keeping cell components from increasing. From data on atrophy, the impression is gained that feedback mechanisms between synthetic and degradative systems attempt to maintain amounts of cell components in a steady state, until the equilibrium is disturbed by prolonged alterations in functional demand.

Conclusions about intracellular mechanisms are hampered by our lack of information about turnover of specific muscle cell components. The turnover rate of such a major contractile protein as myosin is not known. There is some evidence that myosin exists in several pools with different rates of turnover, possibly reflecting different positions within a myofibril. We also do not know how myosin is degraded or lost.

There is no reason to believe that mechanisms of myocardial hypertrophy are different from those responsible for normal myofiber growth. In growth and development each myofiber increases in diameter, presumably because of increased functional demand from increasing organ and body mass; from an increasing vascular volume. Factors that lead to cardiac hypertrophy, such as hypertension, exercise, anemia, anoxia, atherosclerosis, and valvular disease all seem to have in common the requirement that myofibers are involved in more work. The final signal might be increased stress, or frequency of stress per unit cross section of myofiber. The big question is how such a signal might be transmitted to the protein synthesizing machinery to bring about an increased number of myofibrils so that the ratio between work and myofiber cross section is maintained fairly constant.

Myocardial cell division plays no role in either normal heart growth or cardiac hypertrophy. Heteroploidy of nuclei is known to occur in hypertrophy, but the extent of this is controversial at present. A steadily increasing cytoplasmic volume and number of myofibrils in the face of slight, or no increase in nuclear volume, and with no increase in numbers of nuclei might pose some problems.

Where cell division occurs, an organ increases in size while ratios of cytoplasmic to nuclear volumes are kept low, and all parts of the cytoplasm are not too far from the nucleus. Exchanges between nucleus and cytoplasm occur over short distances, and a given nucleus does not have to provide RNA to an excessively large number of cytoplasmic sites. In the case of myofibers, the optimal cytoplasmic/nuclear ratio is probably found in a healthy young adult. As hypertrophy proceeds, RNA must be transported to increasingly greater distances. There is also the problem of assembling individual myofibrils of considerable length from structural proteins synthesized at different sites which are rather far from nuclei. These factors suggest there may be a limit to the size a myofiber can attain in the absence of nuclear division.

The reactivity of myocardium to functional demand and adaptive growth of the heart are of great importance because they are fundamental to the pathogenesis of all chronic heart disease. The myofiber is also an excellent model for the study of control of intracellular mechanisms by external factors. There are large gaps in our knowledge of the sequence of events leading from an external chemical or physical stimulus to altered rates of translation, transcription, and enzyme activation. With respect to myofibers, we are perhaps at the stage of learning how to ask the appropriate questions.

ADAPTIVE GROWTH WITHOUT MITOSIS

Horton A. Johnson

The myocardium, like skeletal and smooth muscle, responds to an increased work load by increasing its capacity to do work. Since the rate of doing work, or the power output of the heart, is a function of the minute volume of cardiac output and the mean resistance against which blood is pumped, any increase in the minute volume as with exercise or anemia, or an increase in peripheral resistance as in hypertension increases the demand for power output and has the same physiological effect at the cellular level. An increase in functional capacity requires an increase in contractile protein and an increase, through synthesis of more mitrochondrial membrane, in the capacity to generate ATP. The synthetic response to a demand for increased power output is striking in experimental cardiac hypertrophy. Soon after the surgical induction of aortic stenosis the rate of protein synthesis increases two to four times, and the myocardial mass increases some 10% in 24 hr (Meerson, 1962; Gudbjarnason *et al.*, 1964).

The question is often raised as to how the heart can grow as much as it does in view of the scarcity of mitotic activity. It may be more provocative to put the question in reverse: Why should nuclei divide? The demand for greater power output is a demand for more cytoplasm, not more nuclei. An increased work load demands an expansion of the protein mass of the cytoplasm in the form of energy-producing elements and contractile structures. What is the role of the nucleus in this adaptive process and why should there be a need for more nuclei? The main function of the nucleus in compensatory growth is the maintenance of an outflow of messenger RNA sufficient to support the increased rate of protein synthesis in the cytoplasm. This also seems to be true in the case of adaptive growth of other organs. In both the liver and kidney, the response to the demand put upon the remaining tissue after partial extirpation results in an almost immediate increase in synthesis of RNA and protein (McArdle and Creaser, 1963; Braun *et al.*, 1962; Johnson and Vera Roma, 1966), apparently as a means of enlarging the functional capacity of the cytoplasm (Johnson and Amendola, 1968). After some hours of generalized cytoplasmic growth, mitotic figures begin to appear in a small fraction of the nuclei, probably in those cells in which cytoplasmic growth has outstripped the ability of the nucleus to support it (Johnson, 1969). It appears that adaptive growth in response to an increased functional demand calls forth an increase in cytoplasmic mass, which, after all, is the part of the cell that is directly responsible for its specialized function. Nuclear division in this context is a secondary response to a nucleocytoplasmic imbalance.

From this point of view, how can one account for the fact that in the process of doubling its mass, a remnant of liver shows considerable mitotic activity, a kidney shows a slight mitotic response, and the myocardium shows no nuclear division whatever? The implication here is that doubling the ratio of cytoplasmic to nuclear mass induces less functional imbalance in the kidney than in the liver and still less in cardiac muscle. The potential demand on the nucleus for synthesis of messenger RNA is probably related, among other factors, to the number of ribosomes in the cytoplasm. If two different cells have messenger RNA of similar mean half-lives, one might then expect the cell with the greater ribosomal number to place a greater demand upon the nucleus for transcription of messenger RNA. Conversely, the cell with fewer ribosomes has a greater nuclear reserve, that is to say, a greater number of transcription sites per ribosome. In general, the latter cell should tolerate a greater increase in ribosome number and accelerated protein synthesis without overloading nuclear transcription sites. For a given degree of cytoplasmic growth it should have less likelihood of requiring nuclear replication. Since the total RNA of the cell is largely ribosomal, the total RNA per cell should be a rough index of the ease with which a cell tends to nucleocytoplasmic imbalance. According to this line of reasoning, the liver should have the least nuclear reserve, or the greatest amount of RNA per nucleus, so that cytoplasmic growth has a high probability of overtaxing the nucleus and requiring nuclear replication. The kidney should show less RNA per nucleus and the heart least of all. Measurements of RNA/DNA ratios show just this correlation: approximately 4, 2, and 1 for rat liver, kidney, and heart, respectively (Leslie, 1955). This suggests that the heart could increase its cytoplasmic complement of ribosomes and its rate of protein synthesis by a factor of two and still have the same nucleocytoplasmic balance found in the normal kidney. These ratios are for whole tissue and are not entirely appropriate, since they include interstitial cells as well as parenchymal cells. Even if correct, this correlation does not represent a definite explanation of why heart muscle grows without nuclear division. It is presented simply as a heuristic argument. However, it does tend to support the concept that any compensatory growth in response to an increased work load is primarily a matter of cytoplasmic growth and that nuclear division is a secondary and obligatory consequence of cytoplasmic hypertrophy.

References

Braun, G. A., Marsh, J. B., and Drabkin, D. L. (1962). *Metab. Clin. Exp.* **11**, 957.
Gudbjarnason, S., Telerman, M., Chiba, C., Wolf, P. L., and Bing, R. J. (1964). *J. Lab. Clin. Med.* **63**, 245.
Johnson, H. A. (1969). *Amer. J. Pathol.* **57**, 1.
Johnson, H. A., and Amendola, F. (1968). *Amer. J. Pathol.* **54**, 35.
Johnson, H. A., and Vera Roman, J. M. (1966). *Amer. J. Pathol.* **49**, 1.
Leslie, I. (1955). *In* "The Nucleic Acids" (E. Chargaff and J. N. Davidson eds.). Academic Press, New York.
McArdle, A. H., and Creaser, E. H. (1963). *Biochem. Biophys. Acta.* **68**, 561.
Meerson, F. Z. (1962). *Circ. Res.* **10**, 250.

Part II
The Effects of Endocrines on the Growth of Heart Muscle

EFFECTS OF HYPOPHYSEAL HORMONES ON CARDIAC GROWTH AND FUNCTION

William V. Whitehorn

Introduction

It seems quite appropriate that this chapter on the the effects of endocrines on the growth of heart muscle should follow the previous section on adaptive growth. The hormones are regulators of growth and metabolism and it would be logically expected that this regulation might include these processes in cardiac muscle. Studies on the effects of hormones on cardiac growth and function have been complicated, however, by the use of a great variety of experimental preparations, varying methods of inducing endocrine effects or imbalances, the use of endocrine preparations of varying potency and purity, and other technical and experimental considerations. Furthermore, since the hormones do produce significant changes in the metabolic activity of many tissues, and since these noncardiac effects may result in modifications of circulatory parameters and cardiac work, the interpretation of data relevant to endocrine effects on cardiac growth and function may be complicated. This differentiation between direct and indirect endocrine effects on the heart is a matter of primary importance.

I should like to begin with some observations on the role of hypophyseal hormones in cardiac growth and function. Since the trophic hormones of the hypophysis exert their physiological actions, with minor exceptions, through their target glands, and since the effects of some of these other endocrines is the topic of the following chapters, these observations will be limited to consideration of the role of the growth hormone (GH) or somatotropic hormone (STH) of the hypophysis.

The work reported upon includes a study done some time ago and previously reported (Whitehorn *et al.*, 1962) and portions of more recent experiments not yet published in detail. In all of these studies the albino rat is the experimental animal. The procedure followed was to perform an endocrine manipulation, allow a period of about 3 weeks for observation and/or treatment, and then remove the heart for experimental study. Chemical analyses were performed on the combined ventricles; mechanical studies were carried out on isolated surviving left ventricular papillary muscles. The fundamental question asked was: Does the somatotropic factor of the hypophysis exert a direct influence on the size of the heart and/or modify the chemical composition and basic properties of the cardiac muscle?

Results and Discussion

The effects of hypophysectomy and administration of STH on body and ventricular weights are presented in Table I. In the dosage used, STH restored the growth rate of hypophysectomized rats to normal. As expected, hypophysectomy was associated with reduction of ventricular weight both absolutely and relative to body weight. More significantly, the ventricular weights and the ventricle–body weight ratios of the hypophysectomized animals were significantly less than those predicted for controls of similar weight from regression equations developed in our laboratory. A true cardiac "atrophy" was demonstrated. STH in dosage sufficient to produce a normal rate of growth in hypophysectomized animals did not return these values to normal, and administration of STH to normal animals did not result in significant modification of ventricle–body weight ratios. A direct "cardiotrophic" action of STH was therefore not demonstrated. The effects of hypophysectomy and administration of STH on the chemical composition of rat ventricles are shown in Table II. When corrections are made for slight differences in water content, total protein concentration did not differ from group to group. However, there were differences in the concentrations of ventricular actomyosin (myosin B). Hypophysectomy (Hypx) resulted in slight but significant increases in actomyosin concentration, whether expressed as percentage of wet ventricular weight or percentage of total protein. Administration of STH tended to return these concentrations to normal. Thus, it appeared that absence of STH did not impair an adequate production of cardiac contractile protein.

The contractile protein of the hypophysectomized animals was characterized by a modified response to the administration of ATP (ATP sensitivity). These data are presented in Table III. There were no significant differences in viscosity per unit of protein, but ATP sensitivity was consistently less in the hypophysectomized groups. The administration of STH tended to increase the ATP sensitivity both in hypophysectomized and normal animals. These modifications of concentration and properties of contractile protein were not accompanied by changes in the ability of isolated left ventricular papillary muscles from any of the groups to develop tension. Maximum developed isometric tension was not affected by hypophysectomy or the addition of STH.

TABLE I

BODY AND VENTRICLE WEIGHTS[a, b]

Group	No.	Body wt (gm)		Ventricular wt (mg)		Ventricle/Body wt (mg/gm)	
		Initial	Terminal	Actual	Predicted[c]	Actual	Predicted[c]
Group 1							
Control	8	–	191.5 ± 5.3	532 ± 17.0	565	2.78	2.94
Hypx	10	–	122.6 ± 1.2	284 ± 11.7	426	2.32	3.47
Group 2							
Control	10	181 ± 2.2	213.3 ± 5.1	601 ± 13.9	595	2.83	2.80
Control + GH	8	184 ± 2.9	223.4 ± 2.6	620 ± 10.8	615	2.78	2.75
Hypx	16	153 ± 2.1	157.8 ± 3.2	356 ± 5.2	492	2.26	3.12
Hypx + GH	15	155 ± 2.1	181.5 ± 2.1	393 ± 5.2	535	2.17	2.96

[a] Data from Whitehorn *et al.* (1952).
[b] Means ±S.E.
[c] Predicted ventricle weight = 197.2 + 1.87 (body weight).

TABLE II

WATER CONTENT, TOTAL PROTEIN, AND ACTOMYOSIN CONCENTRATIONS OF VENTRICULAR MUSCLE[a, b]

Group	No.	Total protein (% wet ventricle)	No.	Actomyosin (% wet ventricle)	No.	Actomyosin (% total protein)	No.	Dry heart wt (% wet)
Control	9	20.2 ± 0.27	8	2.16 ± 0.11	7	10.8 ± 0.61	9	23.7 ± 0.36
Control + GH	8	20.2 ± 0.25	8	2.06 ± 0.09	8	10.2 ± 0.44	8	23.8 ± 0.19
Hypx	15	18.9 ± 0.13	15	2.48 ± 0.09	15	13.1 ± 0.46	16	22.2 ± 0.25
Hypx + GH	11	18.7 ± 0.28	9	2.31 ± 0.14	9	12.4 ± 0.91	14	21.9 ± 0.21

[a] Data from Whitehorn *et al.* (1962).

[b] Mean values ± S.E.

TABLE III

VISCOSIMETRIC DATA[a, b]

Group	No.	Viscosity No. (Zn)	Viscosity No. after ATP (Zn ATP)	ATP sensitivity (%)
Control	6	0.218 ± 0.014	0.119 ± 0.008	82.6 ± 3.8
Control + GH	6	0.251 ± 0.011	0.127 ± 0.008	97.6 ± 3.2
Hypx.	13	0.233 ± 0.006	0.145 ± 0.006	60.7 ± 4.1
Hypx + GH	8	0.253 ± 0.010	0.140 ± 0.006	73.6 ± 5.8

[a] Data from Whitehorn *et al.* (1962).
[b] Means ±S.E.

The experiments described above (Whitehorn *et al.*, 1962) were conducted on rapidly growing animals. It seemed of interest to determine whether removal of hypophyseal factors in older rats would result in similar findings. Hypophysectomy was therefore performed on rats with body weights of 300, 325, and 370 gm. These data are summarized in Tables IV–VI. As shown in Table IV, hypophysectomy resulted in reduction in ventricular mass and ventricle–body weight ratios. Significantly, ventricular weights in the hypophysectomized animals were less than the predicted values at the time of operation indicating that a true regression of cardiac mass had occurred. The data of Table V are similar to those previously described. Ventricular actomyosin concentration expressed as a percentage of ventricular protein tended to increase in the absence of the hypophysis. Also in agreement with observations on younger animals, the data of Table VI substantiate the reduction in ATP sensitivity in ventricular actomyosin of hypophysectomized animals. These data are also in agreement with other observations from this laboratory (Grimm *et al.*, 1965), indicating a general relationship between ventricular size and the ATP sensitivity of extracted actomyosin. In further agreement with the earlier observations, no changes were observed in the isometric length–tension relationships nor the maximum developed isometric tensions of the groups in these experiments. The results obtained in the case of rapidly growing animals were accordingly confirmed in these observations on older animals.

The experiments summarized to this point were followed by additional studies with two principal objectives. First, the work of Beznak (1963) indicated that many of the effects of hypophysectomy on cardiac growth could be prevented by the administration of thyroid hormones. Studies were therefore conducted to clarify the relationship between hypophyseal growth hormone and thyroxine. Second, additional data relative to the mechanical

TABLE IV

BODY AND VENTRICLE WEIGHTS[a]

Group	No.	Body wt (gm)		Ventricular wt (mg)			Ventricle/Body wt (mg/gm)	
		Initial	Terminal	Predicted at Hypx[b]	Terminal Actual	Terminal Predicted[b]	Actual	Predicted[b]
Control	10	300	383 ± 6.2	758	938.8 ± 18.6	913	2.45	2.38
Hypx	10	300	270 ± 3.6	758	584.2 ± 12.4	702	2.16	2.60
Control	7	325	388 ± 12.0	795	953.7 ± 36.9	933	2.46	2.40
Hypx	8	325	255 ± 9.8	795	610.1 ± 39.4	664	2.37	2.60
Control	10	370	427 ± 21.6	889	1001.4 ± 92.6	996	2.37	2.34
Hypx	10	370	314 ± 25.0	889	702.2 ± 56.7	804	2.24	2.56

[a] Means ± S.E.

[b] Predicted ventricle weight = 197.2 + 1.87 (body weight).

TABLE V

WATER CONTENT, TOTAL PROTEIN, AND ACTOMYOSIN CONCENTRATION OF MYOCARDIUM

Body wt at Hypx	Group	No.	Total protein % (wet ventricle)	*P*	No.	Actomyosin % (wet ventricle)	*P*	No.	Actomyosin (% total protein)	*P*	No.	Dry heart wt (% wet)	*P*
300	Control	10	21.4 ± 0.18	Not	10	2.99 ± 0.14	Not	10	14.1 ± 0.62	<0.05	8	21.4 ± 1.0	<0.05
	Hypx	11	20.6 ± 0.51	sig.	11	3.23 ± 0.16	sig.	11	15.5 ± 0.62		9	24.4 ± 1.3	
325	Control	6	19.9 ± 1.4	Not	6	3.32 ± 0.10	Not	6	16.8 ± 3.3	not	–	–	–
	Hypx	5	19.1 ± 1.3	sig.	6	3.58 ± 0.11	sig.	5	18.7 ± 1.8	sig.	–	–	–
370	Control	10	22.2 ± 1.4	Not	9	3.08 ± 0.31	Not	9	14.7 ± 1.8	<0.01	8	22.9 ± 1.7	Not
	Hypx	10	20.1 ± 1.1	sig.	10	3.49 ± 0.32	sig.	10	17.5 ± 1.4		9	21.8 ± 2.2	sig.

TABLE VI

VISCOSIMETRIC DATA

Body size at time of Hypx (gm)	Control		Hypophysectomy		
	No.	ATP sensitivity (%) S.E.	No.	ATP sensitivity (%) S.E.	*P*
300	10	127.6 ± 5.9	11	105.3 ± 4.6	<0.01
325	5	140.8 ± 17.0	6	110.8 ± 9.7	>0.05
370	8	129.9 ± 10.9	10	111.8 ± 16.0	<0.05

properties of cardiac muscle following hypophysectomy and selective hormonal replacement then seemed desirable.

Experiments were conducted on hypophysectomized, thyroidectomized albino rats obtained through the kind cooperation of Dr. Robert Scow of the National Institutes of Health and Dr. Neena B. Schwartz, Department of Physiology, University of Illinois College of Medicine. The animals were divided into five groups: (1) an unoperated control group; (2) hypophysectomized (Hx), thyroidectomized (Tx) untreated animals; (3) double-operated animals to whom STH was administered in a dosage of 0.5 mg per day; (4) double-operated animals who received thyroxine (T_4) in a dosage of 1.25 ug per day; and (5) double-operated animals receiving both STH and thyroxine.

The data of Table VII summarize the findings with respect to body growth

TABLE VII

BODY AND VENTRICLE WEIGHTS

Group	No. of animals	Body wt (gm)	Ventr. wt (mg)	Predicted ventr. wt
Normal	15	208	558	585
HxTx	2	81	200	349
HxTx + STH	6	147	304	472
HxTx + T_4	6	95	342	375
HxTx + STH + T_4	6	210	543	590

and ventricular weight. As expected, the double-operated untreated animals did not grow and demonstrated ventricular weights significantly less than those expected on the basis of their body weights. In agreement with the previous experiments, administration of STH to the double-operated animals resulted in an increase in body weight and ventricular weight. Ventricular weights, however, were still significantly lower than those predicted on the basis of the increase in body weight. The administration of thyroxine to the double-operated animals resulted in some increase in body weight and restored ventricular–body weight ratios to normal. Administration of STH and thyroxine to double-operated animals produced normal values of body weight, ventricular weight, and ventricle–body weight ratio.

These data therefore support the conclusion that the disproportionate reduction of ventricular size following hypophysectomy is related to the deficiency in thyroid hormone level associated with that condition and can be corrected by administration of thyroxine, even in the absence of the somatotrophic hormone of the hypophysis.

The concentration of ventricular actomyosin (myosin B) in double-operated treated and untreated animals is presented in Table VIII. There were no significant deviations in any of the groups.

The data of Table IX summarize observations on maximum force development and time-to-peak contraction in isometric contractions of left ventricular papillary muscles from the normal and experimental animals. Muscles were prepared and studied according to the method of Ullrick and Whitehorn

TABLE VIII

VENTRICULAR ACTOMYOSIN CONCENTRATIONS

Group	No.	% Actomyosin	Actomyosin/total protein × 100
Normal	15	3.56	16.5
HxTx	2	3.46	16.6
NxTx + STH	6	3.38	18.0
HxTx + T_4	6	3.71	18.1
HxTx + T_4 + STH	6	4.01	18.5

TABLE IX

MECHANICAL PROPERTIES

Group	No.	Body wt	Muscle cross section (mm^2)	Max force (gm/mm^2)	Time-to-peak (msec)
Normal	8	209.0 ± 98	1.33 ± 0.13	2.55 ± 0.88	96.8 ± 7.1
HxTx	7	74.6 ± 10.6	0.73 ± 0.10	2.90 ± 0.46	105.5 ± 4.5
HxTx + T_4	4	94.5 ± 4.2	1.33 ± 0.24	1.35 ± 0.25	84.0 ± 3.9
HxTx + STH	5	142.0 ± 17.5	1.11 ± 0.30	2.56 ± 0.48	110.0 ± 5.0
HxTx + STH + T_4	5	195.4 ± 24.2	1.41 ± 0.32	2.36 ± 0.47	99.2 ± 4.8

(1956). The bath temperature was 37.5° C. Muscles were driven with square-wave stimuli of 6-msec duration at a frequency of 1 stimulus per second. Isometric force–time curves were recorded on a model 5 Grass polygraph or photographed from the screen of a Textronix model type 502 dual-beam oscilloscope. In agreement with previous studies, no significant change in maximum isometric force was observed in muscles from untreated double-operated animals nor in muscles from animals treated with STH or with STH plus thyroxine. The muscles of double-operated animals treated with thyroxine alone, however, developed significantly less force per cross-sectional area than did those of the normal or other groups. It should be particularly noted that the cross-sectional area of these muscles was identical with that of the normal controls and in the same range as the cross-sectional area of muscles of the other groups, with the exception of the untreated double-operated animals. The time to the peak of the contraction was significantly longer than normal in the double-operated untreated group and in the double-operated animals treated with STH. On the other hand, administration of thyroxine alone to double-operated animals produced a significant shortening of contraction time.

The results of these data indicate that although hypophysectomy does not significantly influence the maximum force development of cardiac muscle under the conditions studies, there are significant changes in the rate phenomena of cardiac muscle contraction. They also indicate that these disturbances are not related to deficiency of somatotrophic factor but are due to the reduction in thyroid activity associated with hypophysectomy and can be corrected by the administration of thyroxine alone. These findings are in general agreement with the earlier observations of Beznak and her co-workers (1963).

The marked reduction in maximum isometric force development found in the muscles of double-operated animals treated with thyroxine is in agreement with earlier reports of depression of force production in endocrine-intact thyroxine-treated animals (Whitehorn *et al.*, 1959) and with the observations of Korecky and Beznak in this volume. They are in some apparent conflict with the observation of Buccino (Buccino *et al.*, 1967), but the differences may well be explained on the basis of species variations and differences in the temperature and frequency of stimulation of the experimental preparations.

Summary and Conclusions

In summary, it may be concluded that the absence of hypophyseal hormonal function results in a reduction of cardiac size which is out of proportion to the defect in somatic growth. Administration of growth hormone alone does not remedy this defect but normal ventricular weight–body weight ratios can be reestablished by the administration of thyroxine.

Removal of the hypophysis does not prevent the synthesis of the myocardial contractile proteins and may result, in fact, in a slight increase in the concentration of ventricular actomyosin. The reduction in cardiac size, however, is associated with a modification of the viscosimetric response of the cardiac myosin B to administration of ATP (ATP sensitivity). This relationship has been previously noted (Grimm *et al.*, 1965) but its explanation is not clear at present.

The maximum isometric force developed by isolated left ventricular papillary muscles was not modified by hypophysectomy or STH administration under the conditions of these experiments. However, contraction times were significantly prolonged after hypophysectomy. Administration of STH did not influence this finding but administration of thyroxine plus STH returned these values to normal.

Thyroxine administration to double-operated animals produced the effect of a marked reduction of isometric contraction time. Maximum isometric force production was significantly less than normal under these conditions.

References

Beznak, M. (1963). *Circ. Res.* **12**, 333.

Buccino, R. A., Spann, J. F., Jr., Pool, P. E., Sonnenblick, E. H., and Braunwald, E. (1967). *J. Clin. Invest.* **46**, 1669.

Grimm, A. F., Kubota, R., Lorber, M., and Whitehorn, W. V. (1965). *Proc. Soc. Exp. Biol. Med.* **119**, 356.

Ullrick, W. C., and Whitehorn, W. V. (1956). *Circ. Res.* **4**, 499.

Whitehorn, W. V., Ullrick, W. C., and Andersen, B. R., (1959) *Circ. Res.* **7**, 250.

Whitehorn, W. V., Grimm, A. F., and King, T. M. (1962). *Circ. Res.* **10**, 853.

RELATIONSHIP BETWEEN HORMONES AND MUSCULAR WORK IN DETERMINING MUSCLE SIZE

Alfred L. Goldberg

In skeletal muscle as in cardiac muscle, increased work leads to growth of the muscle fibers. For the past several years, we have been investigating this growth process in skeletal muscle in an attempt to elucidate the mechanism through which physiological demand influences muscle size. For such investigations skeletal muscle offers numerous technical advantages over cardiac muscle. Various experimental approaches can be applied to skeletal muscle which are impossible on the heart. Information learned about skeletal muscle hypertrophy, however, should greatly facilitate understanding of the analogous growth process in the heart. It is worth remembering that most of our sophisticated knowledge about cardiac function, e.g., our concepts of contractile mechanisms or impulse propagation, was gained by applying to the heart results first obtained with skeletal muscle. An essential first step in studying compensatory hypertrophy was the development of a simple experimental system for inducing such growth in reproducible fashion. The development of a reliable technique for inducing hypertrophy (Goldberg, 1967a) has enabled us to define more precisely the phenomenon of compensatory growth, i.e., to clarify the relationship of compensatory growth process to other growth phenomena (Goldberg, 1967a, 1968b) and to study some of the biochemical events which underlie work-induced growth (Goldberg, 1968a, 1969a; Goldberg and Goodman 1969c).

Our first experiments were designed to elucidate the relationships between work-induced growth of muscles and the increase in muscle size that occurs during normal development. It has long been known that developmental growth requires the presence of pituitary growth hormone (Smith, 1930; Knobil, 1961). After hypophysectomy, muscle growth stops abruptly, whereas treatment with hormone reinitiates the growth process (Evans *et al.* 1948; Bigland and Jehring, 1952). Experiments were therefore designed to determine whether work-induced growth of muscle also required the presence of pituitary hormones (Goldberg, 1967a).

Earlier studies on the heart (Beznak, 1964) and on the kidney (Goss, 1964) have claimed that compensatory growth of these organs requires growth hormone. Beznak found that hypophysectomy prevented the compensatory growth of the heart which follows artificial coarctation of the aorta. Several workers observed that unilateral nephrectomy which causes compensatory growth of the remaining kidney does not do so in hypophysectomized animals (Goss, 1964). The interpretation of these findings, however, is complicated by the many systemic effects of hypophysectomy and the fact that pituitary hormones drastically affect the work load of these organs. As a result, these earlier conclusions are open to question. No previous studies have been carried out on skeletal muscles, in which these complicating factors can be better controlled.

For these experiments, the following simple technique was developed to induce rapid hypertrophy of two skeletal muscles in the hind limb of the rat. In this animal, three muscles act synergistically to extend the ankle and to support the body weight. The tendons of the large gastrocnemius and the much smaller soleus fuse to form the achilles tendon, while the intermediate-sized plantaris muscle has its own tendon, which also serves to extend the foot. When the gastrocnemius portion of the achilles tendon is sectioned on one limb, the remaining plantaris and soleus muscles must alone support the body weight on that side and undergo rapid compensatory growth.* The contralateral limb received a sham operation, and the corresponding muscles of this limb served as controls. With practice, these operative procedures take about 10 min to perform. The animals actively move about the cage immediately after anesthesia. They exhibit no tendency to avoid walking, although initially after operation, they walk without extending the ankle of the tenotomized limb. This difference between the two limbs is no longer apparent several days after surgery. To increase further the work load of these muscles, the water bottles are raised to the tops of the cages, so that the animals must stand on their hindlimbs in order to drink.

The effects of this operation on the sizes of the soleus and plantaris muscles of normal 100-gm rats are shown in Fig. 1. While the muscles of the control

* This technique for inducing hypertrophy constitutes an incomplete version of the surgical procedure performed upon Achilles by Paris during the Trojan War and described by Homer in the *Iliad*. Nevertheless, I have encountered appreciable difficulty with editors of physiological journals in trying to give credit to Homer's much earlier report. Probably as a result of Homer's account, medical authorities long believed that cutting the achilles tendon had rather serious consequences. In fact, Hippocrates wrote "This tendon, if bruised, or cut, causes the most acute fevers, induces choking, deranges the mind, and at length brings death." In our series of several hundred Charles River rats, we have never encountered such a response to tenotomy of the gastrocnemius.

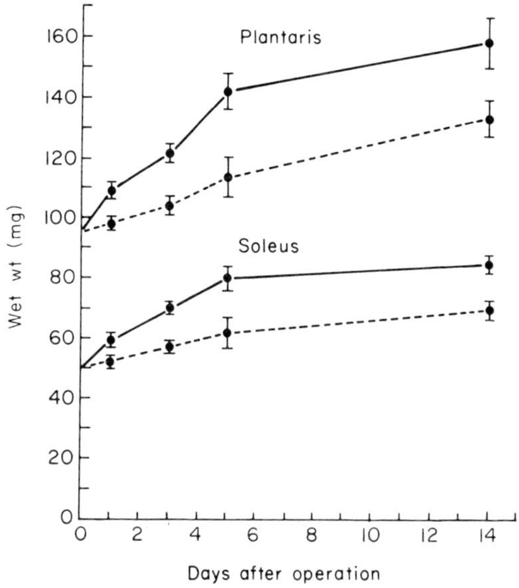

FIG. 1. Sizes of soleus and plantaris muscles after section of the gastrocnemius tendon in normal rats. During the first 5 days, the muscles of the tenotomized limb show an accelerated growth rate presumably in response to their increased work load. Each point represents the average of five animals. Standard errors are indicated. (—), Operated limb; (- - -), control.

limb grew at their normal rate, the muscles of the tenotomized limb grew at a markedly accelerated pace. This compensatory growth occurred surprisingly rapidly. It was already apparent 24 hr after operation, and by the end of five days, it was essentially complete. After this period of time, the muscles of the two limbs continued growing at about the same rate, in line with overall body growth.

Although the data presented in Fig. 1 and in the subsequent figures are for muscle wet weight, parallel changes occurred in the dry weight and in the protein content of the muscles. Histological studies demonstrated that this increase in muscle mass occurred through an increase in the average diameters of the muscle fibers, without any change in the number of fibers. (During hypertrophy, an increase in muscle DNA is found, although our recent autoradiographic experiments indicate that this increase occurs within the connective tissue elements and not within the muscle cells.)

To determine whether growth hormone plays an essential role in work-induced hypertrophy, we performed this same operation in hypophysectomized rats (Fig. 2). In these animals, total body growth was arrested following removal of the pituitary, and the weight of the muscles of the control limb remained constant during the period studied. Nevertheless, the soleus and plantaris of the operated limb underwent compensatory growth in a manner

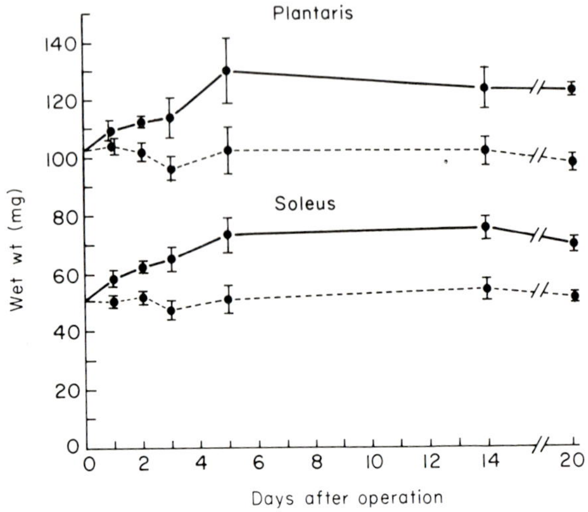

FIG. 2. Sizes of soleus and plantaris after section of the gastrocnemius tendon in hypophysectomized rats. Rapid growth of the muscles of the tenotomized limb is evident. (—), Operated limb; (---), control.

similar to that seen with normal animals. Following the 5-day period of rapid hypertrophy, the soleus and plantaris muscles of the hypophysectomized animals did not grow further. Thus in these rats, compensatory growth has been distinguished from normal developmental growth. When hypertrophy is expressed as the ratio of the weights of the rapidly growing muscles to that of their contralateral controls, it becomes apparent that compensatory growth proceeds to a similar extent and at similar rates in normal and hypophysectomized animals (Goldberg, 1967a).

These experiments thus demonstrated that pituitary growth hormone is not essential for work-induced hypertrophy. Since developmental growth does not occur in the hypophysectomized rat, such animals offer the possibility of studying compensatory hypertrophy as an isolated growth process. The rapidity and magnitude of the hypertrophy obtainable with the present procedures make it a highly useful system for studies of the biochemical events and physiological effects of work-induced growth. A variety of biochemical studies of hypertrophying muscles have been carried out and will be described subsequently (Goldberg, 1968a; 1969a; Hamosh *et al.*, 1967) (see page 301).

Like growth hormone, insulin is believed to be essential for normal growth of skeletal muscle. In its absence, protein synthesis in skeletal and cardiac muscle is significantly reduced, and muscle wasting becomes evident. On the other hand, insulin added *in vitro* to the muscles of diabetic animals causes a stimulation of protein synthesis (Korner, 1967; Wool, 1965). In addition, insulin appears essential for the anabolic effects of pituitary growth hormone (Knobil and Hotchkiss; 1964) and even for the differentiation of muscle cells from embryonic precursors (De la Haba *et al.*, 1967).

Experiments analogous to those described above were therefore carried out to determine whether insulin is also required for work-induced hypertrophy. Normal rats were treated with alloxan to make them severely diabetic, as evidenced by hyperphagia, polydipsia, polyuria, glucosuria, and failure of normal growth. Tenotomy of the gastrocnemius in such animals, however, caused rapid hypertrophy of the soleus and plantaris. In fact, the average percent of hypertrophy in the diabetic animals was similar to that observed in controls (Table I). By contrast, total body growth and the normal increase in muscle mass did not occur in such animals unless they were administered large doses of insulin.

TABLE I

EFFECTS OF TENOTOMY OF THE GASTROCNEMIUS ON THE SIZE OF THE SOLEUS IN DIABETIC AND NORMAL RATS[a]

	Weight of soleus (mg wet wt/100 gm body wt)		
Experimental groups	Control limb	Tenotomized limb	Average % hypertrophy[b]
Normal rats	42 ± 3	56 ± 3	33 ± 4
Diabetic rats	40 ± 1	54 ± 2	37 ± 3

[a] Muscle size was measured 6 days after tenotomy of the gastrocnemius. Values given are the means ±SEM for six diabetic animals and seven controls. The finding that the control soleus muscles did not differ in size per gm body weight indicates that the cessation of body growth in the diabetic rats (Table I) included cessation of growth of the soleus. In both diabetic and normal rats, the plantaris muscles of the tenotomized limb were 15–23% heavier than the contralateral muscles.

[b] Average percent increase in weight of hypertrophied muscle relative to contralateral muscle.

These experiments thus indicate that work-induced hypertrophy is independent of insulin. Subsequent biochemical studies further suggest that increased muscular activity has effects similar to insulin in promoting protein synthesis (Goldberg, 1968a) and amino acid transport into muscle (Goldberg and Goodman, 1969c).

These studies indicated that two types of muscle growth can be distinguished: (1) developmental growth, which is dependent upon growth hormone and insulin, and (2) work-induced hypertrophy. In recent experiments, we have even shown that the compensatory growth process can occur in animals deprived of food and in negative nitrogen balance. Tenotomy of the gastrocnemius was performed in a series of rats 2 days after food was removed from their cages. During the subsequent 5 days, the animals decreased in weight by up to 30%, including a decrease in total muscle mass (Table II). Nevertheless,

TABLE II

EFFECTS OF TENOTOMY OF GASTROCNEMIUS ON THE SIZE OF SOLEUS IN FOOD-DEPRIVED AND NORMAL ANIMALS[a]

	Food-deprived rats	Normal rats
Initial body wt	202 ± 4 gm	197 ± 6 gm
Final body wt	163 ± 7 gm	226 ± 5 gm
% change[b]	−19 ± 4%	+16 ± 2%
Control soleus	79 ± 6 mg	95 ± 5 mg
Hypertrophied soleus	107 ± 5 mg	127 ± 7 mg
Average % hypertrophy[c]	+36 ± 3%	+34 ± 4%

[a] Animals were sacrificed 5 days after tenotomy of the gastrocnemius and 6 days after food deprivation. Values given are the means ±SEM for six animals and are for tissue wet weight. Three additional animals not included in these data died during the period of inanition. In both food-deprived and normal animals, the plantaris muscle also underwent compensatory growth.

[b] Average percent change in wet weight of rats (each animal relative to its initial weight).

[c] Average percent increase in weight of hypertrophied muscle relative to contralateral control.

the soleus and plantaris of the tenotomized limbs showed both an absolute and relative increase in mass. Thus, while depleting muscle protein reserves, the organism appeared to permit the overworked muscles to increase in size and to compensate for the increased demand upon them.

Together these findings suggest that a definite hierarchy exists among the various factors regulating muscle growth. Compensatory hypertrophy clearly takes precedence over hormonal growth and even over endocrine signals for muscle depletion. Recent unpublished studies in our laboratory on compensatory hypertrophy of the heart and kidney have yielded similar conclusions.

The significance of work-induced growth and developmental growth to the organism are clearly different. Compensatory hypertrophy is specific to the organ involved (e.g., the heart) and occurs more rapidly than the growth process that normally accompanies development. The latter process takes place in many organs simultaneously and therefore probably must depend upon hormones to integrate the anabolic responses of the various tissues. Under many conditions, it would appear of selective advantage to the organism to give greater priority to the compensatory growth of an overworked muscle or the heart or to other types of adaptive growth (e.g., the regeneration of liver or wound healing) than to normal body growth.

Effects of Growth Hormone on Muscle Size

In addition to the above studies of work-induced hypertrophy, related experiments were performed in an attempt to characterize more precisely the hormone-induced growth process (Goldberg and Goodman, 1969a). Although it has long been realized that growth hormone is essential for normal growth, and that treatment with large doses of hormone can lead to an overgrowth of body musculature, surprisingly little is known concerning the mechanisms of this effect. The finding that work-induced hypertrophy does not require growth hormone raised the related question: Does the response to growth hormone require muscle work?

To answer this question we examined the effects of growth hormone on unused denervated muscles. These experiments, and all others to be described, employed hypophysectomized rats, in order that the effects of growth hormone might be investigated as isolated events. As shown in Figs. 3(a) and (b), treatment with growth hormone significantly decreased the rapid loss of weight of the denervated muscles, or even caused net growth of these unused muscles. Thus, the hormone-induced growth process can take place independently of normal work.

Although treatment with growth hormone decreased the absolute loss of weight of the denervated muscle, it did not, however, alter the ratio of the weight of the denervated muscles to that of the contralateral control (Fig. 4). In other words, growth hormone appeared to increase the sizes of both denervated and innervated muscles proportionately. For example, after a 10-day treatment with hormone the innervated soleus grew by 31% while the denervated soleus of the hormone-treated rats also became approximately 31% larger than the analogous muscle of the control animals. Although treatment with growth hormone for longer periods produced further absolute growth of the innervated soleus and plantaris muscles and although with time the extent of atrophy of the denervated muscles increased, in no case did treatment with growth hormone significantly change the ratio of the weights of the denervated muscles to the contralateral control (Fig. 5).

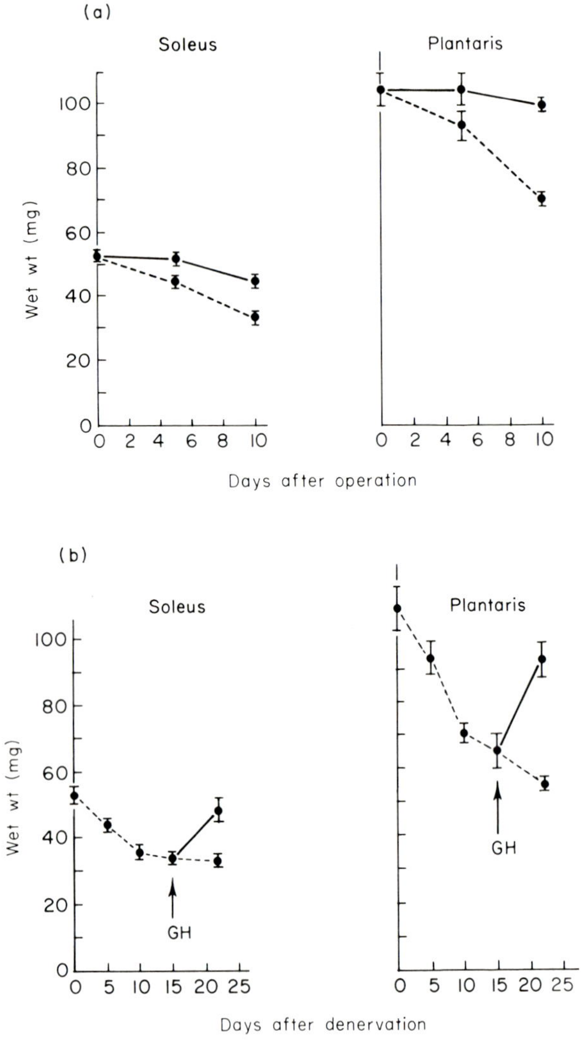

FIG. 3(a). Effects of growth hormone on denervated soleus and plantaris muscles in hypophysectomized rats. Rats received 1 mg/day of ovine growth hormone (NIH-GH-S-7) injected subcutaneously on each day following section of the sciatic nerve. Each point represents the mean ±S.E. of the mean of six animals. After 10-day treatment with hormone, the rats had grown by 20 ± 3%. (- - -), Saline; (—), growth hormone. (b), Effects of growth hormone on denervated soleus and plantaris. Experiments performed in identical manner to Fig. 1, except that hormone therapy was initiated 15 days after nerve section and continued for 7 days. Therapy with hormone resulted in 29 ± 4% increase in body weight. GH represents growth hormone.

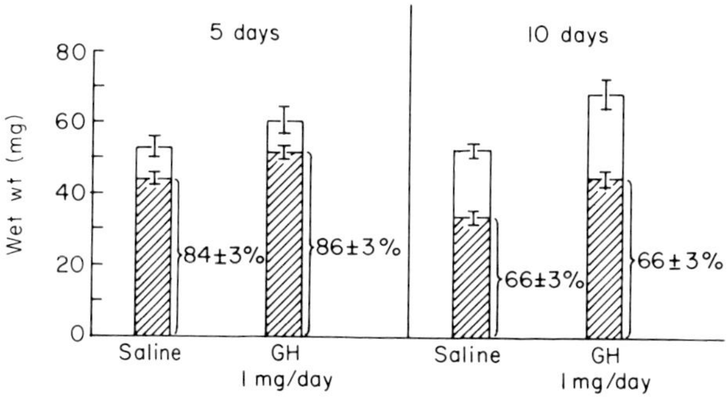

FIG. 4. Relative effects of growth hormone on denervated and innervated plantaris. Both mean size of muscles and mean ratio of weights of contralateral muscles are presented. Animals are the same ones studied in Fig. 3(a). In no case are the ratios of the weights of the contralateral muscles different. Hatched areas, denervated; open areas, control.

These data thus suggest that growth hormone increased the sizes of muscles proportionately, whether they were denervated or innervated. Analogous experiments were carried out to compare the effects of the hormone on control muscles and on contralateral muscles undergoing work-induced hypertrophy. These experiments similarly indicated that growth hormone increased the sizes of hypertrophying and control muscles proportionately.

Thus, although the pituitary hormone can produce growth in the absence

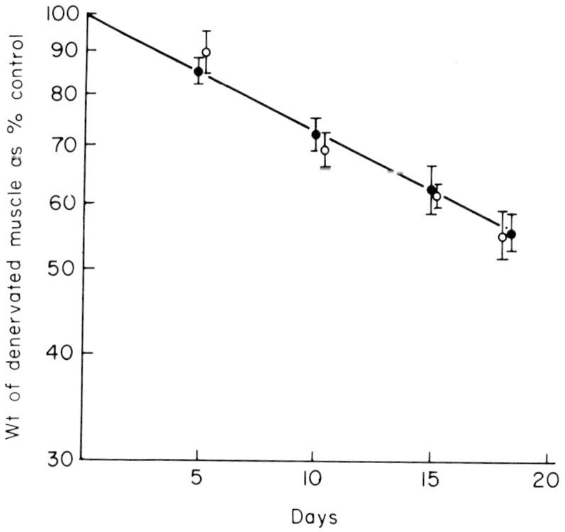

FIG. 5. Effects of growth hormone on atrophy of plantaris of hormone treated and control hypophysectomized rats: 18 days after denervation, and after 18 days of hormone therapy, the rats increased in weight by 54–58%. Filled circles, control; open circles, growth hormone.

of normal function, the effects of the hormone on muscle size are not independent of muscular work. In the various experimental situations studied, the hormone served to increase muscle size without altering the relative sizes of the muscles of the two limbs. Only the amount of use or disuse appeared to determine the relative weights of the contralateral muscles. Growth hormone appears to increase the sizes of skeletal muscles by the same numerical factor whether they are atrophying from denervation or hypertrophying from increased work.

Hence, this action of growth hormone appears analogous to a "gain control" on an oscilloscope or to an "amplifying system" of a phonograph, which influences the absolute intensity of the sound but does not affect the relative intensity of the different instruments playing on the record. Growth hormone appears to determine the absolute but not the relative changes in muscle size which result from changes in muscular work. This view of growth hormone as a sort of "linear amplifier" for other determinants of growth is in accord with clinical observations on "pure growth hormone deficiency in man" (Rimoin *et al.*, 1966). In this form of dwarfism, body proportions and sexual development are normal; only absolute body size is reduced.

The biochemical basis for such an "amplifying" effect is presently unknown. Any complete biochemical explanation of how the hormone promotes muscle growth must be able to account for these proportionate effects on atrophying, control, and hypertrophying tissues. Presently, we favor the view that in the various muscles growth hormone merely proportionately increases the basal rates of protein synthesis in muscle, which in turn are determined by the amount of muscular work (Goldberg, 1967b, 1968a). Although both the hormone and increased work increase protein synthesis in muscle, the two growth processes appear to differ in their effects on protein turnover in cells and eventually on the composition of the muscle (Goldberg, 1969a). Extended studies of the effects of these two types of growth on the biochemical and physiological properties of muscles remain to be carried out.

Effects of Cortisone on Muscle Size

Although these findings with growth hormone represent an interesting model for the interaction of hormones and physiological demand in determining muscle size, this type of interaction probably is not true in general of other hormones. For example, quite different results were found with cortisone. In large doses, cortisone and other adrenal steroids cause a net loss of body weight and marked muscle wasting (Leathem, 1964; Munro, 1964). Physiologically, the stimulation of net catabolism in muscle by glucocorticoids serves in time of need to make amino acids from muscle available to the liver for gluconeogenesis (Engel, 1950; Long *et al.*, 1940). In excessive doses, as seen for example in Cushing's syndrome, cortisone leads to a marked redistribution of body mass, in which the size of the liver is increased while the mass of skeletal muscle is decreased. The mechanisms through which cortisone induces muscle atrophy are as yet unclear, and represent an interesting related problem in the regulation of organ size. We undertook analogous studies to clarify the interaction of cortisone and muscular work in determining muscle size (Goldberg and Goodman, 1969b).

Treatment of hypophysectomized rats with cortisone caused a rapid decrease in body weight, and marked wasting of limbs was grossly evident. As shown in Fig. 6, the weight loss was not uniform in different muscles. For example, the pale plantaris muscle decreased in weight by approximately 40% within 10 days, but no significant loss of weight was demonstrable in the red soleus muscle. Two other pale muscles, the gastrocnemius and the anterior tibialis, also were reduced by 40% after 10 days' treatment with cortisone. These data thus suggested a selective effect of cortisone on the pale muscles, in clear contrast with our findings with growth hormone, which had parallel effects on the sizes of the soleus and plantaris.

Figure 6 also suggests that after denervation, the soleus and plantaris muscles became more susceptible to the effects of cortisone than were innervated controls. This possibility was tested by an analysis similar to that used in the studies with growth hormone (Fig. 7). If cortisone produced loss of weight proportionately in denervated and innervated muscles, the average

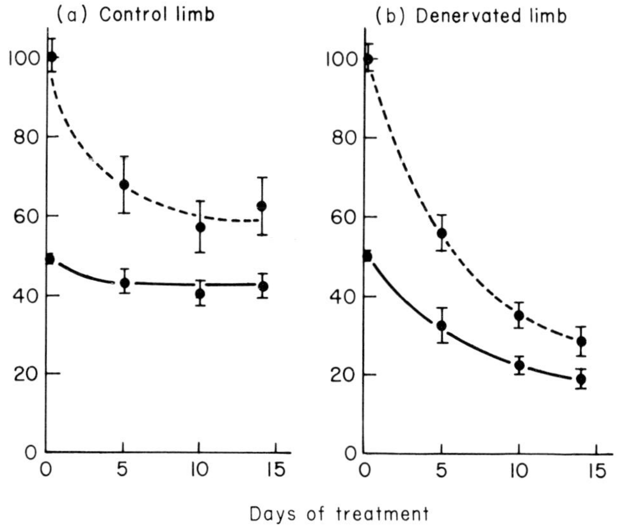

FIG. 6. Effects of cortisone acetate on muscle size in hypophysectomized rats. Each value is the mean ±S.E. of the mean of at least six rats. (---), Plantaris; (—), soleus rats.

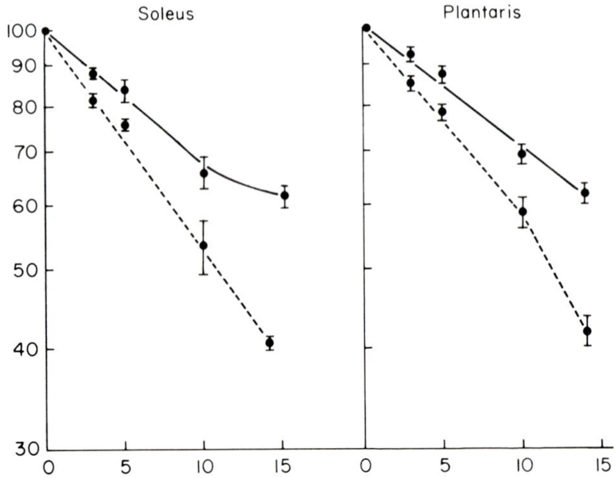

FIG. 7. Effects of cortisone on the rate of denervation atrophy, relative to contralateral innervated muscles. Animals are the same ones studied in Fig. 6. (- - -), Cortisone; (—), control.

ratio of the denervated muscle to its contralateral control should be identical in hormone-treated and untreated rats. The denervated soleus and plantaris, however, were consistently smaller, relative to internal controls, in those animals receiving hormone. Again, the findings with cortisone are clearly different from those with growth hormone.

During normal activity, dark (tonic) muscles are used more frequently by the organism than the pale (phasic) ones (Henneman and Olson, 1965). The observations that pale muscles atrophy to a greater extent than the dark soleus and that denervated muscles atrophy to a greater extent than innervated ones suggest that the effects of cortisone may be influenced by the level or muscular work (Engel, 1950). To further test this possibility the work load of the plantaris muscle of one limb was increased and compensatory hypertrophy was induced by tenotomy of the synergistic gastrocnemius. When such animals were treated with cortisone, the muscles of both limbs lost weight. However, cortisone treatment increased the ratio of the weight of the hypertrophied plantaris to that of the contralateral control (Goldberg and Goodman, 1969b). Thus, the relative amount of atrophy which occurred in the control plantaris must have exceeded that in the hypertrophying muscle.

The present experiments have demonstrated that cortisone in producing muscle atrophy does not affect skeletal muscle uniformly. Susceptibility of muscle to the catabolic levels of this hormone appears to be related to the level of muscular work. This finding may be of some importance in the management of muscle wasting in patients with Cushing's syndrome. This apparent specificity of corticosteroids for the less active muscles may also have important physiological significance. It would appear of selective advantage to the organism, in time of need, to mobilize protein reserves from skeletal muscle nonuniformally, since the atrophy of certain muscles would probably be of greater physiological consequence to the organism than would atrophy of others. The finding that cortisone had little effect on the tonic soleus or hypertrophying plantaris suggests that cortisone spares those muscles which are used most frequently by the organism. On the other hand, cortisone promoted marked wasting in the phasic or denervated muscles whose functional loss is probably less crucial.

The biochemical basis for the differences in sensitivity to cortisone remains to be determined. It is of interest that the catabolic effects of cortisone appear greatest in those muscles, which appear least active in protein synthesis (Goldberg, 1968a; 1967b; 1969b). Cortisone-induced atrophy appears to proceed through both decreased protein synthesis and increased protein catabolism (Goldberg, 1969e). Although formally these changes are analogous to those occurring during disuse atrophy, these two atrophy processes have different effects on the various muscle components (Goldberg, 1969b).

Finally, these observations on the effects of cortisone on muscle size are in sharp contrast to our earlier findings with growth hormone. In the analogous experiments, treatment with growth hormone not only increased the sizes of the soleus and plantaris but increased them proportionately whether they were functioning normally, atrophying from denervation, or hypertrophying from increased work. The very different effects of these two hormones suggest that cortisone and growth hormone are not simply biochemical antagonists, but influence protein metabolism in muscle in qualitatively different ways. Our recent biochemical studies on protein catabolism in skeletal muscle support this conclusion (Goldberg, 1969a,b).

Summary and Conclusions

Experiments were designed to clarify the relationship between work-induced hypertrophy and the growth process that accompanies development. A simple technique was developed for inducing rapid compensatory hypertrophy of the soleus and plantaris muscles of one hind limb of a rat. Within 1 week of tenotomy of the gastrocnemius, the weight of the soleus of the operated limb was 40% greater, and that of the plantaris was 20% greater than their contralateral controls. This experimental technique offers many technical advantages for investigating the mechanisms and effects of work-induced hypertrophy (see page 301).

Work-induced growth can occur in hypophysectomized rats, in which normal growth is arrested. Similarly work-induced hypertrophy can be induced in diabetic nongrowing animals. Thus, hypertrophy, unlike developmental growth does not require growth hormone or insulin. Work-induced hypertrophy can even be induced in animals deprived of foods and in negative nitrogen balance.

On the other hand, treatment with growth hormone induced net growth of denervated muscles, which suggests that hormone-induced growth can occur independently of muscle work. Growth hormone, however, did not alter the weight of the denervated muscles relative to its contralateral control, i.e., the hormone increased the sizes of denervated and control muscles proportionately. It is suggested that growth hormone determines the absolute changes in muscle size which in turn result from changes in muscular work.

By contrast, the effects of cortisone on muscle size appear to be critically dependent upon the level of muscular work. Large doses of cortisone caused marked atrophy of the plantaris and other pale muscles but had little effect on the size of the tonic red muscles. Denervation increased the sensitivity of the soleus and plantaris to the catabolic effects of the hormone, while increased work made the plantaris muscle less sensitive. Since the catabolic effects of cortisone are more pronounced in the less active muscles, it is suggested that in mobilizing body protein for gluconeogenesis, the hormone spares those muscles physiologically most active.

Growth hormone and cortisone thus represent two distinct models for the interaction of muscular work and hormones in determining muscle size. The biochemical basis of these interactions is a challenging problem, which we are presently pursuing (see page 301). The effects of other hormones, such as thyroxine or the androgens, remain to be investigated in a systematic fashion. This type of analysis constitutes a necessary step toward understanding the physiological significance of the various determinants of muscle size.

Acknowledgments

These studies have been supported through grants from the Berkshire County Chapter of the Massachusetts Heart Association and from the Milton Fund of Harvard University. Most of the experiments described herein were carried out in the laboratory of Dr. H. M. Goodman. The author is deeply grateful to Dr. Goodman for his expert advice and encouragement.

References

Beznak, M. (1964). *Circ. Res.* **5**, Suppl. 2, 141.

Bigland, B. and Jehring, B. J. (1952). *J. Physiol. (London)* **116**, 129.

De la Haba, G., Cooper, G. W., and Elting, V. (1967). *Proc. Nat. Acad. Sci. U.S.A.* **56**, 1719.

Engel, F. L. (1950). *Rec. Prog. Horm. Res.* **6**, 277.
Evans, H. G., Simpson, M. E., and Li. C. H., (1948). *Growth*, **12**, 15.
Goldberg, A. L. (1967a). *Amer. J. Physiol.* **213**, 1193.
Goldberg, A. L. (1967b). *Nature (London)* **216**, 1219.
Goldberg A. L. (1968a). *J. Cell Biol.* **36**, 653.
Goldberg, A. L. (1968b). *Endocrinology* **83**, 1071.
Goldberg A. L., (1969a). *J. Biol. Chem.* **244**, 3217.
Goldberg, A. L. (1969b). *J. Biol. Chem.* **244**, 3223.
Goldberg, A. L., and Goodman, H. M. (1969a). *J. Physiol.* **200**, 655.
Goldberg, A. L., and Goodman, H. M. (1969b). *J. Physiol.* **200**, 667.
Goldberg, A. L., and Goodman, H. M. (1969c). *Amer. J. Physiol.* **216**, 1111.
Goss, R. J. (1964). "Adaptive Growth." Logos Press, London.
Hamosh, M., Lesch, M., Baron, J., and Kaufmann, S. (1967). *Science* **159**, 35.
Henneman, E. and Olson, C. B. (1965). *J. Neurophysiol.* **28**, 581.
Knobil, E. (1961). "Growth in Living Systems" (M. Zarrow, ed.). Basic Books, New York.
Knobil, E., and Hotchkiss, J. (1964). *Annu. Rev. Physiol.* **26**, 4774.
Korner, A. (1967). *Progr. Biophys.* **17**, 61.
Leathem, J. H. (1964). *In* "Mammalian Protein Metabolism" (H. N. Munro and J. B. Allison, eds.), Vol. I, p. 343. Academic Press, New York.
Long, C. N. H., Katzen, B., and Fry, E. G. (1940). *Endocrinology* **26**, 309.
Munro, H. N. (1964). *In* "Mammalian Protein Metabolism" (H. N. Munro and J. B. Allison, eds.), Vol. I, p. 382. Academic Press, New York.
Rimoin, D. L., Merimee, T. J., and McKusick, V. A. (1966). *Science* **152**, 1635.
Smith, P. E. (1930). *Amer. J. Anat.* **45**, 205.
Wool, I. G. (1965) *In* "Actions of Hormones on Molecular Processes" (P. Karlson, ed.), p. 99. Academic Press, New York.

*EFFECT OF THYROXINE ON GROWTH AND FUNCTION OF CARDIAC MUSCLE**

B. Korecky and M. Beznak

Introduction

Experimental hyperthyroidism is one of the techniques used to produce a model of cardiac hypertrophy. If compared with other techniques (aortic constriction, physical exercise) it has certain advantages. The hypermetabolism may be evoked gradually, may be controlled, and if desired, discontinued completely. The particular factor that stimulates the growth of the heart acts upon the heart continuously during the hypermetabolic period. On the other hand, the increased heart rate, decreased peripheral resistance, and higher body temperature create some problems in evaluating the pumping function of the hyperthyroid heart and comparing it with euthyroid controls. Last but not least, operative procedures in hyperthyroid animals, which are performed under artificial respiration and where tissue hypoxia may be expected, may interfere with the function of the hyperthyroid heart more than in euthyroid controls.

Effect of Thyroid Hormones on the Growth of the Heart

Thyroxine and thyroxine-like substances have been used to produce experimental cardiomegaly. If thyroxine (T_4) or triiodothyronine (T_3) is used the degree of cardiomegaly corresponds approximately to the degree of hypermetabolism. For this reason, a relatively high dose has to be administered to lead to marked hypertrophy.

Sandler and Wilson (1959) produced cardiac hypertrophy by intramuscular injections of sodium-L-thyroxine (T_4) in doses of 0.2 mg three times a week for 8 weeks. This method of administration did not evoke tissue necrosis.

* Supported by grants from the Medical Research Council of Canada and the Ontario Heart Foundation.

Beznak (1962) injected thyroxine in aqueous solution subcutaneously in gradually increasing amounts until the overall dose of approximately 5–6 mg was reached in the 7th week. The weight increase of the heart paralleled the oxygen utilization and reached approximately 60% by the 7th week. In a similar experiment of Beznak *et al.* (1969) with a lower dosage of T_4 a three-week administration of T_4 increased the weight of the heart by 22%, 5 weeks by 27%, and 8 weeks by 38%. When this treatment was discontinued, the disappearance of cardiac hypertrophy could be observed to occur within 2 weeks in the last group (Fig. 1). Gemmill (1958) used 15.6 μg T_3 per 100 gm body weight per day for a period of 5–35 days to produce cardiac hypertrophy. Inchiosa and Freedberg (1963) injected 88–330 μg of T_4 or 22–37 μg of T_3/kgm of body weight subcutaneously to growing rabbits for a period of 12–15 days and the heart weight increased by 79% and 61%, respectively.

In experiments where the dry weight/wet weight ratio was reported, no significant differences between the control and experimental animals were observed. The newly synthesized proteins seemed to be responsible for the greatest part of the newly grown tissue. Cardiac hypertrophies in rats produced by different techniques were compared to determine the changes in collagenous and noncollagenous protein in the myocardium (Bartosova *et al.*, 1969). It was found that after T_4, the concentration of hydroxyproline

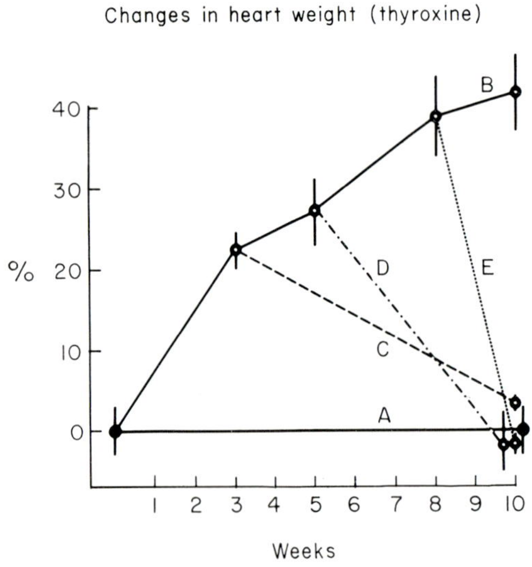

FIG. 1. Percentage changes in the weight of the heart during treatment with thyroxine. Ordinate: percentage changes in the heart weight/body weight ratio compared to a normal rat of the same weight. Abscissa: Experimental period in weeks. (A) normal control; (B) treatment with thyroxine; (C) same as (B) but thyroxine discontinued after 3 weeks; (D) same as (B) but thyroxine discontinued after 5 weeks; (E) same as (B) but thyroxine discontinued after 8 weeks. Mean values ±SEM. (From Beznak *et al.*, 1969.)

decreased as an indicator of collagen synthesis, and the total collagenous stroma of the hypertrophied heart of hyperthyroid rat did not increase. From this point of view it seems that cardiac hypertrophy produced by thyroxine resembles the one produced by low iron diet anemia, and differs from the cardiac hypertrophies produced by the other techniques which seem to stimulate an increased synthesis of hydroxyproline and thus increase of total collagenous stroma of the enlarged myocardium (Fig. 2).

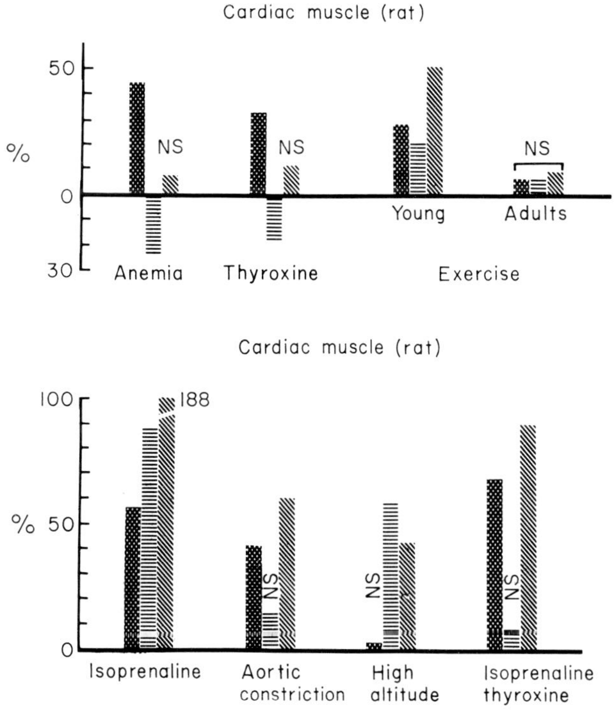

FIG. 2. Changes of the heart weight, myocardial concentration of hydroxyproline, and of total myocardial collagen in cardiac hypertrophies produced by different techniques. Percentage changes of mean values compared to means of control untreated animals. NS means nonsignificant. Double-hatched bars represent heart weight; horizontal, hydroxyproline; diagonal, collagen. (Data from Bartosova *et al.*, 1969.)

Effect of Thyroid Hormones on the Function of the Heart

The function of the hyperthyroid heart has been investigated at different degrees of hyperthyroidism and hypertrophy. The heart was considered as both a pump and a muscle and was investigated at different functional levels: isolated papillary muscle, isolated heart–lung preparation, whole animal.

Isolated Papillary Muscle

In the cat, an increased maximum developed tension, an increased maximum rate of tension development, and a shortened time to maximum tension were reported by Buccino and co-workers (1967). Similar results were described by Pannier (1968) for the same species. In our unpublished experiments a small increase of rate of tension development was also observed in isolated papillary muscles of hyperthyroid rats. However, the time to peak tension shortened and the maximum developed tension did not change in these hyperthyroid rats. With higher degrees of hyperthyroidism, the time to peak tension shortened more than the rate of tension development increased, and consequently the maximum developed tension decreased. Since our experimental arrangement was similar to that in the experiments reported by Buccino *et al.* (1967), the results seem to indicate a species difference. The duration of the active state as indicated by time to peak tension in the rat is only half as long as in the cat. Thus, any decrease of it would be rather detrimental to the developed tension. Since the frequency–strength relationship was not altered by different states of thyroid function in the rat, the reported experiments could not be explained by this factor.

Isolated Heart–Lung Preparation

The effect of different degrees of hyperthyroidism and of the concurrent effect of hypertrophy upon the maximum cardiac work of isolated heart–lung preparation were described by Korecky *et al.* (1966a) and Fig. 3 summarizes these results. The rats were treated with thyroxine in gradually increasing cumulative dosages for a period of 9 weeks. The maximum static work of the left ventricle, the oxygen consumption of the rats, and the degree of cardiac hypertrophy gradually increased during this period. When the maximum work of the left ventricle was recalculated per unit of body surface, it remained practically unchanged. When it was recalculated per unit of left ventricular weight it gradually decreased and in no group was this value higher than in the euthyroid animals. After 5 weeks of treatment, it even became significantly lower.

In the heart–lung preparation the pacemaker remains intact and the heart beats at its intrinsic rate. This rate is dependent on the temperature of the perfusing blood. The body temperature of the hyperthyroid animals ranges between 38°–39.5°C. Since the temperature of the perfusing blood was maintained at 37°C in the above experiments, it was felt that this might have been the factor contributing to the lower maximum cardiac work per unit weight of the left ventricle in hyperthyroid animals. When different temperatures were used, it was found that the hyperthyroid hearts exhibit different sensitivity to temperature than do the euthyroid ones. The maximum cardiac

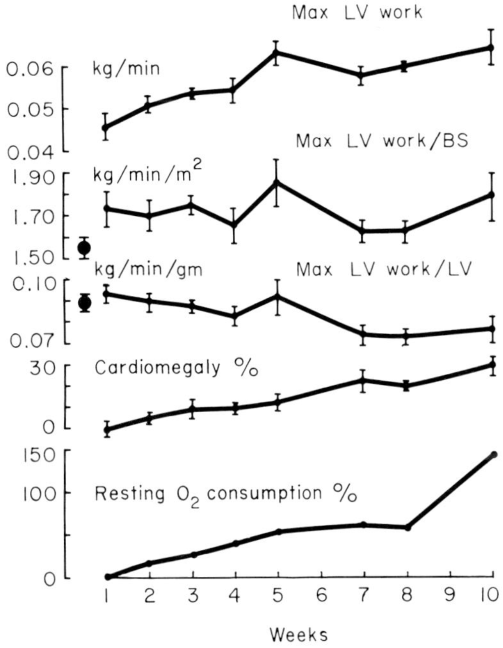

FIG. 3. The hemodynamic values obtained in the heart–lung preparation of rats treated with thyroxine. Mean values ±SEM. Filled circles represent the values obtained from normal euthyroid rats. Oxygen consumption was measured in anesthetized animals and expressed as differences from euthyroid controls.

work of the hyperthyroid animals reached its peak with a perfusion fluid of around 39°C and declined above and below that temperature. On the other hand, very little change was observed in euthyroid animals, where the maximum cardiac work remained unchanged between 36°–39°C (Korecky and Souhrada, 1967). Even at its optimum temperature, the hyperthyroid heart did not perform significantly better than the heart of euthyroid rats.

Whole Animal

The effects of thyroxine administration upon the cardiovascular system of mammals are: tachycardia, increasing cardiac output, increased cardiac work, and decreased peripheral resistance. Beznak (1962) measured the effect of thyroxine on these parameters in the whole anesthetized rats. Cardiac output was measured by the direct Fick principle and simultaneous monitoring of the arterial pressure enabled the calculation of cardiac work. The maximum cardiac output was measured as the highest output that could be achieved by the infusion of polyvinylpyrrolidone before the heart failed.

In rats to which T_4 was administered for a period of 4–8 weeks, both the resting and the maximum cardiac output significantly increased. The calculated static work of the left ventricle also was significantly higher. It was well above the euthyroid range if recalculated per unit of body weight per body surface or per unit of mass of the left ventricle. In our recent experiments the higher cardiac work of hyperthyroid animals could be brought down to normal levels by propranolol. It seems therefore that the thyroid–catecholamine relationship might explain this hyperfunction.

Effect of Thyroxine on the Heart of Hypophysectomized Animals

After hypophysectomy, the growth of the heart is inhibited to a greater extent than the growth of the body. The heart weight to body weight ratio decreases and the hemodynamic functions are depressed. Subsequent treatment with growth hormone can partly restore the growth of the heart and slightly improves its function. Subsequent treatment with T_4 restores the size and hemodynamic function of the heart to normal level. This was shown in whole anesthetized animals (Beznak, 1963) and later, to a certain extent, in isolated heart–lung preparations (Korecky *et al.*, 1966b). The profound changes in the size of the heart, in the weight of the animal, and in the heart rate made it practically impossible to describe the improvement of hemodynamics in terms other than as an increase of the maximum cardiac output and work. The results from the isolated heart–lung preparation indicated that T_4 has a direct effect on the contractile function of the myocardium.

When the descriptive mechanics of isometrically contracting papillary muscles were investigated (Minelli and Korecky, 1969) it was found that after hypophysectomy the maximum tension and the maximum rate of tension development decreased while the time to peak tension was prolonged. These results indicate that the pattern of isometric contraction was profoundly changed and that the contraction became slower and lasted longer. All these changes could be reversed by the administration of T_4 (Fig. 4).

Since the decrease of the maximum rate of tension development was greater than the decrease in maximum tension after hypophysectomy, it was felt that the velocity rather than the force of contraction was impaired. To prove this, the force–velocity relationship of isotonically contracting papillary muscles from hypophysectomized rats and hypophysectomized rats subsequently treated with thyroxine and growth hormone was determined (Korecky and Minelli, 1969). These results summarized in Fig. 5 indicate that after hypophysectomy, the maximum velocity of shortening was more depressed than the maximum tension. Subsequent T_4 administration after hypophysectomy restored both values to normal.

The decrease of maximum velocity of shortening after hypophysectomy

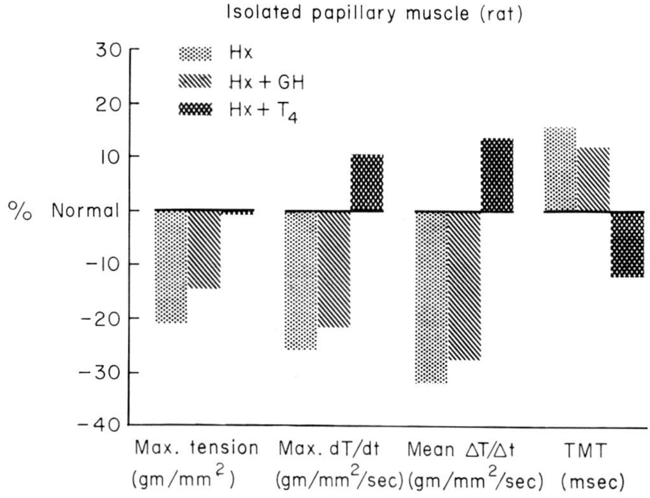

FIG. 4. Effect of hypophysectomy and subsequent hormonal treatment on the descriptive mechanics of myocardial contraction. The percentage differences in mean values between the group of normal control animals and the investigated experimental groups are plotted. Hx, Hypophysectomy; GH, growth hormone; T_4, thyroxine. Pooled results of anterior and posterior muscles of Wistar rats. (Data from Minelli and Korecky, 1969.)

in isotonic contraction was larger than the decrease in maximum rate of tension development in isometric contraction. The maximum rate of tension development reflects the velocity of shortening of the contractile element provided that the modules of elasticity of the series elastic component remained unchanged (Sonnenblick, 1964). Our results indicate, therefore, that the series elasticity might have become stiffer after hypophysectomy. To verify this, the modulus of elasticity was calculated at the point of transition from the isometric to the isotonic part of the afterloaded contraction. It was shown (Fig. 6), that the stiffness of the series elastic component increased after hypophysectomy and that subsequent treatment with T_4 restored it to normal. Since this technique provides indirect estimation of changes in series elasticity, a direct measurement of this component should be used to verify this finding.

Conclusions

The effect of thyroxine upon the growth of the heart has been investigated by several authors in different mammalian species. It seems that both the direct effect on the myocardial protein synthesis and the indirect effect resulting from increased demand for tissue perfusion are factors initiating

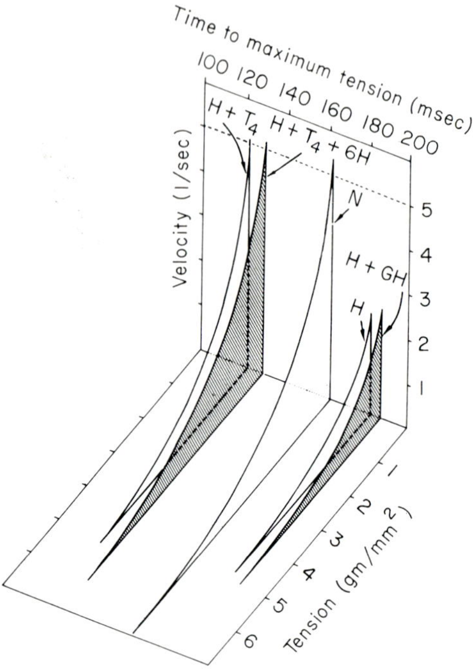

FIG. 5. Force–velocity relationship changes after hypophysectomy and subsequent hormonal treatment. The force–velocity curve was determined in afterloaded isotonic contractions with a small preload (0.2 gm) and the maximum velocity extrapolated. The maximum tension was determined in isometric conditions at the peak of length tension. The force–velocity curves are plotted against the duration of the contraction as expressed by time to maximum isometric tension.

the stimulated growth of the myocardium. There is no significant change in the chemical composition of the hyperthyroid myocardium. The parenchymatous part of the organ seems to be growing faster than the collagenous stroma.

The effect of thyroxine upon the function of the heart as a muscle differs according to species and is dependent on the dosage and experimental conditions. In isolated preparations it seems that the velocity of contraction is affected more than the developed force. This would be more pronounced in species with a slower heart rate. The average duration of contraction seems to be decreased in hyperthyroidism, which may be responsible for the decreased maximum developed tension observed in species with fast-beating hearts, where the velocity of contraction cannot proportionally increase. Tachycardia is maintained in hyperthyroid hearts with intact pacemakers after isolation, and cardiac output is achieved by higher heart rates and lower stroke volumes than in euthyroid animals.

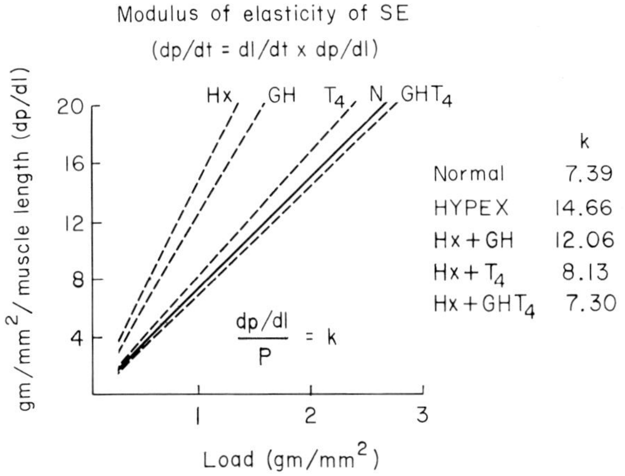

FIG. 6. Modulus of elasticity determined from isotonic afterloaded contractions of rat papillary muscles in normal, hypophysectomized, and hypophysectomized rats subsequently treated with thyroxine and growth hormone. (—), Normal values; (- - -), hypophysectomized (Hx), and hypophysectomized subsequently treated with thyroxine T_4 and GH.

In whole anesthetized animals the cardiac output is also achieved by higher heart rates while the stroke volume remains low. Unlike that of isolated hearts, the maximum cardiac work per unit mass seems to be higher in hyperthyroid animals than in euthyroid controls. Different peripheral readjustment in hyperthyroidism and the thyroid–catecholamine relationship may explain the high hemodynamic performance of hyperthyroid hearts in whole animals.

The effect of thyroxine upon the myocardium can be even more clearly demonstrated in hypophysectomized animals, where the size of the heart decreases and the double function of the heart as a pump and a muscle is impaired. Administration of thyroxine to hypophysectomized animals restores the size of the heart, the heart rate, the myocardial contractility, and the cardiac output to normal values.

REFERENCES

Bartosova, D., Chvapil, M., Korecky, B., Poupa, O., Rakusan, K., Turek, Z., and Vizek, M. (1969). *J. Physiol. (London)* **200**, 285.

Beznak, M. (1962). *Can. J. Biochem. Physiol.* **41**, 1941.

Beznak, M. (1963). *Circ. Res.* **12**, 333.

Beznak, M., Korecky, B., and Thomas, G. (1969). *Can. J. Physiol. Pharmacol.* **47**, 579.

Buccino, R. A., Spann, J. F., Sonnenblick, E. H., and Braunwald, E. (1967). *J. Clin. Invest.* **46**, 1969.

Gemmill, C. L. (1958). *Amer. J. Physiol.* **195**, 385.

Inchiosa, M. A., and Freedberg, A. S. (1963). *Fed. Proc. Fed. Amer. Soc. Exp. Biol.* **22**, 228.

Korecky, B., and Minelli, R. (1969). *The Physiologist* **12**, 273.
Korecky, B., and Souhrada, J. (1967). *Proc. Can. Fed. Biol. Soc.* **10**, 153.
Korecky, B., Beznak, M., and Korecka, M. (1966a). *Can. J. Physiol. Pharmacol.* **44**, 21.
Korecky, B., Beznak, M., and Korecka, M. (1966b). *Can. J. Physiol. Pharmacol.* **44**, 13.
Minelli, R., and Korecky, B. (1969). *Can. J. Physiol. Pharmacol.* **47**, 545.
Pannier, J. L. (1968). *Arch. Int. Physiol. Biochem.* **76**, 477.
Sandler, G., and Wilson, G. M. (1959). **44**, 282.
Sonnenblick, E. H. (1964). *Amer. J. Physiol.* **207**, 1330.

EFFECT OF INDUCED HYPERTHYROIDISM ON CONTRACTILE PERFORMANCE AND CARDIAC MYOSIN IN THE GUINEA PIG

P. T. Thyrum, E. M. Kritcher, R. J. Luchi, and M. J. Goodkind

The thyroid hormone has been shown to control the rates of numerous metabolic processes and also to have subtle and little-understood effects on the action of genes in controlling development and differentiation (Astwood, 1965). The myocardium of hyperthyroid animals is hypertrophied and differs from the normal myocardium in cardiovascular dynamics. Michels *et al.* (1963) demonstrated that thyroxine injected into rats increased the rate of myocardial protein biosynthesis. Buccino *et al.* (1967) showed that papillary muscle from the hyperthyroid cat had an increase in its velocity of shortening and rate of tension development, but a shorter duration of contraction compared to that of euthyroid animals. These changes in the intrinsic contractile state of cardiac muscle were independent of alterations in both norepinephrine and high-energy phosphate stores. Thyroxine thus appears to have a direct effect on the interaction between contractile sites in cardiac muscle. One of the determinants of the speed of contraction of muscle is generally believed to be splitting of ATP by the contractile protein myosin. Bárány (1967) has shown that the speed of contraction in many muscle types is proportional to the ATPase activity of myosin. In a preliminary report by Goodkind *et al.* (1969), it was shown that hyperthyroidism in guinea pigs increased myocardial contractility and cardiac myosin ATPase activity.

The present study was undertaken to determine whether thyroxine injected into guinea pigs affects (1) the ATPase activity of highly purified cardiac myofibrils as well as that of myosin, and (2) the primary and secondary protein structure of the myosin components of cardiac muscle.

Materials and Methods

Male, Hartley-strain guinea pigs weighing 300–400 gm were randomly divided into two groups, marked, and weighed. One group was made hyperthyroid by intraperitoneal injection of 0.25 mg/kg/day of sodium L-thyroxine for a period of 8 days. The second group was injected with a similar volume of saline over the same time period. The animals were killed by a blow on the head and the hearts rapidly removed.

Isometric contractile tension was measured in right ventricular papillary muscles dissected free from the remainder of the heart while immersed in a bath of Krebs–Henseleit solution (NaCl, 118 m*M*; $CaCl_2$, 2.5 m*M*; KCl, 4.8 m*M*; KH_2PO_4, 1.0 m*M*; $MgSO_4$, 1.2 m*M*; $NaHCO_3$, 27.2 m*M*; glucose, 200 mg/100 ml; with a pH of 7.4) oxygenated with a gas mixture of 95% O_2 and 5% CO_2. The muscle was suspended between a muscle holder hook and a Grass Instrument, model FT 0.03C force-displacement transducer in Krebs–Henseleit solution at 28°C. The signals from the strain gauge were recorded by means of an Electronics for Medicine, Inc., DR-8 oscillograph. The muscle was stimulated by field stimulation achieved by two parallel platinum plates connected to an American Electronics Laboratories 104A stimulator. The pulses were 0.2 V greater than threshold and 4 msec in duration. An equilibration period of 1 hr at 12 beats/min was allowed for each muscle. A curve of developed tension–resting tension was then obtained and the tension placed at the beginning of the plateau of maximum developed tension (average value for all muscle, 1 gm) for the remainder of the study. All muscles accepted for this study showed no spontaneous activity, demonstrated a positive staircase effect with increasing frequency of stimulation and were less that 1.0 mm^2 in cross-sectional area.

Myofibrils and myosin were prepared from the ventricles of beating hearts, rapidly excised, and chilled in iced water. Myofibrils were obtained by the method of Perry and Grey (1956). Cardiac myosin was prepared by the lithium chloride–ammonium sulfate fractionation technique described by Luchi *et al.* (1965).

Determinations of ATPase activities were made by measuring the amount of inorganic phosphate liberated over a 5-min period (Luchi *et al.*, 1965). The myofibrils (1 mg/6 ml) were reacted at 37°C with 5 m*M* $MgCl_2$ and 4 m*M* ATP in a 50 m*M* tris buffer at pH 7.4. Additions of 5 m*M* sodium azide did not influence the ATPase activities. The preparations were therefore considered free of mitochondrial contamination. The myosin obtained was reacted at 30°C with 10 m*M* $CaCl_2$ and 1.6 m*M* ATP in a 0.2-*M* tris buffer at pH 6.5 (Luchi *et al.*, 1965). The ATPase activities of both purified myofibrillar and myosin samples from control guinea pigs were also determined after 5-min and 18-hr incubations with thyroxine (10^{-4} to $10^{-7}M$) in

0.4 *M* KCl-borate buffer at 5°C. These *in vitro* additions of L-thyroxine were found not to influence the ATPase activities of the preparations.

Optical rotatory dispersion spectra of the myosin preparations in 0.4 *M* KCl-borate buffer, pH 6.8, were obtained on a Cary model 60 spectropolarimeter using a 5-mm cell. The amplitude of the negative Cotton effect at 233 mμ was used to estimate the percent helix of the protein (Luchi *et al.*, 1969).

The cysteine, tyrosine, and tryptophan content of myosin was determined by relatively simple spectrophotometric techniques. Cysteine was determined by reacting myosin with *p*-chloromercuribenzoate and recording the optical density change at 255 mμ (Luchi *et al.*, 1969). The tyrosine and tryptophan content of the proteins were determined by the spectrophotometric method of Goodwin and Morton (1946). Protein concentrations were measured by the micro-Kjeldahl technique assuming that nitrogen accounts for 16% of the weight of cardiac myosin.

Amino acid composition data were obtained by the method of Moore and Stein (1963) utilizing a Beckman model 120C amino acid analyzer. Acid hydrolysis of myosin was carried out at 110°C for 24, 48, and 72 hr.

Results

The hyperthyroid guinea pigs suffered an average weight loss of 10% and showed a 28% ventricular weight increase over that of controls. Frequency response curves of developed tension were successfully studied from six euthyroid and six hyperthyroid animals. Figure 1 shows the effect of hyperthyroidism on the maximum rate of tension change (dT/dt max) of right

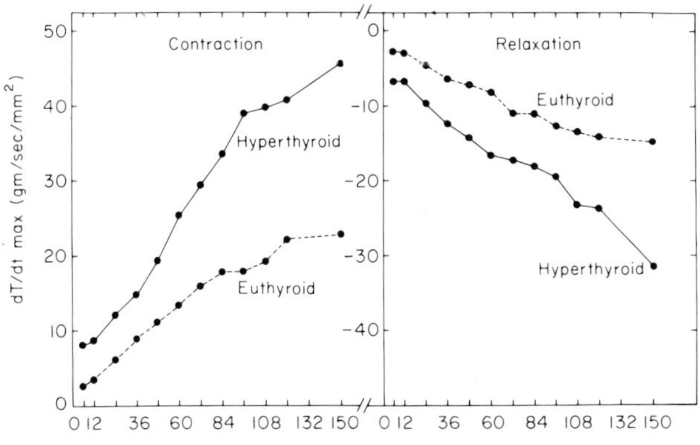

FIG. 1. Effect of frequency of stimulation on the maximum rate of tension change (dT/dt max) during isometric contraction and relaxation of papillary muscle from euthyroid and hyperthyroid guinea pigs.

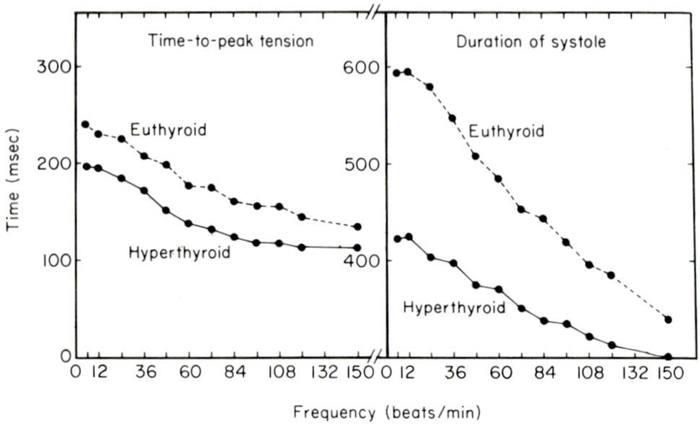

FIG. 2. Effect of frequency of stimulation on the time-to-peak tension and duration of systole of isometric contraction of papillary muscle from euthyroid and hyperthyroid guinea pigs.

papillary muscle during isometric contraction and relaxation at frequencies with a range of 5–150 beats/min. The effect of hyperthyroidism on the time to peak tension and the duration of systole at various frequencies is shown in Fig. 2. The differences in mechanical characteristics between euthyroid and hyperthyroid muscles shown in Figs. 1 and 2 were significant ($p < 0.05$). The alterations in cardiac functions known to be associated with hyperthyroidism (Buccino *et al.*, 1967), were therefore evident in the guinea pigs injected with thyroxine in this study.

The average myofibrillar ATPase activities of three groups each (five animals per group) of euthyroid and hyperthyroid guinea pigs were found to differ ($p < 0.005$). The values obtained are shown in Table I. The myosin ATPase activities of ventricular myosin extracted from 14 groups each (five animals per group) of euthyroid and hyperthyroid guinea pigs are also shown

TABLE I

ATPase Activity of Cardiac Myofibrils and Myosin from Euthyroid and Hyperthyroid Guinea Pigs

Enzyme	ATPase activity[a] (10^{-7} moles P/mg protein × min) Euthyroid	Hyperthyroid	% Change
Myofibrils	0.67 ± 0.04	0.90 ± 0.06	+34
Myosin	8.2 ± 0.7	10.8 ± 1.3	+33

[a] Mean value ± 1 S.D.

in Table I. The 33% greater activity of the hyperthyroid groups was significant at $p < 0.001$.

Purified myosin samples from five groups each (five animals per group) of control and hyperthyroid guinea pigs were analyzed by spectrophotometric methods for their percent helix, cysteine, tyrosine, and tryptophan contents. Myosin from hyperthyroid guinea pigs differed from control myosin in helical content only (28% higher, $p < 0.001$) as shown in Table II.

TABLE II

HELICAL CONTENT AND PARTIAL AMINO ACID COMPOSITION OF CARDIAC MYOSIN FROM EUTHYROID AND HYPERTHYROID GUINEA PIGS DETERMINED SPECTROPHOTOMETRICALLY

		Amino acid content[a] (moles/10^5-gm myosin)		
Thyroid state	% Helix	Cysteine	Tyrosine	Tryptophan
Euthyroid	43 ± 3	7.3 ± 0.5	19 ± 1	4.0 ± 0.2
Hyperthyroid	55 ± 1	7.4 ± 0.4	19 ± 1	4.1 ± 0.1

[a] Mean value ± 1 S.D.

The amino acid composition of myosin samples obtained from 15 pooled euthyroid and 20 pooled hyperthyroid guinea pig ventricles is shown in Table III. Cardiac myosin from hyperthyroid animals was found to have a threonine, serine, lysine, and glutamic acid content significantly different from control myosin. The amino acids have been arranged according to the classification of Havsteen (1966) into promoting, disturbing, and indifferent types with respect to helix formation. The helix-inhibiting amino acids are the prolines and any amino acid having an oxygen atom, sulfur atom, or a disubstitution other than hydrogen, attached to its β-carbon. Glycine is considered indifferent with respect to helix formation and the remaining amino acids helix-promoting.

Discussion

Investigations of the physicochemical properties of cardiac myosin isolated from hyperthyroid guinea pigs have revealed that the administration of thyroxine stimulates the synthesis of a new type of contractile protein. The differences between this myosin and myosin from euthyroid guinea pigs in ATPase activity, helical content, and amino acid composition are shown in Tables I, II, and III, respectively.

TABLE III

AMINO ACID COMPOSITION OF CARDIAC MYOSIN FROM EUTHYROID AND HYPERTHYROID GUINEA PIGS

Amino acid[a]	Moles amino acid/10^5 gm myosin[b] Euthyroid	Hyperthyroid	Significance of observed differences ($p<$)
α-Helix promoting			
Lysine	87 ± 1	94 ± 3	0.01
Histidine	17 ± 1	17 ± 1	
Arginine	49 ± 1	50 ± 1	
Aspartic Acid	84 ± 1	89 ± 4	
Glutamic Acid	150 ± 3	162 ± 7	0.05
Alanine	67 ± 2	72 ± 4	
Methionine	21 ± 1	22 ± 1	
Leucine	80 ± 2	85 ± 5	
Tyrosine	16 ± 1	16 ± 1	
Phenylalanine	28 ± 1	30 ± 3	
α-Helix disturbing			
Threonine[c]	40 ± 1	36 ± 1	0.01
Serine[c]	38 ± 1	34 ± 1	0.01
Proline	24 ± 1	23 ± 1	
Valine	36 ± 1	38 ± 3	
Isoleucine	36 ± 1	37 ± 3	
Indifferent residues			
Glycine	35 ± 1	35 ± 2	
Amide NH_3[c]	93	95	

[a] Classified according to Havsteen (1966) into promoting, disturbing, and indifferent types with respect to helix formation.

[b] Mean ± 1 S.D. of 24, 48, and 72 hr hydrolysis values, except as noted.

[c] Values extrapolated to 0 time to correct for hydrolytic destruction.

The amino acid composition of proteins is known to be of significance in determining protein conformation (Havsteen, 1966). The high helical content of myosin from hyperthyroid guinea pigs can be interpreted as the result of its relatively low content of the helix-disturbing amino acids threonine and serine and its relatively high content of the helix-promoting amino acids lysine and glutamic acid.

The relevance of the altered myosin properties to the *in vivo* muscle changes observed is not yet clear. It is of interest that highly purified myofibrils, which may serve as models of muscle systems under control of factors regulating both contraction and relaxation, also showed a significantly increased ATPase activity (Table I). It has been noted recently (M. J. Goodkind,

G. E. Dambach, and R. J. Luchi, unpublished observations), that the influence of L-thyroxine on most of the mechanical characteristics of isolated guinea pig papillary muscle can be observed 1 day after an intraperitoneal injection as shown in Figs. 1 and 2. Myosin isolated from such animals did not differ from control myosin in ATPase activity. It therefore appears that the thyroid hormone may have a dual effect on the heart. One effect, observable almost immediately, is a change in the intrinsic contractile state of the cardiac muscle. The second effect, occurring later, is an alteration of the enzymatic activity of the contractile protein myosin. This increase in ATPase activity should also augment the speed of contraction of the muscle (Bárány, 1967). The second effect may be the result of a direct influence of thyroxine on genetic action regulating the primary structure of myosin, or an adaptive response to some of the many metabolic alterations known to occur in hyperthyroidism.

Summary

Hyperthyroidism was produced in guinea pigs by intraperitoneal injections of L-thyroxine for 8 days. Isometric contraction measurements demonstrated the expected thyroxine effects on the mechanical properties of the myocardium which apparently precede the effects on the muscle enzymes of interest in this study. Hyperthyroid papillary muscle developed tension at a more rapid rate, but in a shorter period of time than did euthyroid muscle. Both myofibrillar and myosin preparations from the ventricular muscle of hyperthyroid guinea pigs showed more than a 30% increase in ATPase activity over control preparations. Optical rotatory dispersion measurements indicated that myosin from hyperthyroid animals had a 28% higher helical content than that from euthyroid controls. The amino acid compositions of the two types of myosins were dissimilar. The high helical content of myosin from hyperthyroid animals can be interpreted as the result of its relatively low content of the helix-disturbing amino acids threonine and serine and its relatively high content of the helix-promoting amino acids, lysine, and glutamic acid. The results thus demonstrate that the administration of thyroxine to guinea pigs stimulates the synthesis of a new type of cardiac myosin, differing from control myosin in ATPase activity, helical content, and amino acid composition.

References

Astwood, E. B. (1965). *In* "The Pharmacological Basis of Therapeutics" (L. S. Goodman and A. Gilman, eds.), 3rd edition, p. 1466. MacMillan, New York.

Bárány, M. (1967). *J. Gen. Physiol.* **50**, 197.

Buccino, R. A., Spann, J. F., Jr., Pool, P. E., Sonnenblick, E. H. and Braunwald, E. (1967). *J. Clin Invest.* **46**, 1669.
Goodkind, M. J., Dambach, G. E., and Luchi, R. J. (1969). *J. Clin. Invest.* **48**, 30a.
Goodwin, T. W., and Morton, R. A. (1946). *Biochem. J.* **40**, 628.
Havsteen, B. H. (1966). *J. Theor. Biol.* **10**, 1.
Luchi, R. J., Kritcher, E. M., and Conn, H. L., Jr. (1965). *Circ. Res.* **16**, 74.
Luchi, R. J., Kritcher, E. M., and Thyrum, P. T. (1969). *Circ. Res.* **24**, 513.
Michels, R., Cason, J., and Sokoloff, L. (1963). *Science* **140**, 1417.
Moore, S., and Stein, W. H. (1963). Methods Enzymol. **6**, 819.
Perry, S. V., and Grey, T. C. (1956). *Biochem. J.* **64**, 184.

CORTICOSTEROIDS AND THE FUNCTIONAL CAPACITY OF THE MYOCARDIUM

Allan M. Lefer and Richard L. Verrier

In the absence of corticosteroids, the circulatory system undergoes a marked change in functional status. Indeed, adrenal insufficiency is characterized by a state of circulatory collapse. The major factor responsible for this collapse is a marked impairment of myocardial contractility Lefer, 1967, 1968; Lefer *et al.*, 1968, Verrier *et al.*, 1969b). This cardiac impairment occurs in the absence of significant impariments in arterial or venous tone (Verrier *et al.*, 1969a), and without a significant reduction in blood volume (Verrier *et al.*, 1968b).

There is a 10% loss in dry weight of the myocardium (Solomon *et al.*, 1959), as well as alterations in myocardial cell ultrastructure in adrenal insufficiency (Immes and Jones, personal communication; Suzuki, 1967). Nevertheless, these changes do not reveal the intracellular locus responsible for the impairment of myocardial function. In addition, a recent study of the electro-physiological properties of cardiac muscle cell membranes revealed no defects in membrane function (Rovetto and Lefer, 1970. However calcium was able to prevent and/or partially reverse the mechanical defect in cardiac muscle cells. This suggested that perhaps the cardiac dysfunction seen in adrenal insufficiency might be reflected in a defect in contractile proteins of myocardial cells or in excitation–contraction coupling.

Therefore a study was undertaken to determine whether a prolonged administration of corticosteroids is capable of enhancing cardiac performance and of inducing hypertension and/or cardiac hypertrophy in animals with intact adrenals.

Methods

Male Sprague–Dawley rats weighing between 225–250 gm and cats of either sex weighing between 2.5–3.8 kg were used as experimental subjects. All cats were kept in isolation for 10–14 days prior to use and only those judged to be in good health at the end of the quarantine period were accepted as experimental subjects.

The following experimental groups of animals were studied.

Rats

1. Controls: These rats were sacrificed on day 1 of the experiment and received no special treatment.
2. Sesame oil-treated: These rats were given daily injections of 0.2–0.3 ml of sterile sesame oil intramuscularly for 28 days.
3. DOCA-treated: These rats were given 5 mg/kg of deoxycorticosterone acetate (DOCA) (Percorten; Ciba) intramuscularly for 28 days.
4. DOCA-treated, sensitized: These rats were unilaterally nephrectomized on day 1 and were given 0.9% NaCl *ad libitum* as drinking fluid for 28 days. Each animal was also given 5 mg/kg of DOCA intramuscularly daily.
5. Dexamethasone-treated: These rats were injected with dexamethasone (Decadron; Merck, Sharp, and Dohme) 1 mg/kg subcutaneously every day for 28 days.

All rats were fed a diet of Purina rat chow *ad libitum* and were given tap water to drink unless otherwise specified. At the end of 28 days, the rats were anesthetized with ether, weighed on a balance, and a carotid artery was cannulated with a polyethylene cannula for the measurement and recording of mean arterial blood pressure (MABP) with a Statham P-23 pressure transducer and a Beckman type RB Dynograph. After a stable MABP was recorded, a cardiectomy was performed. The hearts were immediately weighed, then placed in a drying oven in tared containers for 72 hr or until a constant weight was obtained at which time the dry weight was recorded.

Cats

1. Controls: These cats were observed for 28 days but were not treated in any way.
2. DOCA-treated: These cats were given 5 mg/kg of DOCA intramuscularly daily for 28 days.
3. DOCA-treated, sensitized: These cats were unilaterally nephrectomized under sterile technique on day 1. They were treated with 50 mg of erythromycin (Gallimycin; Amdal) daily intramuscularly for 2 days after surgery, and 5 mg/kg of DOCA intramuscularly for 28 days. They received 0.9% NaCl *ad libitum* as drinking fluid.
4. Dexamethasone-treated: These cats received 1 mg/kg of dexamethasone subcutaneously every day for 28 days.

All cats were fed a diet of Purina cat chow *ad libitum* and given tap water to drink unless otherwise specified. At the end of 28 days, the cats were anesthetized with pentobarbital sodium (30 mg/kg) administered intravenously. Heparin 1500 U/kg was administered intravenously and 2 ml blood samples were drawn from a venous cannula for determination of plasma sodium and potassium concentrations. MABP, central venous pressure, and heart rate were recorded prior to thoracotomy. The chest was opened and left ventricular function curves were determined by the rapid infusion of Krebs–Henseleit solution according to previously described techniques (Lefer *et al.*, 1968). At the end of this procedure, the hearts were excised, weighed, and dried as described above for rats.

Results

Table I summarizes the results in the five experimental groups of rats. The data show that the sesame oil controls and the DOCA-treated rats showed substantial increases in body weight over the 28-day observation period. The nephrectomized DOCA-treated rats showed a moderate increase in body weight, but the dexamethasone-treated group exhibited a marked decrease in body weight, reflecting the protein catabolic effect of that glucocorticoid.

Only the DOCA-treated sensitized rats exhibited a significant increase in MABP (42 mm Hg higher than the controls). Neither DOCA nor dexamethasone given alone elicited a hypertensive effect. All groups of rats, except the dexamethasone-treated group, exhibited a higher dry heart weight than the controls. The control rats at the time of sacrifice were in the same body-weight range as the other groups on day 28. The heart weight of the dexamethasone-treated rats was not statistically different from that of the control rats.

When one compares the dry heart weight/initial body weight ratio, one finds that the dexamethasone-treated rats are lower than the other groups. However, if one compares the dry heart weight/final body-weight ratio, one can see a significantly higher ratio ($P < 0.01$) than for any other group. Perhaps the most accurate and illustrative designation for the dexamethasone effect on heart size would be a "sparing of cardiac atrophy." When one corrects for growth during the 28-day experimental period, it is found that dexamethasone induced a marked loss in total body weight without any significant alteration in dry heart weight. These data indicate that one must use considerable caution in the use of the term "cardiac hypertrophy." DOCA plus sensitization to salt resulted in hypertension, but no hypertrophy, over the 28-day experimental period.

Table II summarizes the control (preinfusion) hemodynamic values in the four groups of cats studied. Mean arterial blood pressures (MABP) measured

TABLE I

EFFECT OF CHRONIC ADMINISTRATION OF CORTICOSTEROIDS ON BLOOD PRESSURE AND HEART WEIGHT IN ADRENALLY INTACT RATS[a]

Group	N	Body wt change (gm)	MABP (mm Hg)	Dry heart (mg)	Dry heart wt per initial body wt (mg/kg)	Dry heart wt per final body wt (mg/kg)
Control	9	–	124 ± 3.5	174.2 ± 3.3	–	660 ± 11.0
Sesame oil	7	+72 ± 10.6	122 ± 5.3	201.2 ± 7.5	888 ± 35.4	674 ± 6.6
DOCA[c]	8	+90 ± 7.3	130 ± 6.6	213.3 ± 5.4	945 ± 23.4	675 ± 9.1
Nephrex + DOCA[c]	7	+28 ± 6.9	166 ± 10.4[b]	220.2 ± 12.8	874 ± 56.9	788 ± 63.4
Dexamethasone[d]	7	−41 ± 8.7[b]	134 ± 5.1	168.2 ± 3.8	730 ± 14.3	948 ± 35.3[b]

[a] All values are means ± SEM.
[b] $p < 0.01$ when compared with appropriate controls.
[c] Dose of DOCA equals 5 mg/kg daily.
[d] Dose of dexamethasone equals 1 mg/kg daily.

TABLE II

HEMODYNAMIC STATUS OF ADRENALLY INTACT CATS FOLLOWING CHRONIC ADMINISTRATION OF CORTICOSTEROIDS[a]

Group	N	Presurgery MABP (mm Hg)	Open-chest MABP (mm Hg)	Open-chest Aortic flow (ml/min)	Open-chest HR (bpm)	Open-chest TPR (PRU/kg)	Infusion test Peak cardiac power (gm·m/sec)
Control	6	139 ± 4.6	125 ± 14.8	273 ± 33.8	218 ± 14.0	1.20 ± 0.15	24.0 ± 3.6
DOCA	5	137 ± 14.0	115 ± 17.0	333 ± 39.3	218 ± 8.8	1.12 ± 0.19	23.3 ± 1.6
Nephrex + DOCA	4	160 ± 6.3[b]	138 ± 28.0	442 ± 106.8	220 ± 23.5	0.99 ± 0.19	23.9 ± 4.0
Dexamethasone	5	148 ± 10.4	127 ± 6.4	446 ± 51.5[c]	218 ± 14.2	0.98 ± 0.14	26.1 ± 1.1

[a] All values are means ± SEM.
[b] $p < 0.05$ when compared to control values.
[c] $p < 0.02$ when compared to control values.

prior to thoracotomy indicate that the DOCA-treated sensitized cats were hypertensive at the end of the 28-day experimental period. The degree of hypertension was slightly lower than in the rats. As in the rats, DOCA or dexamethasone alone did not produce hypertension. However, after thoracotomy and institution of artificial respiration, the hypertension was diminished. Furthermore, in the open-chest state, heart rate (HR) and total peripheral resistance (TPR) were unchanged in any of the groups of cats. However, aortic flow (cardiac output minus coronary blood flow) was significantly higher in the dexamethasone-treated cats; in spite of this increase in flow, TPR was unchanged. Under these conditions, the peak cardiac power (expressed in gm · m/sec) was unaltered in any of the groups. However, when the peak cardiac power was normalized for left ventricular weight, the dexamethasone-treated cats exhibited a 25% increase in left ventricular power ($p < 0.025$) (Fig. 1). This 25% increase in reserve capacity of the heart was unique for dexamethasone. Treatment with DOCA or DOCA plus unilateral nephrectomy and salt loading failed to affect this increase in cardiac performance. Furthermore, that the dose of DOCA used was effective as a mineralocorticoid is evidenced by the fact that the cats treated with DOCA alone exhibited a significant reduction in plasma potassium (from 4.11 ± 0.24 mEq/liter in control cats to 3.05 ± 0.15 mEq/liter in DOCA-treated cats).

Table III summarizes the effects of the various protocols on heart weight and related calculated functions. In the experimental cats, as opposed to the rats under study, dexamethasone did not reduce body weight significantly.

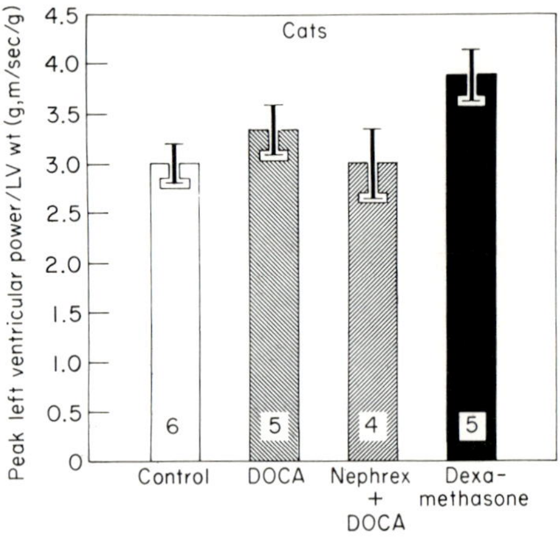

FIG. 1. Bar graph of peak left ventricular power expressed in gram-meters per second normalized per gram of left ventricular wet weight. Only the dexamethasone-treated cats (1 mg/kg for 28 days) showed an increase in cardiac reserve capacity as evidenced by a greater peak cardiac performance. DOCA (5 mg/kg for 28 days) was unable to increase cardiac performance in normal or in salt-loaded unilaterally nephrectomized cats.

TABLE III

EFFECT OF CHRONIC ADMINISTRATION OF CORTICOSTEROIDS ON HEART WEIGHT OF ADRENALLY INTACT CATS[a]

Group	N	Body wt (kg)		Wet heart wt/final body wt (mg/kg)			Dry LV wt/final body wt (mg/kg)
		Initial	Final	Whole heart	Right ventricle	Left ventricle	
Control	6	–	3.55 ± 0.24	3.34 ± 0.21	0.72 ± 0.04	2.22 ± 0.17	508 ± 38.9
Nephrex + DOCA	4	3.05 ± 0.09	3.06 ± 0.34	3.95 ± 0.19	0.83 ± 0.03	2.61 ± 0.13	507 ± 18.4
DOCA	5	2.78 ± 0.21	3.15 ± 0.25	3.47 ± 0.27	0.69 ± 0.07	2.27 ± 0.15	496 ± 40.2
Dexamethasone	5	3.13 ± 0.16	3.03 ± 0.21	3.48 ± 0.14	0.75 ± 0.04	2.25 ± 0.10	513 ± 16.8

[a] All values are means ± SEM.

DOCA alone or DOCA plus sensitization also failed to significantly alter body weight in adult cats. Furthermore, there was no significant alteration in whole heart weight, right ventricular weight, or left ventricular weight normalized for total body weight at the end of the 28-day experimental period. Even when comparing left ventricular dry weight normalized for total body weight, there was no significant change with any steroid regimen studied. Thus, no evidence for a corticosteroid-induced cardiac hypertrophy was found in cats.

Discussion

The data presented in this chapter clearly indicate that DOCA and dexamethasone in relatively high doses do not induce cardiac hypertrophy within a 1-month period. Neither steroid, when given alone, exerted a hypertensive effect. Only when DOCA was administered to salt-loaded unilaterally nephrectomized rats and cats did hypertension occur as de Champlain *et al.* (1969) have shown. Therefore, DOCA appears to induce hypertension more readily than cardiac hypertrophy. Fregly and Arean (1959) also were unable to induce cardiac hypertrophy in rats given DOCA daily for 9 weeks, even though hypertension resulted. Hall and co-workers (Hall and Hall, 1967; Hall *et al.*, 1962) found that DOCA-induced hypertension and cardiac hypertrophy in salt-loaded unilaterally nephrectomized rats, but they used a dose almost five times that used in this study (Hall and Hall, 1967) and administered the steroid for longer periods of time (Hall, *et al.*, 1962). Ueda *et al.* (1967) found that DOCA produced moderate cardiac hypertrophy in rats, but only many weeks after marked hypertension occurred. These findings were associated with severe cardiac lesions confirming the findings of Hall and Hall (1967). Recently Beznak *et al.* (1969) have shown that the DOCA-induced cardiac hypertrophy is reversible since it recedes after steroid and salt withdrawal.

Other mineralocorticoids such as aldosterone exert a smaller degree of hypertension and a moderate degree of cardiac hypertrophy (Gornall *et al.*, 1960; Hall and Hall, 1967) or no cardiac hypertrophy (Fregly and Arean, 1959; Gaunt *et al.*, 1957). Halogenated synthetic mineralocoritcoids such as 2-methyl-9α-fluorocortisol are capable of inducing cardiac hypertrophy associated with cardiac lesions. Undoubtedly, the resultant cardiac hypertrophy is a result of the hypertension.

In the present study, high doses of the synthetic glucocorticoid, dexamethasone, failed to induce hypertension or cardiac hypertrophy over a period of 1 month in rats and cats. Dexamethasone did, however, increase myocardial power in cats and prevented cardiac atrophy in rats. This is in agreement with the findings of Bertazzoli *et al.* (1952) and Northup *et al.* (1967), who also failed to demonstrate cardiac hypertrophy with high doses of cortisone. These doses of cortisone are considerably lower than the present dose of dexamethasone when normalized for glucocorticoid potencies (i.e., liver glycogen deposition, or depression of eosinophils). However, Ogawa *et al.* (1965) were able to induce hypertension with dexamethasone, but no data for cardiac weights are given in their study. The dose of dexamethasone used in this study and the duration of steroid treatment were equal to or slightly greater than those used by Ogawa *et al.* (1965). Nevertheless, we were unable to reproduce their results. Hence, it appears that glucocorticoids in general do not induce cardiac hypertrophy, probably because they are unable to exert a significant hypertensive effect.

The data in this report indicate that some degree of caution must be used in the interpretation of cardiac hypertrophy data. Table I indicates that dexamethasone actually decreased cardiac weight relative to initial body weight in rats. However, this artifact results from the fact that whereas all the other groups of rats gained weight, the dexamethasone-treated rats lost considerable weight. When one compares the cardiac weight relative to the final body weight, dexamethasone appears to induce a cardiac hypertrophy. Again, this is deceptive since the hearts did not actually gain weight; rather, they lost less weight than did the rest of the body. Hence, a more appropriate term for this phenomenon would be "atrophy-sparing."

In summary, the absence of the corticosteroids as occurs in adrenalectomized animals, is characterized by a large decrease in myocardial function and a small decrease in heart size. These changes are readily reversed by administration of corticosteroids (Lefer 1967, 1968; Lefer *et al.*, 1968). Administration of large doses of mineralocorticoids alone to animals with intact adrenals does not appear to increase either myocardial performance or cardiac size. In sensitized animals (i.e., salt-loaded unilateral nephrectomized rats), DOCA induces hypertension but not cardiac hypertrophy within a period of 1 month. More prolonged administration of DOCA may result in cardiac hypertrophy secondary to a well-established hypertension. Glucocorticoids, such as dexamethasone exert only a modest positive inotropic effect in the whole animal with intact adrenals. It appears that some mechanism exists which acts to protect the heart against an excessive corticosteroid concentration, despite the necessity of corticosteroids in normal cardiac function. This does not necessarily mean that corticosteroids exert permissive effects on the heart; rather, physiological control mechanisms place a ceiling on the cardiotonic or inotropic effects of corticosteroids.

Acknowledgments

This work was supported in part by Research Grant No. HE-09924 by the National Heart Institutes. The excellent technical assistance of Thomas F. Inge, Jr., and Asher J. Conn is gratefully acknowledged. The authors also wish to thank Dr. J. J. Chart of Ciba Pharmaceutical Co., Summit, New Jersey for a generous supply of DOCA (Percorten), and Dr. Walter B. Gall of Merck, Sharp, and Dohme Research Laboratories, Rahway, New Jersey for a generous supply of dexamethasone (Decadron).

References

Bertazzoli, C., Cavallero, C., and Sala, G. (1952). *Nature* (*London*) **170**, 43.

Beznak, M., Korecky, B., and Thomas, G. (1969). *Can. J. Physiol. Pharmacol.* **47**, 579.

Bois, P., Beznak, M., and Jasmin, G. (1961). *Can. J. Biochem. Physiol.* **39**, 335.

de Champlain, J., Krakoff, L., and Axelrod, J. (1969). *Circ. Res.* **24**, Suppl. 1, 1–75.

Fregly, M. J., and Arean, V. M. (1959). *Acta Physiol. Pharmacol* **8**, 162.

Gaunt, R., Ulsamer, G. J., and Chart, J. J. (1957). *Arch. Int. Pharmacodyn.* **110**, 114.

Gornall, A. G., Grundy, H. M., and Koladich, C. J. (1960). *Can. J. Biochem. Physiol.* **38**, 43.

Hall, C. E., and Hall, O. (1967). *Acta Endocrinol.* **54**, 399.

Hall, C. E., Rennels, E. G., and Hall, O. (1962). *Lab. Invest.* **11**, 594.

Lefer, A. M. (1967). *In* "Factors Influencing Myocardial Contractility" (R. D. Tanz, F. Kavaler, and J. Roberts, eds.) pp. 611–631. Academic Press, New York.

Lefer, A. M. (1968). *Amer. J. Physiol.* **214**, 518.

Lefer, A. M., Verrier, R. L., and Carson, W. W. (1968). *Circ. Res.* **22**, 817.

Northup, D. W., Van Liere, E. J., and Hunnell, J. E. (1967). *Experientia* **23**, 1061.

Ogawa, H., Tadokoro, S., Kiribara, R., Kawakami, K., and Shibata, K. (1965). *Gunma J. Med. Sci.* **14**, 107.

Rovetto, M. J., and Lefer, A. M. (1970). *Amer. J. Physiol.* **218**, 1015

Solomon, N., Travis, R. H., and Sayers, G. (1959). *Endocrinology* **64**, 535.

Suzuki, T. (1967). *Tohoku J. Exp. Med.* **91**, 239.

Ueda, H., Nishimura, H., and Yasuda, H. (1967). *Jap. Heart J.* **8**, 43.

Verrier, R. L., O'Neill, T. J., and Lefer, A. M. (1969a). *Amer. J. Physiol.* **217**, 341.

Verrier, R. L., Rovetto, M. J., and Lefer, A. M. (1969a). *Amer. J. Physiol.* **217**, 1559.

Part III
The Composition of the Hypertrophied Heart

RELATIONSHIPS BETWEEN MECHANICAL AND CHEMICAL PHENOMENA IN THE MYOCARDIUM

Arnold M. Katz

It is now possible to define several important relationships between the mechanical parameters of muscle activity and those biochemical and biophysical processes that give rise to the contractile process (Katz, 1970). These relationships are most clearly demonstrated in skeletal muscle, where the rapid onset of the active state and the ability to generate a sustained tetanus permit accurate measurements of maximum shortening velocity and maximum isometric tension. A correlation between the well-known differences in the maximal shortening velocities (V_{max}) of various types of skeletal muscles and the rate of ATP hydrolysis by the contractile proteins isolated from these muscles, suggested by several investigators (Engle, 1962; Seidel *et al.*, 1964; Bárány *et al.*, 1965; Katz *et al.*, 1966; Maddox and Perry, 1966) was clearly shown by M. Bárány (1967). On comparing the myosin and actomyosin ATPase activities of a large number of muscles which differed in their V_{max}, Bárány showed an almost perfect correlation between enzymatic activity and maximal shortening velocity (Bárány, 1967). The maximal tetanic tension (P_0) of a skeletal muscle, however, is not related to the rate of ATP hydrolysis by the contractile proteins, but is instead correlated with the number of potential interacting sites between actin and myosin (Huxley and Niedergerke, 1954; M. Bárány, 1967). This latter relationship is seen most clearly in the length–tension relationship of the sarcomere, where, at muscle lengths greater than rest length, P_0 is dependent on sarcomere length in a manner that directly reflects the number of actin sites than can interact with the myosin cross-bridges (Gordon *et al.*, 1966).

In the myocardium, where the active state is slow in onset and it is not possible to elicit tetanic contractions, considerable uncertainty exists as to the accuracy to which P_0 and V_{max} can be measured (see Brady, 1966 for a review of this subject). This lack of precise mechanical data makes it more difficult to correlate changes in the contractile properties of the hypertrophied heart with specific biochemical and biophysical phenomena. Changes in mechanical behavior which have been observed in the hypertrophied myocardium are considered elsewhere in this volume so that the present chapter will center on the potential correlations between alterations in contactile performance, expressed in terms of shortening velocity and tension generation, and the properties of the contractile proteins described in the preceding paragraph.

It might appear reasonable to conclude (1) that changes in V_{max} of hypertrophied muscle reflect an alteration in the properties of the hydrolytic site of myosin or in the ability of actin to activate myosin ATPase activity, and (2) that changes in P_0 will result from a change in the number of interactions between actin and myosin. Such reasoning, however, represents an oversimplification that does not account for potential changes in the composition of the muscle that may occur during hypertrophy. It is clear that P_0, which is expressed as force generated per unit of muscle cross-sectional area, will decrease if the fraction of this cross-sectional area that is occupied by the contractile proteins is reduced. Thus, an increase in the water content of the muscle (edema), or mitochondrial or connective tissue proliferation can reduce P_0 without any primary alteration in the contractile proteins. Furthermore, P_0 can be reduced by changes in the orientation of the contractile proteins, e.g., in the heart by an increase in the branching of the fibers so that less of the force generated will be parallel to the fiber axis. Thus it is not possible, even in a skeletal muscle where P_0 can be measured with precision, to attribute an impairment of the ability to generate tension directly to an alteration in the properties of the contractile proteins.

Variations in V_{min}, which are expressed per unit of muscle length, can also result from changes in muscle composition. Changes in the orientation of muscle bundles towards an arrangement that is less parallel with the fiber axis can reduce measured V_{max} without creating a true change in the shortening velocity of the individual myofibrils. Fibrosis can also reduce the velocity of shortening if there is fibrous replacement of the myofibrillar units in series with active tissue, and processes like fibrosis, mitochondrial proliferation, and edema could reduce V_{max} by increasing the viscous resistance to shortening. Thus, changes in the mechanical behavior of a hypertrophied muscle cannot be attributed to one or another specific alteration in the properties of the contractile proteins without additional information about the anatomical state of the muscle.

With the recent elaboration of the role of calcium ion in the excitation–contraction coupling of skeletal muscle (see Katz, 1970; Sandow, 1965; and Ebashi and Endo, 1968, for reviews of these findings), it now appears that the actomyosin interactions which effect the contractile process are set in motion when Ca^{2+} is bound to troponin, the calcium receptor protein of the myofibril. Although the availability of Ca^{2+} does not appear to play a major role in the physiological variations of skeletal muscle contractile performance, there is considerable evidence to suggest that the physiologically significant variations in myocardial contractility are due to changes in the amount of this ion made available for binding to cardiac troponin during systole (Katz, 1970). Thus, it is possible that changes in the tension developed by hypertrophied cardiac muscle may be due to an impairment of this calcium-release mechanism (Gertz *et al.*, 1967).

It has often been assumed that a reduction in the amount of calcium made available to the contractile proteins of the hypertrophied heart during excitation–contraction coupling might account for a decrease in both P_o and V_{max}. There is no reason to doubt that impairment of excitation could reduce the number of active interactions between actin and myosin and thereby cause a decrease in P_o, but it does not follow that a lessened amount of calcium released during excitation–contraction coupling in the hypertrophied heart would cause a fall in maximal shortening velocity. Contrary to observations in isolated actomyosin systems, in which ATPase activity shows a graded response to free Ca^{2+} concentration, the contractile proteins in the intact muscle probably respond to calcium by an "off–on" type of mechanism (Katz, 1970). Therefore, actin–myosin interactions will either be active (when the troponin–tropomyosin complex is bound to calcium, see Katz, 1970) or blocked (when the calcium-binding site on troponin is not bound to calcium), so that variations in the availability of this cation can modify the number of active actin–myosin interactions (P_o) but not the rate at which each such interaction (V_{max}) can proceed. For this reason, an abnormality in excitation–contraction coupling would not be expected to directly modify the maximal shortening velocity of the hypertrophied heart. Because of the apparent high internal viscosity of the myocardium, however, variations in force-generating ability might be manifest as changes in apparent V_{max} (see Katz, 1970).

Finally, some mention should be made of the mechanical consequences that are probably caused by intracellular acidosis, a state that may be present in the hypertrophied myocardium. Evidence that hydrogen ion competes with calcium ion for the binding site which controls the actin–myosin interaction has recently been reviewed (Katz, 1970, Katz and Hecht, 1970). Because of this apparent competition, a decrease in intracellular pH would impair the ability of calcium to bind to troponin, thereby reducing the number of active actin–myosin interactions at any level of intracellular free calcium ion concentration. Evidence that aerobic metabolism may be impaired in the hypertrophied heart has been reviewed elsewhere in this symposium. Should this be the case, and should the rate of anaerobic glycolysis be increased in the hypertrophied myocardium, the resultant release of hydrogen ion could directly impair contractile performance.

In conclusion, although there is excellent reason to believe that the maximal tension generated by a muscle reflects the number of active interactions between actin and myosin, and that maximal shortening velocity is correlated with the maximal rate at which myosin can hydrolyze ATP, changes in the mechanical parameters seen in the myocardium after hypertrophy cannot be attributed directly to biochemical or biophysical alterations without additional data that describe the anatomical state of the hypertrophied heart.

Acknowledgments

Supported by Research Grants HE-11734 from the U.S. Public Health Service, G5-G-61 from the American Heart Association, N68-41 from the Chicago and Illinois Heart Associations, and a Fund in memory of William A. Gist.

References

Bárány, M. (1967). *Gen. Physiol.* **50**, 197.

Bárány, M., Bárány, K., Reckard, T., and Volpe, A. (1965). *Arch. Biochem. Biophys.* **109**, 185.

Brady, A. J. (1966). *J. Physiol.* **184**, 560.

Ebashi, S., and Endo, M. (1968). *Progr. Biophys. Mol. Biol.* **18**, 123–183.

Engle, W. K. (1962). *Neurology* **12**, 778.

Gertz, E. W., Hess, M. L., Lain, R. F., and Briggs, F. N. (1967). *Circ. Res.* **20**, 477.

Gordon, A. M., Huxley, A. F., and Julian F. J. (1966). *J. Physiol.* (*London*) **184**, 170.

Huxley, A. F., and Niedergerke, R. (1954). *Nature* (*London*) **173**, 971.

Katz, A. M. (1970). *Physiol. Rev.* **50**, 63.

Katz, A. M., and Hecht, H. H. (1970). *Amer. J. Med.* **47**, 497.

Katz, A. M., Repke, D. I., and Rubin, B. B. (1966). *Circ. Res.* **19**, 611.

Maddox, C. E. R., and Perry, S. V. (1966). *Biochem. J.* **99**, 8P.

Sandow, A. (1965). *Pharmacol. Rev.* **27**, 265.

Siedel, J. C., Sreter, F. A., Thompson, M. M., and Gergely, J. (1964). *Biochem, Biophys. Res. Commun.* **17**, 662.

CARDIAC MUSCLE:
A Comparative Ultrastructural, Anatomical View

Joachim R. Sommer and Paul H. Jewett

The fine structure of the cardiac muscle cell is not the same in the hearts of different animals nor necessarily is it the same from one location to another in the same heart. The heart muscle cell (myofiber) is one that contains striated contractile material which defines the cell of concern in this review.

In adult mammals, at least two major populations of myofibers can be distinguished structurally (Johnson and Sommer, 1967; Sommer and Johnson, 1968a): (1) atrial and ventricular fibers with transverse tubules that may be conveniently termed working fibers, and (2) atrial and ventricular fibers that do not have transverse tubules (along with other discrete but highly variable and species-dependent characteristics) and which may be conveniently termed conducting fibers. Mammalian atrial myofibers, both with and without transverse tubules, can be further characterized as having prominent specific granules (Jamieson and Palade, 1964) which are not seen in the myofibers of ventricles. In the chicken, two discrete populations of myofibers also exist that can be clearly distinguished, as they must, by other criteria, despite their lack of transverse tubules (Sommer and Johnson, 1969). The diameter of the working fibers in the chicken (and the frog) is between 5 to 10 times less than that of corresponding mammalian fibers. In the frog only one structurally discrete fiber population seems to exist whose fibers are quite like the working myofibers in chickens: They are of similar diameter, have no transverse tubules, no prominent M line, and they contain specific granules throughout the myocardium, i.e., including the ventricles.

The working fibers in the ventricles of various adult mammals appear to be of rather similar structure (Figs. 1–4) (Fawcett and McNutt, 1969; McNutt and Fawcett, 1969; Simpson and Rayns, 1968; Sommer and Johnson, 1968a). The contractile material is organized into sarcomeres containing myosin and actin filaments, which together with the Z-line material and the M-line densities form the typical band pattern characteristic of striated muscle. The

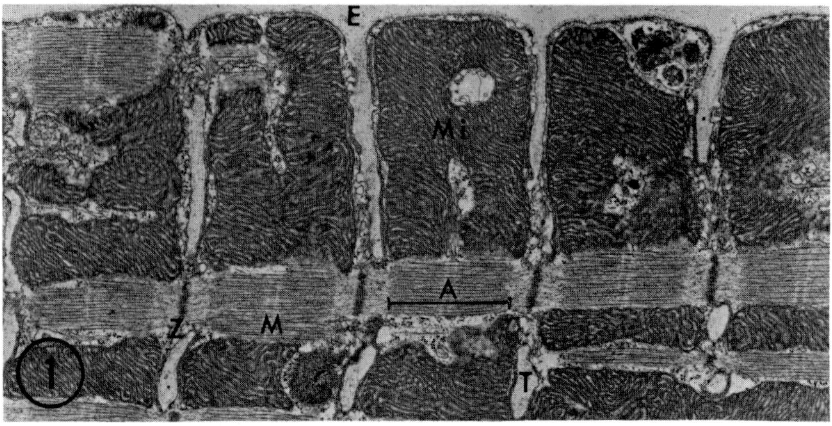

FIG. 1. Dog working myofibers. Epon section. Extracellular space (E) extends folds around mitochondria (Mi). From these folds emanate transverse tubules (T, cf. X in Fig. 2) that penetrate deeply into the myofibers. The M line is rarely seen in avian and frog cardiac muscle, where usually only a light zone is visible in the center of the A band (cf. Figs. 6 and 7; however, cf. Fig. 9). Magnification: ×12,000.

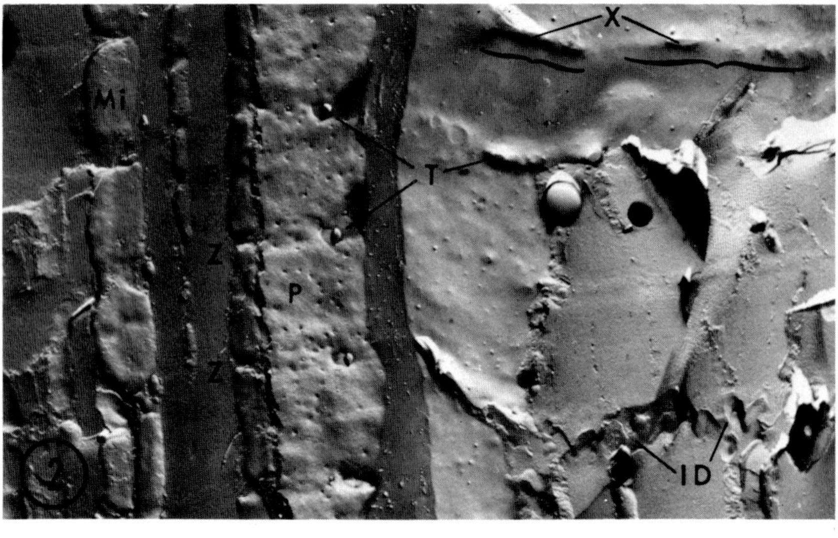

FIG. 2. Freeze-etch preparation of dog working myofibers. The plane of fracture splits myofibrils (F) longitudinally, faintly revealing Z lines (Z), with some I bands vaguely showing on either side. The fracture plane exposes the surface of mitochondria (Mi), rather than splitting them through the middle. Elsewhere, the fracture plane reveals some outer aspect of the sarcolemma showing many pinocytotic vesicles (the letter P is ringed by such vesicles). Then, to the right, the fracture plane ascends to another plane where some inner (juxtacytoplasmic) aspect of the sarcolemma is exposed, which is clearly demonstrated by the reversal of the bulge of both transverse tubules (T) and pinocytotic vesicles. An intercalated disc is present (ID). The brackets indicate sarcolemmal folds (Z grooves, cf. Fig. 1) from which the transverse tubules emanate (X). Magnification: ×5,000.

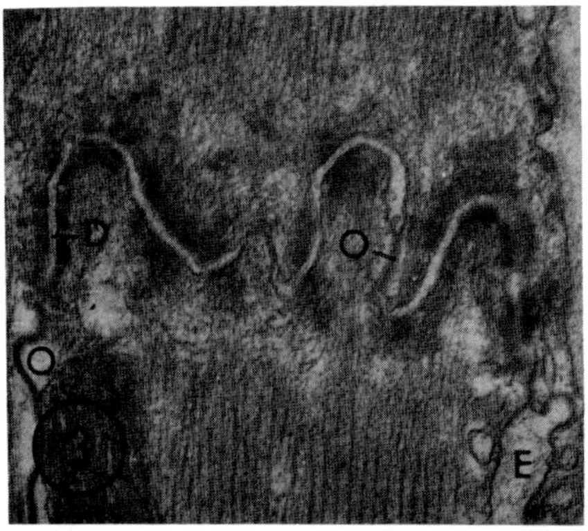

FIG. 3. Dog working myofiber. Epon section. Intercalated disc. The bulk of this junctional complex connecting myofibers end-to-end is made up of ff. adherentes that are occasionally interrupted by desmosomes (D) and gap junctions (0). Magnification: ×30,000.

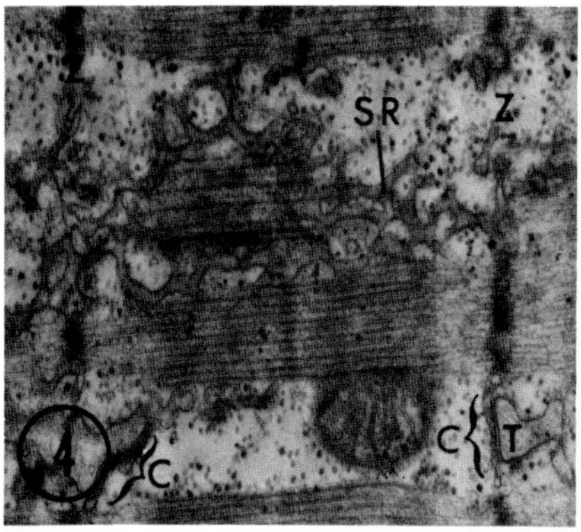

FIG. 4. Rabbit working myofiber. Maraglas section. The SR is a delicate network of tubules which freely cross from one sarcomere to another (i.e., across Z lines, Z). Couplings (C) are present at transverse tubules (T). Magnification: ×22,000.

myofibers also contain nuclei, mitochondria, Golgi regions, profiles related to the lysosome complex, glycogen, some ribosomes (free and attached), an occasional microtubule, and the sarcoplasmic reticulum (SR) which varies in its degree of differentiation. In this very general way, cardiac muscle and skeletal muscle are quite similar structurally. However, considerable differences exist between these two kinds of muscle with respect to the size of the fibers, the structural substrata for the process of excitation (functional syncitium versus individual innervation), the number and location of mitochondria, the location of the nuclei, the specializations of the plasma membrane (transverse tubules), the intercellular membrane contacts, and the extent and differentiation of the SR.

The working myofibers in mammalian hearts are attached to one another by junctional complexes: gap junctions, desmosomes, and fasciae adherentes (structural and, presumably, functional relatives of the desmosome); the latter form the bulk of the intercalated disc (Fig. 3). The gap junctions presumably serve to establish low resistance pathways between cells (Barr *et al.*, 1965; Dreifuss and Girardier, 1966), whereas the other junctional complexes are mainly involved, for all we know, in physical adhesion between cells. Because of their discrete morphology, which is clearly polarized (Revel and Karnovsky, 1967), the gap junctions have invited further inquiry into their architecture by taking advantage of the freeze-etching technique (Kreutziger, 1968; McNutt and Weinstein, 1969; Bullivant, 1969; Sommer and Steere, 1970; Sommer and Johnson, 1970), a method that was originally described by Steere (Steere 1957). The gap junctions are surrounded by a halo of clear cytoplasm and they are always oriented in a plane parallel to the axis of the myofibrils, which is probably the position of least stress for these essentially free-floating junctional complexes (free floating in contrast to the ff. adherentes and desmosomes which are attached to fibrillar cellular elements). It remains to be seen whether the phosphatase that has been localized on the gap junction (Sommer and Spach, 1964), and that seems to be much more sensitive to inhibition by glutaraldehyde than by formaldehyde has any functional significance.

Chicken cardiac muscle fibers have similar junctional complexes; however, the gap junctions are as small as they are exceedingly uncommon (Sommer and Johnson, 1969). Most junctional complexes in frog hearts are very similar to the ff. adherentes in mammals and chickens, but they do not appear to be identical to them. Gap junctions have not conclusively been demonstrated in frog myofibers (Staley and Benson, 1968; Sommer and Johnson, 1969; however cf. Barr *et al.*, 1965).

The working myofibers in mammals are lined by sarcolemma, the plasma membrane, which has fingerlike invaginations of large diameter (the transverse tubules, approx. 0.2 μ in diameter) that penetrate the myofiber transversely at the Z lines (Figs. 1 and 2) as far as the center of the cell. Branches of transverse tubules seem to exist, some of which may run in longitudial direction (i.e., parallel to the axis of the myofiber) for short distances (Fawcett and McNutt, 1969). In contrast, Purkinje fibers (P-fibers) in all animals studied so far have not revealed any transverse tubules. Recently arguments have been presented that suggest, everything else being equal and given the large diameter of the cardiac transverse tubules, that the presence or absence of transverse tubules would influence the conduction velocity of action potentials in such fibers; the absence of transverse tubules favors faster conduction (Sommer and Johnson, 1968b). Myofibers with and without transverse tubules can be found also in the atria (McNutt and Fawcett, 1969; Sommer and Johnson 1968a); the fibers without transverse tubules are situated toward the endocardium, whereas the fibers with transverse tubules, where present (e.g., in pectinate muscles), are located toward the epicardium (Sommer, 1968).

Atrial myofibers (with and without transverse tubules) of all animals studied contain specific granules (Fig. 5) the nature of which remains obscure (Jamieson and Palade, 1964). They are electron-dense material lined by a unit membrane, and they occur predominately in the Golgi region, but also elsewhere in the cell. Similar granules are virtually absent in myofibers of mammalian ventricles, but they are present in ventricular myofibers of chicken (Sommer and Johnson, 1969) and frog hearts (Staley and Benson, 1968).

Very considerable are the structural differences among the so-called Purkinje fibers (P-fibers) of different animals (Truex and Smythe, 1965). Light microscopists have been frustrated by the failure to discover certain fibers in several small mammals that correspond to the microscopic description given originally by Purkinje, despite the fact that fibers were investigated that by gross description and topography were clearly equivalent to those identified and studied by Purkinje. Thus, many of the criteria used for the

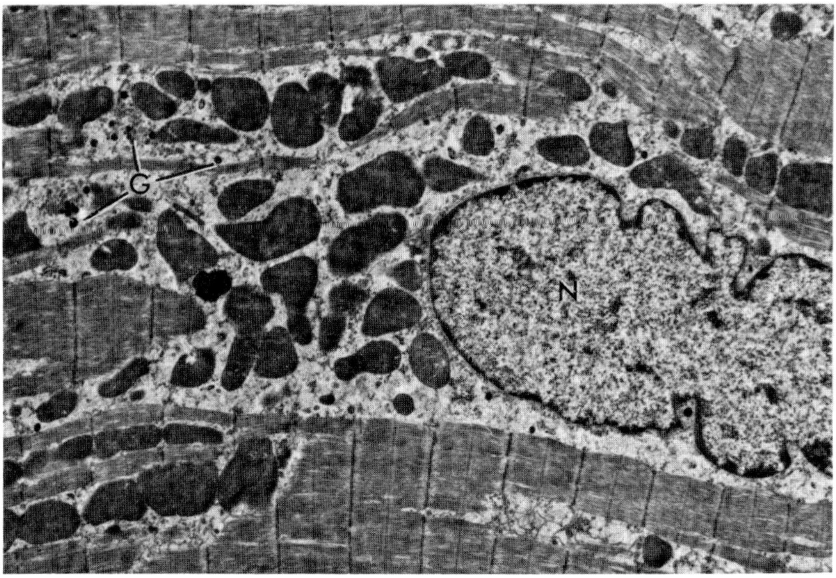

FIG. 5. Atrial myofiber of dog heart. Epon section. Note specific granules (G) closely associated with the Golgi region, but also elsewhere in the cell. Magnification: ×5,000.

microscope identification of Purkinje fibers, such as the large fiber diameter, the large amount of glycogen, the paucity of myofibrils, the perinuclear halo, etc., must suffer modification when applied to one animal or another. However, regardless of the species studied, the one singular anatomical feature that fibers taken from locations where Purkinje took his fibers have in common, is the absence of transverse tubules (Johnson and Sommer, 1967). If indeed the Purkinje fibers represent the morphologic substrata of the conduction system, and assuming further that a conduction system does in fact exist in those animals that do not readily reveal "classical" Purkinje fibers, then, clearly, other criteria have to be established that tend to be more credible the less they are in conflict with physiologic observations, e.g., the fast conduction velocity of Purkinje fibers when compared with the working fibers. Difficulties of nomenclature are well illustrated in the case of the Purkinje fibers of the dog. These fibers seem to conform to the original histological criteria of Purkinje if one considers, as seen in some cells, only the clear zone in the center of such fibers and the peripheral location of myofibrils in that region. However, closer scrutiny discloses that this clear zone, in contrast to the classical Purkinje fibers of the ungulates where it is present throughout the cell, is confined to the perinuclear region and, in addition, seems to have a somewhat different fine structure. In any event, transverse sections through these fibers in the dog show that unlike the classical Purkinje fibers of the ungulates, the cell diameters are comparable to those of the working myofibers of the heart and that, again unlike the classical Purkinje fibers, these fibers are filled to capacity with contractile material. However—and significantly—they do share with the classical Purkinje fibers the absence of transverse tubules.

It should, perhaps, be emphasized that while all P-fibers lack transverse tubules, not all heart muscle fibers without transverse tubules are P-fibers. In small adult mammals, however, and in the absence of other distinguishing features (Sommer and Johnson 1968a) the presence or absence of transverse tubules is the only tangible criterion for distinguishing P-fibers from working fibers. In chicken hearts in which the working fibers have no transverse tubules, the P-fibers are morphologically different from the working fibers, and they also have a much larger diameter than the latter, say, 5 times or more. In the newborn puppy heart transverse tubules are absent in both working and P-fibers, and measurements show that the cross-sectional area of the P-fibers in the puppy heart (unpublished observations) is not only larger than that of the working fibers by a factor of 2 or so, but the P-fibers, in addition and in contrast to the loosely assembled working fibers, are tightly packed into bundles not unlike the P-fibers seen in the ungulates and other large mammals. In contemplating the physiological properties of these fibers, one must consider not only the fine structure of the individual cells, but also the geometry of cell apposition when such cells combine to form bundles or strands, as this is likely to influence the conduction velocity of action potentials within such bundles (Sommer and Johnson, 1968a). Thus, everything else being equal and irrespective of species and anatomical variations, morphology in every case favors that the P-fibers have faster conduction velocity.

The sarcoplasmic reticulum (SR), too, is quite different in extent and differentiation as one compares the hearts of different animals and, within one heart, different myofibers. The working fibers of mammals and some birds have a rather well-developed SR (Figs. 4 and 9), usually in the form of an interconnected network that, in contrast to skeletal muscle is continuous from one sarcomere to the next. The SR of Purkinje fibers is more poorly developed, regardless of the location of such fibers (atria or ventricles), and irrespective of the animal studied. The development of the SR in the frog heart is much less complex than it is, for example, in the working myofibers of mammals.

The SR in the hearts of mammals and chickens, as well as in some birds (finch and hummingbird), has sharply defined regions of structural specialization. We have called these portions junctional SR (subsarcolemmal cisternae, Fawcett and McNutt, 1969), since they are tightly apposed to the sarcolemma of either the transverse tubules or the sarcolemma covering the surface of the cells. This anatomical and presumably functional unit between sarcolemma and SR seems to figure prominently in excitation–contraction coupling. These units are seen, *mutatis mutandis*, in skeletal and cardiac muscle alike, and we have called them couplings (Johnson and Sommer, 1967), (Figs. 6–8), regardless of whether they occur at transverse tubules (skeletal and cardiac muscle) or at the peripheral sarcolemma (cardiac muscle only). The couplings have an appearance that is quite similar in the hearts of both mammals and chickens, as well as in some birds (finch and hummingbird). They seem to be absent in the frog heart, although segments of SR are seen occasionally in close apposition to the sarcolemma. However, the junctional SR of the couplings in chicken cardiac fibers shows additional features not seen in mammalian myofibers. In the chicken, many couplings display a markedly distended junctional SR that contains electron-dense material, especially in adult chickens (Figs. 9–11). Electron-dense material is also seen elsewhere in the remainder of the SR throughout the cell (Fig. 9), occasionally appearing as dense casts of segments of SR. Dense granules are also present in the SR of frog cardiac fibers and similar material has recently been found in the skeletal muscle of a crustacean (Rosenbluth, 1969). The topography of this dense material is not in conflict with the notion that it represents part of a process of at least intermittent exocytosis, a mechanism known to occur in secretory cells.

Couplings are present also in the finch (Fig. 6) and in the hummingbird

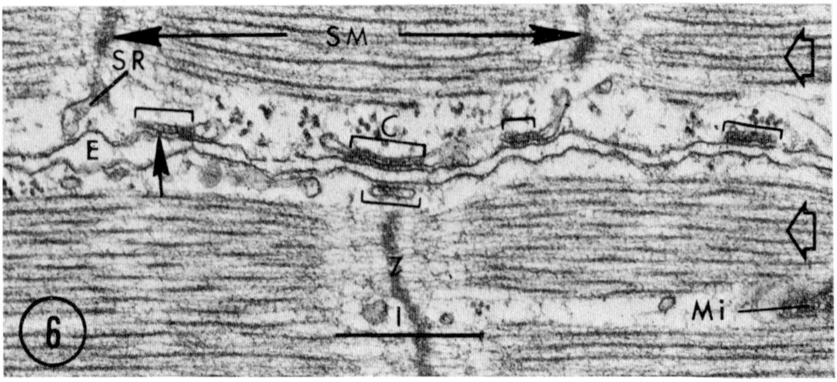

FIG. 6. Chicken working myofibers (open arrows), epon section. Several couplings (brackets) are seen on either side of the extracellular space (E). The junctional SR, limited by the brackets (cf. C) contains in its center an interrupted dense line (central membrane or junctional granules). Periodic densities between the junctional SR and the plasma membrane (junctional processes) are indicated by arrow. In the chicken there is usually one coupling on either side of the Z line, although more than two couplings per sarcomere (SM) are sometimes seen as in the upper cell in Fig. 6 (three couplings). The location of a coupling straddling the Z line, their preferred location in finches and hummingbirds, is uncommon in the chicken. (I), I band; (Mi), mitochondrion.

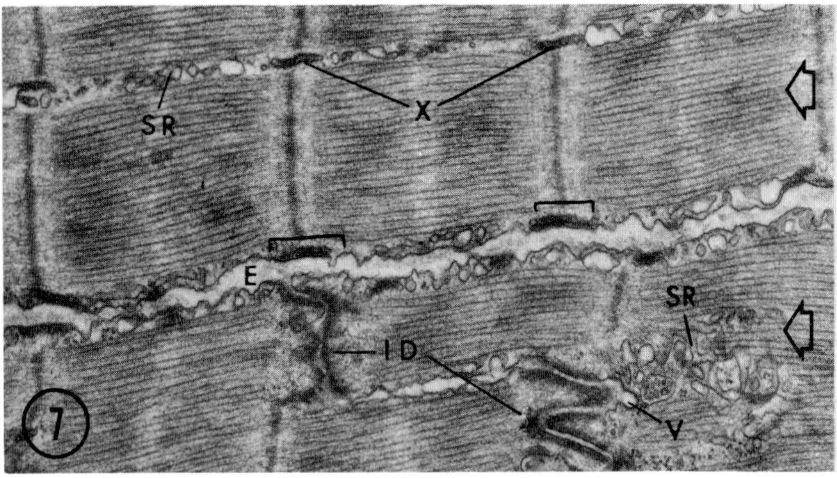

FIG. 7. Working myofibers (open arrows) of the finch heart, maraglas section. The couplings at the sarcolemma are indicated by brackets. Profiles indistinguishable from junctional SR with its central membrane (junctional granules) are seen between myofibrils at Z lines and away from the sarcolemma (X). Note absence of transverse tubules. (ID), Intercalated disc; (V) pit; (E), extracellular space. Magnification: ×24,000.

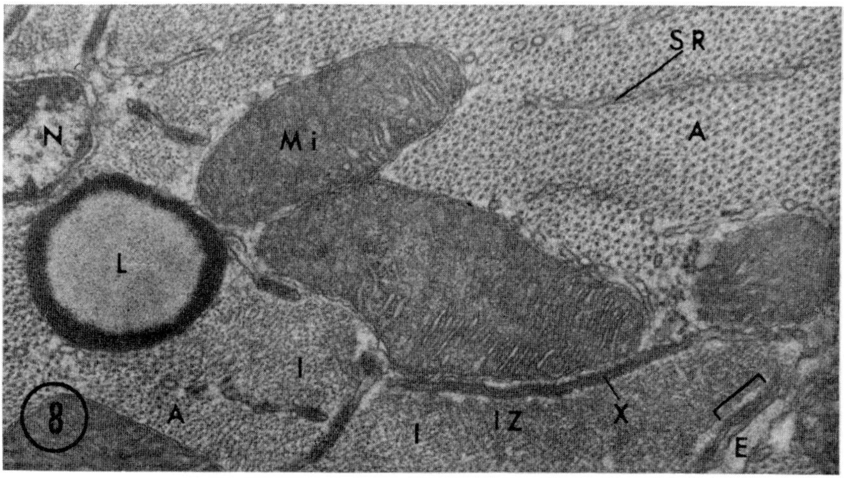

FIG. 8. Working myofiber of hummingbird. Transverse Epon section. Note smooth sarcoplasmic reticulum (SR) at A bands (A), and extended junctional SR (X) at I bands (I) and where the I band fuses with the Z lines (IZ). The bracket indicates what is presumably a coupling at the sarcolemma. The extended junctional SR is often seen to entirely surround I-band material. (L), lipofuscin granules; (Mi), mitochondrion; (N), nucleus; (E), extracellular space. Magnification: × 33,000.

(Fig. 7). However, in the hearts of these birds, structural profiles that are indistinguishable from the junctional SR of couplings (the latter having sarcolemma as one of their invariant components by definition) are found elsewhere in the cells, that is, unassociated with sarcolemma. These profiles are of unusual length and are rather like structures that we have observed previously in the atria and also occasionally in the Purkinje fibers of the dog (Sommer, 1968) where they often form lamellar stacks of tubules, or sheets (Figs. 12, 13). In the hearts of the finch and the hummingbird these structurally discrete segments of the SR, which we have named extended junctional SR, are invariably associated with the I band, especially the Z lines (Figs. 7, 8).

The question of whether or not the SR is open to the extracellular space is an important one. This question has been discussed more recently in great detail (Forssmann and Girardier, 1966; Sommer and Johnson 1968a). If one studies the continuity between the SR and the extracellular space by introducing from the extracellular space electron-dense tracers, such as ferritin (Page, 1964; Huxley, 1964), lanthanum (Revel and Karnovsky, 1967) or exogenous peroxidase (Karnovsky, 1965), such electron-dense material marks all spaces that are continous with the extracellular space, presumably by simple diffusion. In experiments using these techniques, usually only the transverse tubules are marked. In fact, these techniques have been instrumental in proving the continuity of the lumens of transverse tubules

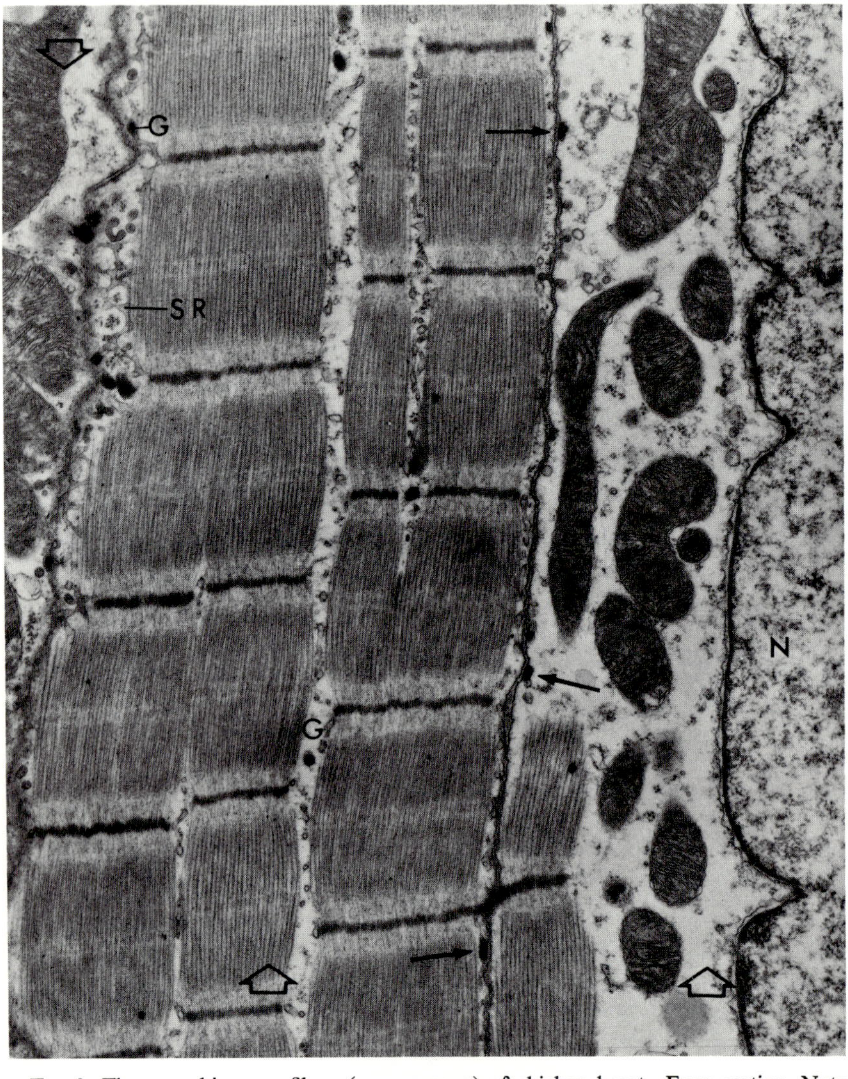

FIG. 9. Three working myofibers (open arrows) of chicken heart. Epon section. Note the well-developed SR (SR) containing dense material (G) in the junctional SR and elsewhere in the cells. Arrows indicate couplings at sarcolemma. Magnification: ×14,000.

with the extracellular space (Page, 1964; Huxley, 1964; Girardier and Pollet, 1964; Sommer and Johnson 1968b). Thus, one definition of transverse tubules is a phenomenological one; the transverse tubules are tubules that can be filled with contrast material from the extracellular space. On the other hand,

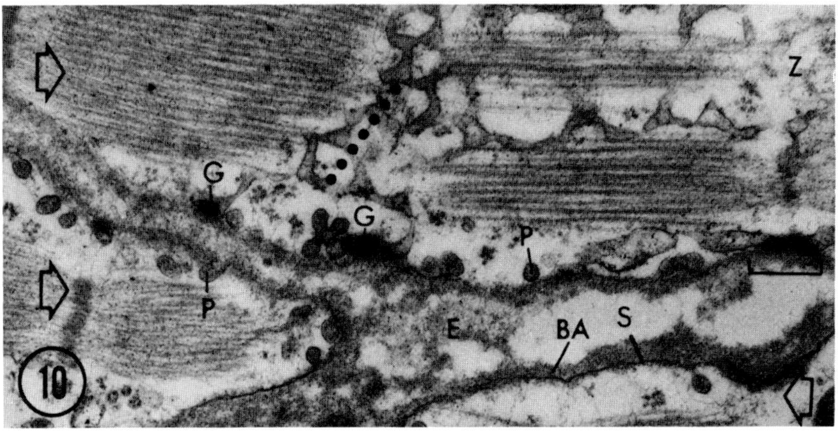

FIG. 10. Working myofibers (open arrows) of chicken heart. Note the well-developed SR in the region of the Z line which is just out of the plane of sectioning. The couplings are in their typical position on either side of that imaginary Z line (dotted line) and contain electron-dense material (G) within the junctional SR which imperceptibly blends with the basement membrane. Electron-dense material with or without a surrounding unit membrane is not seen in the extracellular space beyond the basement membrane except where there is evidence of faulty tissue preparation as well. Note the ramifications of the SR in longitudinal direction. (P), Pinocytotic vesicle. Magnification: × 30,500.

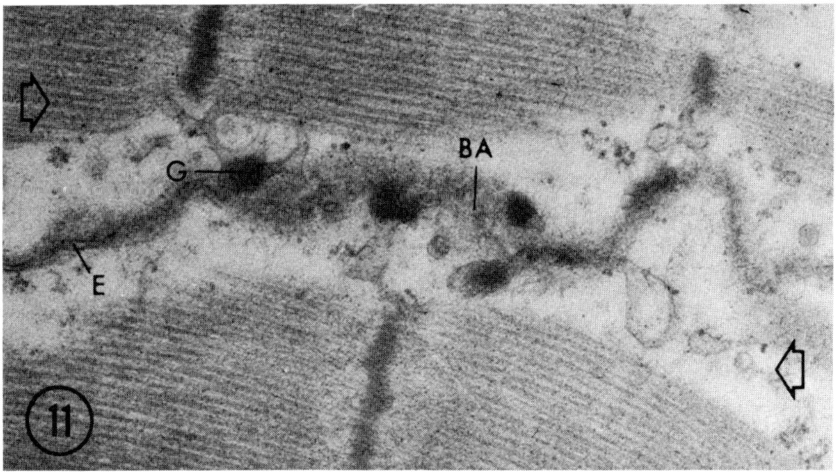

FIG. 11. Same tissue as in Fig. 10. Note electron-dense mass inside the junctional SR of the coupling at (G) and elsewhere. (E), Extracellular space between two cells (open arrows); (BA), grazing section through basement membrane. Some of the dense material in fortunate sections shows circular substructures with a center-to-center spacing of approximately 15 to 20 mμ. Magnification: × 32,000.

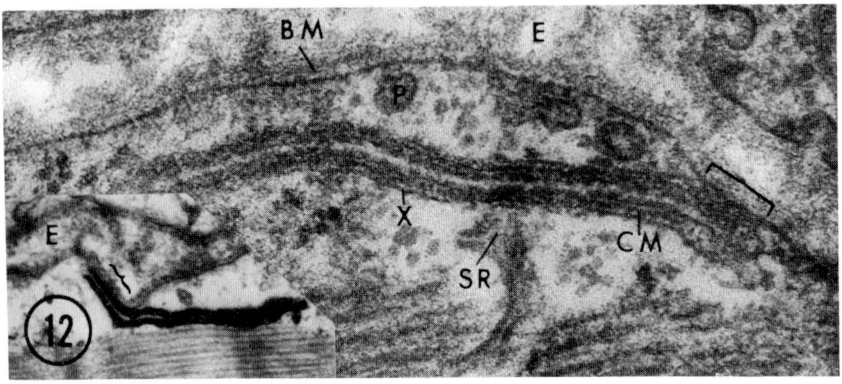

FIG. 12. Atrial myofiber of dog heart. Specialized SR (X)—see text—of considerable length and containing central membrane (CM). One of these profiles forms a coupling (bracket). (E), Extracellular space; (BM), basement membrane covering sarcolemma; (P), pinocytotic vesicle; (SR), sarcoplasmic reticulum. Magnification: × 65,000. Inset: Similar profiles of specialized SR, one of which forms a coupling at the bracket, are clearly filled with lanthanum following perfusion fixation with glutaraldehyde. Magnification: × 26,500.

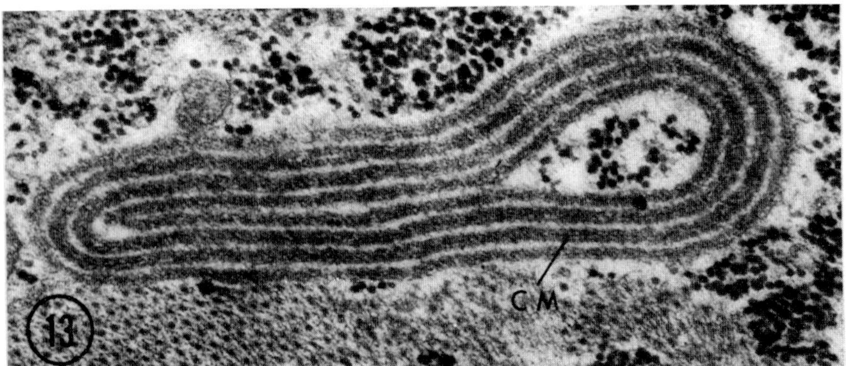

FIG. 13. Structures similar to those in Fig. 12 forming lamellae in a Purkinje fiber of dog cardiac muscle. Most of the black granules are glycogen; some others may be ribosomes. Magnification: × 54,000.

a merely morphologic definition may be attempted, despite the fact that such has been found unsatisfactory because of structural similarity between transverse tubules and the tubules of the SR, at least in a skeletal muscle (Page, 1964). Nevertheless, in cardiac muscle in which the transverse tubules can become very much attenuated, as has been suggested (Forssmann and Girardier, 1966), the basement membranes will not be clearly identifiable any longer, and thus the anatomical separation of transverse tubules from the SR becomes ever more difficult if not impossible. Therefore, in cardiac muscle one is also tempted to rely more on the phenomenological definition of transverse tubules in order to distinguish between them and the SR. Unfortunately, sometimes the SR too is marked by an extracellular tracer (Fig. 14). One is thus faced with the choice of either viewing the transverse tubules as a network much more extensive (Forssmann *et al.*, 1968) than one would have suspected on previous evidence, or of concluding that the SR is patent to the extracellular space, including the transverse tubules; in the latter case, one is faced with yet another problem, namely to decide where the transverse tubules begin and where the SR ends. Perhaps this dilemma may be resolved by simply assuming that transitory open connections between the SR and the extracellular space exist, as for example, in contractile vacuoles. Thus, our considerations and those of Forssmann and Girardier (Forssmann and Girardier, 1966) are entirely compatible in many respects, in spite of the fact that we reject their evidence (Sommer and Johnson, 1968a), since under most circumstances of tissue preparation, open connections between the SR and the extracellular space cannot be demonstrated safely, and if indeed connections are indicated by tracer studies, their possible artifactual nature cannot be overlooked. To be sure, the perfusion of the heart with the fixative just prior to exposure to lanthanum may succeed in instantaneously stopping the process of exocytosis (as it may actually create such openings), and in so doing, manage to preserve an opening through which the subsequently applied tracer may gain access to the SR; moreover, once such a connection has been made permanent by the fixative, the time course of the tracer experiment (minutes) would not prevent the tracer from expanding through the entire SR through that one opening. *In vivo* communications between the SR and the extracellular space, however, are expected to be short-lived (fractions of seconds). Thus, because of the dynamic nature of biological membranes, even under ideal circumstances of *in vivo* experiments with demonstrably inoffensive substances, tracers introduced from the extracellular space fall short of conclusively proving, or for that matter ruling out, *in vivo* transitory openings between the SR and the extracellular space, especially since the entrance of the tracer into the SR may have to be accomplished against a pressure gradient; the *vis a tergo* of that gradient can be provided by a secretory process culminating in exocytosis. The use of artificial tracers moving from the inside of the SR toward the extracellular space would avoid these difficulties, but such a tracer is not available. However, accepting the electron-dense material in the SR of chicken myofibers as a quasi-endogenous tracer, one may propose that our findings in chicken cardiac muscle provide fairly conclusive indirect evidence that *in vivo* the SR and the extracellular space do communicate at least intermittently. Moreover, these

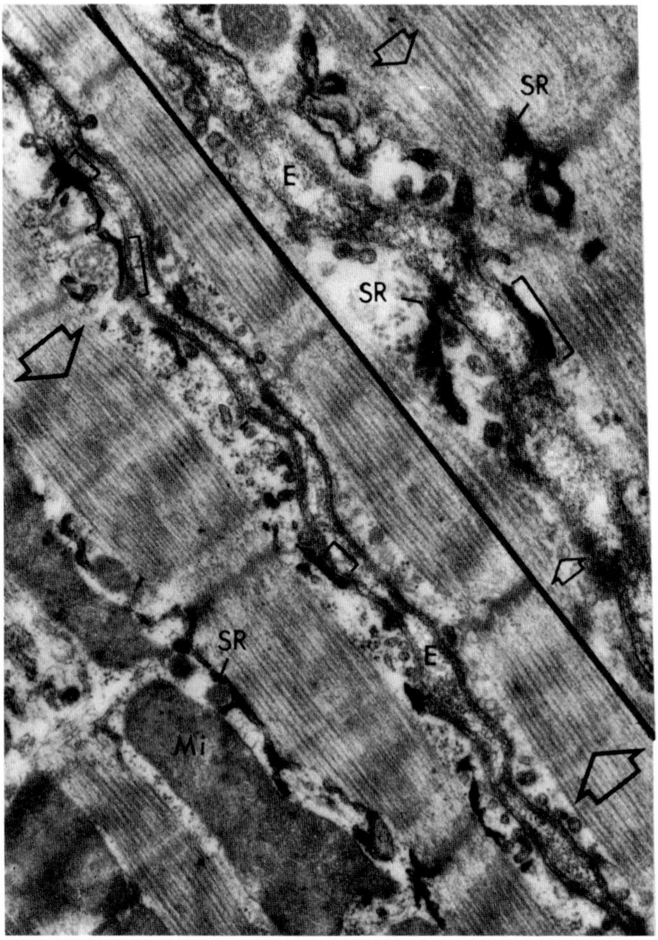

FIG. 14. Atrial myofibers (open arrows) of the dog heart. Epon section. The heart was perfused with glutarldehyde followed by exposure to lanthanum. The junctiona SR (brackets) as well as other SR tubules (SR) are filled with the tracer. (E), Extracellular space; (Mi), Mitochondria. Magnification: ×24,000. Inset: A similar preparation at higher magnification. The scalloped appearance of the junctional SR (bracket) is presumably a result of the filling of junctional processes by lanthanum from inside the SR. Magnification: ×33,000.

findings seem to provide needed additional and independent information for an at least reasonable interpretation of earlier unpublished observations, an interpretation that tends to reconcile artifact and reality; both combine to create the observable phenomenon (Fig. 14). Underscoring the dynamic nature of the relationships between sarcolemma and the SR are the findings of Fawcett and McNutt (1969) regarding the fusion of coated vesicles with the SR; in spite of the fact that our knowledge of the essence of these vesicles is rather limited, they may have something to do with protein uptake from the outside of the cell (Roth and Porter, 1964).

The nature of the electron-dense material in chicken and frog hearts is as yet obscure, nor can it be said that the dense material in various locations is necessarily identical in nature. However, the significance of finding this material within the SR is that it affords an insight into a possible function of the SR in addition to, and perhaps even complementary to that associated with the calcium pump of Hasselbach (Hasselbach and Makinose, 1968), an ion pump that is central to relaxation of muscle; the evidence favors the notion that the SR is presumably involved in exocytosis of a secretory product. The success of such a hypothetical process would depend on at least transitory communications of the SR with the outside of the cell. Thus, the expulsion of other substances (e.g., calcium), even if not related to the primary secretory intent, may become possible, if only incidentally. Secretory processes seem to be dependent on respiratory energy (Jamieson and Palade, 1968). That ATPase of the SR which is unassociated with calcium uptake *in vitro* and which may be demonstrable (although inseparable from the calcium-dependent one) cytochemically in cardiac and skeletal muscle (Schulze and Wollenberger, 1967; Sommer and Spach 1964; Sommer and Hasselbach, 1967), but for which no function has been found thus far, might be related to the process of exocytosis.

Unfortunately, anatomical studies including comparative ones, have thus far not provided any insight into so obvious an anatomical reality as myocardial hypertrophy if only as regards its formal genesis. Clearly, myocardial hypertrophy results in an increase in contractile material and at first glance one might expect to find morphological evidence under appropriate experimental conditions that might permit one to reconstruct the formal genesis of at least new sarcomeres. So far, no satisfactory morphological information regarding that process has been produced, although some observations that may or may not be pertinent to the problem have been reported (Bishop, 1969; Johnson and Sommer, 1967). Abnormal Z-line material in animals with myocardial hypertrophy has been thought to possibly be related to that process (Bishop, 1969). This conflicts with observations regarding the occurence of similar material in cardiac muscle of presumably normal animals (Fawcett, 1967), (Fig. 15), although this conflict is not necessarily prohibitive. With respect to the presence of abnormal Z-line material in Purkinje fibers, it should perhaps be noted that such fibers seem not to participate in the process of hypertrophy.

Because of the large diameter of skeletal muscle fibers, transverse tubules

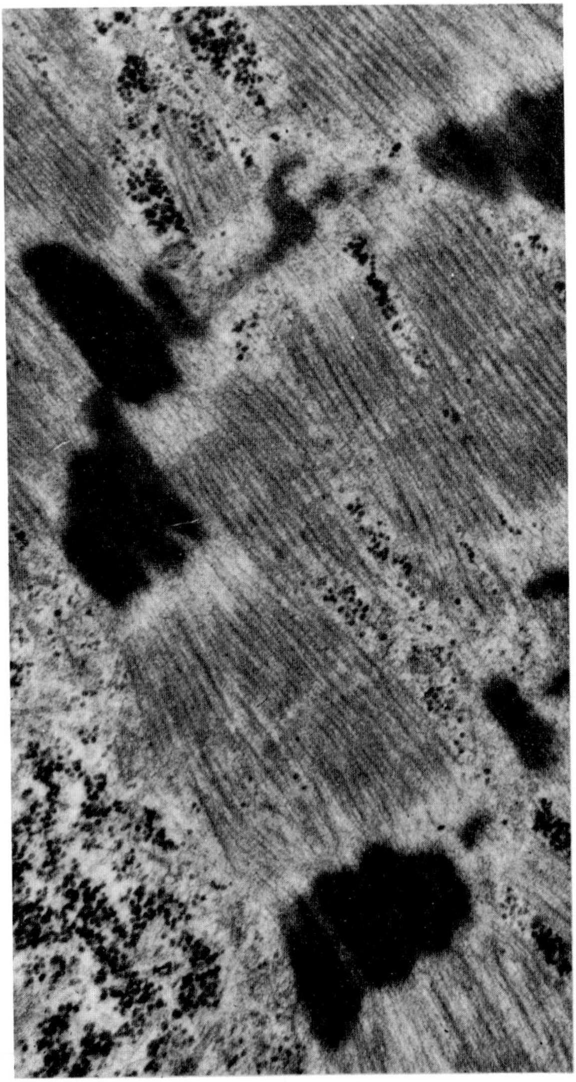

FIG. 15. Purkinje fiber of dog heart, maraglas section. Note large irregular patches of Z-line material (having a substructure similar to Z lines). Magnification: × 51,500.

(Anderson-Cedergren, 1959) appear to be useful in overcoming diffusion problems (Hill, 1948). The working fibers of mammalian hearts have transverse tubules despite the fact that the fibers are of very small diameter, which would tend to obviate the need for such tubules. However, this would no longer be true were these fibers to change their diameter, as is apparently the case in myocardial hypertrophy. It is an intriguing speculation to look upon the transverse tubules in mammalian cardiac muscle as an evolutionary feature upon which the development of hypertrophy might depend, and it would be interesting to see if cardiac hypertrophy comparable to that occurring in mammals can be produced experimentally in animal hearts whose myofibers do not have transverse tubules, such as in the chicken, several other birds, and the amphibians.

It is quite clear that the increased interest in comparative investigations has been informative toward a better understanding of structure–function relationships in cardiac muscle. The emphasis in this chapter has been on the comparative structure of the sarcoplasmic reticulum. The latter was shown, on the one hand, to be differentiated in various ways in different animals, whereas some components such as the couplings may be regarded homologous, mutatis mutandis, in cardiac muscle of different animals, and in skeletal muscle as well. Although at the moment the lumping of certain fiber populations into several anatomically and topographically discrete groups is possible and useful, additional regional differences within the myocardium may be discovered in the future as has previously been pointed out (Simpson and Rayns, 1968). The evidence concerning a possible secretory function of the SR in the chicken* seems to have implications concerning the overall functions of the SR in general and, more specifically, concerning the translocation of calcium in the course of the contraction–relaxation cycle. Although it is impossible to prove from static electron micrographs the dynamic process of exocytosis, the impressive anatomical evidence is not in conflict with such a process as being operative *in vivo* and should be taken into account when movements of calcium from one compartment to another are considered. For this reason, inquiries into this process of possible exocytosis and into the nature of the substances being transported by that route (e.g., protein–polysaccharide complexes, catecholamines) are imperative.

Acknowledgments

Mr. Isaiah Taylor again has contributed his best to the technical preparation of this communication. The freeze-etch preparation of Fig. 2 was made in collaboration with Dr. Russel L. Steere. This research was supported, in part, by NIH grant HE12486-01, and in part, by NIH grant 5-T01-HD00132.

* Preliminary observations show that the SR of mammalian cardiac muscle also occasionally contains some discrete globular electron-dense material.

References

Anderson-Cedergren, E (1959). *J. Ultrastruct. Res. Suppl.* **1**, 1.
Barr, L., Dewey, M. M., and Berger, W. (1965). *J. Gen. Physiol.*, **48**, 797.
Bishop, S. P. (1969). *Fed Proc. Fed. Amer. Soc. Exp. Biol.* **28**, 728.
Bullivant, S. (1969). *Proc. 27th Annu. Mtg. Electron Microsc. Soc. Amer. St. Paul, Minnesota* 1969, p. 330. Claitor's Publishing Div., Baton Rouge.
Dreifuss, J. J., and Girardier, L. (1966). *Pflueger Arch. Gesamte Physiol. Menschen Tiere* **292**, 13.
Fawcett, D. W. (1967). *J. Cell Biol.* **36**, 266.
Fawcett, D. W., and McNutt, N. S. (1969). *J. Cell Biol.* **42**, 1.
Forssmann, W. G., and Girardier, L. (1966). *Z. Zellforsch. Mikrosk. Anat.* **72**, 249.
Forssmann, W. G., Matter, A., Daldrup, J., and Girardier, L. (1968). *J. Cell. Biol.* **39**, 45a.
Girardier, L., and Pollet, M. (1964). *Helv. Physiol. Pharmacol. Acta* **24**, C72.
Hasselbach, W., and Makinose, M. (1968). *Biochem. Z.* **333**, 518.
Hill, A. V. (1948). *Proc. Roy. Soc. London Ser. B.* **135**, 446.
Huxley, H. E. (1964). *Nature* (*London*) **202**, 1067.
Jamieson, J. D., and Palade, G. E. (1964). *J. Cell Biol.* **23**, 151.
Jamieson, J. D., and Palade, G. E. (1968). *J. Cell Biol.* **39**, 589.
Johnson, E. A., and Sommer, J. R. (1967). *J. Cell Biol.* **33**, 103.
Karnovsky, M. J. (1965). *J. Cell Biol.* **27**, 49A.
Kreutziger, G. O. (1968). *Proc. 26th Annu. Mtg. Electron Microsc. Soc. Amer. New Orleans, Louisiana* 1968, p. 234. Claitor's Publishing Div., Baton Rouge.
McNutt, N. S., and Fawcett, D. W. (1969). *J. Cell Biol.* **42**, 46.
McNutt, N. S., and Weinstein, R. S. (1969). *Proc. 27th Annu. Mfg. Electron Microsc. Soc. Amer. St. Paul, Minnesota*, 1969, p. 330.
Page, S. (1964). *J. Physiol.* **175**, 10.
Revel, J. P., and Karnovsky, M. J. (1967) *J. Cell Biol.* **33**, 67.
Rosenbluth, J. (1969). *J. Cell Biol.* **42**, 534.
Roth, T. F., and Porter, K. R. (1964). *J. Cell Biol.* **20**, 313.
Schulze, W., and Wollenberger, A. (1967). *Histochemie*, **10**, 140.
Simpson, F. O., and Rayns, D. G. (1968). *Amer. J. Anat.* **122**, 193.
Sommer, J. R. (1968). *Fed. Proc. Fed. Amer. Soc. Exp. Biol.* **27**, 357.
Sommer, J. R., and Hasselbach, W. (1967). *J. Cell Biol.* **34**, 902.
Sommer, J. R., and Johnson, E. A. (1968a). *J. Cell Biol.* **36**, 497.
Sommer, J. R., and Johnson, E. A. (1968b). *J. Cell Biol.* **37**, 570.
Sommer, J. R., and Johnson, E. A. (1969). *Z. Zellforsch. Mikrosk. Anat.* **98**, 437.
Sommer, J. R., and Johnson, E. A. (1970). *Amer. J. Cardiol.* **25**, 184.
Sommer, J. R., and Spach, M. S. (1964). *Amer. J. Pathol.* **44**, 491.
Sommer, J. R., and Steere, R. L. (1970). *J. Cell Biol.* **47**, 198a.
Staley, N. A., and Benson, E. S. (1968). *J. Cell Biol.* **38**, 99.
Steere, R. L. (1957). *J. Biophys. Chem. Cytol.* **3**, 45.
Truex, R. C., and Smythe, M. Q. (1965). *Ann. N.Y. Acad. Sci.* **127**, 19.

ULTRASTRUCTURAL ALTERATIONS IN CANINE MYOCARDIAL HYPERTROPHY

Sanford P. Bishop

Hypertrophy is the response of the myocardium to an increased work load. Although adaptive hypertrophy may be beneficial to the host (Badeer, 1967), it is a well-known clinical observation that many patients with myocardial hypertrophy develop signs of congestive heart failure. In the experimental animal, it has been demonstrated that the hypertrophied heart does have a decreased contractility even before the onset of overt myocardial failure (Spann *et al.*, 1967). In addition, certain biochemical alterations such as a decreased level of myofibrillar ATPase activity (Albert and Gordon, 1962; Chandler *et al.*, 1967), decreased catecholamine content (Chidsey *et al.*, 1964), and decreased carnitine content (Wittels and Spann, 1968) have been reported in the hypertrophied heart.

It has been known since the 1925 studies of Karsner, Saphir, and Todd that the myocardial fiber increases in width with hypertrophy, and more recent studies by Laks *et al.* (1969a) have confirmed earlier suspicions (Linzbach, 1960) that the cell also increases in length. With the possible exception of severe hypertrophy, there appears to be little evidence that cellular hyperplasia occurs during cardiac enlargement (Linzbach, 1960). With regard to the increase in cell width, Richter and Kellner (1963) demonstrated that in human myocardial hypertrophy the normal lattice arrangement of the actin and myosin filaments is retained. These authors also suggested that with myocardial hypertrophy there is an increase in the number of myofibrils, resulting in increased width of the myocardial cell. The recent report by Fawcett and McNutt (1969), however, in which the myofibrils are described as a single interconnecting mass of filaments rather than as individual fibrils, would appear to render an evaluation of the number of myofibrils in a cross section of a myocardial cell an impossible task. Nevertheless, in compensated myocardial hypertrophy, there is an increase in the cell width and the normal myofilament area to mitochondrial area is retained (Meerson *et al.*, 1964);

therefore, there must have been an increase in the number of myofilaments. Carney and Brown (1964, 1967) have shown that myosin filaments retain their normal size and morphology in the hypertrophied myocardial fiber. They suggested that myosin and actin filaments may be added to the periphery of the existing myofibrillar structure to produce increased cell width. An increased longitudinal folding of the myofibrillar structure could give the appearance of an increased number of myofibrils, as Richter and Kellner (1963) have suggested. In order for the hypertrophied myocardial cell to increase in length (Laks *et al.*, 1969a), yet have no increase in sarcomere length (Linzbach, 1960; Laks *et al.*, 1969a), there must be an addition of new sarcomeres to the fibrils.

During the ultrastructural study of canine cardiac hypertrophy we have encountered alterations in the Z bands and intercalated discs, which may have a bearing on the mechanism of cardiac hypertrophy and failure (Bishop and Cole, 1969a). The purpose of this chapter is to describe the morphology of these Z band and intercalated disc alterations, to report their occurrence in various types of experimental and naturally occurring canine myocardial hypertrophy, and to discuss their possible significance in cardiac hypertrophy and failure.

Right ventricular hypertrophy (RVH) was produced in the dog by surgically implanting an inflatable rubber cuff around the main pulmonery artery, as previously described (Bishop and Cole, 1969b). The cuff connector was brought out through the ribs, and the injection bulb implanted subcutaneously. The pulmonary artery cuff was distended by percutaneous injections into the bulb at biweekly intervals, resulting in progressive pulmonary artery stenoses and right ventricular hypertrophy. Right ventricular hypertrophy and dilation developed during the course of the experiment, subjectively determined by increase in wall thickness and heart size on radiographs and cineangiocardiograms. Right ventricular free-wall weight to body weight ratio was nearly doubled as shown in Table I. Left ventricle and septum combined weight to body weight ratios were not altered. The development of congestive heart failure (CHF) was determined by elevation of right atrial systolic and right ventricular end-diastolic pressure above 7 mm Hg, decreased exercise tolerance, venous congestion, liver enlargement, and ascites.

In addition to seven animals with experimentally produced RVH and CHF, Table I lists the animals with myocardial hypertrophy secondary to congenital cardiac malformations, chronic mitral valve disease, and dirofilariasis which have been examined by electron microscopy. Tissues were collected from the right and left ventricular free-walls in all animals immediately after death. The tissues were minced either directly in 1% osmium tetroxide or in 2.5% glutaraldehyde followed by postfixation is osmium tetroxide, dehydrated through ascending grades of ethyl alcohol, and embedded in Dow Epoxy

TABLE I

EFFECTS OF EXPERIMENTAL AND NATURALLY OCCURRING MYOCARDIAL HYPERTROPHY IN THE DOG

Group	Age (years)	CHF	RV/BW[a] (gm/kg)	LV/BW[b] (gm/kg)	Altered Z bands RV frequency (severity)[c]	Altered Z bands LV frequency (severity)[c]	Wide intercalated discs RV frequency (severity)[c]	Wide intercalated discs LV frequency (severity)[c]
Control	1–3	No	1.93	5.25	0/5	0/5	0/5	0/5
			(1.66–2.16)	(4.65–5.85)	0	0	0	0
Exp. RVH and	1–6	Yes	3.39	4.70	6/7	4/7	6/7	0/7
CHF			(3.12–3.57)	(4.30–5.48)	++	+	++	0
Dirofilaria immitis								
(Heartworm)	7–10	No-3	3.11	4.93	6/6	2/6	5/6	0/6
RVH		Yes-3	(2.19–5.22)	(3.92–6.06)	+, ++	+	+, ++	0
Congenital	4	No	13.9	14.4	++	++	+	0
pulmonic stenosis	3.5	No	7.4	7.6	+	0	+	0
	7	No	5.5	5.9	0	0	0	0
Congenital subaortic	4	No	–	–	0	++	0	+
stenosis	0.3	No	1.85	7.80	+	+	0	+
Spontaneous mitral	12	No	4.34	9.71	+	+	0	0
valve insufficiency	11	No	1.88	5.96	0	0	0	0
	0.5	No	2.15	7.06	+	+	0	+

[a] RV/BW = Right ventricular free wall weight per total body weight. Average (range) shown.

[b] LV/BW = Left ventricle plus septum weight per total body weight. Average (range) shown.

[c] 0 indicates lesion not present, +, lesion present but not frequent, ++, lesion present and frequent.

Resin (DER). Silver-gray sections, cut with glass knives on a Porter–Blum ultramicrotome and suspended on uncoated 200- or 300-mesh copper grids, were stained with uranyl acetate and lead citrate, and then examined with either a Phillips EM-200 or Hitachi HU-11B electron microscope.

The ultrastructure of the myocardium in the control dogs was similar to that which has been previously described (Moore and Ruska, 1957; Price *et al.*, 1959). Figure 1 illustrates a fiber from a control animal representative of normal canine myocardium. Of particular interest to this study is the even parallel arrangement of myofibrils and the regular lateral register of the Z bands. In general, the mitochondria form single rows between the

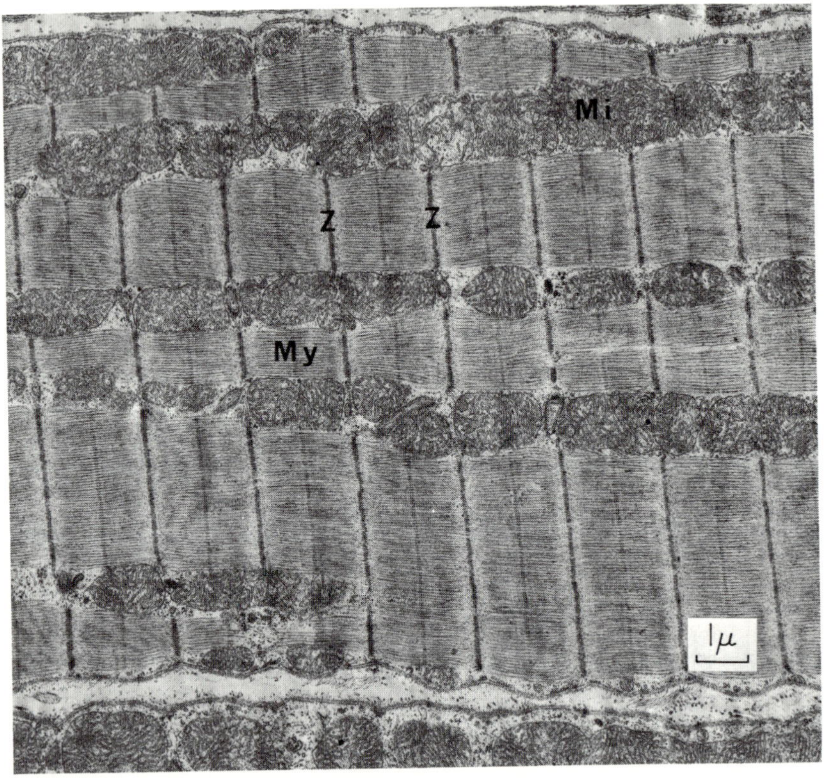

FIG. 1. Myocardial fiber from right ventricle of a control dog. (Z), Z band; (My), myofibril; (Mi), mitochondria. (From Bishop and Cole, 1969a.)

myofibrils and are usually about one sarcomere in length, although longer forms up to seven or more sarcomeres in length occur regularly in normal canine myocardium. The usual accumulations of mitochondria are present at the nuclear poles and variable numbers of lipofuscin granules also occur at this location. Glycogen is abundant throughout the normal canine myocardium. Golgi membranes and rough endoplasmic reticulum are unusual in control tissue.

In the hypertrophied myocardium the size and number of mitochondria were quite variable. In some fibers the mitochondria appeared to pile up on one another (Fig. 2), whereas in others, mitochondria were less numerous than usual. In several animals, numerous small irregularly shaped mitochondria, less than one-half sarcomere in length were found, especially at the nuclear poles. Although long forms of mitochondria have been reported in canine left ventricular hypertrophy (Wollenberger and Schulze, 1961), with the exception of one animal, long forms of mitochondria were quite

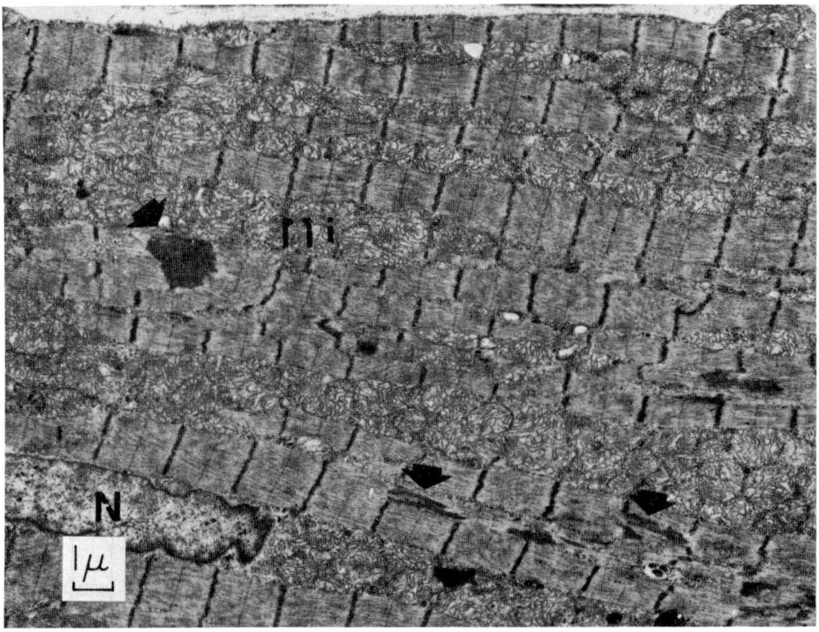

FIG. 2. Right ventricle from dog with experimental right ventricular hypertrophy and congestive heart failure. There is moderate disorientation of myofibrils with Z bands out of register with each other and a tendency for mitochondria (Mi) to occur in aggregations. Altered Z bands are marked by arrowheads. (N), Nucleus. (From Bishop and Cole, 1969a.)

unusual in our material. In the one exception, a dog with experimental RVH, mitochondria in the right ventricle formed long chainlike structures with incomplete pinching off at the Z-band level, suggesting either an incomplete budding or a fusion of adjacent mitochondria. This dog was also the only one with experimental RVH in which altered Z bands (*vide infra*) were not found. Heart weight and hemodynamic data for this dog were similar to others in the group—the explanation for the differences is not clear.

In addition to the mitochondrial alterations noted above, other changes included increased glycogen in the hypertrophied myocardial tissue as previously noted by Laks *et al.* (1969b). Figure 3 illustrates the ribbon-like structure of the nucleolus characteristic of the hypertrophied fibers. Rough endoplasmic reticulum, which appeared to be increased in hypertrophy, occurred in the nuclear pole region of hypertrophied myocardial cells.

In the severely hypertrophied canine myocardium there was often a disorganization of the orderly array of myofibrils and a loss of lateral register of the Z bands in the widened myocardial fibers. Comparison of adjacent myofibrils frequently suggested the presence of an additional sarcomere in a myofibril with resulting loss of lateral register.

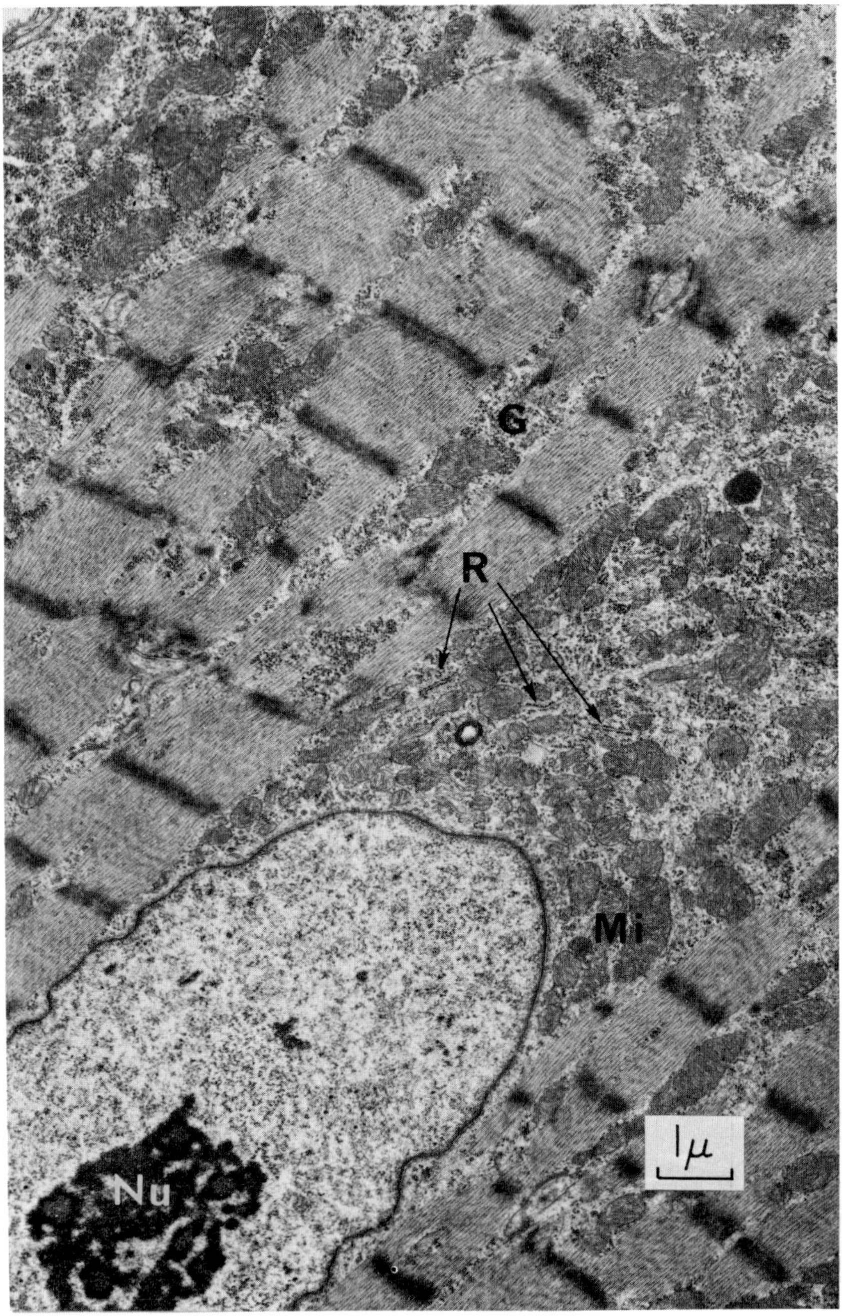

FIG. 3. Myofiber from right ventricle of a dog with experimental right ventricular hypertrophy and congestive heart failure. Many of the mitochondria (Mi) are smaller than in control animals, glycogen (G) is abundant, the nucleolus (Nu) has a ribbon-like appearance, and rough endoplasmic reticulum (R) is present in the nuclear pole region.

Structural alterations were present in the Z-band region of myocardial fibers from dogs with severe cardiac hypertrophy and congestive heart failure. With low magnification, these alterations appeared as electron-dense thickenings of the Z band varying in size from a small focal thickening up to the complete width of a sarcomere (Figs. 2 and 4). The altered Z bands were associated with a distortion of the myofiber and loss of lateral register of sarcomeres. Figures 5 and 6 show the attachment of these dense structures to Z bands and the apparent longitudinal displacement of adjacent sarcomeres. The adjacent sarcomeres were of normal length, and in relaxed fibers an I band was present surrounding the altered Z-band material. The fine actin filaments of the I band appeared to attach to the altered Z-band material. Occasionally, an appearance suggesting the formation of a new myofibril by production of new sarcomere units in series and the longitudinal splitting or folding of a preexisting myofibril was found (Fig. 6).

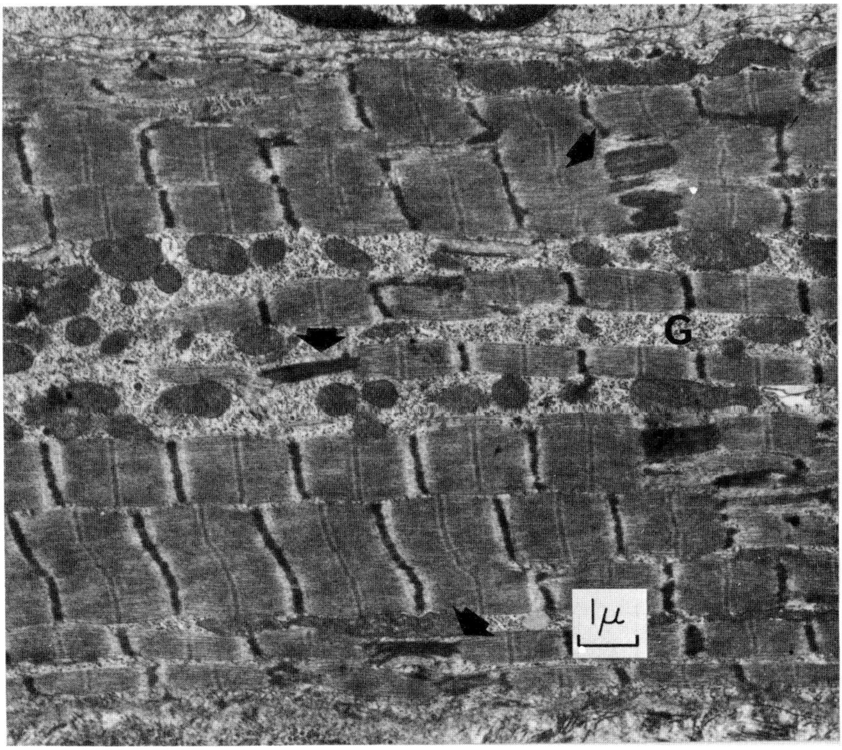

FIG. 4. Myofiber from right ventricle of a dog with dirofilariasis. Numerous altered Z bands (arrowheads) are present resulting in distortion and loss of lateral register of the myofibrils. Glycogen (G) is abundant.

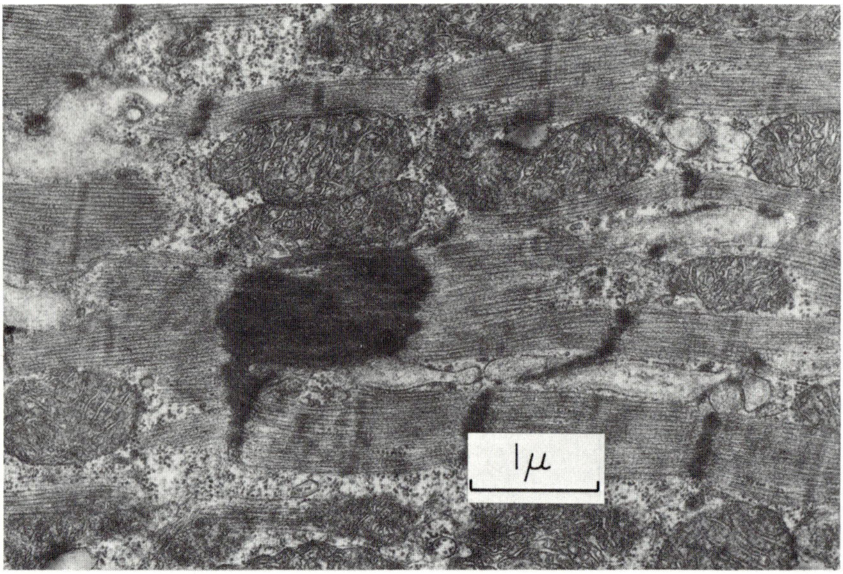

FIG. 5. Right ventricle from a dog with congenital pulmonic stenosis. Part of a Z band has expanded appearing to have resulted in longitudinal displacement of one branch of the myofibril.

High-resolution electron micrographs revealed the altered Z-band material to have a regular repeating period of about 200 Å (Fig. 7). Fine longitudinal striations were also present. Similar striations are present in normal Z bands and there are many similarities with published photographs of crystalline tropomyosin prepared by Huxley (1963) and by Hodge (1959). It has recently been pointed out by Stromer *et al.* (1969), however, that the lattice of normal Z bands has distinct morphologic differences from the lattice of tropomyosin crystals.

Table I summarizes the distribution of these altered Z bands in the myocardia of dogs with various types of hypertrophy. The myocardium of animals with marked hypertrophy and signs of CHF had altered Z bands in nearly all fibers examined, many fibers having numerous altered Z bands. Those animals which were in a compensated state of myocardial hypertrophy had only a few or no altered Z bands present. The nonstressed left ventricles of dogs with RVH and CHF also contained occasional alterations of the Z bands. Altered Z bands have not been found in normal dog myocardium.

From the results of ultrastructural investigations of hypertrophied myocardial tissue, a morphological sequence of events for development of new sarcomere units can be proposed. Under the influence of the proper stimulus, the Z band becomes wider, starting with small focal thickenings, either singly or in several adjacent Z bands (Figs. 2, 4, and 8). The material apparently

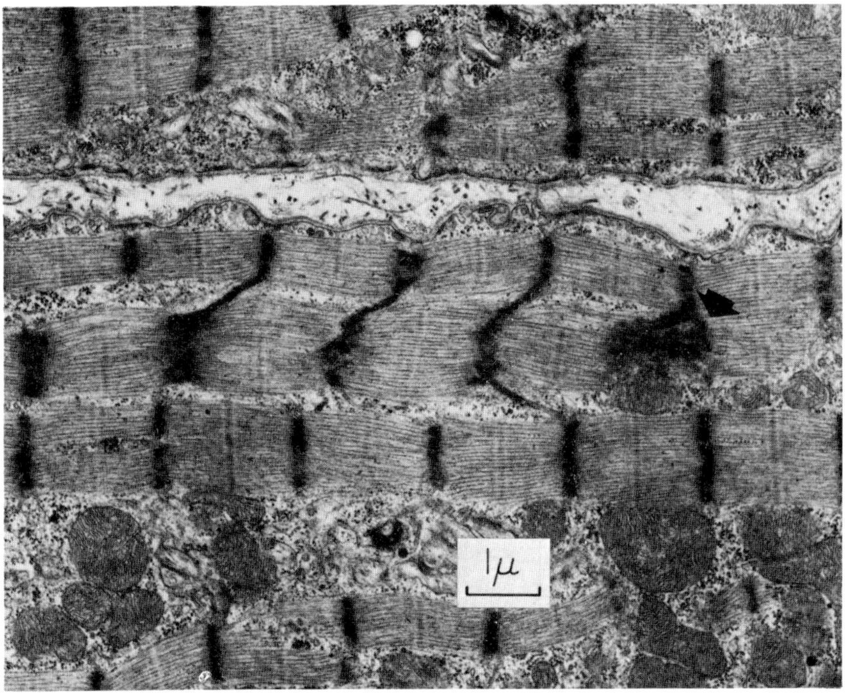

FIG. 6. Right ventricle from a dog with experimental right ventricular hypertrophy and congestive heart failure. Widened Z bands are connected to Z bands of adjacent myofibrils suggesting a longitudinal splitting of the myofibril at right center to produce two myofibrils. The Z band at right center (arrowhead) appears to have expanded, forcing movement of the central myofibril to the left. (From Bishop and Cole, 1969a.)

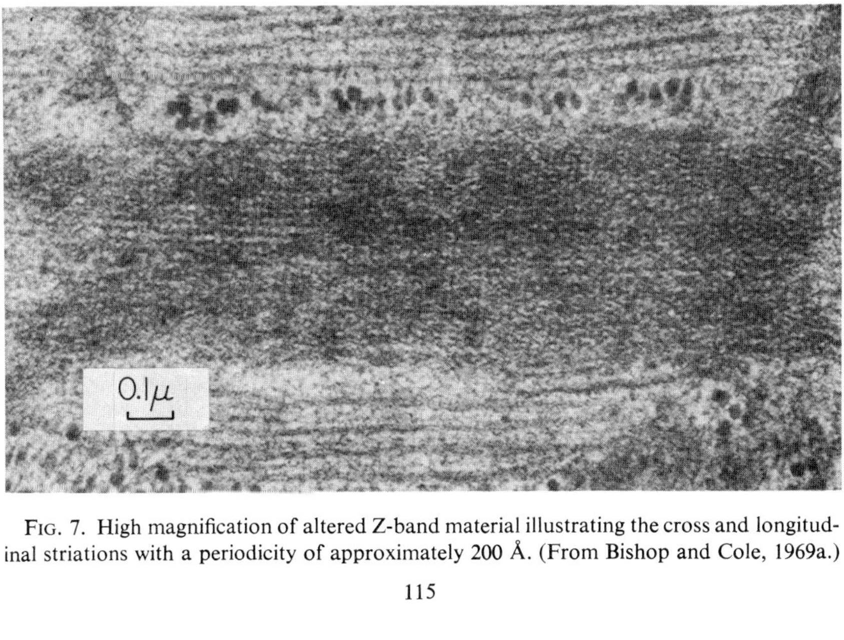

FIG. 7. High magnification of altered Z-band material illustrating the cross and longitudinal striations with a periodicity of approximately 200 Å. (From Bishop and Cole, 1969a.)

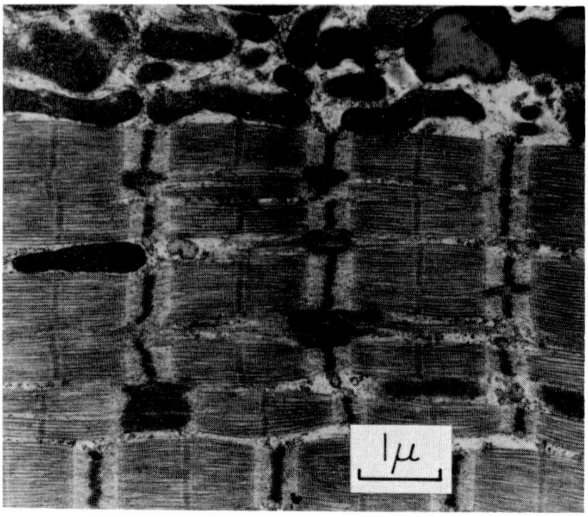

FIG. 8. Altered Z bands in the right ventricular myocardium from a dog with experimental right ventricular hypertrophy and congestive heart failure.

displaces adjacent sarcomeres (Figs. 5 and 6), sometimes resulting in disruption of filament orientation. The Z-band material expands over the entire new sarcomere, possibly acting as a structural support for assembly of actin and myosin filaments. The dark Z-band material thus appears to be removed with formation of a new sarcomere in its place. Myofilaments occurred individually and in bundles in association with altered Z-band material (Fig. 9) and appeared to be in various stages of organization, suggesting the formation of a new sarcomere. In Fig. 10 a number of altered Z bands and sarcomeres in various stages of organization are seen in one myocardial fiber.

According to this proposed sequence, increase in fiber length occurs by replication of the functional unit of muscle, the sarcomere. Increase in width of the myofiber may occur by branching or splitting of new or previously existing myofibrils (Fig. 6). It does not exclude the possibility, however, that actin and myosin filaments may be added to already existing sarcomeres.

The hypertrophied ventricles also had alterations in the intercalated discs. The normal intercalated disc consists of an electron-dense band with a discrete regular wavy appearance and rather uniform width of 0.5–0.8μ (Fig. 11). In hypertrophied ventricles distortion of the intercalated discs occurred with increased longitudinal foldings of an irregular nature, producing an increased width of the disc. The degree of irregularity was proportional to the severity of hypertrophy and varied from a moderate distortion as seen in Fig. 12 to a much more marked and obvious distortion as seen in Fig. 13. Longitudinal folds up to 4 or 5μ in extent were sometimes found. Higher-power examination revealed these folds to consist primarily of myofilament attachment

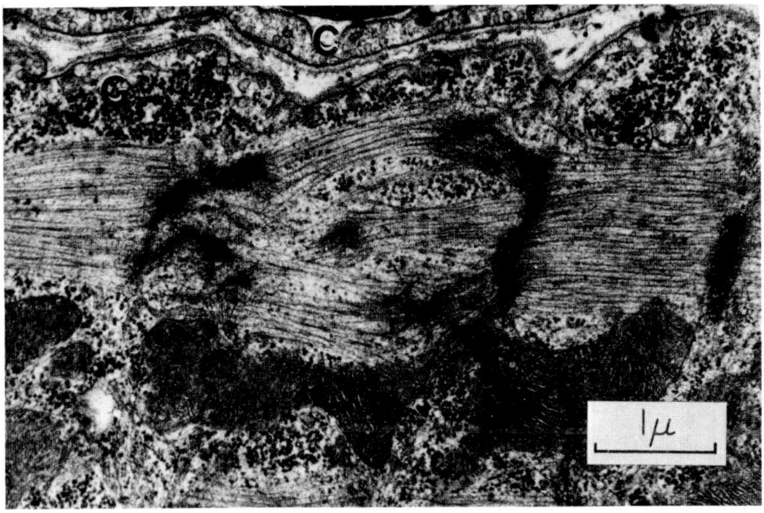

FIG. 9. Disoriented sarcomere in the right ventricle of a dog with experimental right ventricular hypertrophy and congestive heart failure. Note the small bundles of myofilaments within the the disoriented sarcomere. Glycogen granules (G) are numerous; (C), capillary endothelium.

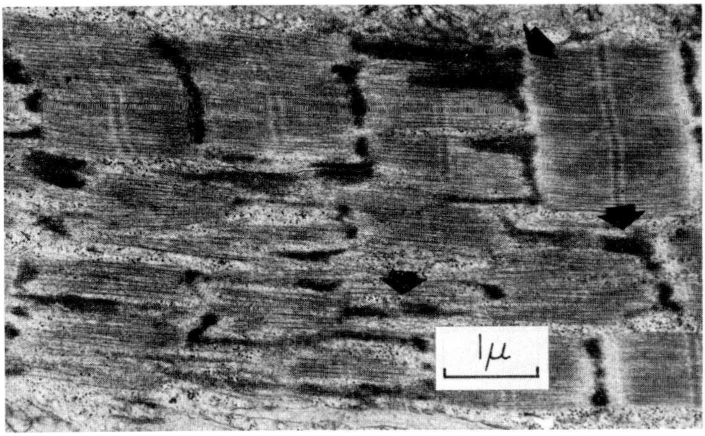

FIG. 10. Right ventricle from a dog with dirofilariasis. Several altered Z bands are present (arrowheads) resulting in disorientation of myofilaments and loss of lateral register of myofibrils.

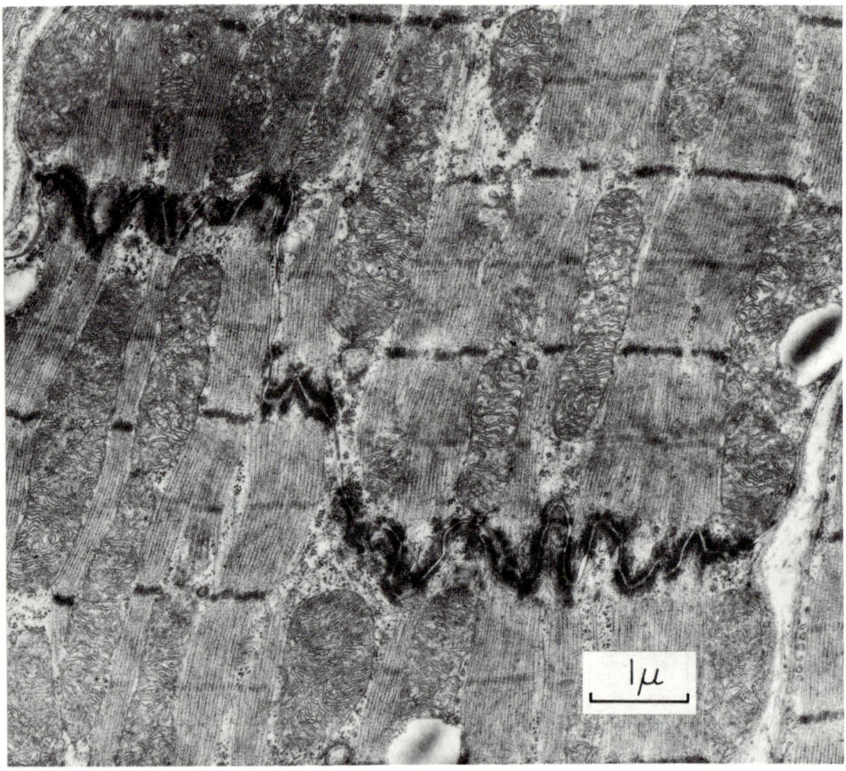

FIG. 11. Normal intercalated disc from right ventricle of control animal. (From Bishop and Cole, 1969a.)

areas and desmosomes (Fig. 14). Disorganized myofilaments were included within the folds, suggesting that new sarcomeres were being formed at the intercalated disc.

One interpretation of the increased folds in the intercalated discs is that altered Z bands, which are producing longitudinal displacement and irregular arrangement of the myofibrils, are producing an irregular push–pull effect on the intercalated disc resulting in its distorted appearance. In support of this interpretation was the consistent finding of altered Z bands and wide, irregular intercalated discs in the same fibers. Cognate with this interpretation is the possibility that asynchronous contraction of the myofibrils containing altered Z bands may produce distortion of their attachment area, the intercalated disc. If asynchronous contraction does indeed occur in hypertrophied myocardial fibers, this could explain the decreased contractility which is characteristic of this tissue. Third, if new sarcomeres are formed at the intercalated disc, as suggested by the presence of myofilaments in various stages of

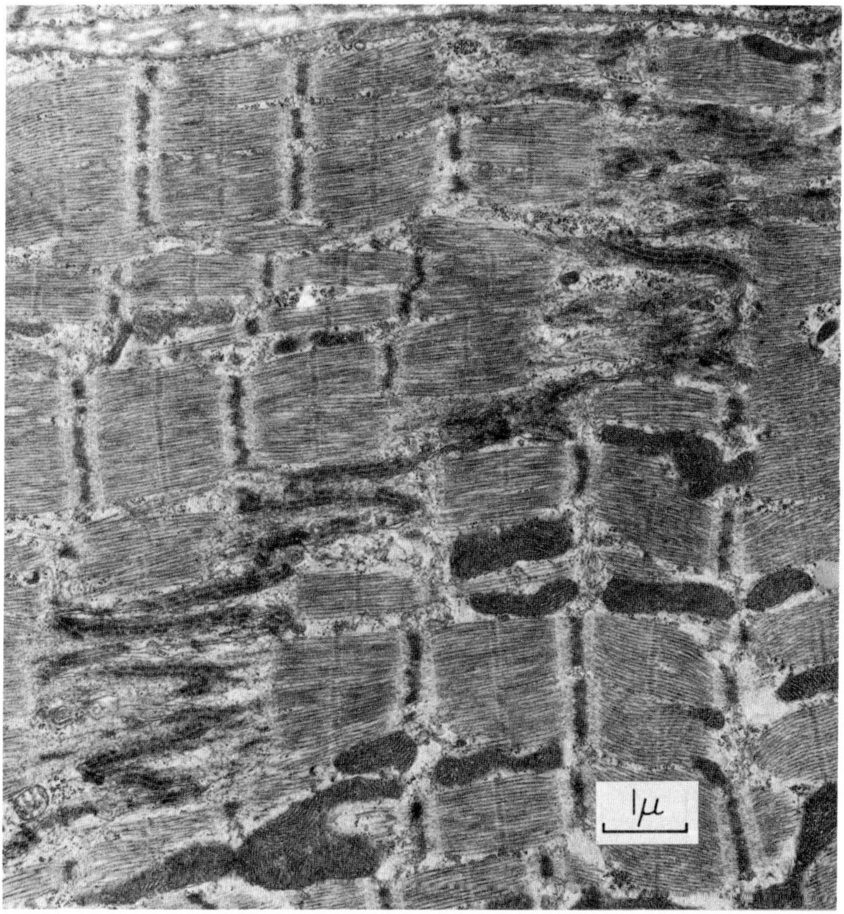

FIG. 12. Widened intercalated disc from right ventricle of a dog with experimental right ventricular hypertrophy and congestive heart failure. Note the increased length of the longitudinal folds (compare with Fig. 11).

organization, they also could be exerting an irregular distorting force on the intercalated disc. A fourth possibility is that an unknown stimulus is producing hypertrophy of the disc disproportionately to the increase in cell width resulting in increased disc surface area, and thus an increased folding to accommodate the disc within the cell.

Structures that are very similar to the altered Z bands found in hypertrophied canine myocardium were first reported to occur in a familial muscular dystrophy of man referred to as nemaline myopathy because of the rodlike structures characteristic of the disease (Shy *et al.*, 1963). Several reports have

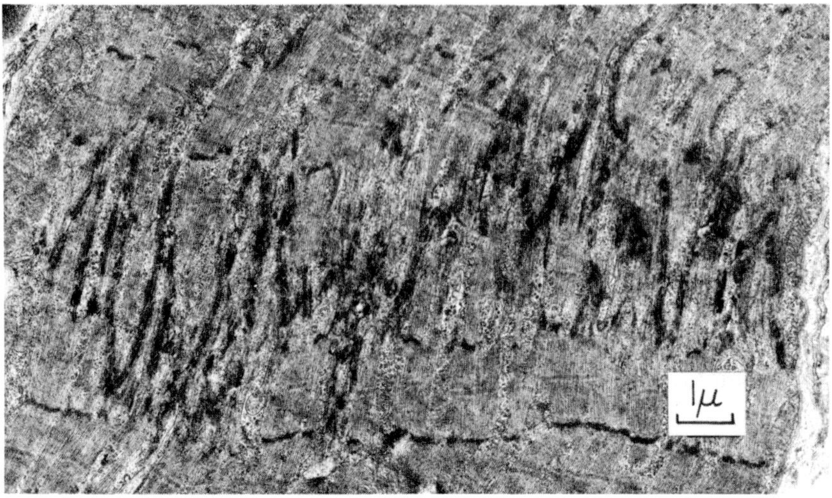

FIG. 13. Extreme widening of an intercalated disc from the right ventricle of a dog with right ventricular hypertrophy and congestive heart failure. Compare with Figs. 11 and 12.

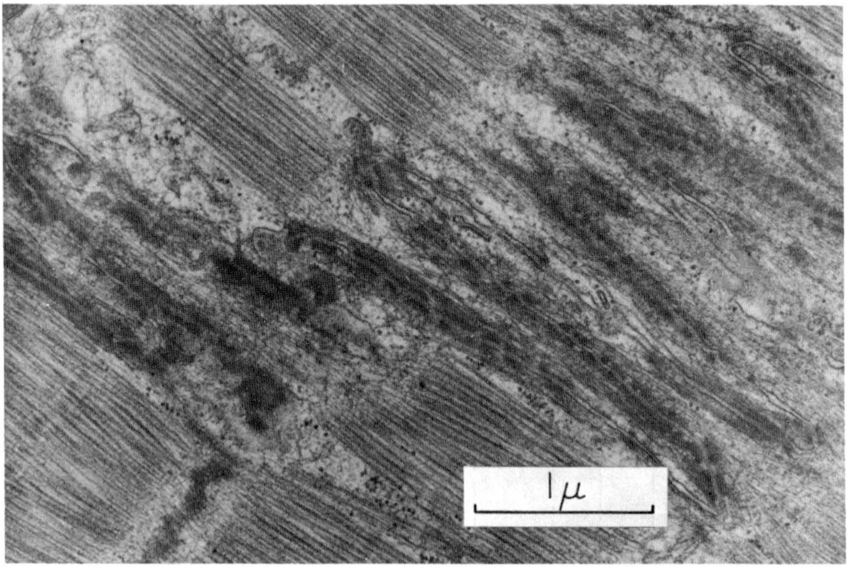

FIG. 14. Higher magnification of a portion of the intercalated disc illustrated in Fig. 12. Note the loosely organized myofilaments within the longitudinal folds of the disc.

appeared in the literature concerning nemaline myopathy and their findings have recently been summarized by Engel (1966). Similarities between the structures in nemaline myopathy and altered Z bands in canine cardiac hypertrophy include (1) direct association with the Z band; (2) apparent structural continuity with adjacent thin filaments in the I band; (3) periodic striations perpendicular to the long axis; and (4) periodic striations parallel to the long axis. The lattice bears many similarities to that found in normal Z bands and the possibility that the structure is identical with crystalline tropomyosin prepared by Huxley (1963) and by Hodge (1959) has been discusssd by Gonatas (1966) and Fawcett (1968). The localization of tropomyosin B in the Z band is still not completely settled, but recent information using fluorescent antitropomyosin antibody (Pepe, 1966) indicates that tropomyosin is more likely located in the I band. In addition, electron microscopic studies by Stromer *et al.* (1969) have demonstrated differences between the crystalline structure of tropomyosin and the normal Z band or "reconstituted" Z band. The identification of the material in altered Z bands of canine hypertrophy and nemaline myopathy awaits further investigation.

In addition to the structures found in nemaline myopathy, similar dense structures have also been identified in skeletal muscle biopsies obtained from patients with a vacuolar myopathy (Rewcastle and Humphrey, 1965), central core disease (Afifi *et al.*, 1965), and diabetes mellitus (Orci *et al.*, 1968). The association of these structures with degenerative diseases of skeletal muscle suggests that an alternative interpretation of the altered Z bands should be examined; that is, that they are associated with degenerative changes in the myocardium. In support of this interpretation, it was found that dogs with the most severe signs of congestive heart failure had the greatest number of altered Z bands, whereas dogs with naturally acquired hypertrophy but which had been in a compensated state without signs of failure for several months had very few altered Z bands. It must be remembered, however, that animals in a compensated state of myocardial hypertrophy would not be expected to produce large amounts of structural protein (Gudbjarnason *et al.*, 1964; Meerson, 1969). In addition, the possibility exists that the electron-dense structures described in the various skeletal muscle diseases could represent an attempt at repair of the cell or compensatory "organelle hyperplasia." Although degenerative changes were uncommon in the hypertrophied myofibers, an occasional fiber with altered Z bands did have disruption of the myofibrils suggesting a possible association with degeneration of the cell.

The finding of occasional altered Z bands in the nonhypertrophied ventricle of dogs with univentricular hypertrophy is evidence against an association with mocyardial degeneration. This finding is further evidence that the unstressed ventricle is affected by changes in the opposite stressed ventricle as has been noted by other investigators with regard to decreased catecholamine levels (Chidsey *et al.*, 1964), depressed myofibrillar ATPase activity (Alpert and Gordon, 1962; Chandler *et al.*, 1967), increased muscle-type lactate dehydrogenase (Bishop and Altschuld, 1970 and this volume), and increased hyproxyproline content (Buccino *et al.*, 1969).

Fawcett (1968) has reported finding structures in the right ventricle of three old male cats which are identical to altered Z bands in canine myocardial hypertrophy. I have also observed their occurrence in the feline normal right ventricle and occasionally in the left ventricle (unpublished observations). The explanation for the presence of altered Z bands in the normal feline myocardium is not apparent. These animals do not have abnormal intercalated discs, and no evidence of myocardial degeneration was found. Challice and DeFelice (1967) have reported the occurrence of similar altered Z band structures in the atrioventricular node of the rabbit.

Munnell and Getty (1968) studied the myocardium of 35 dogs of all ages and found altered Z bands in two old animals. They suggested that the altered Z bands may represent an age-dependent change. There is, however, a very high incidence of atrioventricular valve disease in the old dog (Detweiler and Patterson, 1965); therefore, it appears possible that the lesions reported by Munnell and Getty were actually from dogs with myocardial hypertrophy due to valvular insufficiency.

Developing cardiac and skeletal muscle have been studied ultrastructurally in several species including man (Leak and Burke, 1964), dog (Schulze, 1962), chick (Allen and Pepe, 1965; Fischman, 1957), and frog (Huang, 1967) among others. Recent studies are in agreement that actin and myosin filaments form before the appearance of Z-band material. The actin and myosin filaments very early assume the hexagonal arrangement seen in the adult and line up into sarcomeres forming myofibrils. Z-band structures such as are present in hypertrophied canine myocardium have not been reported in developing myocardial tissue. In our study of hypertrophying myocardial tissue, Z-band alterations sometimes occurred with little disturbance of the myofibrillar structure, apparently as the earliest change. Disoriented bundles of myofilaments occurred simultaneously with altered Z bands, suggesting a later stage in the development of new sarcomeres. If this interpretation proves to be correct, and similar wide Z band structures are not found in normally developing myocardium, then adaptive hypertrophy resulting from an abnormal hemodynamic state in the adult heart would appear to be due to a different mechanism than the increase in cell size which occurs during normal growth. Further investigation is required to clarify this mechanism as well as the role that the intercalated disc may play in myocardial hypertrophy.

ACKNOWLEDGMENTS

This investigation was supported in part by the Ohio Heart Association and USPHS Grants GM 1052 and HE-09884.

REFERENCES

Afifi, A. K. Smith, J. W. and Zellweger, H. (1965). *Neurology* **15**, 371.
Allen, E. R., and Pepe, F. A. (1965). *Amer. J. Anat.* **116**, 115.
Alpert, N. R., and Gordon, M. S. (1962). *Amer. J. Physiol.* **202**, 940.
Badeer, H. S. (1967). *Amer. Heart J.*, **73**, 693.
Bishop, S. P., and Altschuld, R. A. (1970). *Amer. J. Physiol.* **218**, 153.
Bishop, S. P., and Cole, C. R. (1969a). *Lab. Invest.* **20**, 219.
Bishop, S. P., and Cole, C. R. (1969b). *J. Appl. Physiol.* **26**, 659.
Buccino, R. A., Harris, E., Spann, J. F., Jr., and Sonnenblick, E. H. (1969). *Amer. J. Physiol.* **216**, 425.
Carney, J. A., and Brown, A. J., Jr. (1964). *Amer. J. Pathol.* **44**, 521.
Carney, J. A., and Brown, A. L., Jr. (1967). *Lab. Invest.* **16**, 36.
Challice, C. E., and DeFelice, L. J. (1967). *Proc. Electron Microsc. Soc. Amer, p. 204.* Twenty-fifth Meeting, Chicago, Ill., Claitor's, Baton Rouge, Louisiana.
Chandler, B. M., Sonnenblick, E. H., Spann, J. R., Jr., and Pool, P. E. (1967) *Circ. Res.* **21**, 717.
Chidsey, C. A., Kaiser, G. A., Sonnenblick, E. H., Spann, J. F., Jr., and Braunwald, E. (1964). *J. Clin. Invest.* **43**, 2386.
Detweiler, D. K., and Patterson, D. F. (1965). *Ann. N.Y. Acad. Sci.* **127**, 481.
Engel, A. G. (1966). *Proc. Mayo Clin.* **41**, 713.
Fawcettt, D. W. (1968). *J. Cell Biol.* **36**, 266.
Fawcett, D. W., and McNutt, N. S. (1969). *J. Cell Biol.* **42**, 1.
Fischman, D. A. (1967). *J. Cell. Biol.* **32**, 5571.
Gonatas, N. K. (1966). *J. Neuropathol. Exp. Neurol.* **25**, 409.
Gudbjarnason, S., Telerman, M., Chiba, C., Wolf, P. L., and Bing, R. J. (1964). *J. Lab. Clin. Med.* **63**, 245.
Hodge, A. J. (1959) *Rev. Mod. Phys.* **31**, 409.
Huang, C. Y. (1967). *J. Ultrastruct. Res.* **20**, 211.
Huxley, H. E. (1963). *J. Mol. Biol.* **7**, 281.
Karsner, H. T., Saphir, O., and Todd, T. W. (1925). *Amer. J. Pathol.* **1**, 351.
Laks, M. M., Morady, F., and Swan, H. J. C. (1969a). *Circ. Res.* **24**, 705.
Laks, M. M., Van De Velde, S., and Swan, H. (1969b). *Cardiovasc. Res.* **3**, 272.
Leak, L. V., and Burke, J. F. (1964). *Anat. Rec.* **149**, 623.
Linzbach, A. J. (1960). *Amer. J. Cardiol.* **5**, 370.
Meerson, F. Z., Zaletayeva, T. A., Lagutchev, S. S., and Pshennikova, M. G. (1964). *Exp. Cell. Res.* **3**, 568.
Meerson, F. Z. (1969). *Circ. Res.* **25**, Suppl. 2, 88.
Moore, D. H., and Ruska, H. (1957). *J. Biophys. Biochem. Cytol.* **3**, 261.
Munnell, J. F., and Getty, R. (1968). *Lab. Invest.* **19**, 303.
Orci, L., Forssmann, W. G., Matter, A., Pictet, R., and Rouiller, C. (1968). *Z. Zellforsch.* **84**, 24.

Pepe, F. A. (1966). *J. Cell Biol.* **28**, 555.
Price, Z., Eide, B., Printzmetal, M., and Carpenter, C. (1959). *Circ. Res.* **7**, 858.
Rewcastle, N. B., and Humphrey, J. G. (1965). *Arch. Neurol.* **12**, 570.
Richter, G. W., and Kellner, A. (1963). *J. Cell Biol.* **18**, 195.
Schulze, W. (1962). *Z. Mikrosk. anat. Forsch.* **68**, 271.
Shy, G. M., Engel, W. K., Somers, J. E., and Wanko, T. (1963). *Brain* **86**, 793.
Spann, J. R., Jr., Buccino, R. A., Sonnenblick, E. H., and Braunwald, E. (1967). *Circ. Res.* **21**, 341.
Stromer, M. H., Hartshorne, D. J., Mueller, H., and Rice, R. V. (1969). *J. Cell Biol.* **40**, 167.
Wittels, B., and Spann, J. F., Jr. (1968). *J. Clin. Invest.* **47**, 1787.
Wollenberger, A., and Schulze, W. (1961). *J. Biophys. Biochem. Cytol.* **10**, 285.

RECONSTRUCTION OF HEART TISSUE FROM SUSPENSIONS OF EMBRYONIC MYOCARDIAL CELLS: ULTRASTRUCTURAL STUDIES ON DISPERSED AND REAGGREGATED CELLS

D. A. Fischman and A. A. Moscona

Introduction

The finding that single heart cells obtained by trypsin dissociation of embryonic chick myocardium can grow and differentiate in monolayer culture (Cavanaugh, 1955; Cavanaugh and Cavanaugh, 1957), has stimulated much interest in the use of single-cell cultures of heart cells for biochemical, cytological, and physiological studies of cardiac myogenesis (Cedergren and Harary, 1964a, b; DeHaan, 1967; Harary and Farley, 1963; Holtzer *et al.*, 1959; Lieberman, 1967; McCarl *et al.*, 1965; Muscatello *et al.*, 1969; Rumery and Blandau, 1964). The main advantage of a monolayer culture is its apparent simplicity, in that the cytological characteristics of the single cells can be correlated with their electrophysiological properties, thus providing an approach to structure–function relationships which might otherwise be difficult to obtain. However, the apparent simplicity of a monolayer culture is also its major drawback; the disruption of the histological structure of the tissue necessarily destroys those characteristic intercellular relationships which endow the tissue with most of its distinct and interesting structural and functional properties. Furthermore, it is known that cells in monolayer cultures frequently become profoundly modified (Kuroda, 1964; Moscona, 1960, 1964). Thus, even though monolayer cultures are useful in various cell studies, they are not always adequate for examining the nature of cellular interrelationships and interactions in the formation, differentiation, and function of tissues. The procedures of aggregation *in vitro* of dissociated cells in suspension (Moscona, 1961; 1965; A. A. Moscona and Moscona, 1966) have been developed to overcome this difficulty in that they make it possible to study in detail the formation of histogenetic cell contacts, the assembly of cells into multicellular systems, and cell cooperation in forming organized and differentiating tissues.

In our laboratory, we recently adapted the techniques of cell aggregation by rotation to studies on embryonic heart cells (Fischman and Moscona, 1969). Suspension of embryonic heart cells obtained by trypsinization were made to reaggregate and reconstruct intercellular relationships and intracellular structures much more typical of the normal myocardium that can be obtained in the usual monolayer cultures. The contractile activity of the multicellular aggregate more closely resembled the compressive type of contraction in heart tissue than the linear or planar contraction evident in monolayers of single cells.

Methods

The preparation of heart-cell suspensions and their aggregation by rotation was according to previously described methods (Moscona, 1961, 1965; A. A. Moscona and Moscona, 1966). Cell suspensions from the 6-day-old embryonic chick or 14-day-old embryonic mouse ventricular myocardium were prepared by dissociation of the tissue with trypsin. The cells were dispersed in a culture medium which consisted of Eagle's basal medium with 20% fetal bovine serum (sterile unfiltered, Colorado Serum Co), 1% glutamine solution, and 1% penicillin–streptomycin mixture (Microbiol. Assoc.). Cultured in 25-ml Erlenmeyer flasks on a gyratory shaker at 70 rpm at 38°C were 3-ml aliquots of the cell suspensions (Moscona, 1961, 1965; A. A. Moscona and Moscona, 1966). At selected intervals after initiating the cultures, the aggregates were examined microscopically for evidences of contractility and photographed. Material for electron microscopy was fixed in 0.08 *M* phosphate buffered (pH 7.6) 2.5% gluteraldehyde, postfixed in 1% O_sO_4, *en-block* stained with 0.5% uranyl acetate and embedded in Araldite. Thin sections, for electron-microscopic examination, were sequentially stained on grids with uranyl acetate and with lead citrate.

Results

Light and electron micrographs of intact 6-day-old ventricular myocardium are presented in Figs. 1–4. The ultrastructural characteristics of this tissue have been previously described (Challice and Edwards, 1961; Hibbs, 1956; Oliva *et al.*, 1964; Spiro and Hagopian, 1967; Wollenberger, 1964), and will only be summarized here. The 6-day-old chick myocardial cells are generally spindle shaped, basophilic due to their high content of ribosomes, and

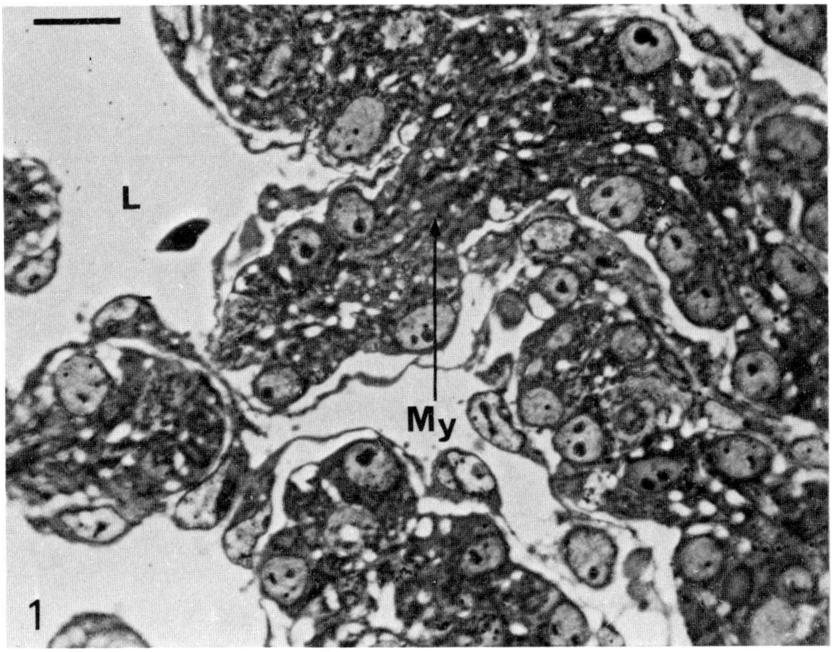

FIG. 1. Light micrograph of a 0.5 μm-thick section of 6-day embryonic chick heart Glutaraldehyde and osmium tetroxide fixation; Araldite section stained with alkaline toluidine blue. The myocardial cells (My) containing cross-striated myofibrils are present within trabeculae in rows or cords separated from the lumen (L) of the ventricle by a thin endothelial layer. A nucleated red blood cell is seen within the lumen. Note the prominent nucleoli within the myocardial cell nuclei. Magnification: ×1,100; calibration bar, 10 μm.

actively contractile. The single, large nucleus in each cell has one or two prominent nucleoli and a finely granular chromatin pattern considered to be characteristic of cells active in ribonucleic acid (RNA) synthesis. Myofibrils course in many directions within the cells, and many are incompletely developed. Free thick (160 Å) and thin (60 Å) filaments (Fig. 3), which are not part of myofibrils, are frequently observed in the cytoplasm. Areas in which two or three separate myofibrils converge on a common Z band (Z center) are seen in embryonic cardiac cells but are never observed in developing chick skeletal muscle cells (Fischman, 1967). Intercalated discs of varying sizes are observed at junctional sites between adjacent myocardial cells (Muir, 1957; Fig. 3). In embryonic chick myocardium, the intercalated discs are composed of both maculae adhaerentes (desmosomes) and zonulae or fasciae adhaerentes (Fawcett and McNutt, 1969). Myofibrils generally insert at the region of electron density associated with the cytoplasmic side of each fascia adhaerens (Fig. 3). No true tight or pentalaminar junctions (Brightman and Reese, 1969)

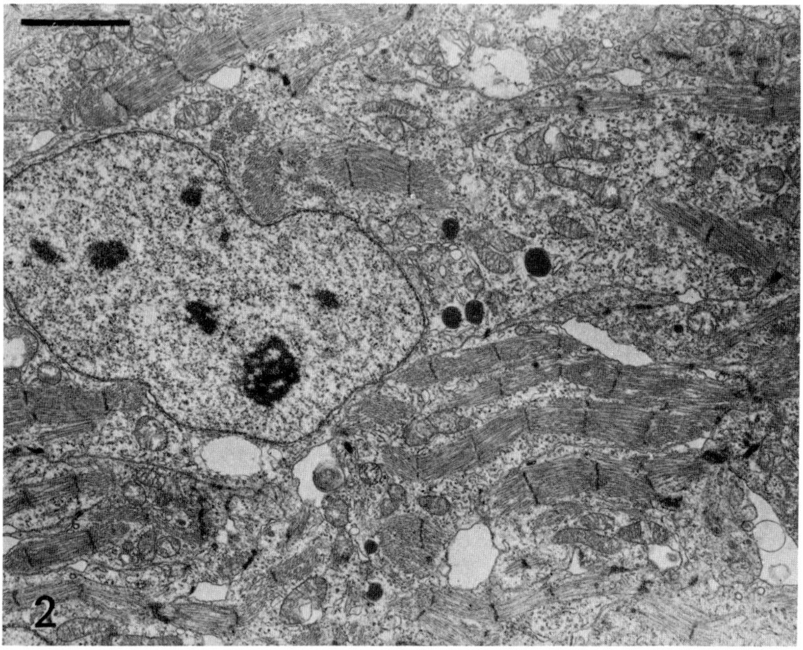

FIG. 2. Electron micrograph of the same material presented in Fig. 1. Numerous free ribosomes, myofibrils of varying size, abundant mitochondria, and a few lipid droplets are all characteristic cytoplasmic features of these embryonic myocardial cells. Nuclei contain one or two prominent nucleoli with a finely dispersed chromatin pattern. Magnification: ×6,000; calibration bar, 2.5 μm.

have been observed in the 6-day-chick material although our studies do not exclude the possibility of focal tight junctions (Hay, 1968) linking adjacent myocardial cells. In contrast to the chick material, numerous pentalaminar junctions were seen in the 13-day embryonic mouse heart, which is at a comparable stage of development. A comparative electron-microscopic study of vertebrate myocardia (Sommer and Johnson, 1699) has shown that adult chick ventricle apparently lacks or contains few pentalaminar junctions between its muscle cells. The interfibrillar regions of the cytoplasm contain large numbers of free ribosomes and ribosomal aggregates (polyribosomes), and although membrane-bound ribosomes are found in these cells, they are not very abundant. Large pools of material assumed to be glycogen are frequently observed in the cytoplasm; these regions appear as electron-translucent, finely granular pockets of cytoplasm which are poorly stained by the methods used in the present study.

With this background material in mind, let us proceed to some of the experimental results. We first analyzed the effects of the dissociation

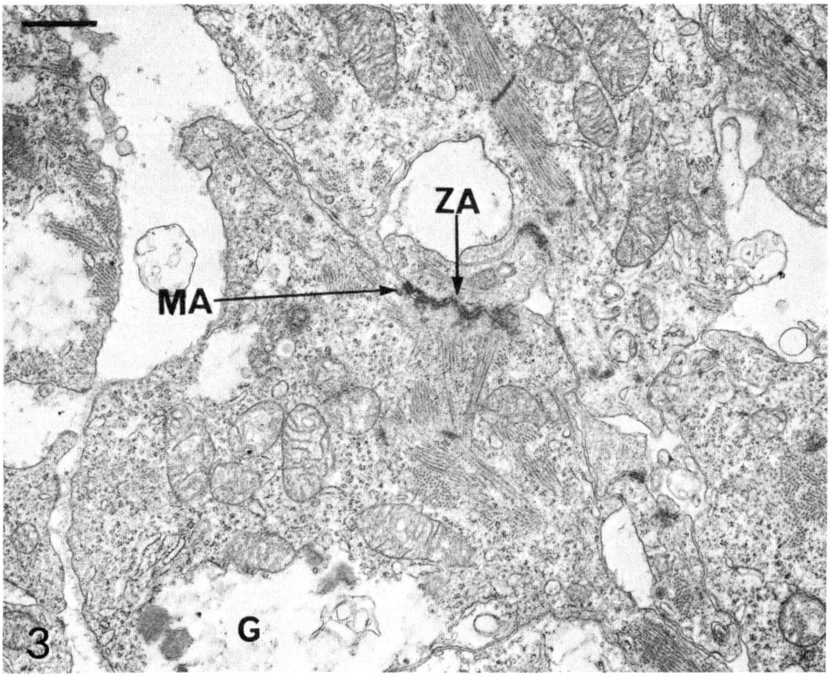

FIG. 3. The intercalated discs in the embryonic chick myocardium are composed of a well-structured desmosome or macula adhaerens (MA) and a more irregular zonula adhaerens (ZA) into which the myofibrils insert. The pale staining region of cytoplasm (G) is believed to be a pool of glycogen probably extracted during the *en block* staining with uranyl acetate. Magnification: ×10,500; calibration bar, 1 μm.

procedure on the structure of the embryonic myocardium. Since dissociation involves treating the tissue with trypsin in a calcium- and magnesium-free* modified Tyrode's solution (CMF), we first tested the effect of this CMF on the myocardial tissue. When small pieces of the 6- or 7-day embryonic chick heart were incubated for 30 min in CMF, we observed no outstanding changes in the ultrastructure of these cells (Fig. 5). Adherent junctions and myofibrillar structures appeared similar to the control tissue incubated for the same period in a fully constituted Tyrode's solution. However, when crystalline trypsin (0.5% final concentration) was added to CMF, there were striking effects on the intercellular junctions within the same 30-minute period (Figs. 6 and 7). Although the intracellular electron-dense material associated with each desmosome appeared well preserved, incubation in the

* Since there was no chelater of divalent cations in the CMF, it is likely that small amounts of Ca^{2+} and Mg^{2+} remained in this solution.

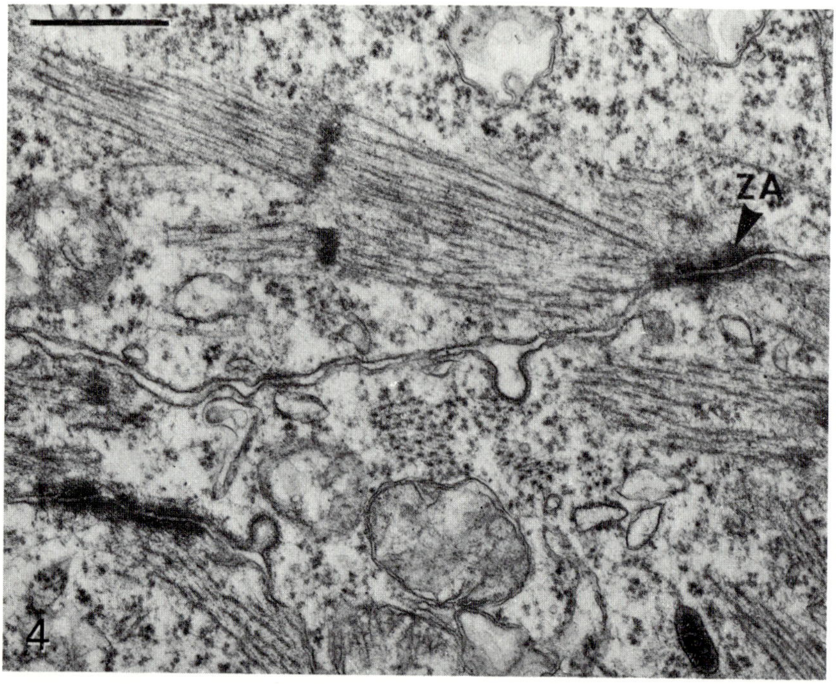

FIG. 4. Higher-magnification micrograph of a zonula adhaerens (ZA) demonstrating the attachment of myofibrils to the cell surface at this site. Note the rather uniform intercellular gap within the zonula adhaerens. Magnification: ×39,000; calibration bar, 0.5 μm.

trypsin-containing solution resulted in a separation and retraction of the hemi- or half-desmosomes, and most of them appeared to have been invaginated into cytoplasmic vesicles. In Figs. 6 and 7 several vesicles (~0.05–0.1 μ in diameter) are seen near the plasma membrane; most of them contain a flat, electron-dense plaque as part of their wall. Since these intravesicular plaques appear to be identical in appearance with the hemidesmosomes, and since numerous infoldings of the cell surface contain these plaques (Fig. 7), it is suggested that the hemidesmosomes produced by cleavage of a whole desmosome are an unstable configuration of the cell surface and are autophagocytosed by the cells which are in the process of separation due to the treatment with trypsin. A similar conclusion has been reached by Overton (1968) in her study of trypsinized epithelia.

These findings do not indicate that the desmosomes are the only means or sites by which these cells adhere to each other, nor do they indicate that trypsin disconnects only these junctions. They demonstrate that the functional integrity of myocardial desmosomes depends on peptide bonds susceptible to trypsin action, and that these and possibly similar bonds elsewhere at

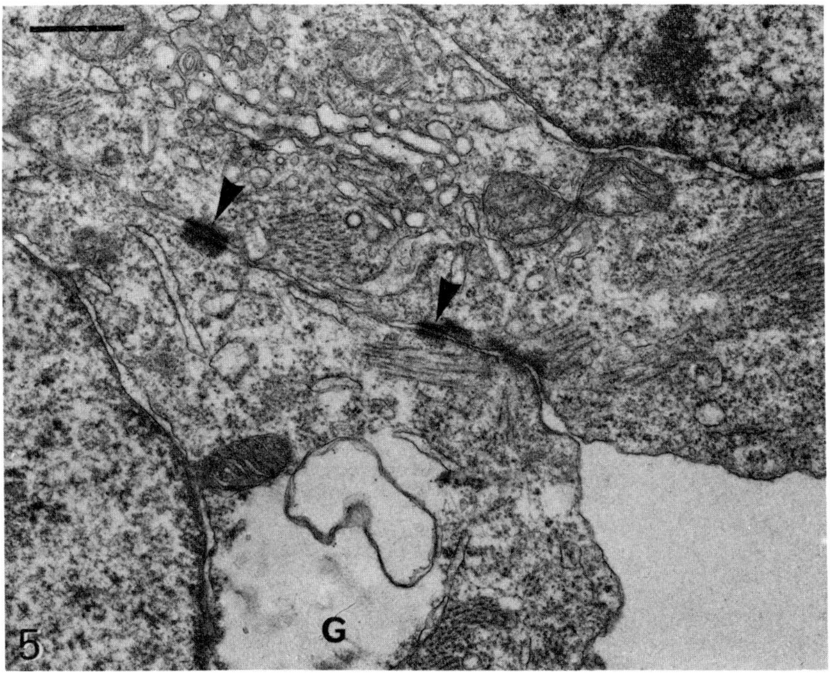

FIG. 5. Electron micrograph of embryonic chick myocardium which has been immersed for 30 min in a Ca^{2+}- and Mg^{2+}-free Tyrode's solution. Both maculae adhaerentes (arrows) and zonulae adhaerentes appear morphologically unaffected by this experimental procedure. Mitochondria and myofibrils also appear normal in structure. Magnification: ×26,000; calibration bar, 0.5 μm.

the cell surface are therefore essential for intercellular adhesion (Moscona, 1962a; M. H. Moscona and Moscona, 1966).

An interesting feature of the cells in these trypsin-treated tissue fragments is the excellent structural preservation of nuclei, mitochondria, lipid droplets, and most myofibrils. There seems to be an increase in the number of free, thick myofilaments in these cells; perhaps these are released from intact myofibrils, but we have not yet attempted to substantiate this impression. As seen in Fig. 7, the hexagonal array of the myofibril, when examined in cross section, appears unaltered.

To obtain single cells in suspension, such trypsin-treated tissue fragments are mechanically dispersed by passing them several times in and out of a fine Pasteur pipette (Moscona, 1961). With 6-day chick or 14-day mouse embryonic myocardium, one obtains thereby an almost single-cell suspension. Residual small cell clumps, which had remained undissociated, are removed by filtration of the suspension through two layers of sterile lens paper or a metal sieve.

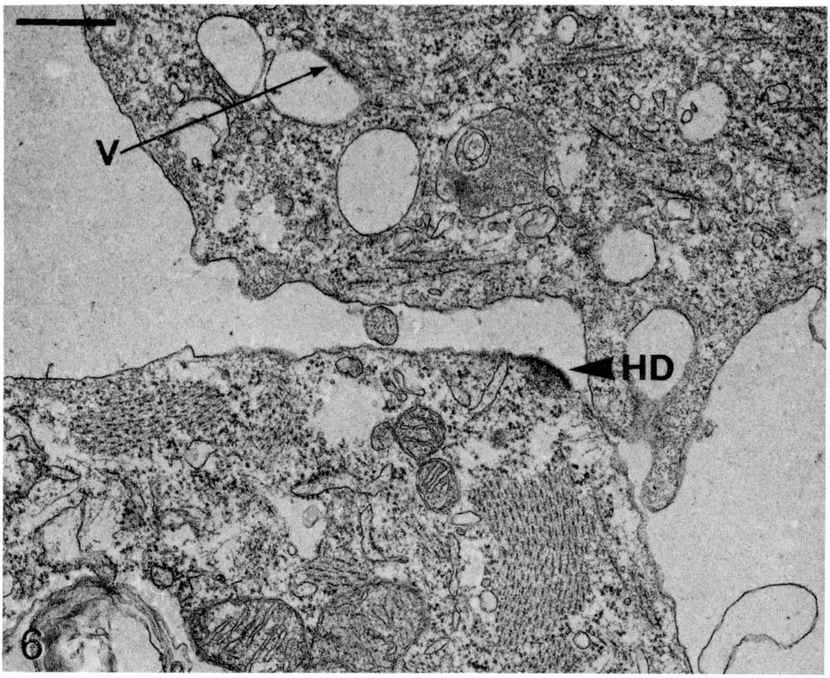

FIG. 6. Electron micrograph of embryonic chick myocardium incubated for 30 min in a divalent cation-free Tyrode's solution containing 0.5% trypsin. The distance between adjacent cells is substantially greater than in any of the preceding micrographs. Adherent junctions are separated with the frequent production of half- or hemidesmosomes (HD). Numerous cytoplasmic vesicles (V) are seen, many of which contain a linear dense plaque along one wall (arrow). Mitochondria appear well preserved. Magnification: ×27,000; calibration bar, 0.5 μm.

An example of single cells obtained by such treatment is shown in Fig. 8. Study of these dissociated cells in suspension reveals four principal features. (1) The shape of the nuclei is often distorted, but within minutes *in vitro* they regain sphericity. (2) The cells possess numerous pseudopodia some of which tend to break off. (3) Almost all the hemidesmosomes are found invaginated within vesicles, and the cell surface possess very few, if any, membrane densities or junctional specializations. (4) Myofibrillar structures are almost totally disrupted into tangled masses of freely dispersed myofilaments. Associated with this breakdown of the myofibrillar architecture is a loss of Z-band density and structure. A similar disruption of myofibrillar structure during trypsin induced dissociation of the myocardium has previously been observed by Wollenberger (1964). The mechanism for this intracellular release of myofilaments from the hexagonal array is unknown. Since the

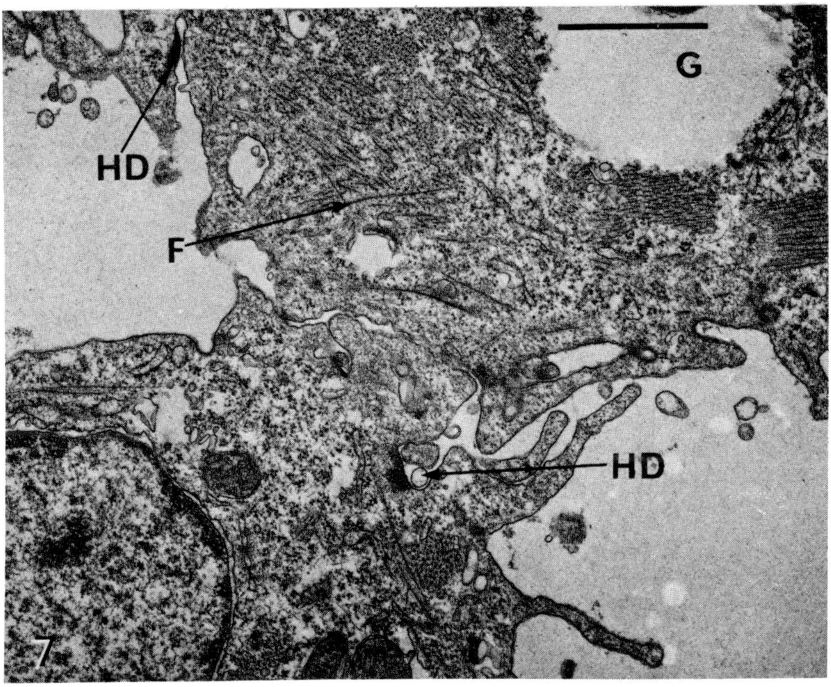

FIG. 7. Another example of trypsin-treated embryonic chick myocardium. The half-desmosomes (HD) are frequently observed within surface invaginations of these cells. Randomly oriented thick (160 Å) myofilaments (F) are often seen after incubation of the tissue in trypsin. A glycogen (G) region is present at the upper right of the micrograph. Magnification: ×20,000; calibration bar, 1 μm.

Z-band is known to be sensitive to trypsin hydrolysis (Stromer *et al.*, 1967), it would be of interest to determine the trypsin content of these cells during the period of fibrillar breakdown. It is conceivable that trypsin from the dissociation medium enters these cells and causes the disruption of myofibrillar architecture; the dissociation procedure may also result in the activation of intracellular proteases; it is also possible that changes at the cell surface due to trypsin action and the rounding of the disconnected cells leads to the breakdown of myofibrillar architecture. (For a discussion of the possible sites of trypsin action in cell dissociation see Moscona, 1962b.)

The appearance of the cell suspension examined in a hemocytometer is shown in Fig. 9. There is an almost complete absence of multicellular clumps, although some blood cells and cytoplasmic fragments are present. When such a cell suspension is placed in an Erlenmeyer flask and rotated at 70 rpm on a gyratory shaker at 38°C (see Methods), the cells aggregate and form multicellular clusters; these cell aggregates are visibly contractile within 2–3 hr

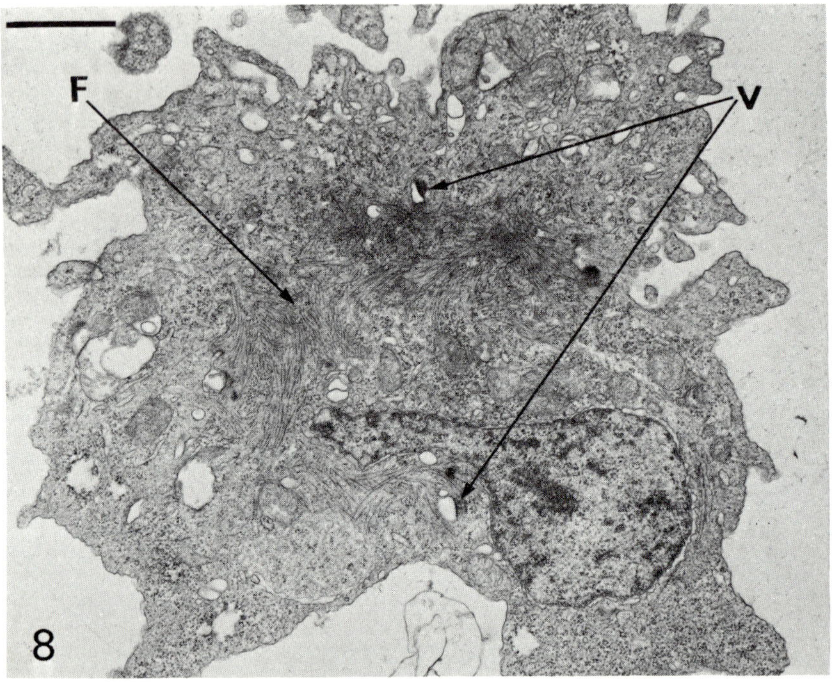

FIG. 8. A dissociated chick myocardial cell fixed in suspension after mechanical dispersion of tissue previously incubated for 30 min in 0.5% trypsin. Note the pear-shaped nucleus, numerous pseudopodia, and the almost total dissolution of the myofibrils into a randomly oriented pool of cytoplasmic filaments (F). Cytoplasmic vesicles (V) containing a dense plaque along one wall are observed in almost all dissociated cells. Presumably, these represent invaginated and subsequently phagocytosed hemidesmosomes. Note the absence of any junctional specializations at the cell surface. Magnification: ×15,000; calibration bar, 1 μm.

after the beginning of aggregation. During the first 2–3 hr the aggregates can be redispersed into single cells by pipetting, but after 24 hr they can be separated into cells only by enzymatic treatment. An example of myocardial aggregates obtained after 20 hr of cell culture by rotation is seen in Fig. 10. The surface of the aggregates is smooth and cells at the periphery of the aggregate are circumferentially oriented. Contractile activity is evidenced by a synchronous compression of the aggregate at an approximate rate of 1 beat every 2–3 sec. Sizes of the aggregates vary, but generally range from 75–200μ in diameter under the condition used in this study.

When aggregates of cardiac myoblasts were examined by electron micro-

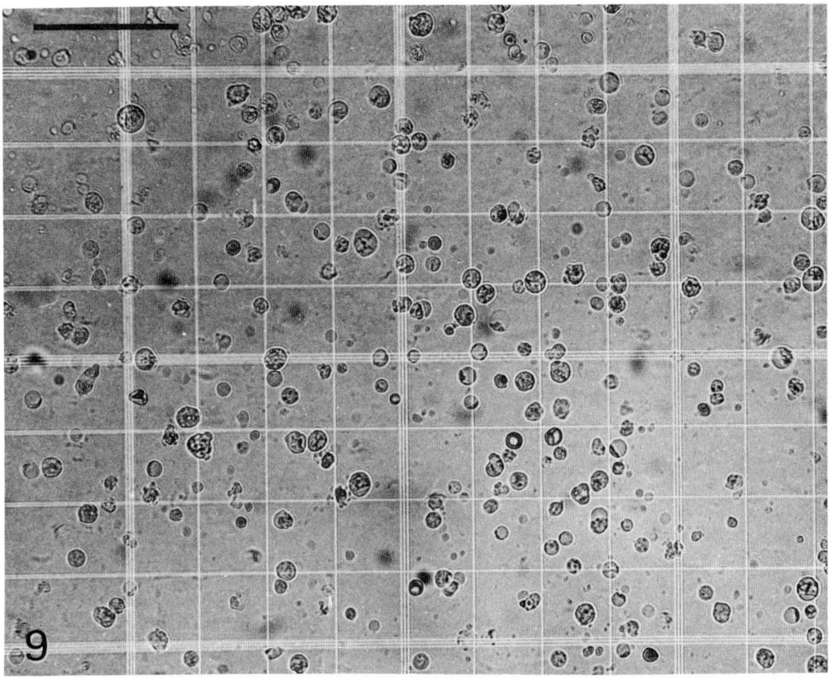

FIG. 9. A cell suspension of dissociated chick myocardium viewed in a hemocytometer. The preparation contains mainly single cells from the musculature, connective tissue, and blood. Some cell fragments are also visible. Magnification: ×190; calibration bar, 100 μm.

scopy, it was found that excellent morphogenesis can take place within the reaggregated structures. Figure 11 is a micrograph of reaggregated mouse heart cells after 72 hr *in vitro*. Zonulae adhaerentes have formed between adjacent cells, myofilaments have organized into typical cardiac myofibrils and numerous polyribosomes are apparent. In general, the cytological and histological appearance of these structures was found to reproduce quite faithfully the tissue of origin.

It is interesting that aggregates of chick heart cells resumed pulsatile activity within 2–3 hr *in vitro*. An electron micrograph of a 3-hr cell aggregate is presented in Fig. 12, where it is shown that, by this time, the cells had already reconstructed the double hexagonal lattice of thick and thin myofilaments which probably accounts for the resumption of contractile activity. The fact that these cells beat synchronously suggests that within 3 hr they had re-established electrical coupling.

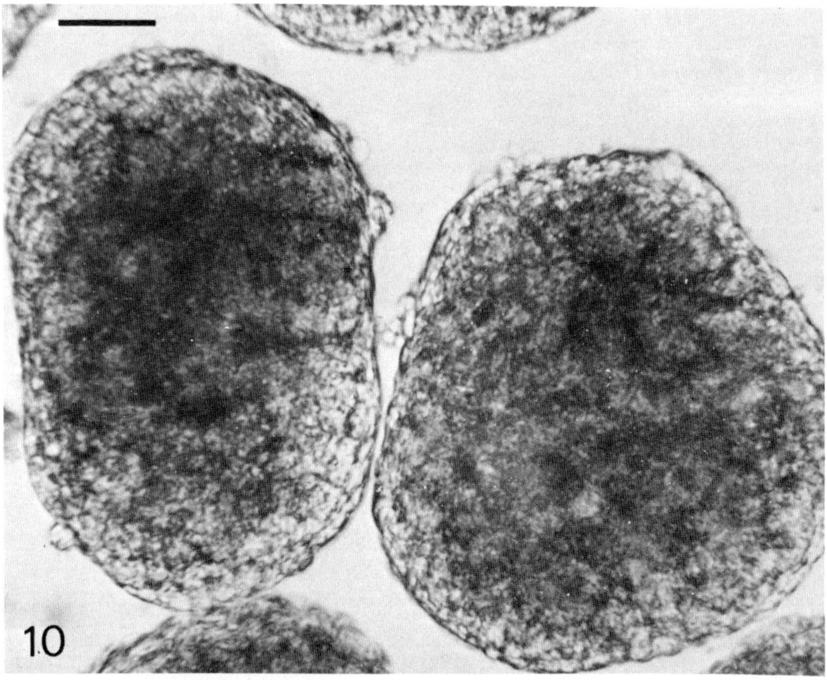
10

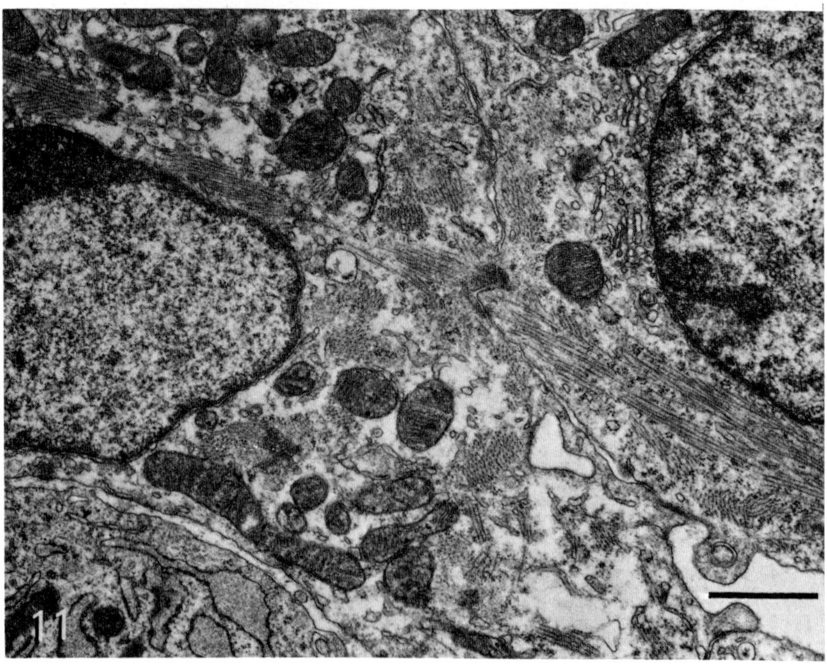
11

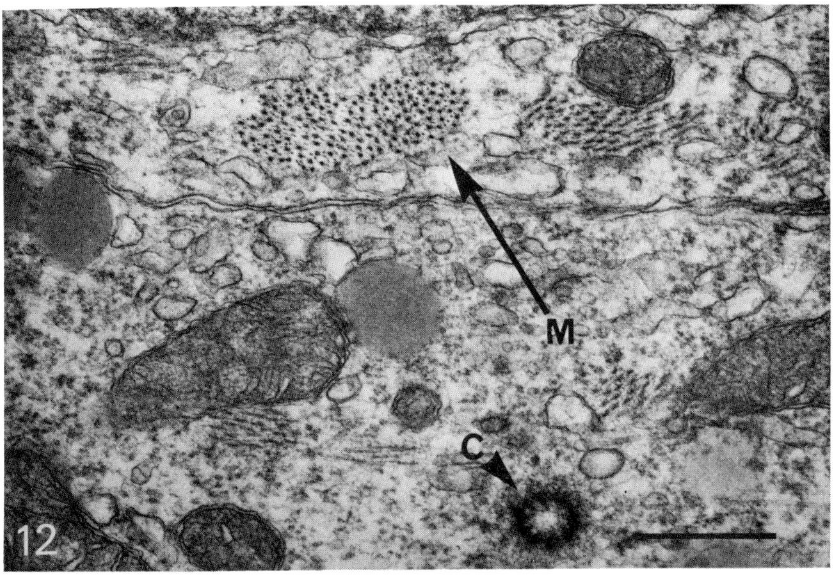

FIG. 12. A reaggregate of chick myocardial cells after 3 hr in rotation culture. The myofibrillar (M) lattice has been reformed from the dissociated filament population seen in Fig. 8. A centriole (C) is seen at the bottom. Magnification: ×39,000; calibration bar, 0.5 μm.

Summary and Conclusions

Aggregation by rotation of suspensions of freshly dissociated embryonic cells involves the assembly of single cells *in vitro* into tissue under controlled and standardized conditions; thus, it is possible to analyze the events and mechanisms involved in the construction of tissue from single cellular units and to study differentiation in terms of intracellular and intercellular processes (Moscona, 1961, 1965; A. A. Moscona and Moscona, 1966). The above-described experiments represent an initial step towards applying these procedures to studies on myocardial differentiation. They have shown that

FIG. 10. Chick myocardial cell aggregates after 20 hr in rotation culture. Cells at the periphery are oriented circumferentially; those in the center are more randomly arranged. Such aggregates exhibit a pulsatile contraction approximately once every 2–3 sec. Magnification: ×270; calibration bar, 50 μm.

FIG. 11. An electron micrograph of reaggregated mouse myocardial cells after 72 hr in rotation culture. Note the reestablishment of adherent junction into which myofibrils insert. The general ultrastructure of these cells is identical to those developing *in vivo*. A fibroblast is shown at the left. Magnification: ×15,000; calibration bar, 1 μm.

reaggregation of dissociated, embryonic heart cells results in the reconstruction of spherical masses of cardiac tissue which resume contractile activity. Under the conditions of aggregation by rotation employed here, most of the single cells become associated within 2–3 hr *in vitro* into loose, irregular clusters that can still be mechanically dispersed. During the next 12–24 hr, these loose multicellular clusters become increasingly coherent, compact, and regularly spherical, and the cells can be redispersed only by enzymatic treatment. Within the reconstructed cardiac tissue, the fine structure of the reaggregated cardiac cells appears remarkably similar to that typical of cells of the same embryonic age developing *in vivo*. In these cell aggregates, myofibrils and characteristic intercellular junctions (intercalated discs) become reconstructed in less than 24 hr *in vitro*; it therefore appears that aggregates of embryonic cells offer a promising system for detailed structural and biochemical studies on myofibrillar synthesis and assembly, cell association, the formation of specialized intercellular junctions, and the establishment of synchronous pulsatile activity.

Acknowledgments

The authors thank Miss Rita Yambot for excellent technical assistance during this study. This research was supported by research grants from the National Science Foundation (GB-7591; G-23852), Chicago and Illinois Heart Association (N-69-32), American Cancer Society (IN-41-1), and National Institute for Child Health and Human Development U.S.P.H.S. (HD-01253).

References

Brightman, M. W., and Reese, T. S. (1969). *J. Cell Biol.* **40**, 648.
Cavanaugh, M. W. (1955). *J. Exp. Zool.* **128**, 573.
Cavanaugh, M. W., and Cavanaugh, D. J. (1957). *Arch. Int. Pharmacodyn.* **110**, 43.
Cedergren, B., and Harary, I. (1964a). *J. Ultrastruct. Res.* **11**, 428.
Cedergren, B., and Harary, I. (1964b). *J. Ultrastruct. Res.* **11**, 443.
Challice, C. E., and Edwards, G. A. (1961). *In* "The Specialized Tissues of the Heart" (A. Paes de Caravallo, W. C. de Mello, B. I. Hoffman, eds.). Elsevier, Amsterdam.
DeHaan, R. L. (1967). *Develop. Biol.* **16**, 216.
Fawcett, D. W., and McNutt, M. S. (1969). *J. Cell Biol.* **42**, 1.
Fischman, D. A. (1967). *J. Cell Biol.* **32**, 557.
Fischman, D. A., and Moscona, A. A. (1969). *J. Cell Biol.* **43**, 37a.
Harary, I., and Farley, B. (1963). *Exp. Cell Res.* **29**, 451.
Hay, E. C. (1968). *In* "Epithelial-Mesenchyme Interactions" (R. W. Fleischmajer, ed.). Williams and Wilkins, Baltimore, Maryland.
Hibbs, R. G. (1956). *Amer. J. Anat.* **99**, 17.
Holtzer, H., Abbott, J., and Cavanaugh, M. W. (1959). *Exp. Cell Res.* **16**, 595.
Kuroda, Y. (1964). *Exp. Cell Res.* **35**, 337.
Lieberman, M. (1967). *Circ. Res.* **21**, 879.

McCarl, R. R., Szuhaj, B. F., and Houlihan, R. T. (1965). Science **150**, 1611.

Moscona, A. A. (1960). *In* "Developing Cell Systems and Their Control" (D. Rudnick, ed.), pp. 45–70. Ronald Press, New York.

Moscona, A. (1961). *Exp. Cell Res.* **22**, 455.

Moscona, A. A. (1962a). *J. Cell Comp. Physiol.* **60**, 65.

Moscona, A. A. (1962b). *Int. Rev. Exp. Pathol.* **1**, 371.

Moscona, A. A. (1964). *In* "The Epidermis" (W. Montagna, ed.), pp. 83–96. Academic Press, New York.

Moscona, A. A. (1965). *In* "Cells and Tissues in Culture" (E. N. Willmer, ed.), pp. 489–529. Academic Press, New York.

Moscona, A. A., and Moscona, M. H. (1966). *Exp. Cell Res.* **41**, 697.

Moscona, M. H., and Moscona, A. A. (1966). *Exp. Cell Res.* **41**, 706.

Muir, A. R. (1957). *J. Biophys. Biochem. Cytol.* **3**, 193.

Muscatello, V., Pasquali-Ronchetti, I., and Barasa, A. (1968). *J. Ultrastruct. Res.* **23**, 44.

Oliva, O. M., Laschi, M. R., and Lucchi, M. L. (1964). *Sperimentale* **114**, 69.

Overton, J. (1968). *J. Exp. Zool.* **168**, 203.

Rumery, R. E., and Blandau, R. J. (1964). *Acta Anat.* **58**, 116.

Sommer, J. R., and Johnson, E. A. (1969). *Z. Zellforsch. Mikrosk. Anat.* **98**, 437.

Spiro, D., and Hagopian, M. (1967). *In* "Formation and Fate of Cell Organelles" (K. B Warren, ed.), pp. 71–98. Academic Press, New York.

Stromer, M. H., Goll, D. E., and Roth, L. E. (1967). *J. Cell Biol.* **34**, 431.

Wainrach, S., and Sotello, J. R. (1961). *Z. Zellforsch. Mikrosk. Anat.* **55**, 622.

Wollenberger, A. (1964). *Circ. Res.* **15**, Suppl. 2, 184.

CONNECTIVE TISSUE OF THE HYPERTROPHIED HEART

James F. Spann, Jr., Edmund H. Sonnenblick, Edward D. Harris, Jr., and Robert A. Buccino

Introduction

The synthesis of contractile protein increases rapidly in the ventricle subjected to an excessive work load. The extent to which collagen, representing the connective tissue stroma of the heart, participates in this increased protein synthesis has not been defined. Data from postmortem studies in hypertrophy of the human heart are conflicting; Blumgart *et al.* (1940) found the collagen concentration to be increased in 9 of 24 hypertrophied human hearts while Monfort and Perez-Tamayo (1962) found no change in the ratio of collagen to muscle protein in the hypertrophied human left ventricle, and Oken and Boucek (1957) showed no increase in left ventricular collagen content in 20 of 22 human hearts with significant hypertrophy. In the present study (Buccino *et al.*, 1969), the changes in connective tissue which accompany ventricular hypertrophy were determined in a controlled experimental animal model of ventricular hypertrophy (Spann *et al.*, 1967a).

The imino acid, hydroxyproline, is found exclusively in collagen and forms a constant percentage of collagen (Neuman and Logan, 1950). Therefore, the concentration of collagen and thus the connective tissue component of the myocardium can be measured by determination of hydroxyproline. Myocardial specimens were obtained from the hearts of 17 normal adult cats and 26 adult cats with right ventricular hypertrophy produced by chronic constriction of the main pulmonary artery (Spann *et al.*, 1967b). Constriction of the main pulmonary artery so that the remaining lumen was approximately 20% of normal was achieved 3–90 days prior to removal of the heart for determination of hydroxyproline; the majority of animals were studied 20–50 days after constriction. All animals in which there was evidence of overt congestive heart failure, such as pleural effusion, ascites, a reduction in cardiac index, or marked elevation in right ventricular end-diastolic pressure or arteriovenous oxygen difference were excluded from the study. Hydroxyproline was determined by a modification of the method of Prockop and Udenfriend (1957) and was expressed in μg/mg of dry weight. The nitrogen concentration of dried tissue was measured by the semimicro-Keldjahl technique and was found to closely parallel dry weight, indicating that there was no measurable change in the concentration of the nonprotein components of the heart during hypertrophy.

Extent of Ventricular Hypertrophy

The atria were removed by dissecting along the atrioventricular groove, and the right ventricular wall was separated from the septum and left ventricle. The right ventricular weight was that of the free wall of the right ventricle, whereas the septum and left ventricle were considered left ventricle for purposes of weighing. However, for determination of hydroxyproline the free wall of each ventricle, excluding the septum, was used.

In 17 normal cats, the right ventricular weight expressed as wet weight in gm/kg body weight averaged 0.55 ± 0.02 (SEM), whereas in the 26 cats with pulmonary artery constriction this value averaged 1.14 ± 0.05 gm/kg body weight ($p < 0.01$). Left ventricular weight was unchanged in the group with right ventricular hypertrophy, averaging 2.13 ± 0.09 gm/kg body weight compared with a value of 2.21 ± 0.06 gm/kg body weight in the 17 normal cats. Samples of each ventricle were weighed as wet tissue, dried to a constant weight for 24 hr at 100°C in a vacuum, and reweighed; there were no changes in the water content of the hearts with hypertrophy. Thus, the increase in right ventricular weight represented a true increase in myocardial tissue and was not caused by an accumulation of interstitial or intracellular fluid. Furthermore, the nitrogen concentration of dried tissue was found to closely parallel dry weight, indicating that there was no measurable change in the concentration of the nonprotein components of the heart during hypertrophy.

Hydroxyproline Concentration of the Normal and Hypertrophied Ventricles

The free wall of both the right and left ventricle, excluding the septum, was divided at a midplane into endocardial–myocardial and epicardial–myocardial specimens for assay of hydroxyproline. In the normal heart, hydroxyproline concentration was found to be significantly higher in epimyocardial than in endomyocardial specimens in both ventricles (Fig. 1). Furthermore, in both the epimyocardium and endomyocardium of the normal

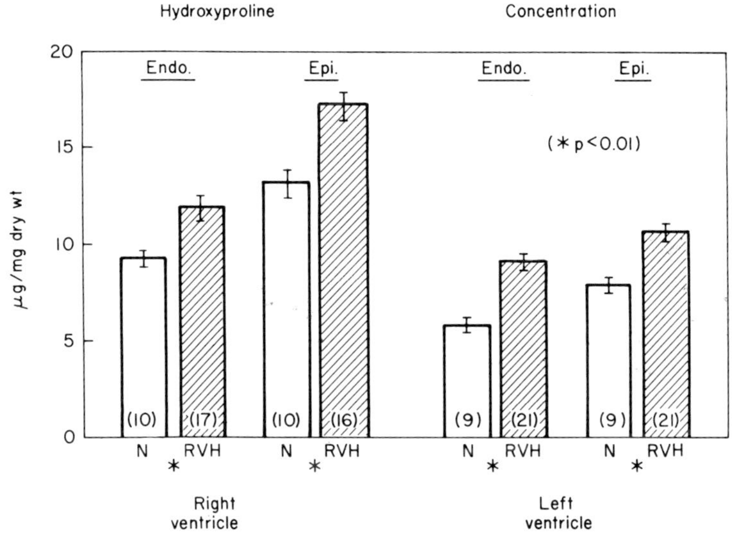

FIG. 1. Hydroxyproline concentrations in endomyocardial and epimyocardial specimens from normal right and left ventricles and from the right and left ventricles of cats with right ventricular hypertrophy resulting from pulmonary artery constriction. Hydroxyproline concentration is expressed as μg dry weight. The columns represent the mean value for each group and the bar represents ±1 SE. The number of the animals in each group is given in parentheses. All differences are statistically significant ($p < 0.01$).

heart, hydroxyproline was significantly higher in the right ventricle than in the corresponding left ventricle.

In the hearts with right ventricular hypertrophy, hydroxyproline concentration in epimyocardial and endomyocardial specimens of both the right and left ventricles were significantly higher than in the corresponding specimens from normal hearts (Fig. 1). The dry weight concentration of hydroxyproline was increased by 39% in the right ventricular endomyocardium and by 31% in the right ventricular epimyocardium of the animals with hypertrophy. Interestingly, in the unstressed and nonhypertrophied left ventricle the concentration of hydroxyproline was increased; the dry weight concentration of hydroxyproline was 57% greater than normal in the left ventricular endomyocardium of animals with right ventricular hypertrophy and 34% greater than normal in the left ventricular epimyocardium.

Since mammalian collagen consists of a constant 13.4% hydroxyproline by weight (Neuman and Logan, 1950), collagen concentration was calculated by multiplying hydroxyproline concentration by 7.46. Thus, in terms of wet tissue weight, the normal right ventricular collagen concentration averaged 2.4%, whereas in the hypertrophied right ventricle, this value was 3.3% of the wet weight. In the left ventricle the connective tissue or collagen increased from 1.4% of the wet weight in the normal animal to 2.0% in the animals with ventricular hypertrophy.

Conclusions

It is concluded that connective tissue does participate in the process of myocardial hypertrophy, and in fact, increases proportionately more than the muscle proteins do themselves. An explanation for an increase in connective tissue which is out of proportion to the increase in contractile proteins in ventricular hypertrophy is not available. However, it is possible to conclude on the basis of the distribution of collagen in the hypertrophied ventricle from a greater concentration in the epimyocardium to a lower concentration in the endomyocardium, that the increase in connective tissue is probably not due to limitations in coronary blood flow, hypoxia or simple mechanical stress. By the law of Laplace, wall stress would be least in the endomyocardium where the radius of curvature is least; this is the reverse of the collagen concentration distribution. Also, limitations in coronary blood flow and hypoxia would be expected to be more marked in the endocardial surface of the heart (Kirk and Honig, 1964); it is therefore unlikely that this collagen increase which is greatest in the epimyocardial portion of the hypertrophied heart is due to limitations in coronary blood flow or hypoxia.

Since collagen is known to be distributed primarily between muscle fibers and along blood vessels, the present findings could reflect the normal distribution of the coronary vasculature; coronary vessels arise from the epicardial surface and diminish in number as they penetrate to the endocardial surface (Bloom and Fawcett, 1962; Wearns, 1928). If collagen follows a similar distribution, the decrease in collagen from the epicardium toward the endocardium would be explained. Since there is histological evidence (Meerson *et al.*, 1963) that collagen fibers around blood vessels in the heart appear to increase in response to a systolic overload, this explanation seems tenable.

It is of interest to consider the possible relationship of the increased collagen concentration to the previously demonstrated reduction in the mechanical performance of the hypertrophied and failing ventricle (Spann *et al.*, 1967a, c; Mason *et al.*, this volume). The contractile force per unit cross-sectional area of hypertrophied and failing heart muscle is reduced 50–75% below normal values, whereas the increased collagen concentration still represents only 3.3% of the total mass of the ventricle compared to a normal value of 2.4%. Thus, it is concluded that the reduced contractile performance of right ventricular cardiac muscle in cats with right ventricular hypertrophy and heart failure due to pulmonary artery constriction cannot be attributed to any significant degree to replacement of contractile elements by connective tissue components.

Perhaps the most interesting finding in the current study is the striking increase in collagen concentration in the nonstressed free wall of the non-hypertrophied left ventricle. It should be pointed out that these animals were studied under controlled experimental conditions—there were no changes in body weight, there was no evidence of overt circulatory failure, the cardiac output was not depressed, there was no increase in oxygen extraction by the peripheral tissues, and there was no congestion of pulmonary or peripheral tissues. Thus, overt heart failure was not present to be a possible cause of stress to the left ventricle and a potential cause of the increase in collagen concentration. A similar alteration in a constituent of the nonstressed, non-hypertrophied left ventricle of animals with right ventricular hypertrophy due to pulmonary artery constriction is the severe depression of left ventricular myocardial norepinephrine concentration observed in pure right ventricular hypertrophy without heart failure (Spann *et al.*, 1967a). Further, a slight reduction in myofibrillar adenosine triphosphatase activity has been observed in the left ventricle of animals with pure right heart failure (Chandler *et al.*, 1967). Explanations for these intriguing contralateral changes in the nonstressed ventricle are completely lacking at present.

References

Bloom, W., and Fawcett, D. W. (1962). "A Textbook of Histology," 8th Ed. p. 720. Saunders, Philadelphia, Pennsylvania.

Blumgart, H., Gilligan, D., and Schlesinger, M. (1940). *Trans. Ass. Amer. Physicians* **55**, 313.

Buccino, R. A., Harris, E., Spann, J. F., Jr., and Sonnenblick, E. H. (1969). *Amer. J. Physiol.* **216**, 425.

Chandler, B. M., Sonnenblick, E. H., Spann, J. F., Jr., and Pool, P. E. (1967). *Circ. Res.* **21**, 717.

Kirk, E. S., and Honig, C. R., (1964). *Amer. J. Physiol.* **207**, 661.

Meerson, F. Z., Beloshapkina, T. D., Lishnikov, E. F., Leikina, E. M., Markovskaya, G. N., and Cheonyshova, G. V. (1963). *Vestn. Akad. Med. Nauk SSSR.* **18**, 667.

Montfort, I., and Perez-Tamayo, R. (1962). *Lab. Invest.* **10**, 1240.

Neuman, R. E., and Logan, M. S. (1950). *J. Biol. Chem.* **184**, 299.

Oken, D. E., and Boucek, R. J. (1957). *Circ. Res.* **5**, 357.

Prockop, D. J., and Undenfriend, S. (1957). *Anal. Biochem.* **1**, 228.

Spann, J. F., Jr., Buccino, R. A., Sonnenblick, E. H., and Braunwald, E. (1967a). *Circ. Res.* **21**, 341.

Spann, J. F., Jr., Buccino, R. A., and Sonnenblick, E. H. (1967b). *Proc. Soc. Exp. Biol. Med.* **125**, 1967.

Spann, J. F., Jr., Covell, J. W., Eckberg, D. L., Sonnenblick, E. H. Ross, J., Jr., and Braunwald, E. (1967c). *Circulation* **36**, Suppl. 2, 241.

Wearns, J. T. (1928). *J. Exp. Med.* **47**, 273.

EFFECTS OF ACUTE HYPERTROPHY ON THE CONTRACTILE PROPERTIES OF SKELETAL MUSCLE

Michael Lesch

Although hypertrophy is a characteristic response of both skeletal and cardiac muscle to an increased work load, relatively little is known about this process in skeletal muscle in contrast to the rather extensive literature that exists on the biochemical and physiological correlates of work-induced cardiac hypertrophy. Studies concerned with the definition of these correlates in skeletal muscle hypertrophy have recently appeared in the literature (Goldberg 1968, 1969; Hamosh *et al.*, 1967) and a major reason for this new-found interest in skeletal muscle hypertrophy appears to be the recent introduction of an adequate experimental model of the process.

It has long been recognized that tenotomy of all the tendons except one in a synergistic muscle group will result in compensatory hypertrophy of the remaining intact muscle. Jewell and Zaimis (1954) produced hypertrophy in the cat soleus by tenotomy of the synergistic plantaris and gastrocnemius muscles and reported on changes in the neuromuscular junction of the hypertrophied muscle. Recently, Goldberg (1968) demonstrated the feasibility of this operative procedure in the rat, and the adaptation of this procedure to a small laboratory animal has made feasible various studies of hypertrophied skeletal muscle which were hitherto impossible. In 1968, we (Lesch *et al.*) utilized this model to study the contractile properties of the hypertrophied rat soleus muscle. The purpose of this chapter is to briefly review these studies.

Methods

Male rats weighing 30–50 gm were anesthetized with intraperitoneal chloral hydrate. The plantaris and gastrocnemius tendons were dissected free through a small skin incision and either severed or left intact as sham-operated controls, depending upon the particular experimental protocol.

To determine the time course of the hypertrophy process, a group of 38 animals was utilized. In these animals, the gastrocnemius and plantaris tendons of the left and right leg were dissected free. These tendons were severed in the left leg but not in the right leg so that the right leg acted as an internal, sham-operated control. Groups of nine or ten animals were sacrificed at 1, 2, 4, and 6 days postoperative, the solei removed, and wet and dry weights determined.

Only one soleus per animal could be used for mechanical studies due to limitations as regards the time required for adequate dissection and mounting of the muscle in the myograph. In order to circumvent this problem, the following protocol was devised. In one group of animals, the gastrocnemius and plantaris tendons of the left leg were dissected free and severed (hypertrophied group), while in a second group a sham-operative procedure was performed on the left leg (sham-operated group) and a third group of unoperated animals acted as normal controls. In these three groups of animals, the right leg was not surgically manipulated. At 1, 2, 4, and 6 days postoperative, six or more animals from each group were sacrificed and the mechanical properties of the left soleus muscle were studied in the myograph. At the time of sacrifice, the wet weight of the unoperated right leg was determined and at the end of any myograph study the wet weight of the muscle studied was determined. In this manner, the percent hypertrophy, on a wet weight basis, of any muscle studied mechanically was measured relative to its contralateral normal control. Control studies demonstrated that the muscles studied in the myograph did not accumulate significant amounts of water from the bath. The myograph, force transducers, isotonic lever system, stimulator, and methods of recording and calculation have been adequately described elsewhere (Lesch *et al.*, 1968). Tetanic stimuli (5-msec duration and 100/sec with a voltage 20% above threshold) were delivered for 1 sec at intervals of 1 min. Single stimuli of the same duration and voltage were used in studies of twitch tension.

Results

Development of Hypertrophy

Figure 1 depicts the percent hypertrophy of the soleus muscle from the tenotomized limb on a dry and wet weight basis relative to that of the soleus from the sham-operated contralateral limb. At day 1 postoperative, a $29.7 \pm 1.7\%$ increase in wet weight and a $12.6 \pm 1.7\%$ increase in dry weight was found in the hypertrophied muscles. Maximum hypertrophy was found at 4 days with a $48 \pm 6.0\%$ increase in wet weight and a $27.0 \pm 5.0\%$ increase in dry weight. A small but significant decrease in percent dry weight was

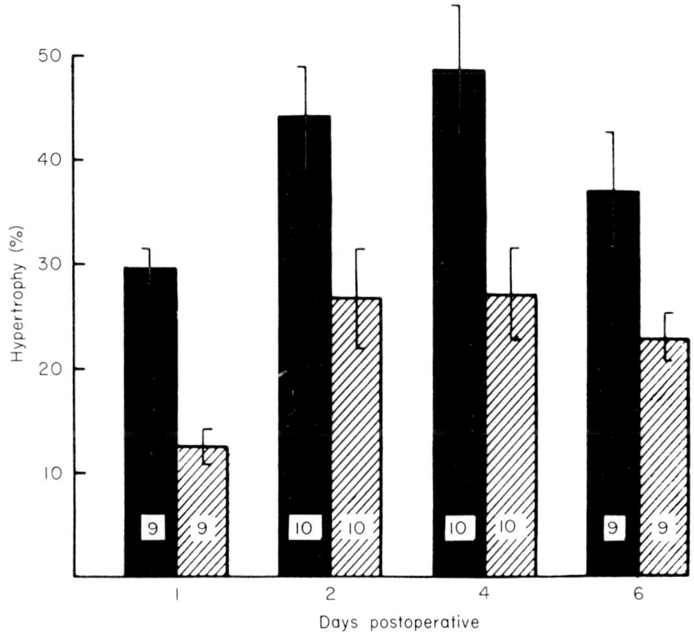

FIG. 1. Average percent increase in wet and dry weights of a separate group of hypertrophied muscles compared to their contralateral sham-operated controls. N denotes the number of muscles in each group with results expressed as the mean ±SEM. None of these muscles were studied in the myograph. Filled bars represent wet weight; hatched, dry weight. Reprinted from Lesch *et al.* (1968).

found in the hypertrophied groups as compared to the sham-operated groups, the former averaging 20.2 ± 0.2%, the latter 23.0 ± 0.2% ($P < 0.01$). The average percent dry weight of soleii from unoperated normal rats in this laboratory is 23.9 ± 0.1%, a value slightly but significantly larger than that of the sham-operated animals of the present study, attesting to the minor amount of operative edema.

CONTRACTILITY STUDIES

Tetanic Tension

Maximum tetanic tension (P_o), and the maximum rate of tetanic tension development corrected for cross-sectional area for the hypertrophied muscles were significantly reduced at 1, 2, 4, and 6 days postoperative as compared to the sham-operated controls (Fig. 2). Since some depression of function was noted in the sham-operated group relative to the unoperated controls,

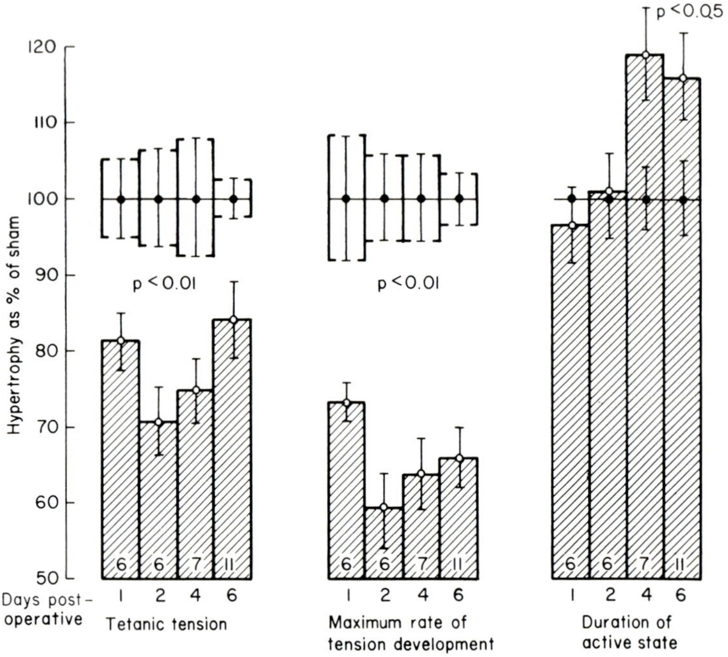

FIG. 2. Tetanic tension (gm/mm²), maximum rate of tension development normalized for cross-sectional area (gm/sec/mm²) and duration of maximum active state (msec) of the hypertrophied muscle groups expressed as a percent of the corresponding sham-operated groups. The mean ±SEM and number of muscles in each group are indicated. Dot-filled bars represent sham-operated; hatched, hypertrophy; temp., 20°C. (Reprinted from Lesch *et al.*, 1968.)

data from the hypertrophied muscle groups are compared only to the sham-operated controls to negate any effects of the operative procedure. Similarly, at 6 days postoperative, maximum twitch tension per millimeter cross-sectional area and the maximum rate of twitch tension development were significantly reduced in the hypertrophied group as compared to the sham operated controls (Fig. 3). Despite the decrease in twitch tension the ratio P/P_0 was not significantly different in the hypertrophied and sham-operated groups.

Since only one soleus from any given animal could be mechanically studied, it was impossible to directly compare total tetanic tension output between a hypertrophied or sham-operated muscle to that of the contralateral normal control muscle. In order to circumvent this problem, an index of the total tetanic tension generated by the three muscle groups was calculated by normalizing the total tetanic force developed by the muscle under study for the cross-sectional area of the contralateral normal, unoperated soleus. Assuming similarity of the right and left soleus in a given animal prior to the

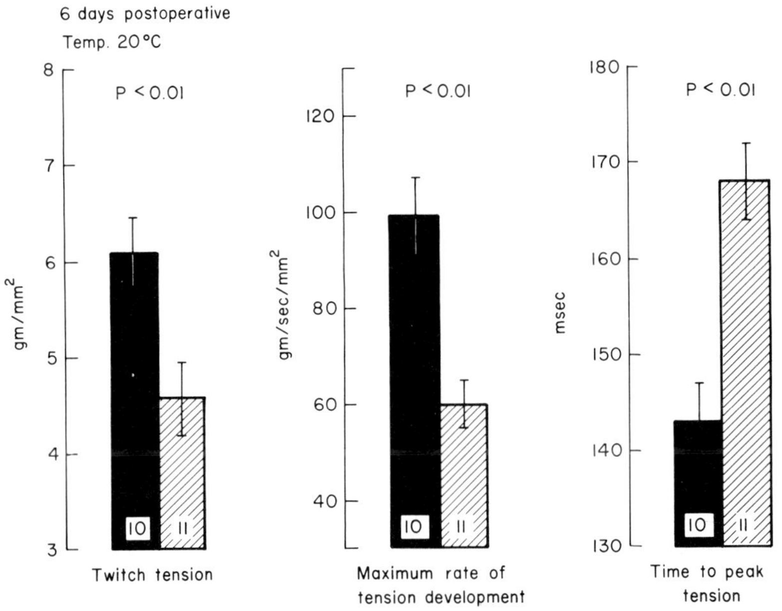

FIG. 3. Twitch tension, maximum rate of twitch tension development, and time to peak tension of the hypertrophied and sham-operated muscles 6 days postoperatively. The number of muscles in each group is shown with results expressed as the mean ±SEM. Filled bars represent sham-operated; hatched, hypertrophy. (Reprinted from Lesch *et al.*, 1968.)

operative procedure, this index provides a better measurement than total tension alone, since it is unaffected by variation in animal size. Thus, any difference of this index between hypertrophied and control groups reflects the direct effect of hypertrophy on total tension development. According to this index, the total tension generated by the hypertrophied muscles remained stable through the fourth postoperative day, but increased significantly ($P < 0.05$) on the sixth postoperative day (Fig. 4).

Duration and Decay of Active State

There was no alteration in the duration of the maximum intensity of active state in the hypertrophied muscles at 1 and 2 days postoperative, whereas a significant prolongation of the maximum intensity of active state was noted on the fourth and sixth postoperative day (Fig. 2). In contrast, the exponential decline in tetanic tension during the relaxation phase of contraction was the same for all muscle groups at all times. Concomitant with the prolongation of the duration of active state in the tetanic contractions, the time from stimulation to peak isometric twitch tension was prolonged at 6 days postoperative from 143 ± 5 to 168 ± 4 msec ($P < 0.01$) (Fig. 3).

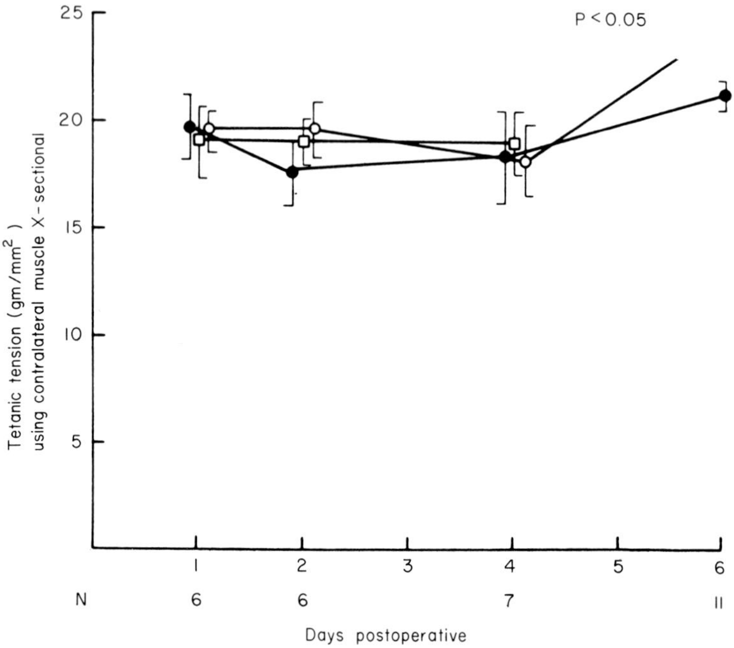

FIG. 4. As an index of total tension development, the force developed by each muscle was corrected by dividing by the cross-sectional area of the normal contralateral soleus. See text for explanation. Open squares represent normal; filled circles, sham-operated; open circles, hypertrophy; temp., 20°C. The number of muscles in each group is shown with results expressed as the mean ±SEM. (Reprinted from Lesch *et al.*, 1968.)

Force–Velocity Relations

Force velocity curves were determined for the hypertrophied and sham-operated solei at 6 days postoperative (Fig. 5). At any given load, the velocity of shortening for the hypertrophied muscles was significantly reduced. V_{max}, calculated from a linear form of the Hill equation (Sonnenblick) was reduced from 1.82 ± 0.03 in the sham-operated group to 1.69 ± 0.02 muscle lengths/sec in the hypertrophied group ($P < 0.05$). Similarly, P_o was reduced from 20.0 ± 0.4 in the sham-operated group to 16.9 ± 0.9 g/mm^2 ($P < 0.01$) in the hypertrophy group.

Effect of Cross-Sectional Area on Tension Development

In vitro studies of muscle function in nonperfused preparations are valid only if the diffusion of oxygen is sufficient to maintain normal oxygen supply into the muscle core. Since the reduction in function in the hypertrophied muscles was always associated with an increased cross-sectional area, it was possible that part, if not all, of the decreased function noted in

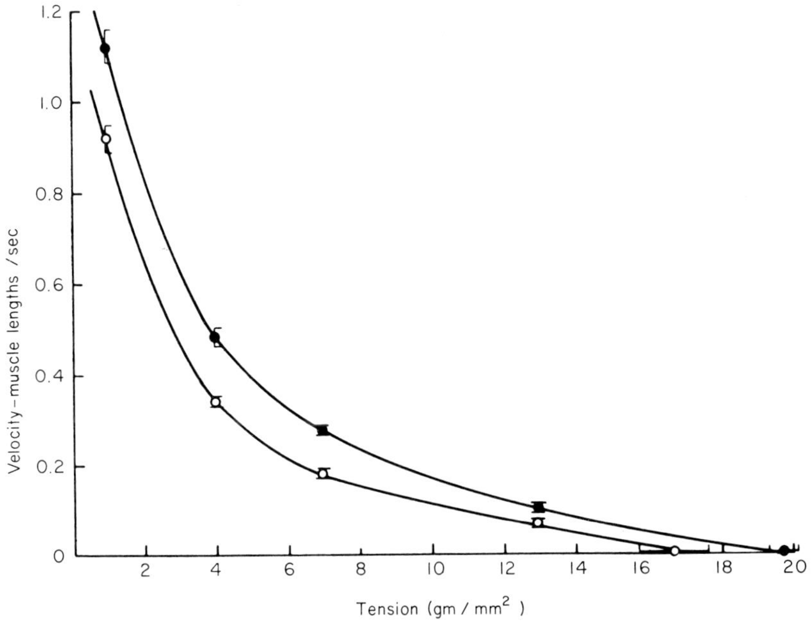

FIG. 5. Normalized force-velocity curves for the hypertrophied and sham-operated muscles 6 days postoperatively. The number of rat soleus muscles in each group with the results expressed as the mean ±SEM is denoted by filled circles, 10 sham-operated; unfilled circles, 11 hypertrophy; 6 days postoperatively; temp., 20°C. (Reprinted from Lesch *et al.*, 1968.)

the hypertrophy group was due to a limitation of oxygen diffusion into the muscle core. To rule out this possibility normal solei, with varying cross-sectional areas, obtained from rats of different weights, were studied and maximum generated tetanic tension was plotted as a function of cross-sectional area. Muscles with a cross-sectional area as great as 3.9 mm^2 were studied, and the plot of tension versus cross-sectional area was linear ($r = 0.90$, $P < 0.001$) indicating that the cross-sectional area of the muscle did not influence the results of the mechanical studies. This is especially so since the cross-sectional area of the hypertrophied muscles in this study ranged from only 1.36 to 2.78 mm^2.

Discussion

These studies demonstrate that the rat soleus which has acutely hypertrophied in response to tenotomy of its synergistic plantaris and gastrocnemius is characterized by the following mechanical properties. (1) Total tetanic tension output remains stable through the fourth postoperative day and is increased by the sixth postoperative day. (2) Contractility of the hypertrophied muscle, i.e., measurements of muscle function normalized per unit mass, is uniformly depressed throughout the 6-day postoperative period. (3) The intrinsic speed of contraction of the acutely hypertrophied rat soleus muscle at 6 days postoperative is reduced as indicated by the reduction in V_{max}, the increased time to peak twitch tension, and the prolonged duration of active state.

The specific significance of these findings as regards the physiologic process of work-induced skeletal muscle hypertrophy as it may occur in the trained athlete, or the more generalized significance apropos of other types of muscle hypertrophy, i.e., cardiac hypertrophy, is a direct function of the validity of the experimental model. Work-induced skeletal muscle hypertrophy as a physiological process is characterized by the following. (1) It is a positive adaptation and is not a primary pathological process as contrasted to cardiac hypertrophy; (2) it develops slowly; and (3) it is usually the result of periods of intense hyperfunction interspersed with periods of rest. Obviously the tenotomy-soleus preparation is an extreme model that bears little resemblance to the physiologic situation. Therefore, the data reported in this paper must not be considered adequate to describe the mechanics of hypertrophied muscle in general, but rather these data describe what can occur mechanically to skeletal muscle when it is acutely subjected to a continuous period of intense hyperfunction.

Significant hypertrophy was present on the first postoperative day and Fig. 4 thus demonstrates that work-induced skeletal muscle hypertrophy is not invariably associated with improved muscle function. More specifically, since the hypertrophied soleus muscle has an increased total myofibrillar protein content at 2 and 4 days postoperative (Hamosh *et al.*, 1967), it is clear that a temporal dissociation may exist between an increase in myofibrillar protein mass and the ability to generate measured force.

The reduction in V_{max} at 6 days postoperative associated with the prolonged duration of active state and increased time-to-peak twitch tension indicate that the intrinsic speed of contraction of the acutely hypertrophied soleus muscle is decreased. Factors that have been correlated to an altered intrinsic speed of contraction in skeletal muscle include age (Buller *et al.*, 1960a), myosin ATPase activity (Barany *et al.*, 1965), source of neural inervation (Buller *et al.*, 1960b), and the pattern of muscular activity and/or neural impulse activity (Fishbach and Robbins, 1969). Despite these correlations, it is presently impossible to determine the exact mechanism by which the intrinsic speed of contraction of a given skeletal muscle is determined. However, in experiments in which changes in the intrinsic speed of skeletal muscle contraction have been correlated to other factors, the time required before alterations in muscle contraction speed could be identified has been of the order of weeks. In contrast, our data indicate that under the appropriate conditions the intrinsic contractile properties of skeletal muscle can rapidly be altered.

In conclusion, the rapid hypertrophy of the rat soleus resulting from tenotomy of its synergistic muscles results in a depression of both tension development per unit mass and intrinsic velocity of shortening, although overall total tension development is maintained.

Acknowledgments

This work was performed in collaboration with Dr. E. H. Sonnenblick, Dr. W. W. Parmley, Dr. S. Kaufman, and Dr. M. Hamosh during the time that the author was a Research Associate in the Laboratory of General and Comparative Biochemistry, National Institute of Mental Health.

References

Barany, M., Barany, K., Reckard, T., and Volpe, A. (1965). *Arch. Biochem. Biophys.* **109**, 185.
Buller, A. J., Eccles, J. C., and Eccles, R. M. (1960a). *J. Physiol. (London)* **150**, 399.
Buller, A. J., Eccles, J. C., and Eccles, R. M. (1960b). *J. Physiol. (London)* **150**, 417.
Fishbach, G. D., and Robbins, N. (1969). *J. Physiol. (London)* **201**, 305.
Goldberg, A. L. (1968). *J. Cell Biol.* **36**, 653.
Goldberg, A. L. (1969). *J. Biol. Chem.* **244**, 3217.
Hamosh, M., Lesch, M., Baron, J., and Kaufman, S. (1967). *Science* **157**, 935.
Jewell, P. A., and Zaimis, E. J. (1954). *J. Physiol. (London)* **124**, 429.
Lesch, M., Parmley, W. W., Hamosh, M., Kaufman, S., and Sonnenblick, E. H. (1968). *Amer. J. Physiol.* **214**, 685.
Sonnenblick, E. H. (1962). *Fed. Proc. Fed. Amer. Soc. Exp. Biol.* **21**, 975.

NUCLEIC ACID CHANGES AND NUCLEAR RNA POLYMERASE ACTIVITY IN EXPERIMENTAL CARDIAC HYPERTROPHY

K. G. Nair, D. Grove, R. Zak, A. Cutilletta, and M. Rabinowitz

The development of myocardial hypertrophy appears to be a fundamental adaptive mechanism of the heart in response to an increased work load. However, the precise manner by which a mechanical stimulus such as pressure or volume overload is translated into a well-ordered biochemical and cellular response is, as yet, not clear. During the last few years, our laboratory has been studying the biochemical and cellular phenomena associated with cardiac hypertrophy produced by acute supravalvar aortic stenosis in rats.

This chapter deals chiefly with the changes in the nucleic acids and the DNA-dependent RNA polymerase of heart muscle during acutely induced cardiac hypertrophy. Our standard system for producing cardiac hypertrophy consists of banding of the ascending aorta of a mature female Sprague-Dawley rat by means of a specially designed silver clip. In this model system, we obtain increases in heart weight and in DNA and RNA content of the left ventricle of the order of 20–50% within 48 hr of surgery. Sham-operated litter mates serve as controls. The details of the surgery and the various methods used in the estimation of hypertrophy and the nucleic acid content of the myocardium have been published recently by Nair *et al.* (1968).

Changes in RNA Content of the Left Ventricle

There is a very early increase in the RNA content of the heart (micrograms per total ventricle) and in the RNA "concentration" (μg/mg wet weight) of the left ventricular muscle. These changes occur within 24 hr of aortic banding (Fig. 1). On the second day, maximal increases in RNA concentration (30%) and total ventricular RNA (65%) are seen over that of sham-operated controls. For about 2 weeks thereafter, these changes maintain a

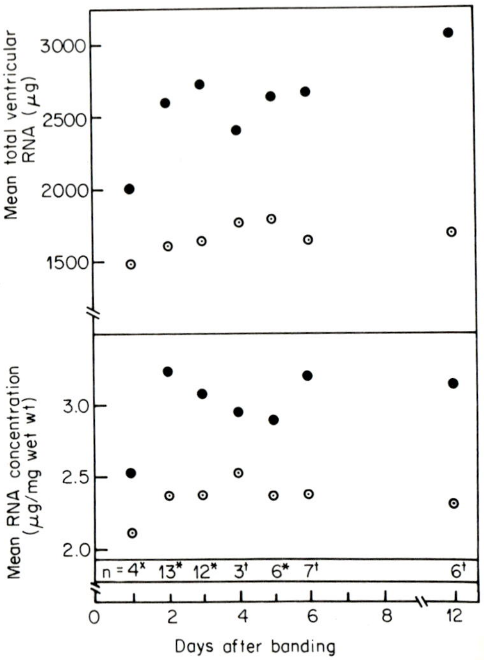

FIG. 1. Changes in RNA concentration and total ventricular RNA at 1–12 days after surgery in banded rats (solid circles) and sham-operated rats (open circles). *$P < 0.005$; †$P < 0.05$; ˣ$P < 0.20$. (Reproduced by kind permission from *Circ. Res.*; Nair *et al.*, 1969.)

plateau value. A few months later, there is a definite tendency for the RNA concentration to fall (Nair *et al.*, 1969). In Fig. 2, we have plotted the percentage of increase in heart weight over controls versus the percentage of increase in RNA. Note that the hearts that manifested the greatest degree of hypertrophy had also the greatest increment in RNA content.

The radioactivity profile and the optical density pattern of the left ventricular RNA synthesized during a 1-hr pulse of ^{32}P (12–24 hr after aortic constriction) was analyzed by sucrose density-gradient centrifugation (Koide and Rabinowitz, 1969). In Fig. 3, we note that the radioactive profile does not quite overlie the optical density pattern. There appears to be a region of elevated specific radioactivity in the zone to the left of the 28-S peak. This may be a reflection of the synthesis of ribosomal-precursor RNA. In our experience as well as that of Fanburg and Posner (1968), the RNA in the 4–18 S region remains highly labeled over the next few hours. It has been suggested that this may be a reflection of the synthesis of messenger RNA for

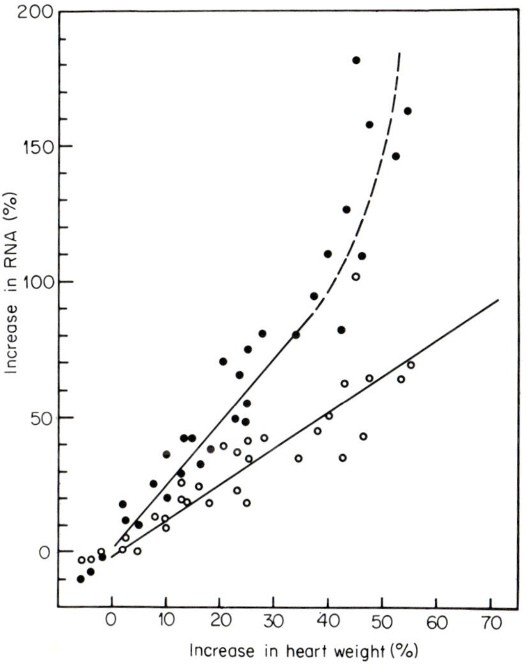

FIG. 2. Relation between the percentage of increment in RNA concentration and in heart weight after aortic banding. Data are expressed as percentage of increase over sham-operated controls. Determinations were made 7–8 days after banding. Open circles represent changes in RNA concentration; solid circles, changes in total Ventricular RNA. (Reproduced by kind permission from *Circ. Res.*; Nair *et al.*, 1968.)

myosin. These studies need further confirmation, e.g., by RNA-DNA hybridization.

Of considerable interest is the demonstration by Koide and Rabinowitz (1969), that there is an early expansion of the uridine nucleotide pool during cardiac hypertrophy. By contrast, the specific activity of the adenine pool does not change significantly. Whether these changes in the uridine nucleotide pool represent an early need for specific uridine nucleotides such as UDP glucose (which is required in glycogen synthesis), or are related to an increased utilization of uridine nucleotide for RNA synthesis remains conjectural for the present time.

The base composition of the RNA synthesized during cardiac hypertrophy does not show any appreciable changes from those of sham-operated controls. In both cases, the RNA base composition is as follows: adenine 19.7 ± 2.8, guanine 32.2 ± 0.3, uridine 17.0 ± 2.5, and cytosine 31.2 ± 0.5. Nair *et al.* (1959) found essentially similar values for RNA synthesized by an *in vitro* system using purified nuclei from normal and hypertrophied hearts.

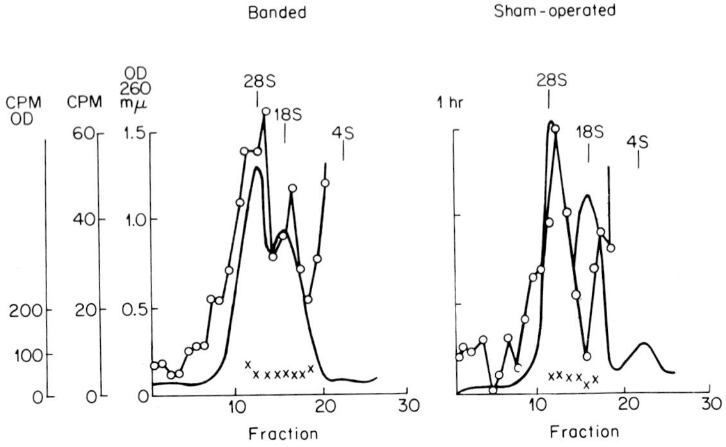

FIG. 3. Pattern of labeling of myocardial RNA with ^{32}P. Sucrose density gradient profile of RNA 1 hr after labeling (1 mC ^{32}P per rat). Optical density at 260 mμ (solid line), counts per minute (open circles), and specific radioactivity (*x*'s). (Reproduced by kind permission from *Circ. Res.*; Koide and Rabinowitz, 1969.)

Changes in RNA Polymerase Activity

It is now known from experimental evidence in bacterial and mammalian systems that DNA-dependent RNA polymerase is the key enzyme that regulates genetic transcription. Because changes in protein synthesis may be due to alterations in the activity of this enzyme, we prepared pure nuclear fractions from heart muscle by a modification of the method of Widnell and Tata (1964) for liver cells (Nair *et al.*, 1968).

The constituents of the assay system are as follows: System I (low ionic strength condition). The 0.5-ml incubation mixture consists of 50 μmoles tris-HCl buffer, pH 7.5, 2.5 μmoles $MgCl_2$ 10 μmoles freshly neutralized glutathione, 5 μmoles phosphoenolpyruvate (Sigma), 10 μg or pyruvate kinase (Sigma), 3 μmoles of NaF, 0.4 μmoles each of GTP, CTP, and ATP (Sigma), 0.024 μmole of UTP-$\alpha^{32}P$, and 0.1 ml of nuclear suspension containing 100–200 μg DNA. The specific radioactivity of the UTP is generally 200–300 μCi μmole. In System II (high ionic strength conditions), the incubation mixture is essentially similar to the one above, except that it contains in addition, 300 μmoles of $(NH_4)_2SO_4$ adjusted to pH 7.5 with NH_4OH, and Mn^{2+} replaces the Mg^{2+} ion in the assay. Incubations are carried out in duplicate or triplicate for 5 min at 37°C. The details of the extraction of RNA and the counting procedure are given in an earlier paper (Nair *et al.*, 1967).

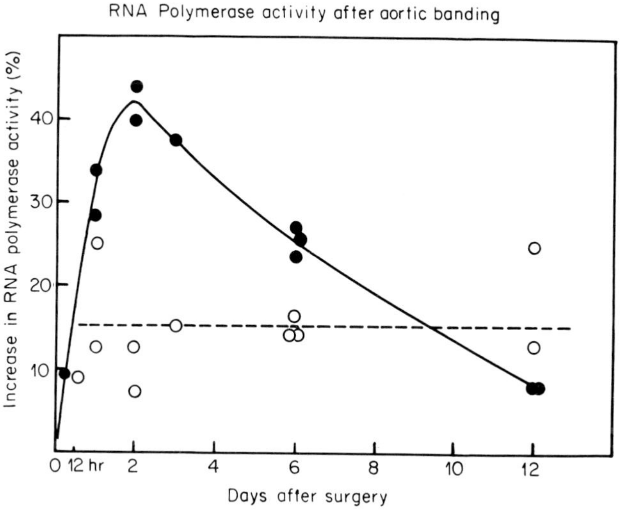

FIG. 4. Time course of changes in nuclear RNA polymerase nuclear RNA activity following aortic banding. Each point represents the results from duplicate assays using nuclei from two pooled hearts. Data are expressed as percentage of changes over values obtained from sham-operated controls. Filled circles and solid lines represent System I; open circles and broken lines, System II. (Reproduced by kind permission from *Circ. Res.*; Nair *et al.*, 1968.)

Figure 4 shows the profile of the changes in RNA polymerase activity from heart muscle nuclei following aortic banding. An early increase is noted within 12 hr. Schrieber *et al.* (see page 213, this volume), noted similar increases in activity of this enzyme within 1 hr following cardiac overloading in a perfused preparation. Peak activity with a 40% increase over that of controls is seen within 2 days following aortic narrowing. Thereafter, the enzyme activity gradually diminishes and tends to return to normal levels by the end of the second week.

The base composition of the RNA synthesized in System I is similar to ribosomal RNA (58% GC content), and in System II is DNA-like RNA. These base composition studies were made by the method of Josse *et al.* (1961) and have been reported in detail earlier (Nair *et al.*, 1967).

Changes in DNA Content during Hypertrophy

We now turn our attention to the changes in DNA content of the left ventricle during cardiac hypertrophy. Since mature heart muscle is a well-differentiated tissue, we should not expect any mitotic activity in muscle

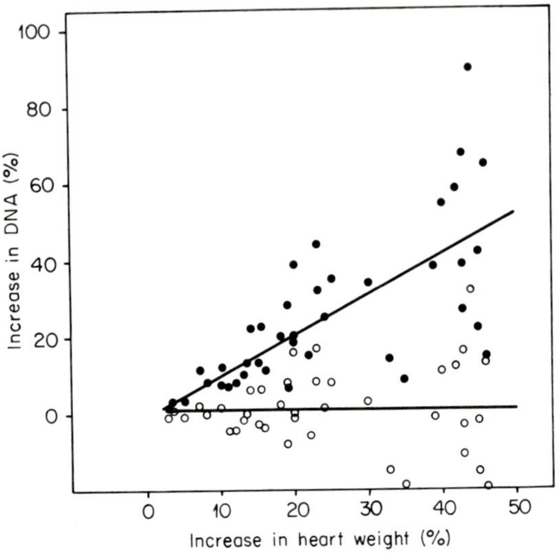

FIG. 5. Relation of changes in DNA concentration, and total ventricular DNA, to changes in heart weight after aortic constriction. Data are expressed as percentage of increase over sham-operated controls. Determinations were made 2–12 days after banding. The slopes of the lines were calculated by the method of least squares. Filled circles represent total ventricular DNA; unfilled circles, DNA concentration. (Reproduced by kind permission from *Circulation Res.*; Grove *et al.*, 1969a.)

cells. Yet, in Fig. 5, we see that the total DNA content of the myocardium does increase during cardiac hypertrophy and the DNA "concentration" per milligram wet weight does not decrease with increasing muscle mass in the early stages. Thus "dilution" of a fixed amount of DNA does not occur. The theoretical causes that might produce changes in DNA content may be listed under (1) an increase in polyploidy of nuclei (2n = diploid; 4n, 8n, or 16n = polyploid), (2) mitosis, (3) karyokinesis without cytokinesis, (4) polyteny, (5) infiltration by round cells from the blood stream, and (6) increase in mitochondrial DNA.

It is important to realize that data pertaining to changes in DNA content of the heart should be analyzed with regard to the maturity of the animal and the duration and intensity of the hypertrophic process. Our data refer to the changes in DNA content of the hearts of mature Sprague-Dawley rats during the acute phase of cardiac hypertrophy. These changes are shown graphically in Fig. 5. It is evident that the DNA concentration (μg DNA/mg wet weight) in the heart does not fall as the muscle mass increases and that therefore the total DNA content of the heart is increased.

The results of a detailed study of the different contributory factors that could give rise to an increase in myocardial DNA content have been published by Grove *et al.* (1969a) from our laboratory. We have found no evidence for infiltration by inflammatory cells. A survey of the frequency of polyploidy, using the microspectrophotometric method of Swift and Rasch (1956), indicates that although the degree of polyploidy increases from about 2–5% in muscle cells, this magnitude of change could hardly account for more than 1–2% of the increment in DNA content.

Mitotic figures were seldom seen in the mature normal heart of rats. In the acutely hypertrophying heart, however, it was possible to identify mitotic figures. If one defines the mitotic index as the number of mitoses per 10,000 nuclei, the mitotic index in the hypertrophied heart was on the average about tenfold as high as that in the controls. Extensive survey of the histological sections failed to reveal unequivocal evidence for mitotic activity in a clearly identifiable muscle cell. We have confirmed this by autoradiography (Grove *et al.* 1969b). Cellular proliferation appears to be restricted to the connective tissue cells, the endothelial cells of blood vessels and other "nonmuscular" cell elements (Fig. 6). These are also the findings of Crane and Dutta (1963), Meerson and Alekhina (1967) and Morkin and Ashford (1968). Thus, during acutely induced cardiac enlargement by an imposed work overload the muscle cells increase in mass, without proliferation

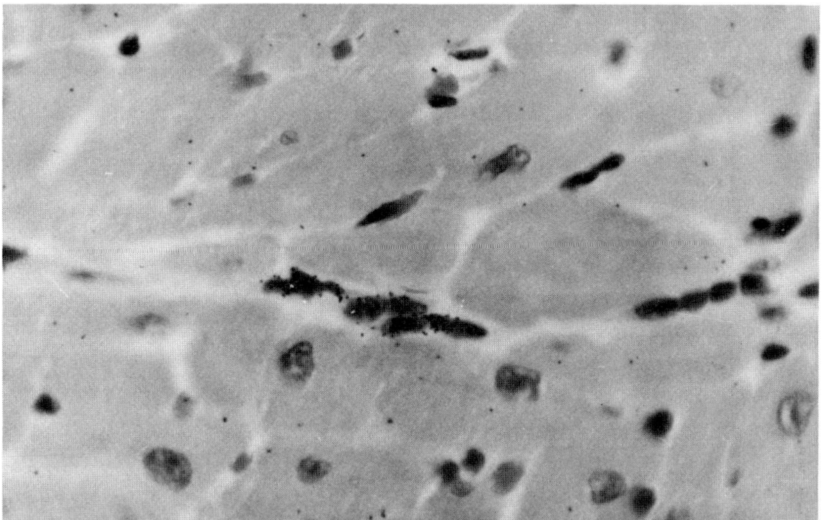

FIG. 6. Connective tissue nuclei labeled by autoradiography with ^{3}H-thymidine. Labeling of muscle cell nuclei was extremely rare. (Reproduced by kind permission from *Circ. Res.*; Grove *et al.*, 1969b.)

(hypertrophy), whereas the nonmuscular cells undergo proliferation (hyperplasia). This is in accord with the generally well-known biological phenomenon that well-differentiated cells to not undergo mitosis after reaching maturity and that less differentiated cells usually respond to the process of growth by hyperplasia.

We have made some preliminary studies on the relative contribution of mitochondrial DNA to the net increase in DNA content of the heart during cardiac hypertrophy. Although it is highly probable that mitochondrial DNA is replicating at the early stage of hypertrophy, the net contribution of this particular species of DNA to the mass of DNA can be regarded as negligible.

Estimations of the hydroxyproline concentration in heart muscle during cardiac hypertrophy show an initial decrease on the second day followed by a rise to above control values by the eleventh day. The total hydroxyproline content (μg/gm heart) also increased by the eleventh day because of the total increase in cell mass. These studies have been reported in detail by Grove *et al.* (1969b) and further substantiate the data concerning increase in myocardial content.

Discussion and Summary

In our studies, we have clearly shown that one of the earliest manifestations of cardiac hypertrophy at the biochemical level is an increase in RNA synthesis. The increase is proportional to the degree of hypertrophy during the acute period. We have also shown in purified nuclear preparations that the activity of DNA-dependent RNA polymerase is increased within 12 hr of banding. Schreiber *et al.* have reported elsewhere in this symposium similar results in perfused hearts subjected to a work overload. It is not yet known whether the increased activity of this key enzyme is due to (1) activation of the enzyme, (2) removal of an inhibitor, (3) derepression of the DNA template, making new sites available for RNA transcription, or (4) synthesis of new units of RNA polymerase. Studies with various inhibitors of the enzyme system are in progress in our laboratory with a view to elaborating the precise mechanism by which enzyme activation takes place.

A detailed biochemical and cellular study of the organization of growth during myocardial hypertrophy has shown that the DNA content of the heart does increase with growth, but that in the mature animal nearly all of the DNA increase can be accounted for by the proliferation of the connective tissue cells and other "nonmuscular" elements such as the endothelium. Thus, in conformation with the general observations on well-differentiated tissues, heart muscle cells enlarge by hypertrophic growth, whereas the rest of the cells which are less well differentiated undergo hyperplasia. In the immature heart, where less differentiated muscle cells exist, one can see evidence for mitotic activity (Klinge and Stocker, 1968), but in the mature rat heart we have seen only a very rare cell that shows any evidence for mitosis (Grove *et al.*, 1969b). Autoradiographic studies using tritiated thymidine have confirmed the view that the bulk of the increase in DNA content is from cells other than heart muscle. The contribution by polyploidy, binucleate cell formation and by increase in mitochondrial DNA to the total DNA content appears to be negligible.

An unresolved problem is the identity of the cells demonstrating an increase in RNA polymerase activity. Attempts to separate muscle cell nuclei from connective tissue cell nuclei by sucrose density gradient centrifugation have not been successful in our laboratory. Yet another intriguing problem is whether there are embryonic muscle cells in the mature heart which retain the ability to undergo cell differentiation and multiplication by cell division. The ultimate problem, of course, is to understand how a mechanical stimulus is translated into a biochemical response—a problem fundamental to many biological systems.

References

Crane, W. A. J., and Dutta, L. P. (1963). *J. Pathol. Bacteriol.* **86**, 83.

Fanburg, B. L., and Posner, B. I. (1968) *Circ. Res.* **23**, 123.

Grove, D., Nair, K. G., and Zak, R. (1969a). *Circ. Res.* **25**, 463.

Grove, D., Zak, R., Nair, K. G., and Aschenbrenner, V. (1969b). *Circ. Res.* **25**, 473.

Josse, J., Kaiser, A. D., and Kornberg, A. (1961). *J. Biol. Chem.* **236**, 864.

Klinge, O., and Stocker, E. (1968). *Experientia* **24**, 167.

Koide, T., and Rabinowitz, M. (1969). *Circ. Res.* **24**, 9.

Meerson, F. Z., and Alekhina, G. M. (1967). *Dokl. Akad. Sci. S.S.R.* **173**, 122.

Morkin, E., and Ashford, T. P. (1968). *Amer. J. Physiol.* **215**, 1409.

Nair, K. G., Cutilletta, A. F., Zak, R., Koide, T., and Rabinowitz, M. (1968). *Circ. Res.* **23**, 451.

Nair, K. G., Rabinowitz, M., and Tu. M. (1967). *Biochemistry* **6**, 1898.

Swift, H., and Rasch, E. (1956). *In* "Physical Techniques in Biology Research" (G. Oster and A. W. Pollister, eds.), p. 354. Academic Press, New York.

Widnell, C. C., and Tata, J. R. (1964). *Biochemical J.* **92**, 313.

ESTIMATION OF THE AMOUNT OF SARCOPLASMIC RETICULUM IN CARDIAC MUSCLE

F. Norman Briggs, R. John Solaro, and Edward W. Gertz

Subcellular Structures in Cardiac Muscle: Effect of Their Proportions on Contractility

One of the most important questions that can be asked about cardiac hypertrophy is whether the various subcellular components of the cell are proliferated in the proportions in which they exist in the normal cell. We became particularly aware of this question when we began to consider how a drug like quinidine could potentiate the contraction of skeletal muscle and inhibit that of cardiac muscle. When we examined the effect of quinidine on calcium uptake by isolated fragments of sarcoplasmic reticulum from skeletal and cardiac muscle (Fuchs *et al.*, 1968) we found both to be inhibited. It is easy to understand how this action of quinidine would tend to prolong the duration of the active state in skeletal muscle and thereby potentiate the twitch of skeletal muscle. Prolongation of the active state in cardiac muscle on the other hand should have little effect on developed tension and certainly should not inhibit tension development. We began to consider, therefore, what other possible consequences there might be of inhibiting uptake of calcium by the sarcoplasmic reticulum. For example, where might the calcium released from the reticulum go if it were not completely recovered by the reticulum? Two sinks came to mind, one the mitochondrion, the other the sarcolemma. If uptake of calcium by these sinks is to explain the different action of quinidine on cardiac and skeletal muscle it is necessary to argue that their ability to compete for calcium in cardiac muscle is considerably different than in skeletal muscle. This would be possible if the proportions of these structures were not the same in cardiac and skeletal muscle. Electron microscopy has shown that the relative amounts of mitochondria are much greater in cardiac muscle, but they do not reveal anything about the amount of sarcolemma relative to the amount of sarcoplasmic reticulum. Although the amount of sarcolemma can be estimated from cell size, there are unfortunately no estimates of the amount of reticulum in cardiac muscle.

Estimation of the Amount of Sarcoplasmic Reticulum from Calcium Oxalate Capacities

It occurred to us that the amount of sarcoplasmic reticulum could be estimated from measurements of the calcium oxalate capacity of whole muscle and isolated fragmented sarcoplasmic reticulum (FSR). This approach to the determination of the volume of sarcoplasmic reticulum depends upon the assumption that all parts of the reticulum accumulate calcium oxalate. Electron microscope examination by Costantin *et al.* (1965) of skinned muscles exposed to calcium, oxalate, and ATP have shown that the terminal cisternae accumulate calcium oxalate. The experiments of Pease *et al.* (1965) and Hasselbach (1964) have shown that the tubular elements also accumulate calcium oxalate. Hasselbach also observed that the amount of oxalate accumulated parallels the development of the sarcoplasmic reticulum. When the reticulum is isolated from muscle by homogenization and differential centrifugation and exposed to calcium solutions containing oxalate and ATP, an insoluble precipitate of calcium oxalate is deposited within the vesicles of the isolated FSR (Hasselbach, 1964).

Figure 1 shows in diagrammatic form how the accumulation of calcium oxalate can be used to estimate the volume of sarcoplasmic reticulum in muscle.

To apply this technique, it is necessary to devise methods that limit the calcium uptake by the homogenate to the sarcoplasmic reticulum and to isolate the sarcoplasmic reticulum in pure form. To ensure that calcium uptake by nonsarcoplasmic structures is trivial, the free calcium concentration has been set at a low level by addition of EGTA, azide has been added to the incubation solution to depress calcium uptake by the mitochondria, and oxalate has been added to amplify calcium uptake by the sarcoplasmic reticulum. The composition of the incubation mixture was as follows: 104 m*M* KCl; 18 m*M* imidazole pH 7.0; 5 m*M* $MgCl_2$; 5 m*M* ATP; 6 m*M* creatine phosphate; 1.8 m*M* potassium oxalate; and 0.6 m*M* $^{45}CaCl_2$. The amount of calcium taken up after various incubation periods was measured by the loss of ^{45}Ca from the incubation medium after separation of the homogenate or sarcoplasmic reticulum by filtration with 0.45-μ Millipore filters.

The only structures which are known to accumulate calcium are myofibrils, mitochondria, and sarcoplasmic reticulum. To show that the conditions

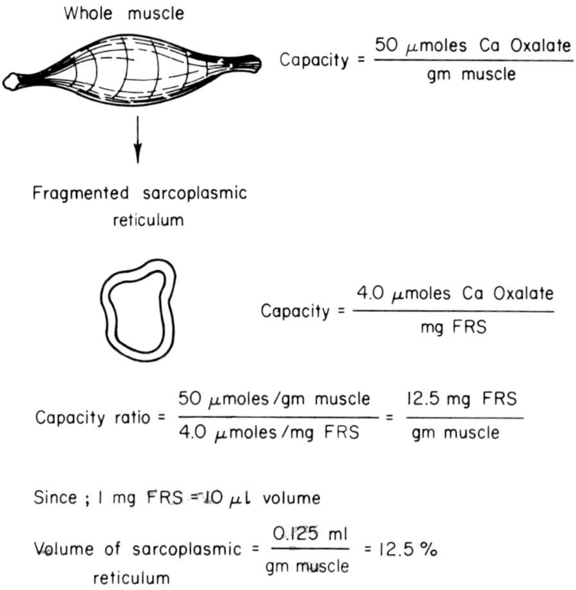

FIG. 1. Schematic of method for utilizing calcium oxalate capacities to estimate the volume of sarcoplasmic reticulum.

we have chosen severely limit the uptake of calcium by mitochondria, we have studied calcium uptake by mitochondria isolated from homogenates of dog myocardium. The homogenates were prepared by homogenizing, for 40 sec, one part of muscle with four parts of ice cold 0.3 *M* sucrose buffered with 10 m*M* imidazole. The mitochondrial fraction was separated by a 10-min spin at 6,300 g from a supernatant obtained with a 1,020-g spin. This pellet was suspended in sucrose and recentrifuged for 10 min at 6,300 g. Figure 2 shows that calcium uptake is severely limited by the presence of EGTA and azide. The uptake was about 0.01 μmoles of calcium per mg of mitochondrial protein. Since there are about 30 mg of mitochondrial protein per gram of heart, the mitochondrial portion of the homogenate of 1 gm of heart would accumulate about 0.3 μmoles of calcium. As will be shown later, this amount of calcium uptake is trivial. Calcium binding by myofibrils, at low calcium concentration, would amount to about 2 nmoles/mg of myofibrillar protein. Since there are about 80 mg of myofibrillar protein per gram of cardiac muscle, this source of calcium binding would represent about 0.16 μmoles of calcium per gram of cardiac muscle. This, too, is trivial compared with the capacity of the sarcoplasmic reticulum for calcium when oxalate is present as a trap.

To ensure that the cellular fraction designated the sarcoplasmic reticulum

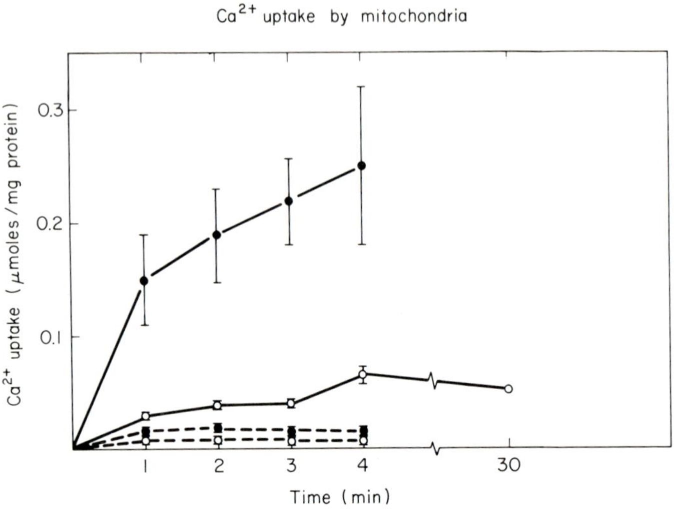

FIG. 2. Ca^{2+} uptake by mitochondria. ●—●, $9 \times 10^{-6} M$ Ca (control); ●- - -●, $9 \times 10^{-6} M$ Ca, 5 mM azide; ○—○, 1.3×10^{-7} Ca (control); ○- - -○, 1.3×10^{-7} Ca, 5 mM azide.

is free of myofibrillar proteins, the fraction was washed with 0.6 M KCl. To minimize contamination by mitochondrial fragments, the FSR fraction was isolated from cardiac homogenates after centrifugation of the homogenate at 13,200 g for 25 min and by taking the pellet obtained after 70 min of centrifugation at 90,000 g. The extent to which the cardiac sarcoplasmic reticulum fraction is contaminated by mitochondrial fragments has been estimated by measuring the specific activities of mitochondrial succinic dehydrogenase and cytochrome oxidase, and by determining the activities of these enzymes in the reticulum fraction. The results of this investigation are shown in Table I and reveal that the reticulum fraction is contaminated to

TABLE I

OXIDATIVE ENZYME ACTIVITIES OF CARDIAC HOMOGENATES AND SUBCELLULAR FRACTIONS

Enzyme	Expt.	Homogenate (μl O_2/gm wet muscle)	Mitochondria μl O_2/mg/hr	FSR μl O_2/mg/hr	% Contamination of FSR by mitochondria
Succinic dehydrogenase activity	1	24,480	1,043	70	6.7
	2	30,600	708	30	4.2
	3	32,250	930	44	4.7
Cytochrome oxidase activity	1	99,000	2,044	74	3.6
	2	135,000	1,876	120	6.4
	3	131,000	2,142	259	12.0

the extent of about 5% by mitochondria. This level of contamination would not seriously limit the validity of any conclusions drawn from studies with this sarcoplasmic reticulum fraction (FSR).

Skeletal Muscle

The calcium oxalate method of estimating the volume of the sarcoplasmic reticulum was first applied to frog skeletal muscle, since the volume of this reticulum has been estimated by the independent method of electron microscopy. A typical study with a muscle homogenate and a FSR preparation is shown in Fig. 3. The homogenate accumulated 53 μmoles of calcium per gm weight of muscle and the FSR accumulated 3.96 μmoles/mg FSR protein. Azide, a potent inhibitor of mitochondrial calcium uptake, decreased calcium uptake in the homogenate by 8%. In this experiment, azide inhibited calcium uptake by the FSR preparation only by 3%. The results of three calcium uptake studies with 15 frogs is summarized in Table II. The volume of the FSR, estimated from the azide-poisoned preparations averaged 12.1%, a value in close agreement with the 13% volume estimated by electron microscopy (Peachey, 1965). It is noteworthy that the yield of FSR, 1.2 mg/gm, in these experiments represents only about 10% of the total FSR (12.1% = 121 μl/gm = 12.1 mg/gm) in the muscle. This is a much lower yield than most investigators have assumed when extrapolating their studies with isolated FSR to the function of the FSR in the intact muscle.

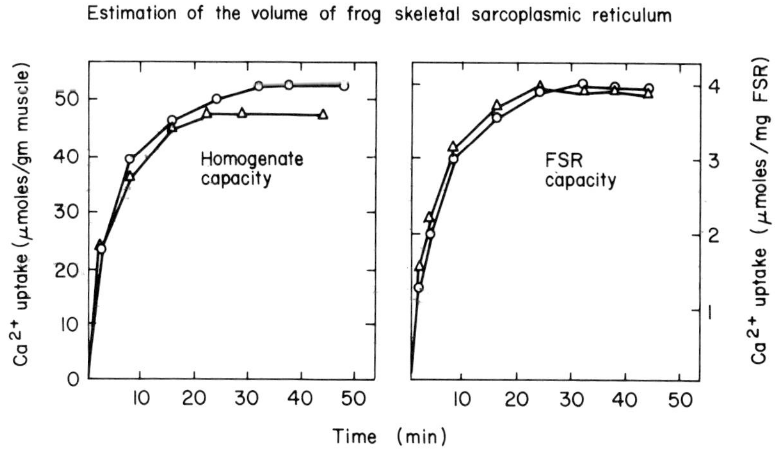

Fig. 3. Calcium uptake by frog skeletal muscle homogenate and fragmented sarcoplasmic reticulum (FSR). See methods section for experimental conditions. Control, O—O; 5 mM azide, △—△.

TABLE II

HOMOGENATE AND FSR CAPACITIES OF FROG SKELETAL MUSCLE

Expt.	No. frogs	Yield of FSR (mg FSR/gm wet muscle)	Homogenate capacity (μmoles Ca/gm wet muscle)		FSR capacity (μmoles Ca/protein)		FSR vol % of muscle volume	
			Control	5 m*M* azide	Control	5 m*M* azide	Control	5 m*M* azide
1	3	1.0	52.5	50.9	4.30	4.30	12.2	11.8
2	6	1.4	53.0	47.9	3.96	3.87	13.4	12.4
3	6	1.3	51.0	50.2	4.15	4.10	12.3	12.2
Average							12.6	12.1

CARDIAC MUSCLE

We then applied the calcium oxalate capacity method to the estimation of the volume of sarcoplasmic reticulum in canine ventricle. Figure 4 provides a typical record of calcium uptake by a homogenate and FSR preparation. The amount of calcium accumulated by the homogenate plateaued after about 24 min of incubation at 19–20 μmoles/gm wet weight of heart. The time course of calcium uptake by the FSR preparation is also shown in Fig. 4. Accumulation plateaued after 30 min at 3.3 μmoles/mg FSR. Table III summarizes the data obtained from six experiments. The capacity of the homogenate averaged 19 μmoles/gm of heart. Azide produced no depression of this uptake. The capacity measurements give a volume for the canine cardiac sarcoplasmic reticulum of 6.9%. The yield of FSR averaged 10% of that calculated to be in the homogenate.

Discussion

These estimates of the amount of reticulum in skeletal and cardiac muscle permit one, in a crude and imperfect fashion, to estimate the difference in the proportions (surface area) of sarcolemma to sarcoplasmic reticulum in cardiac and skeletal muscle. The bases for this comparison are shown in Table IV.

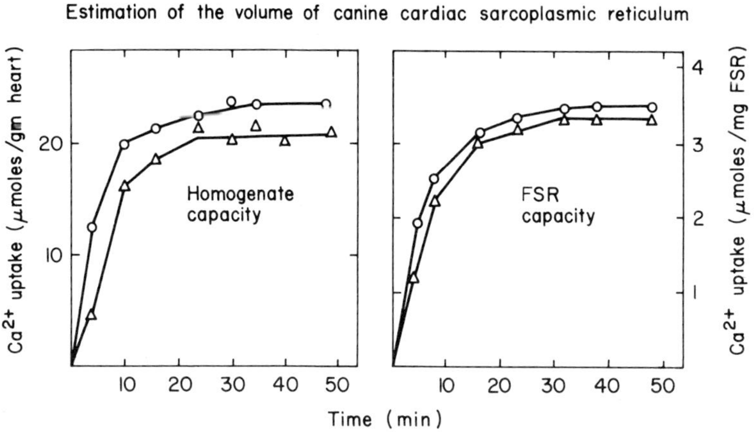

FIG. 4. Calcium uptake by canine cardiac muscle homogenate and fragmental sarcoplasmic reticulum (FSR). See methods section for experimental conditions. Control, O—O; 5 mM azide, △—△.

TABLE III

HOMOGENATE AND FSR CAPACITIES OF CANINE CARDIAC MUSCLE

Dog no.	Yield of FSR (mg FSR/gm wet muscle)	Homogenate capacity (μmoles Ca/gm wet muscle)		FSR capacity (μmole Ca/mg FSR)		FSR volume	
		Control	5 m*M* azide	Control	5 m*M* azide	Control	5 m*M* azide
1	0.5	18.9	19.2	2.97	2.95	6.4	6.5
2	0.7	18.2	17.2	2.39	2.41	7.6	7.3
3	0.5	15.0	15.7	2.50	2.49	6.0	6.3
4	0.7	23.4	21.1	3.45	3.30	6.8	6.4
5	0.8	21.7	24.7	2.75	2.76	7.9	8.5
6	0.6	21.4	19.2	3.13	3.0	6.8	6.4
Average						6.9	6.9

TABLE IV

ESTIMATE OF THE MAGNITUDE OF COMPONENTS INVOLVED IN CALCIUM METABOLISM

	Skeletal	Cardiac
Fiber diameter	80	10
Surface area[a] per gm muscle	525 cm^2	4000 cm^2
Amount of SR[b] per gm muscle	12.0 mg	6.0 mg

[a] Assuming right cyclinders.
[b] We assume that the surface area is proportional to the amount of material.

Since there is eight times as much sarcolemmal area per gram of muscle in cardiac muscle as in skeletal and only one-half as much sarcoplasmic reticulum membrane, on this basis there would be 16 times as much chance of losing calcium from the sarcoplasmic reticulum in cardiac muscle as in skeletal muscle. If the calcium pump rates in the sarcolemma or sarcoplasmic reticulum of the two types of muscle are different then the chance of losing calcium would be modified by the appropriate ratios of rates. For example, it appears that the calcium transport rate of skeletal sarcoplasmic reticulum may be two to four times faster than cardiac muscle. If this is the case, then the chance that cardiac muscle would lose calcium would be increased to 32–64 times. Final analysis of this problem will require accurate information on the calcium pump rates of the sarcolemma as well as the sarcoplasmic reticulum.

ACKNOWLEDGMENTS

R. John Solaro and Edward W. Gertz were supported by PHS Training Grant No. GM 01404 from General Medical Sciences. F. Norman Briggs is the recipient of Research Career Award (1 K6-HE-5290) from the National Heart Institute. This work was supported by research grant 68-781 from the American Heart Association and HE-06782 from the National Institutes of Health.

REFERENCES

Costantin, L. L., Franzini-Armstrong, C. F., and Podolsky, R. J. (1965). *Science* **147**, 158.
Fuchs, F., Gertz, E. W., and Briggs, F. N. (1968). *J. Gen. Physiol.* **52**, 955.
Hasselbach, W. (1964). *Progr. Biophys. Mol. Biol.* **14**, 167.
Peachey, L. D. (1965). *J. Cell Biol.* **25**, 209.
Pease, D. C., Jenden, D. J., and Howell, J. N. (1965). *J. Cell. Comp. Physiol.* **65**, 141.

STRUCTURE AND FUNCTION OF MYOSIN

Lewis C. Gershman and Paul Dreizen

Introduction

The sliding together of thick and thin filaments during contraction of striated muscle is linked with the enzymatic splitting of ATP by myosin, the contractile protein of the thick filament (Hanson and Huxley, 1955). In this chapter, we shall describe work from our laboratory on the structure of myosin and the relationship between this structure and the enzymatic properties of myosin. Much of the work is very actively under way, and this chapter should be considered a progress report, the conclusions of which may well be modified as further evidence is accumulated.

Details of the experimental procedures have been described previously (Dreizen *et al.*, 1966; Gershman *et al.*, 1966, 1969; Gershman and Dreizen, 1970).

Subunit Structure of Myosin

Molecular Weight of Myosin

Determination of the molecular weight of myosin has been controversial for nearly two decades. In recent years, most investigators have reported molecular weight values between 500,000 and 600,000 for rabbit skeletal myosin (see Stracher and Dreizen, 1966, for review). The molecular weight values of 600,000 are referable to preparations of myosin obtained by ammonium sulfate fractionation (Kielley and Harrington, 1960; Woods *et al.*, 1963); this procedure has been found to enhance irreversible aggregation of myosin (Stracher and Dreizen, 1966; Dreizen *et al.*, 1967). Although the monomer weight of myosin might be expected to be closer to 500,000 than 600,000, it remained uncertain as to whether aggregation of myosin in the absence of ammonium sulfate fractionation might have contributed to reported weight-average molecular weight values of ~500,000 (Holtzer and Lowey, 1959; Mueller, 1964; Tonomura *et al.*, 1966). This point is by no means inconsequential—a precise molecular weight value for myosin turns out to be critical to the determination of subunit structure.

Our work on this problem involved the use of several ultracentrifugal methods, namely, low-speed sedimentation equilibrium, high-speed sedimentation equilibrium, and Archibald method, all of which provide information on monomer weight and the extent of aggregation (Gershman *et al.*, 1966, 1969; Dreizen *et al.*, 1967; Gershman, 1968). In order to minimize irreversible aggregation of myosin in these experiments, the protein was purified without ammonium sulfate treatment, stored in 0.05 *M* inorganic phosphate at 4°C (Holtzer and Lowey, 1959), and analyzed within several days of purification. The low-speed sedimentation equilibrium experiments indicated progressive increase in weight–average molecular weight during prolonged ultracentrifugation, consistent with the occurrence of continuous aggregation throughout. Data from one such experiment show a linear increase in weight–average molecular weight from 520,000 at the expected equilibrium time of 40 hr to nearly 800,000 after 160 hr of centrifugation (Fig. 1). Assuming a simple kinetic model for aggregation, these data would indicate a monomer weight for myosin between 450,000 and 480,000, and a rate constant of 1.3×10^{-4} sec^{-1} for dimerization of myosin (Gershman, 1968; Gershman *et al.*, 1969).

In approach-to-equilibrium experiments (Archibald method) on similar preparations of myosin, the weight–average molecular weight at the meniscus region decreased from ~530,000 initially, to 470,000 after several hours of centrifugation (Gersham *et al.*, 1969). These findings indicate that dimers or other low *n*-mers of myosin may be present even in "good" preparations of myosin, and that such low *n*-mers are selectively depleted from the meniscus during sedimentation, leaving behind almost pure myosin monomer.

However, the most precise determination of molecular weight for myosin was obtained in high-speed sedimentation equilibrium experiments (Yphantis, 1964), where myosin *n*-mers were selectively sedimented so that monomer weight could be determined directly from the concentration distribution of nonaggregated myosin at low radial distances and low protein concentrations. The data indicated a molecular weight of 468,000 (±10,000) for myosin, based on somewhat more than 2,000 comparator readings from a series of experiments (Gershman, 1968; Gershman *et al.*, 1969). The value for monomer weight remained constant for at least 72 hr of centrifugation, despite the slow aggregation of myosin that was evident at high radial distances and high protein concentrations. The monomer weight was invariant to rotor speed over a twofold range in ultracentrifugal field strength consistent with weight-homogeneity of myosin. In a way, the Yphantis

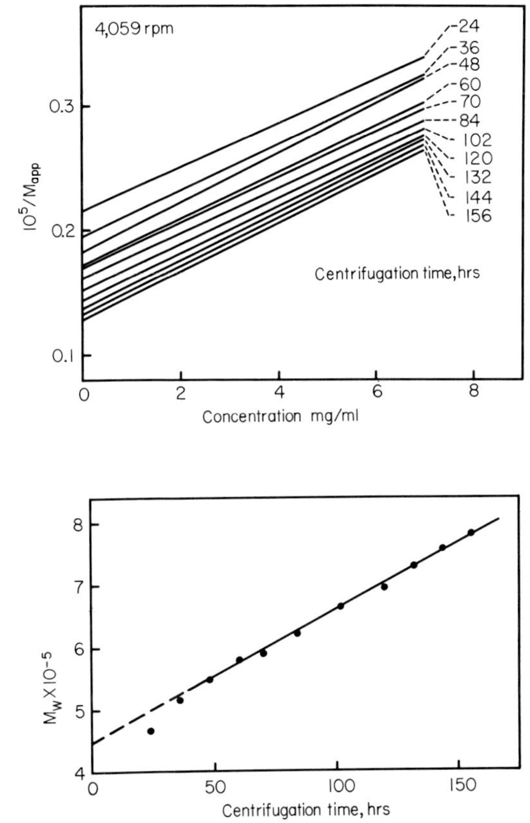

FIG. 1. Sedimentation equilibrium of myosin at 1.7, 2.9, and 6.5 mg/ml in 0.4 *M* KCl–0.05 *M* KH_2PO_4, pH 6.5, 4°C, at 4,059 rpm. Apparent molecular weight (M_{app}) was calculated over the whole column at intervals from 24 to 156 hr of centrifugation; expected equilibrium time 40 hr. Upper, reciprocal of apparent molecular weight plotted against initial protein concentration; lower, weight average molecular weight (M_w) from extrapolation to zero-concentration in upper graph, plotted against time of centrifugation. From Gershman *et al.* (1969).

method (1964) is more accurate for heavier molecules such as myosin, than for lighter molecules, since the conditions for meniscus depletion are achieved at relatively low field strength (10,000–15,000 rpm) where effects from Wiener skewing are negligible and optical artifacts in the interference fringes minimal. Consequently, we believe that the present determination approaches the precision of 2 or 3% that may be obtained by physical chemical methods, and that any significant improvement in the molecular weight determination will probably require analysis of the primary structure of myosin.

Light and Heavy Polypeptide Chains

It was first shown by Tsao (1953) that myosin releases light and heavy components on prolonged treatment in urea or guanidine solutions and at pH 11; subsequent investigators reported that heat denaturation (Locker, 1956; Yasui *et al.*, 1960), alkaline treatment (Kominz *et al.*, 1959; Connell and Olcott, 1961), and urea treatment (Szent-Györgyi, 1960; Wetlaufer and Edsall, 1960) liberate low molecular weight material from myosin preparations. But the apparent absence of light component on dissociation of purified myosin in 5 *M* guanidine (Kielley and Harrington, 1960; Small *et al.*, 1961; Woods *et al.*, 1963) led to the belief that any low molecular weight component, if present, represented contaminant proteins or proteolytic fragments of myosin. From ultracentrifugal experiments indicating a weight–average molecular weight slightly less than 200,000 for myosin in 5 *M* guanidine, it was concluded that myosin is composed of three weight-equivalent polypeptide chains (Kielley and Harrington, 1960; Woods *et al.*,1963).

The homogeneity of myosin in 5 *M* guanidine is critical to the three-stranded model for myosin, and a reinvestigation in this laboratory indicated sedimentation and diffusion data that were essentially identical with the earlier findings on myosin in 5 *M* guanidine. However, more detailed analysis of these data revealed that myosin is in fact heterogeneous in 5 *M* guanidine, with a predominantly heavy component and a slowly sedimenting (or rapidly diffusing) component (Dreizen *et al.*, 1966, 1967). The heavy component shows a strong concentration dependence of sedimentation, resulting in poor resolution of light and heavy components on sedimentation of myosin in 5 *M* guanidine; failure to recognize this problem would appear to account for the earlier confusion on the heterogeneity of myosin in 5 *M* guanidine.

The nature of the heterogeneity was explored in sedimentation equilibrium experiments on myosin in 5 *M* guanidine, in which equilibrium was successively reached at different rotor speeds over a ten-fold range in ultracentrifugal field strength. As shown in a representative experiment (Fig. 2), this procedure permitted analysis of molecular weight (MW) and proportion of light and heavy components. Data from a number of experiments performed on native myosin and ammonium sulfate-treated myosin, with and without reduction and carboxymethylation, showed dissociation of myosin by 5 *M* guanidine into a heavy component of 200,000 to 220,000 MW, and a light component of $\sim$21,000 MW that comprises 10–15% of the total protein (Dreizen *et al.*, 1966, 1967). Following removal of the light component, sedimentation equilibrium experiments on the purified heavy component indicated a molecular weight of 212,000 ($\pm$5,000) for the heavy chains of myosin (Gershman *et al.*, 1966, 1969).

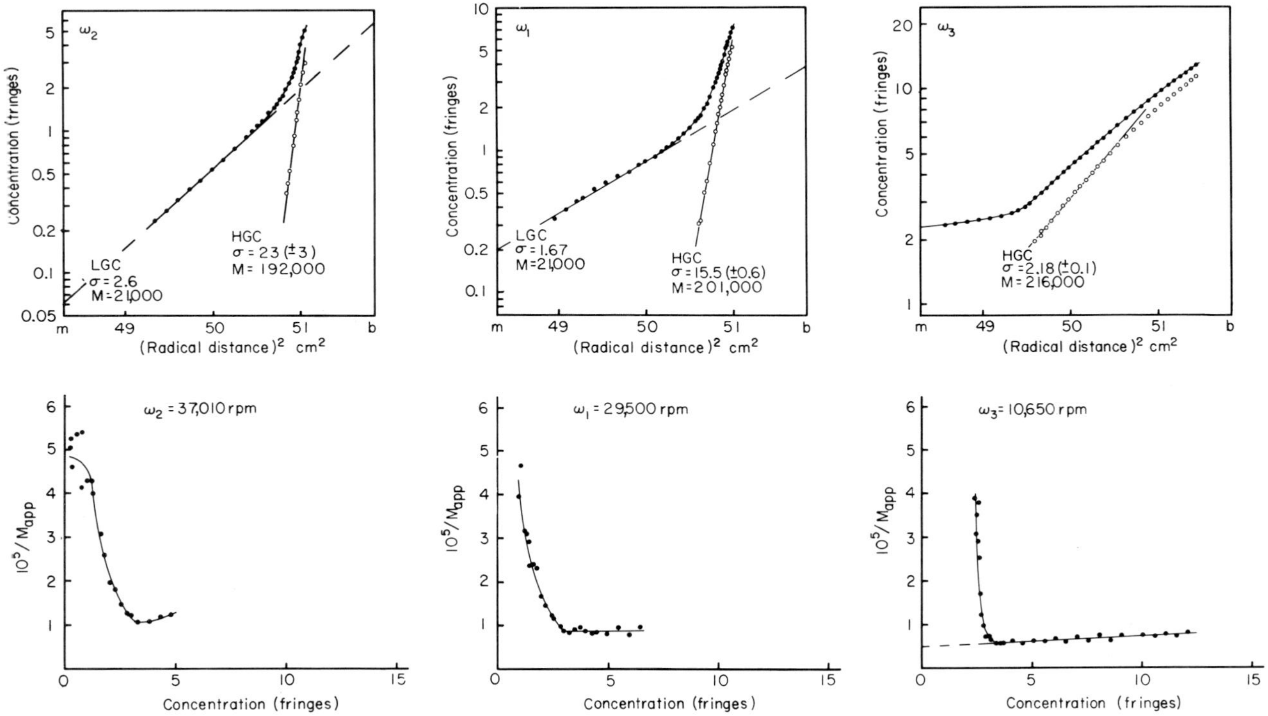

FIG. 2. Sedimentation equilibrium of myosin (ammonium sulfate preparation, reduced and carboxymethylated) at 2.5 mg/ml in 5 *M* guanidine·HCl–0.4 *M* KCl, pH 5.5, 4°C, at 29,500 rpm (ω_1), 37,010 rpm (ω_2), and 10,650 rpm (ω_3). (LGC), Light guanidine component; (HGC), heavy guanidine component; (m), meniscus; (b), bottom. From Dreizen *et al.* (1967).

These results indicate that myosin contains two heavy chains (212,000 MW) and several light chains of average molecular weight ~ 21,000; but it was not possible to ascertain the exact proportions of light and heavy components in sedimentation velocity or sedimentation equilibrium experiments on myosin in 5 *M* guanidine. This technical problem prompted experiments to determine the subunit composition of alkaline-dissociated myosin (Gershman *et al.*, 1966, 1969; Gershman, 1968). Sedimentation velocity experiments indicated that at pH ~ 10.5, myosin is dissociated into a heavy component, with a sedimentation coefficient close to that of native myosin, and a light component that comprises 12.0% of the total protein. Multispeed sedimentation equilibrium experiments indicated 11.5% of the light component and molecular weight values of 420,000 for the myosin core and 20,200 for the light component (Table I). These results indicate approximately 2.7 (±0.3) light

TABLE I

SUBUNIT DISSOCIATION OF RABBIT SKELETAL MYOSIN UNDER DIFFERENT SOLVENT CONDITIONS[a]

Solvent	Sed. velocity: Light component %	Sed. equilibrium: Light component %	Sed. equilibrium: Light component MW	Sed. equilibrium: Heavy component $MW \times 10^{-5}$		Light chains dissociated per myosin molecule
5 *M* guanidine	–	~12.5	21,000	2.12	(±0.05)	~2.8
pH 11	12.0	11.5	20,200	4.2	(±0.2)	2.7
2 *M* guanidine	12.0	12.0	21,400	4.3	(±0.3)	2.7
30°–40°C		~10	20,000[b]	6.2[c]		
4 *M* LiCl	12.3	11.6	20,600[b]	9.0[c]		2.7
1 *M* KSCN	12.5	11	~23,600	4.1	(±0.3)	
4.7 *M* NH_4Cl						
1 hr	4.0					0.9
24 hr	6.0	~ 6.0	20,600[b]	5.2[c]		~1.4

[a] Based on data from Gershman *et al.*, 1966, 1969; Dreizen *et al.*, 1967; Gershman, 1968; Gershman and Dreizen, 1970.

[b] About one-third to one-half of the light component has aggregated to ~90,000 MW.

[c] Limiting molecular weight; much of the heavy component has aggregated to and beyond dimer level.

chains per myosin molecule (468,000 MW), and the stoichiometry is confirmed by the difference in molecular weight between native myosin and the heavy chain core.

Extensive studies were conducted in Alfred Stracher's laboratory on the effect of chromatography on myosin; the proportion of light component in myosin is not significantly lowered by single chromatographic passage on DEAE-cellulose or cellulose phosphate (Hartshorne and Stracher, 1966; Gershman *et al.*, 1969). However, three chromatographic cycles on cellulose phosphate result in extensive denaturation of myosin, and the residual soluble myosin (only 10% of the original unchromatographed myosin) contains about 1.9 light chains and retains 60% of control ATPase activity (Gershman *et al.*, 1969).

It has also been shown that light chains are dissociated from the heavy chain core on treatment of myosin in 2 *M* guanidine (Gershman *et al.*, 1969) and in concentrated salt solutions, pH 7, 4°C (Gershman, 1968; Gershman *et al.*, 1968a; Gershman and Dreizen, 1969a, 1970). The salt effect is highly specific, and anions and cations may be listed in a Hofmeister series with respect to their dissociating effect on myosin. Thus, light chains are fully dissociated from myosin by 1 *M* KSCN and 4 *M* LiCl, but not at all dissociated from myosin by KCl or NaCl solutions at salt concentrations to saturation. In some instances, as in treatment of myosin in 4.7 *M* NH_4Cl, pH 7, 4°C (Gershman and Dreizen, 1969a, 1970) and in 0.4 *M* KCl, pH 7, at temperatures above 10°C (Gershman *et al.*, 1968a, 1969), there is incomplete, time-dependent dissociation of the light component from myosin, accompanied by the aggregation of both dissociated light chains and of the residual myosin.

Light and heavy components are largely reassociated during dialysis against 0.4 *M* KCl at pH 7 following the dissociation of myosin at pH 11, in 2 *M* guanidine and in concentrated salt solutions, provided that the period of denaturation was short and thiol groups were protected. Light and heavy components both aggregate during prolonged treatment under dissociating conditions and also on storage in 0.4 *M* KCl, pH 7, especially in the absence of prior carboxymethylation (Gershman *et al.*, 1969; Gershman and Dreizen, 1970; Dreizen and Gershman, 1970a). We have suggested previously that aggregation phenomena might account at least in part for the molecular weight values ~30,000 that have been reported for the light alkali component of unmodified myosin, based on sedimentation-diffusion (Kominz *et al.*, 1959; Connell and Olcott, 1961) and viscosity and light-scattering measurements (Frederiksen and Holtzer, 1968).

Subunit Composition of Proteolytic Fragments

Digestion of myosin with trypsin yields two major fragments, light meromyosin and heavy meromyosin (Mihályi and Szent-Györgyi, 1953; Lowey and Holtzer, 1959), that are arranged end-to-end in the intact molecule (Rice, 1964). Light meromyosin undergoes reversible association at low ionic strength and forms the axial core of the thick filament, whereas heavy meromyosin retains ATPase activity and forms the cross-bridges and peripheral part of the thick filament core (Mihályi and Szent-Györgyi, 1953; Huxley, 1963). Sedimentation velocity and sedimentation equilibrium experiments on the alkaline-treated meromyosins indicate that light meromyosin contains a remnant of the heavy chain core and no light chains, at least in measurable proportion, and that heavy meromyosin contains the entire light component and two-thirds of the heavy chain core (Gershman *et al.*, 1966).

Heavy meromyosin, or native myosin directly, may be digested with trypsin (Mueller and Perry, 1962) or papain (Kominz *et al.*, 1965) into a smaller particle, Subfragment-1, that retains ATPase activity. That each myosin molecule yields two Subfragment-1 particles was suggested on stoichiometric grounds (Stracher and Dreizen, 1966; Nauss and Gergely, 1967), and shown directly on electron microscopy of myosin (Slayter and Lowey, 1967). With treatment at pH 11 and in 5 *M* guanidine, papain-prepared Subfragment-1 is dissociated into a heavy component of 85,000 MW, and a light component of 18,000 MW, in close to molar ratio (Trotta *et al.*, 1968). C-terminal analyses confirm the presence within Subfragment-1 of the light-chain end-group isoleucine in molar ratio (Trotta *et al.*, 1968).

Figure 3 summarizes our present concept of the myosin structure and the subunit interactions on which this proposed structure is based. Native myosin comprises an axial core of two 210,000 MW heavy polypeptide chains, that terminate in a globular region also containing 2.7 ($\pm$0.3) light polypeptide chains, of average weight 20,200. Each Subfragment-1 particle contains remnants of one light chain and one heavy chain; the additional light chain appears to be less tightly bound to myosin, as indicated by the partial dissociation of the light component from myosin on short treatment in 4.7 *M* NH_4Cl and during three chromatographic cycles on cellulose phosphate.

Light Chain Heterogeneity

The light component dissociated from carboxymethylated myosin at pH 11 yields three or four different bands on cellulose acetate electrophoresis (Gershman *et al.*, 1966), and comparable heterogeneity has been described for light-component dissociation from myosin on acetylation (Locker and Hagyard, 1967a). However, it remained uncertain from these experiments as to whether the electrophoretic heterogeneity represented structural differences in the light chains or merely artifacts resulting from light chain aggregation or charge differences in the number of carboxymethylated (or acetylated) groups within identical polypeptide chains.

In order to resolve this uncertainty, we carried out electrophoretic experiments on light component dissociated from myosin at pH 11, in 2 *M*

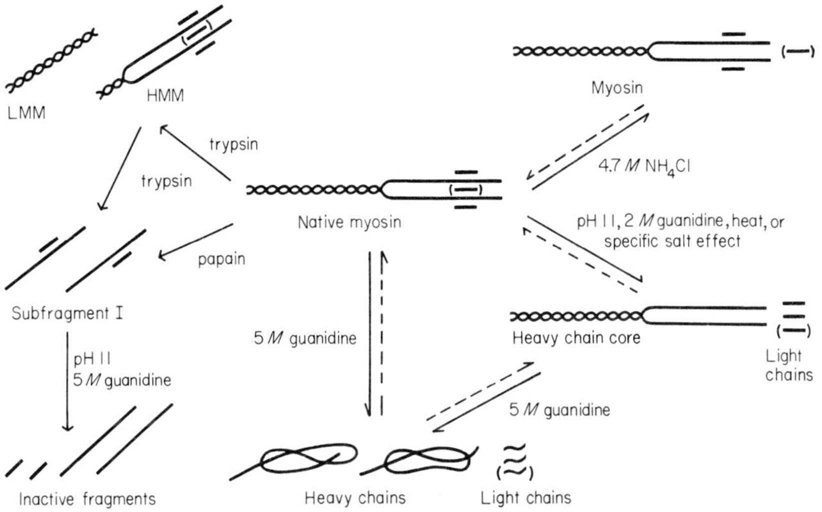

FIG. 3. Schematic diagram of subunit structure and interactions of rabbit skeletal myosin. Chain lengths are drawn proportional to atomic mass, and differ from the actual dimensions of rodlike and globular portions of myosin as determined from electron microscopy. According to Rice (1964), the rodlike portion of myosin is 1350 Å in length and 20 Å in diameter and the globular region is 210 Å in length and 50 Å in diameter; light meromyosin is 900 Å long and the rodlike part of heavy meromyosin is about 400 Å long. The globular head appears to be bilobed in a considerable proportion of myosin molecules (Slayter and Lowey, 1967), and a similar structural arrangement has been shown for the globular head of heavy meromyosin (Zobel, 1967). From Dreizen and Gershman (1970a).

guanidine, 4 *M* LiCl, and 1 *M* KSCN, all performed in the absence of chemical modification of myosin (Gershman and Dreizen, 1969c, 1970). Purification procedures were carried out simultaneously so as to minimize possible effects from genetic variations in myosin, irreversible denaturation of myosin, or the electrophoretic procedure itself. Figure 4 shows electrophoretic patterns obtained on light component dissociated from myosin at pH 11 and in 4 *M* LiCl; in both cases, there are four major bands and one or two minor bands of comparable mobility. The light components dissociated from myosin in 2 *M* guanidine and in 1 *M* (or 2 *M*) KSCN show very similar electrophoretic heterogeneity, with minor differences in relative intensity of the different bands. We would conclude from these data that electrophoretic heterogeneity arises from actual structural differences among the light chains of myosin.

The effect of irreversible denaturation on the light chains is shown in an experiment in which the myosin preparation indicated in Fig. 4 was stored for 1 week in 0.4 *M* KCl, pH7, and then treated in 4 *M* LiCl for periods

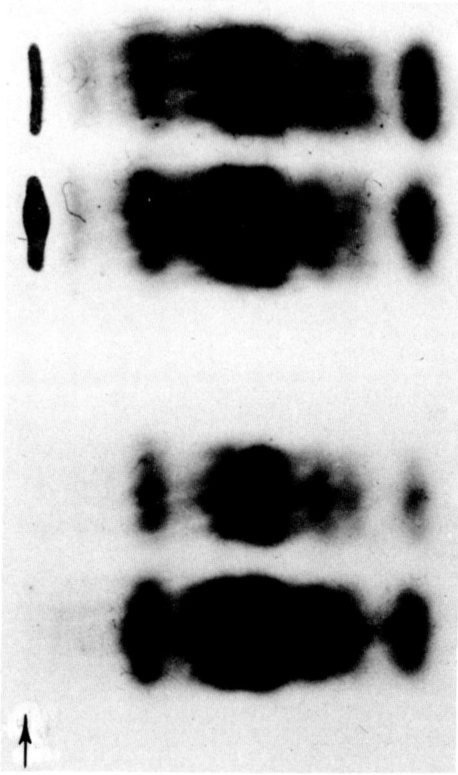

FIG. 4. Cellulose acetate electrophoresis of myosin light component in 0.75 *M* sodium barbital, pH 8.6. (a, b) 4 *M* LiCl-citrate supernatant; (c, d) pH 11-dilution supernatant. Arrow indicates origin; anode to right in this and other experiments. From Gershman and Dreizen (1970).

of 5 min to 72 hr prior to salting out in 60% saturated potassium citrate. On electrophoresis the supernatant fraction from 5 min LiCl treatment (Fig. 5a) showed less of the discrete band pattern evident 1 week earlier (Fig. 4), and the residual light component (dissociated at pH 11 from the precipitate fraction) migrated as a slow band extending back to the origin (Fig. 5b). After prolonged LiCl treatment, the supernatant fractions showed progressively slower electrophoretic components (Fig. 5 c, e, g), and the precipitate fractions showed concomitant increase in the proportion of trailing material, presumably aggregated protein (Fig. 5 d, f, h). Similar

Cellulose acetate electrophoresis was performed on light component from supernatant and precipitate fractions (after solubilization in 0.4 *M* KCl and fractionation by alkali-dilution). (a), Supernatant, 5 min LiCl; (b), precipitate, 5 min LiCl; (c), supernatant, 1 hr LiCl; (d), precipitate, 1 hr LiCl; (e), supernatant, 24 hr LiCl; (f), precipitate, 24 hr LiCl; (g), supernatant, 72 hr LiCl; (h), precipitate, 72 hr LiCl.

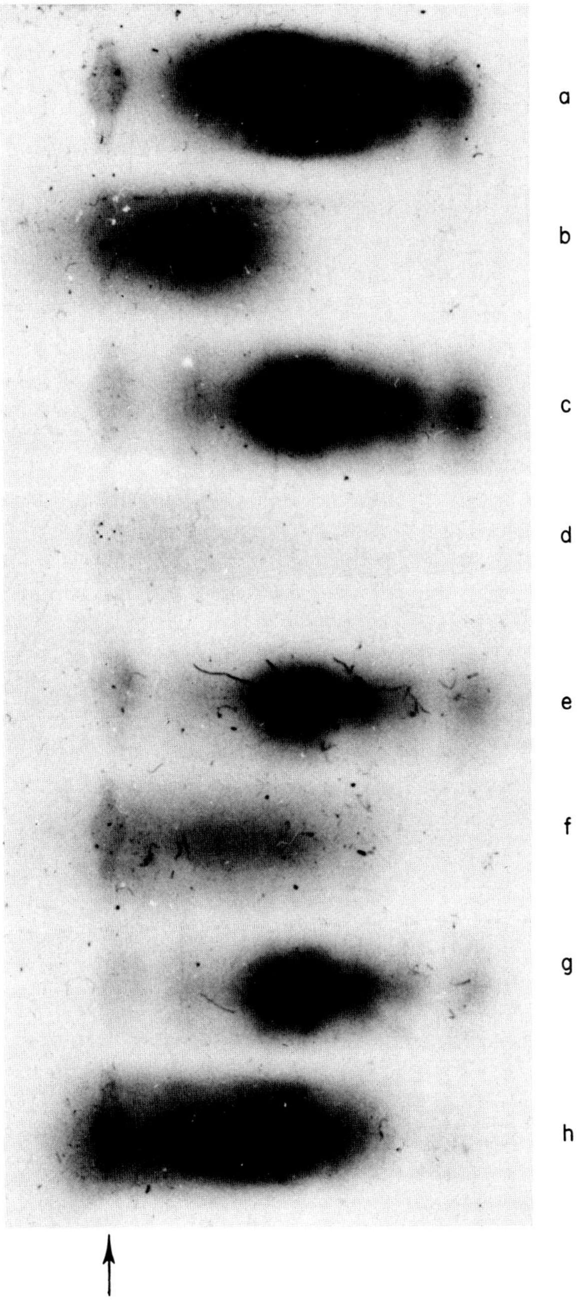

FIG. 5. Effect of aging and prolonged LiCl treatment on light component of myosin. The same preparation of myosin as used in Fig. 4 stored for 1 week, then titrated in 4 *M* LiCl for times indicated prior to citrate salting out. Final volumes were equivalent for all samples, and total dye intensity is roughly proportional with the yield of recovered protein.

experiments on light component isolated on prolonged alkaline treatment of aged preparations of myosin showed transformation of the discrete band pattern into a diffuse distribution, without formation of additional discrete bands. In general, the loss of discrete electrophoretic bands was more pronounced in the absence of thiol protection, but occurred despite the presence of dithiothreitol during purification and/or the electrophoretic procedure.

A fraction of the light component is dissociated from myosin on short treatment in 4.7 *M* NH_4Cl (page 182), and, as noted below (page 195), the dissociation of 3% light component by NH_4Cl treatment of myosin does not result in significant loss of Ca-ATPase or ADP binding by the residual myosin. This would indicate that part of the light component is not essential for ATPase activity or substrate binding (Gershman and Dreizen, 1969a,c; Dreizen and Gershman, 1969b, 1970b), and one questions whether or not NH_4Cl dissociation of myosin represents selective dissociation of light chains from myosin. Accordingly, electrophoretic experiments were done on light component isolated by ammonium sulfate fractionation of myosin in 4.7 *M* NH_4Cl. Interestingly, the supernatant fraction from 5-min treatment in 4.7 *M* NH_4Cl and salting out with 50% saturated $(NH_4)_2SO_4$ contains mostly protein of the fast electrophoretic band (Fig. 6c), whereas the precipitate fraction contains some fast component and the other electrophoretic components (Fig. 6d). On solubilization of the precipitate in 4.7 *M* NH_4Cl and salting out by 100% saturated $(NH_4)_2SO_4$, there is additional dissociation of light component from one of the slower electrophoretic bands (Fig. 6d). The same two bands are also dissociated from myosin on prolonged NH_4Cl–50% saturated $(NH_4)_2SO_4$ salting out and by 3.5 *M* LiCl-citrate salting out (Fig. 6e), conditions under which about half of the total light component is dissociated from myosin.

Myosin preparations exhibit trace myokinase activity, and this activity may be recovered in the supernatant fraction from rapid NH_4Cl–50% $(NH_4)_2SO_4$ salting out (Gershman and Dreizen, 1969a, 1970). Although rabbit skeletal myokinase (Noda and Kuby, 1957) has almost the same molecular weight as that of the myosin light chains, myokinase migrates more slowly than the fast electrophoretic component (Fig. 6f), and for other reasons as well cannot be identified with the predominant part of the NH_4Cl dissociated light component (Gershman and Dreizen, 1969a,c; 1970).

Locker and Hagyard (1967b) have shown that the light component dissociated from myosin by acetylation exhibits different electrophoretic bands in preparations isolated from red, white, and cardiac muscle. Our own experiments confirm that light chains dissociated from myosin by alkaline or salt treatment (in the absence of any chemical modification of the protein) differ in preparations obtained from red, white, and intermediate muscle

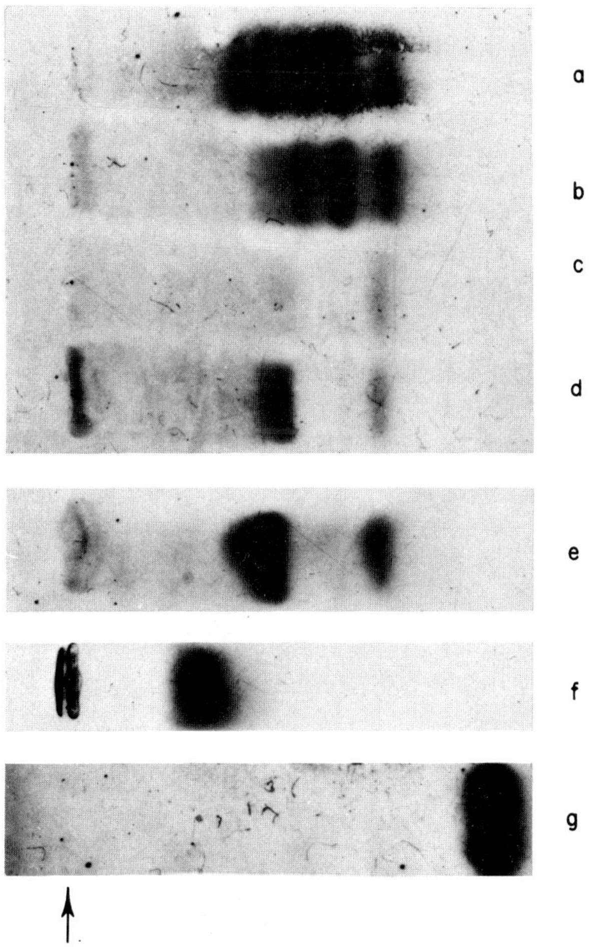

FIG. 6. Selective dissociation of light component from myosin. (a) Precipitate fraction from 5 min 4.7 *M* NH_4Cl–50% saturated $(NH_4)_2SO_4$ salting out; (b) precipitate from (a) was dissolved in 4.7 *M* NH_4Cl and salted out with 100% saturated $(NH_4)_2SO_4$; (c) supernatant fraction, same experiment as (a); (d) precipitate fraction, same experiment as (b); (e) supernatant fraction from 5 min 3.5 *M* LiCl-citrate salting out; (f) rabbit skeletal myokinase (Sigma); (g) bovine serum albumin (Armour).

fibers. For example, although the light component from white and intermediate muscle myosin shows the same fast migrating band, its trailing bands differ (Fig. 7). In conjunction with the results of recombination experiments described below (page 195), our present interpretation is that native myosin contains two essential light chains which are sampled from a population of three or more electrophoretically different light chains, the

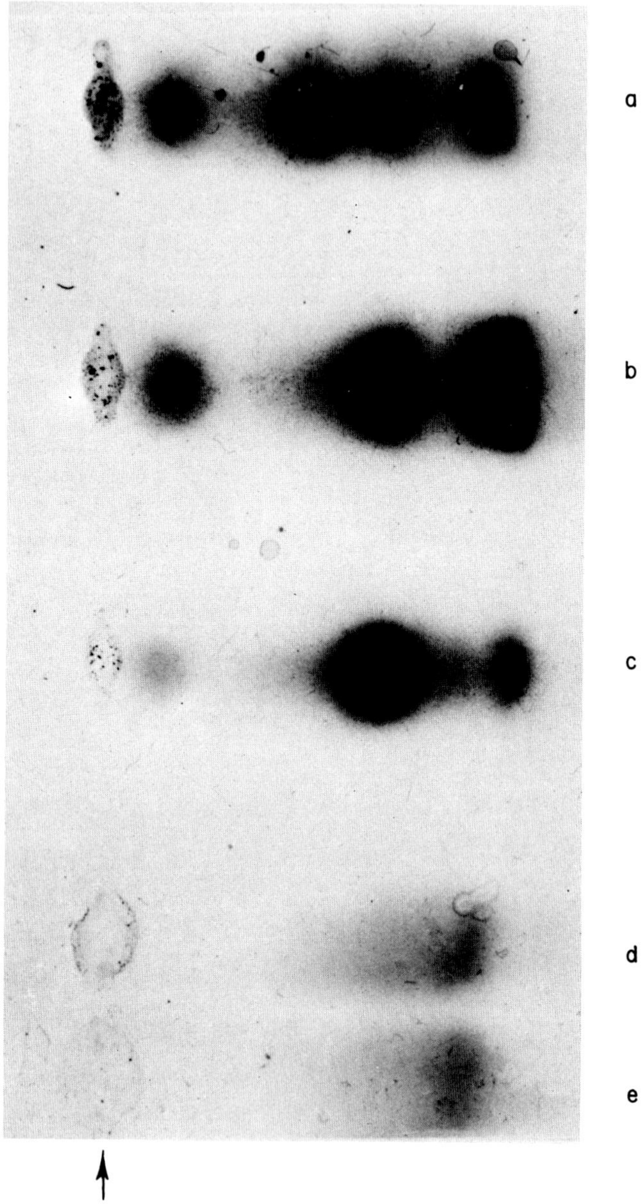

FIG.7. Heterogeneity of light component in myosin isolated from white (back) and intermediate (leg) rabbit skeletal muscle. (a) Supernatant, pH 11-dilution, intermediate muscle; (b) supernatant, pH 11-dilution, white muscle; (c) precipitate, 5 min 4.7 *M* NH_4Cl–50% saturated $(NH_4)_2SO_4$ salting out, white muscle; (d) supernatant, same experiment as (c); (e) supernatant, 5 min NH_4Cl–50% saturated $(NH_4)_2SO_4$ salting out, intermediate muscle.

exact distribution of which varies in myosin from red, white, and intermediate muscle. An additional light chain that does not appear to be essential for the enzymatic activity of myosin migrates as a distinct (fast) electrophoretic component.

Myosin–Nucleotide Interaction

Effect of Dissociating Conditions on Myosin ATPase

The presence of light and heavy chains within the enzymatically active portion of myosin (Gershman *et al.*, 1966; Trotta *et al.*, 1968) raises the question whether light chains, heavy chains, or both, are involved in the ATPase property of myosin. Our intent was to explore the possible dependence of ATPase activity on subunit composition by means of ATPase assays following alkaline or guanidine dissociation of myosin and subunit recombination in varying proportion; however, both alkaline and guanidine treatment were found to be accompanied by irreversible inactivation of Ca-ATPase (Gershman *et al.*, 1966, 1968a,b; Dreizen *et al.*, 1967). This prompted an examination of the relationship between subunit dissociation and irreversible ATPase inactivation during denaturation of myosin, and a concomitant search for methods of dissociating myosin into light and heavy components without total loss of ATPase activity.

Heat Denaturation

Treatment of myosin at temperatures above 25°C results in irreversible inactivation of ATPase (Oellet *et al.*, 1952) and dissociation of the light component (Locker, 1956). Both phenomena follow first-order kinetics, with similar values for activation enthalpy (about 55 kcal/mole) and activation entropy (~100 eu); however, the overall rate for ATPase inactivation exceeds that for light chain dissociation (Gershman, 1968; Gershman *et al.*, 1968a, 1969). Hence, heat denaturation does not provide a useful way to carry out recombination experiments on myosin ATPase, but the kinetic parameters do indicate that ATPase inactivation and subunit dissociation are thermodynamically comparable denaturation phenomena characterized by disruption of enthalpic bonds and loss of ordered structure.

Alkaline Denaturation

On alkaline titration of myosin in 0.4 *M* KCl, the light component is fully dissociated from the heavy chain core on increase from pH 10 to pH 11 (Fig. 8, upper). Despite nearly complete reassociation of light and heavy compounds on return to pH 7, titration of myosin above pH 10 leads to

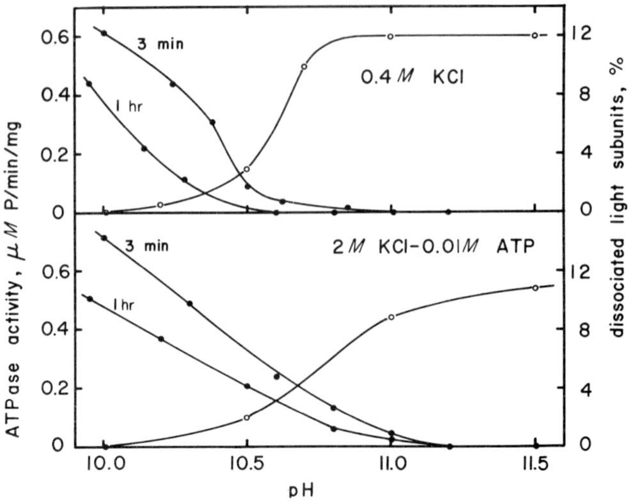

FIG. 8. pH dependence of light chain dissociation and irreversible inactivation of Ca-ATPase. Myosin in 0.4 *M* KCl (upper) or 2 *M* KCl–0.01 *M* ATP (lower) was titrated to a set pH with K_2CO_3–KOH solution, 4°C. The percentage dissociation of light component (O) was determined from sedimentation velocity experiments initiated promptly after alkaline titration. Ca-ATPase (●) was assayed on samples at alkaline pH for 3 min and 1 hr, respectively, prior to dialysis against 0.4 *M* KCl, 0.005 *M* $NaHCO_3$, pH 7. From Gershman *et al.* (1969).

irreversible inactivation of Ca-ATPase (Fig. 8, upper). Thus, at pH 10.5, there is partial dissociation of light chains and time-dependent ATPase inactivation, while at pH 11.0, ATPase activity is totally lost within several minutes (Gershman, 1968; Gershman *et al.*, 1968a, 1969). The use of dithiothreitol, EDTA, and inorganic phosphate was found to be unsuccessful in protecting myosin ATPase from alkaline denaturation. However, about 10% of the original ATPase activity was recovered following brief treatment of myosin in 2 *M* KCl–0.01 *M* ATP, pH 11.0, and dialysis to 0.4 *M* KCl, pH 7 (Fig. 8, lower). The effect of 2 *M* KCl–0.01 *M* ATP appears to involve stabilization of the myosin structure to alkaline dissociation, as the transition for light chain dissociation is also shifted upwards by 0.25–0.5 pH units.

It should be noted that data on alkaline denaturation of myosin ATPase are somewhat controversial at present. Most investigators have described time-dependent inactivation of myosin ATPase on alkaline treatment above pH 10.0 (Mommaerts and Green, 1954; Stracher, 1961; Seidel, 1967; Gaetjens *et al.*, 1968); however, Frederiksen and Holtzer (1968) have reported that myosin titrated to pH 7 and back-titrated to pH 7 retained 50–80% control ATPase, the extent of enzymatic recovery being independent of duration of alkaline treatment for periods up to 100 min. We have reinvestigated the discrepancy in results and were unable to account for it by minor differences in pH or the method of alkaline treatment, but we did find that traces of inorganic phosphate in the myosin preparation may lead to spurious "ATPase" values, unless inorganic phosphate is sequentially determined during reaction of alkaline-treated myosin with ATP (Dreizen and Gershman, 1970a). This artifact would not be picked up by the customary procedure (used by Frederiksen and Holtzer) of basing "ATPase" on a 5-min determination of inorganic phosphate, but whether or not this kind of effect was contributory to the Frederiksen–Holtzer data is, of course, unknown.

Guanidine Denaturation

The light component is fully dissociated from the intact heavy-chain core on increase from 1 to 2 *M* guanidine, and myosin dialyzed back to 0.4 *M* KCl after 5 min guanidine treatment shows total loss of ATPase activity, despite thiol protection with 0.001 *M* dithiothreitol (Gershman *et al.*, 1969).

Salt Denaturation

Subunit dissociation of myosin in concentrated salt solutions, pH 7, 4°C, is also characterized by irreversible inactivation of Ca-ATPase (Gershman, 1968; Gershman *et al.*, 1968a,b; Dreizen and Gershman, 1970b). Thus, upon treatment of myosin in salt solutions like NaCl or KCl in which the subunit structure remains intact at salt concentrations up to saturation, there is complete or nearly complete recovery of Ca-ATPase on dialysis back to 0.4 *M* KCl. In contrast, on treatment of myosin in those salt solutions in which the light chains are fully dissociated from myosin, there is irreversible inactivation of Ca-ATPase at or slightly below the transition concentration for light chain dissociation. For example, on treatment of myosin in LiCl solutions (Fig. 9), the light component is dissociated on increase from 3 to 4 *M* LiCl; after dialysis back to 0.4 *M* KCl the recovery of Ca-ATPase is sharply decreased over the same range of LiCl concentration, despite nearly complete reassociation of light and heavy components. Although the rate of ATPase inactivation is somewhat diminished in the presence of 0.001 *M* dithiothreitol, the occurrence of some ATPase inactivation even with thiol protection would implicate inclusion of groups other than sulfhydryl groups in the irreversible denaturation of myosin ATPase. On treatment of myosin at LiCl concentrations below 3 *M*, there is also slow denaturation of Ca-ATPase, presumably from reaction of the same (or other) groups within the intact myosin molecule.

Thus, a number of very different solvent conditions, including heat treatment, alkaline pH, guanidine solutions, and concentrated salt solutions, are all manifest by a close relationship between the dissociation of myosin into

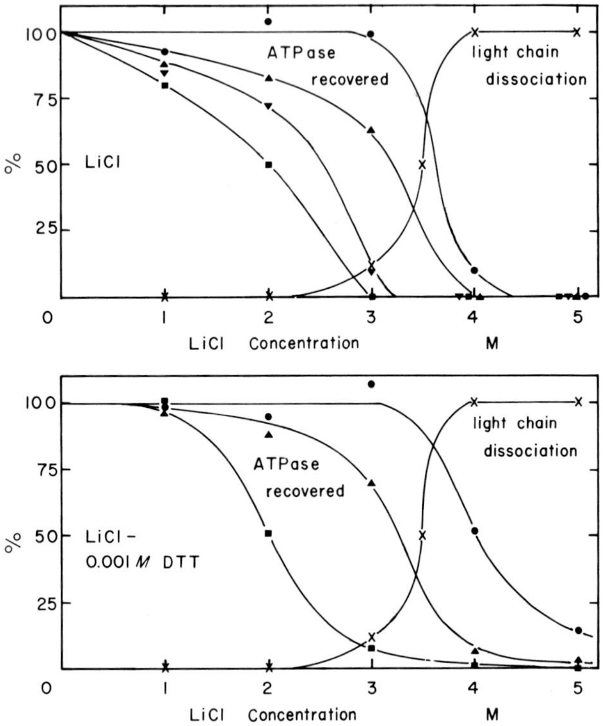

FIG. 9. Denaturation profile for myosin in LiCl solutions, pH 7, 4°C. % Dissociation of light component (×) from sedimentation velocity experiments initiated promptly after adjustment of salt concentration; Ca-ATPase was assayed on samples treated in specified salt solutions for 5 min (●), 2 hr (▲), 8 hr (▼), and 24 hr (■) prior to dialysis against 0.4 *M* KCl, 0.005 *M* $NaHCO_3$, pH 7. From Dreizen and Gershman (1970b).

light and heavy components and the rapid irreversible inactivation of Ca-ATPase. The simplest explanation for this relationship would be that sulfhydryl groups and/or other side-chain groups at or near the hydrolytic site undergo covalent reaction(s) during subunit dissociation under denaturing conditions. The relationship between light chain dissociation and ATPase loss also suggests that some kind of interaction between light and heavy chains may be involved in myosin ATPase (Dreizen *et al.*, 1967; Gershman, 1968; Gershman *et al.*, 1968a,b).

The interpretation is complicated, however, by the ratio of close to three light chains to two heavy chains, and the further evidence that some of the light component is not required for ATPase activity (Gershman and Dreizen, 1969a,c; Dreizen and Gershman, 1970b). Myosin stored in 4.7 *M* NH_4Cl undergoes irreversible inactivation of Ca-ATPase according to first-order kinetics. This effect is presumably due to reaction of heavy metal contaminants in the NH_4Cl reagent with critical sulfhydryl groups on myosin, since the rate of enzymatic inactivation is appreciably lower in the presence of 0.001 *M* EDTA or 0.001 *M* dithiothreitol. Extrapolation to zero-time of NH_4Cl treatment indicates almost full recovery of Ca-ATPase, despite irreversible dissociation of 3% light component from myosin. As noted above (page 188), the NH_4Cl dissociated light component contains a single (fast) electrophoretic band, and would thus appear to include a distinct polypeptide chain that is not essential for myosin ATPase.

Recombination Experiments

The partial recovery of myosin ATPase after alkaline treatment in 2 *M* KCl–0.01 *M* ATP permitted recombination experiments to be done in which myosin in 2 *M* KCl–0.01 *M* ATP was titrated to pH 11.0 and promptly salted out with potassium citrate (Gaetjens *et al.*, 1968); the precipitate and supernatant fractions were recombined in different proportions, and dialyzed against 0.4 *M* KCl, pH 7, for ATPase assays or against 0.4 *M* KCl, 0.1 *M* Na_2CO_3, pH 11.0, for determination of subunit composition by sedimentation velocity or sedimentation equilibrium. Fully reconstituted myosin retained 0.1 μM P_i/min/mg ATPase activity. Samples containing less than 12% light component showed a decrease in ATPase activity, and purified but otherwise identically treated heavy and light components showed negligible ATPase activity (Dreizen and Gershman, 1969a; Gershman *et al.*, 1969).

Similar experiments were performed in which myosin in 4 *M* LiCl was promptly salted out with 60% saturated potassium citrate; and supernatant and precipitate fractions were recombined in different proportions (Dreizen and Gershman, 1969a,b; 1970b). With dithiothreitol present throughout, fully reconstituted myosin showed 0.49 μM P_i/min/mg Ca-ATPase, that is, about 70% of control ATPase activity. There was a sharp decrease of ATPase activity in protein reconstituted with less than 8% light component (Fig. 10), and Ca-ATPase was totally lost in protein reconstituted with only 2% light component and in light component alone. In recombination experiments performed without dithiothreitol or EDTA, only 0.12 μM P_i/min/mg Ca-ATPase was recovered in reconstituted myosin, but significantly less Ca-ATPase was recovered in samples with 6–8% light component (Fig. 10). Recombination experiments based on LiCl-citrate fractionation of the precipitate obtained from 5 min NH_4Cl–50% saturated $(NH_4)_2SO_4$ salting out in 0.001 *M* dithiothreitol yielded results comparable with those described on native myosin (Fig. 10). In parallel experiments based on chromatographic fractionation of myosin in 4 *M* LiCl, Stracher (1968) has described recovery of 30% control ATPase activity in reconstituted myosin, and no activity in the purified light or heavy components.

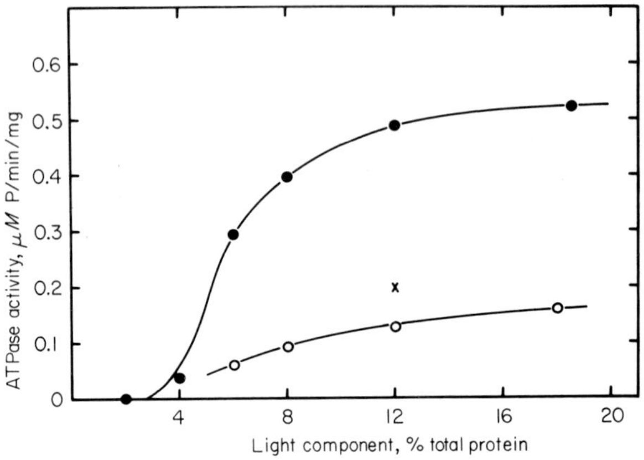

FIG. 10. Ca-ATPase plotted with respect to proportion of light component in protein, from experiments based on 4 *M* LiCl-citrate fractionation of myosin and subunit recombination in different proportions. (●) 0.001 *M* dithiothreitol present throughout; (×) 0.001 *M* EDTA present during 4 *M* LiCl-citrate salting out; (O) neither dithiothreitol nor EDTA present. From Dreizen and Gershman (1970b).

The overall findings provide strong support for the conclusion that myosin proper contains two enzymatically active protomers, each comprising one heavy chain and one essential light chain, and that an interaction between essential light and heavy chains is implicated in the ATPase activity of myosin. This interaction might possibly involve the participation of residues from essential light and heavy chains at or near the hydrolytic site. Alternatively, one subunit, e.g., the heavy chain, might contain the hydrolytic site and the adjacent subunit (essential light chain, according to this model) might stabilize the unique heavy chain conformation required for enzymatic activity.

Although the recombination experiments on Ca-ATPase leave this important question unsettled, additional insight into the nature of the myosin–nucleotide interaction is gleaned from recombination experiments on substrate binding. Myosin contains 1.3 to 1.8 ADP binding sites per molecule (Kiely and Martonosi, 1969; Lowey and Luck, 1969), whereas each subfragment-1 particle contains 1 ADP binding site (Young, 1967). In order to delineate which subunits may be involved in ADP binding, equilibrium dialysis was performed on ADP (0.1–2.0 μM) against reconstituted myosin in 0.4 *M* KCl, 0.001 *M* $MgCl_2$, 0.001 *M* dithiothreitol, after LiCl-citrate fractionation and subunit recombination in varying proportion (Dreizen and Gershman, 1969b, 1970a,b). The experiments indicated approximately 1.6 ADP binding sites per molecule of reconstituted myosin, with or without the

NH_4Cl dissociated light chain present. The number of ADP binding sites was diminished in samples containing less of the essential light chains, and there was no evident binding to heavy chain core or light chains alone. The apparent free energy for binding was 6.8 ($\pm$0.3) kcal/mole ADP, irrespective of the ratio of light chains to heavy chains. These findings indicate that ADP binding also involves some kind of interaction between essential light and heavy chains. The simplest explanation by far would be that ADP directly bridges essential light and heavy chains within each protomer, but the present experiments do not of course exclude the possibility of weak interaction ($<$4 kcal/mole) of ATP with essential light or heavy chains alone.

With respect to the additional light chain that does not seem to be essential for Ca-ATPase activity or ADP binding by myosin, the evidence on this matter is not yet certain, but our present interpretation (Gershman and Dreizen, 1969a,c, 1970; Dreizen and Gershman, 1970a,b) is that the nonessential light chain (fast electrophoretic band) represents a distinct protein, termed *myonin*, that is closely associated with myosin proper. There is preliminary evidence that this component binds Ca^{2+}, but not as strongly as does troponin A (Hartshorne and Dreizen, unpublished data).

Triphosphate Bridging Hypothesis

The myosin structure appears to be somewhat more stable on alkaline treatment in 2 *M* KCl–0.01 *M* ATP than in 0.4 *M* KCl (Fig. 8). Even more striking evidence of subunit stabilization by ATP in concentrated salt solutions is obtained on LiCl denaturation of myosin in 0.01 *M* ATP, where the transition for light chain dissociation is increased from 3.5 *M* to 5.0 *M* LiCl (Dreizen and Gershman, 1969a,b, 1970a). One questions which groups of ATP are responsible for stabilization of the myosin structure. In 0.01 *M* triphosphate, the transition for light-chain dissociation is also increased from 3.5 to 5.0 *M* LiCl; ADP and pyrophosphate result in somewhat less stabilization of myosin to LiCl denaturation, and inorganic phosphate exerts no significant effect on the denaturation transition. In 0.01 *M* AMP and 0.01 *M* adenosine tetraphosphate, there is a decrease in the transition for light chain dissociation to 2.5 *M* LiCl. Adenosine, adenine, and ribose have no effect on the denaturation transition; and ITP, CTP, and GTP result in less stabilization of the myosin structure than is obtained with ATP.

Thus, stabilization of the subunit structure of myosin to LiCl denaturation derives predominantly from interaction with the terminal phosphate groups of ATP. Maximal stabilization is obtained with the triphosphate moiety, and the nucleotide base exerts only minor modification of this effect. In a crude sense, one may consider the myosin–nucleotide interaction as a kind

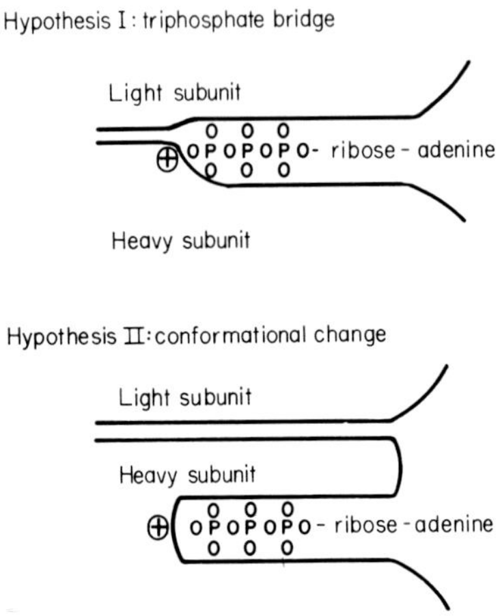

FIG. 11. Alternative models for nucleotide binding to myosin protomer. Representation is schematic and does not show the nonlinearity of the phosphate chain owing to the tetrahedral orientation of σ orbitals of phosphorous, nor the possibility of free rotation about the ester and/or β-glycosidic linkages of ribose (Szent-Györgyi, 1957).

of lock-and-key arrangement, where triphosphate provides optimal fit and the nucleotides base acts in a regulatory role.

Figure 11 illustrates two plausible ways in which the stabilization data may be reconciled with the recombination experiments on Ca-ATPase and ADP binding. Hypothesis I involves bridging by the triphosphate part of ATP between essential light and heavy chains in the region of the active site. According to this hypothesis, both subunits would be required for ATP splitting and substrate binding ($\Delta F^\circ \sim 6.8$ kcal/mole), and the protomeric structure is stabilized by electrostatic interactions along the phosphate chain. Hypothesis II involves an allosteric relationship between nucleotide binding and subunit interactions, in which nucleotide is bound to one subunit (shown here as a heavy chain) at a site not too distant from the contact zone between light and heavy subunits. According to hypothesis II, there would be a linkage phenomenon between nucleotide (or triphosphate) binding and some energetically favorable conformational state of the protomer. Although decisive evidence favoring hypothesis I or II (among others) is not yet available, the absence of catalytic activity or substrate binding ($\Delta F^\circ \sim 6.8$ kcal/mole) in light and heavy subunits alone, and the spectral effect of chain phosphates and nucleotides on the subunit interactions of myosin appear more suggestive of a nucleotide bridge (hypothesis I) than a simple two-state allosteric model (hypothesis II).

In recent experiments we have tested the overall interpretation by determining the electrophoretic components dissociated from myosin by 4 *M* LiCl–0.01 *M* triphosphate. Interestingly, the fast electrophoretic band is selectively dissociated under these conditions, confirming that triphosphate stabilizes the interaction of the heavy chain core with essential light chains, but not the nonessential light chain (NH_4Cl dissociated light component).

Conclusions

On the basis of ultracentrifugal data on native myosin and its proteolytic fragments under different dissociating conditions (pages 180-183), electrophoretic experiments on the light component of native myosin (page 184), and denaturation and recombination experiments on ATPase and ADP binding (page 195), it would appear that myosin contains two enzymatically active protomers, each comprising one heavy chain (210,000 MW) and one essential light chain (20,000 MW) that is sampled from a population of three or more electrophoretically different light chains. An interaction between essential light and heavy chains is involved in Ca-ATPase and ADP binding, and it has been proposed from several lines of evidence that the triphosphate part of ATP directly bridges light and heavy chains within each protomer. That essential light chains differ electrophoretically in myosin preparations isolated from red, white, and intermediate rabbit skeletal muscle would suggest that myosin has multiple molecular forms and presumably represents an isozyme system. Preparations of native myosin also contain trace amounts of myokinase and a light chain (fast electrophoretic band) that is not essential for Ca-ATPase or ADP binding and tentatively may be considered a distinct protein (*myonin*) that is closely associated with myosin proper.

The general implications of this work with respect to the role of myosin in muscular contraction have already been discussed (Dreizen and Gershman, 1970a).

This volume is devoted to cardiac hypertrophy and we have not yet referred to hypertrophy, nor even to the heart. Although the work here presented was done on rabbit skeletal myosin, comparable features are found in myosin isolated from rabbit and dog cardiac muscle (unpublished data) and also human skeletal muscle (Gershman and Dreizen, 1969b). We would be amiss not to speculate that cardiac hypertrophy and possibly heart failure itself may involve subtle variations of the subunit composition of myosin. The enzymatic splitting of ATP plays a unique role in the contractile process, and the evidence for light-chain heterogeneity reveals obvious potential for other changes that might occur in disease states.

Acknowledgments

We gratefully acknowledge the technical assistance of Aida L. Capulong and Dennis H. Richards. We also thank M. S. Drapkin, P. J. Edelson, S. C. Kimler, R. M. Levy, R. Mann, L. M. Russakoff, and L. E. Shapiro for their contributions, both direct and indirect, and we thank Alfred Stracher and the others in his laboratory for the many helpful and heated discussions.

Supported by research grants from the National Institutes of Health (AM-06165), the Health Research Council of New York City (U-1365), and the New York Heart Association.

LCG was recipient of a Fellowship from the Life Insurance Medical Research Fund, and PD is Career Investigator of the Health Research Council of New York City.

References

Connell, J. J., and Olcott, H. S. (1961). *Arch. Biochem. Biophys.* **94**, 128.

Dreizen, P., and Gershman, L. C. (1969a). *Biophysical J.* **9**, A236.

Dreizen, P., and Gershman, L. C. (1969b). *Abstr. 3rd Int. Biophys. Congr., Cambridge*, p. 183.

Dreizen, P., and Gershman, L. C. (1970a). *Trans. N.Y. Acad. Sci.* **32**, 170.

Dreizen, P., and Gershman, L. C. (1970b). *Biochemistry* **9**, 1688

Dreizen, P., Hartshorne, D. J., and Stracher, A. (1966). *J. Biol. Chem.* **241**, 443.

Dreizen, P., Gershman, L. C., Trotta, P. P., and Stracher, A. (1967). *J. Gen. Phys.* **50**, part 2, 85.

Frederiksen, D. W., and Holtzer, A. (1968). *Biochemistry* **7**, 3935.

Gaetjens, E., Bárány, K., Bailin, G., Oppenheimer, H., and Bárány, M. (1968). *Arch. Biochem. Biophys.* **123**, 82.

Gershman, L. C. (1968). Ph.D. Thesis. State University of New York Downstate Medical Center, Brooklyn, New York.

Gershman, L. C., and Dreizen, P. (1969a). *Biophys. J.* **9**, A235.

Gershman, L. C., and Dreizen, P. (1969b). *Clin. Res.* **17**, 241.

Gershman, L. C., and Dreizen, P. (1969c). *Abstr. 3rd Int. Biophys. Congr., Cambridge*, p. 183.

Gershman, L. C., and Dreizen, P. (1970). *Biochemistry* **9**, 1677.

Gershman, L. C., Dreizen, P., and Stracher, A. (1966). *Proc. Nat. Acad. Sci. U.S.* **56**, 966.

Gershman, L. C., Stracher, A., and Dreizen, P. (1968a). *Symp. Fibrous Proteins, Austral 1967*, Butterworths, Australia, p. 150.

Gershman, L. C., Stracher, A., and Dreizen, P. (1968b). *Bull. N.Y. Acad. Med.* **44**, 1115.

Gershman, L. C., Stracher, A., and Dreizen, P. (1969). *J. Biol. Chem.* **244**, 2726.

Hanson, J., and Huxley, H. E. (1955). *Symp. Soc. Exp. Biol.* **9**, 228.

Hartshorne, D. J., and Stracher, A. (1966). *Biochem. Z.* **345**, 70.

Hartshorne, D. J., and Dreizen, P. (unpublished data).

Holtzer, A., and Lowey, S. (1959). *J. Amer. Chem. Soc.* **81**, 1370.

Huxley, H. E. (1963). *J. Mol. Biol.* **7**, 281.

Kielley, W. W., and Harrington, W. F. (1960). *Biochim. Biophys. Acta* **41**, 401.

Kiely, B., and Martonosi, A. (1969). *Biochim. Biophys. Acta* **172**, 158.

Kominz, D. R., Carroll, W. R., Smith, E. N., and Mitchell, E. R. (1959). *Arch. Biochem. Biophys.* **79**, 191.

Kominz, D. R., Mitchell, E. R., Nihei, T., and Kay, C. M. (1965). *Biochemistry* **4**, 2373.

Locker, R. H. (1956). *Biochim. Biophys. Acta* **20**, 514.

Locker, R. H., and Hagyard, C. J. (1967a). *Arch. Biochem. Biophys.* **120**, 241.
Locker, R. H., and Hagyard, C. J. (1967b). *Arch. Biochem. Biophys.* **122**, 521.
Lowey, S., and Holtzer, A. (1959). *Biochim. Biophys. Acta* **34**, 470.
Lowey, S., and Luck, S. M. (1969). *Biochemistry* **8**, 3195.
Mihályi, E., and Szent-Györgyi, A. G. (1953). *J. Biol. Chem.* **201**, 211.
Mommaerts, W. F. H. M., and Green, I. (1954). *J. Biol. Chem.* **208**, 833.
Mueller, H. (1964). *J. Biol. Chem.* **239**, 797.
Mueller, H., and Perry, S. V. (1962). *Biochem. J.* **85**, 431.
Nauss, K. N., and Gergely, J. (1967). *Fed. Proc. Fed. Amer. Soc. Exp. Biol.* **26**, 727.
Noda, L., and Kuby, S. A. (1957). *J. Biol. Chem.* **226**, 551.
Ouellet, L., Laidler, K. J., and Morales, M. F. (1952). *Arch. Bioch. Biophys.* **39**, 37.
Rice, R. V. (1964). *In* "Biochemistry of Muscular Contraction" (J. Gergely, ed.), p. 41. Little Brown, Boston, Massachusetts.
Seidel, J. C. (1967). *J. Biol. Chem.* **242**, 5623.
Slayter, H. S., and Lowey, S. (1967). *Proc. Nat. Acad. Sci. U.S.* **58**, 1612.
Small, P. A., Harrington, W. F., and Kielley, W. W. (1961). *Biochim. Biophys. Acta* **49**, 462.
Stracher, A. (1961). *J. Biol. Chem.* **236**, 2467.
Stracher, A. (1969). *Bioch. Biophys. Res. Commun.* **35**, 519.
Stracher, A., and Dreizen, P. (1966). *Curr. Topics Bioenerget.* **1**, 153.
Szent-Györgyi, A. (1957). "Bioenergetics". Academic Press, New York.
Szent-Györgyi, A. C. (1960). *In* "Proteins of the Myofibril" (G. H. Bourne, ed.), Vol. II, p. 1. Academic Press, New York.
Tonomura, Y., Appel, P., and Morales, M. F. (1966). *Biochemistry* **5**, 515.
Trotta, P. P., Dreizen, P., and Stracher, A. (1968). *Proc. Nat. Acad. Sci. U.S.* **61**, 659.
Tsao, T. C. (1953). *Biochim. Biophys. Acta* **11**, 368.
Wetlaufer, D. B., and Edsall, J. T. (1960). *Biochim. Biophys. Acta* **43**, 132.
Woods, E. F., Himmelfarb, S., and Harrington ,W. F. (1963). *J. Biol. Chem.* **238**, 2374.
Yasui, T., Hashimoto, Y., and Tonomura, Y. (1960). *Arch. Biochim. Biophys.* **87**, 55.
Young, M. (1967). *J. Biol. Chem.* **242**, 2790.
Yphantis, D. A. (1964). *Biochemistry* **3**, 297.
Zobel, C. R. (1967). *Biochim. Biophys. Acta* **140**, 222.

HIGH-ENERGY PHOSPHATE COMPOUNDS AND LDH ISOENZYMES IN THE HYPERTROPHIED RIGHT VENTRICLE

Arthur C. Fox

High-Energy Phosphate Compounds

The importance of ATP in muscular contraction prompted our examination of this and other high-energy phosphate compounds in the failing heart. It seemed possible that there might be a defect in energy storage or utilization during failure, as substrate uptake remains normal while cardiac performance declines (Blain *et al.*, 1956). Since hypertrophy of the chronically afterloaded heart precedes failure, and since the performance of the hypertrophied heart has been described both as normal or mildly impaired (Geha *et al.*, 1966; Spann *et al.*, 1967), we made the same measurements in hearts that were hypertrophied but not yet in failure.

Our experimental model was one in which right ventricular hypertrophy and failure could be sequentially produced in dogs by progressive tightening of a ligature in place around the main pulmonary artery (Fox *et al.*, 1965). With this preparation, the left ventricle can serve as a control for the chronically afterloaded right ventricle. To produce hypertrophy, right ventricular systolic pressures were kept at 75 mm Hg for periods of 3–14 weeks; there was no marked increase in end diastolic pressures, a–v O_2 was normal, and there was no edema or ascites. In the hypertrophied hearts, the ratios of the weights of the free walls of the RV/LV increased to 1/1 (normal, 0.6/1) and the RV's constituted 34% of the total ventricular mass (normal, 26%). To produce failure, RV systolic pressures were kept close to 100 mm Hg during repeated tightening of the pulmonary artery ligatures. The evidence for severe failure consisted of marked ascites and edema with great increases in heart size, right ventricular end-diastolic pressure, and in a–v O_2. The hearts were rapidly extirpated while beating or immediately after induction of cardiac arrest by injection into the cross-clamped aorta of 5 cc of 5%

TABLE I

NUCLEOTIDE CONTENT OF NORMAL AND FAILING RIGHT VENTRICLES REMOVED WHILE BEATING[a]

Sample	Total adenine nucleotides	ATP	ADP	AMP	UTP	GTP	NAD	UDP	GDP	CTP
16 normal hearts										
Mean	29.6	25.0	4.26	0.38	0.61	0.75	0.47	0.96	0.87	0.35
SE ±	0.63	0.59	0.14	0.03	0.06	0.08	0.11	0.09	0.12	0.02
8 failing hearts										
Mean	26.3	22.0	3.98	0.35	0.88	1.17	0.70	1.36	0.99	0.41
SE ±	0.53	0.47	0.16	0.04	0.09	0.16	0.16	0.24	0.13	0.07

[a] Right ventricle: μmoles/gm of fat-free, dry muscle.

potassium citrate @ pH 9, and were then plunged into liquid nitrogen. Large samples of both ventricles were carefully trimmed of adventitious tissue, and homogenized in 0/6 *N* P.C.A. The use of large samples rather than small biopsy specimens permitted better approximations of mean levels in the whole heart. Nucleotides were separated by gradient elution from Dowex 1 (Cl) X-10 resin columns and were measured by spectrophotometry. Creatine phosphate (CrP) was measured by two methods, with determination of free inorganic phosphate (I.P.) and creatine base (Cr) both before and after acid hydrolysis of CrP.

Nucleotide content was measured in 16 normal hearts and in eight failing hearts removed while beating. There were no significant differences between RV and LV in the normal hearts or between LV's from failing hearts. Table I compares the nucleotides of normal and failing RV's. The 12% decrease in ATP in the failing RV was significant with $p < 0.001$. It was unlikely that hydrolysis of ATP during extirpation had produced this difference, since levels of ADP and AMP were not increased. Levels of ATP were the same in hearts removed while beating or after induction of arrest.

Since CrP is much more labile than ATP, it was necessary to measure the phosphagen in hearts that were removed while in arrest. Table II shows that

TABLE II

CREATINE, CREATINE PHOSPHATE (BY TWO METHODS), INORGANIC PHOSPHATE AND TOTAL ACID-SOLUBLE PHOSPHATE IN NORMAL, HYPERTROPHIED, AND FAILING RIGHT VENTRICLES[a]

Sample	Total creatine	Free creatine	CrP (by base)	CrP (by P_i)	P_i	TASP
Normal (14)	130	79	51	52	21	198
Hypertrophied (6)	125	76	50	52	19	205
Failing (7)	82[b]	53[b]	29[b]	35[b]	20	173[b]

[a] Measured in μmoles/gm of fat-free dry weight.
[b] $P < 0.001$.

there were no differences between normal and hypertrophied RV's in Cr, CrP, P_i, or total acid soluble phosphate (TASP). Since CrP was normal in the hypertrophied hearts, it was unlikely that levels of ATP, which are maintained at the expense of CrP, were altered, and nucleotides were therefore not measured in hypertrophied hearts. In the failing hearts, there were marked decreases in Cr (−33%), CrP (−38%), and TASP (−12%). It is unlikely that these changes were a result of artifactual hydrolysis of CrP in the failing hearts, since levels of P_i were not changed and the ratios of CrP/total Cr were not changed (Fig. 1).

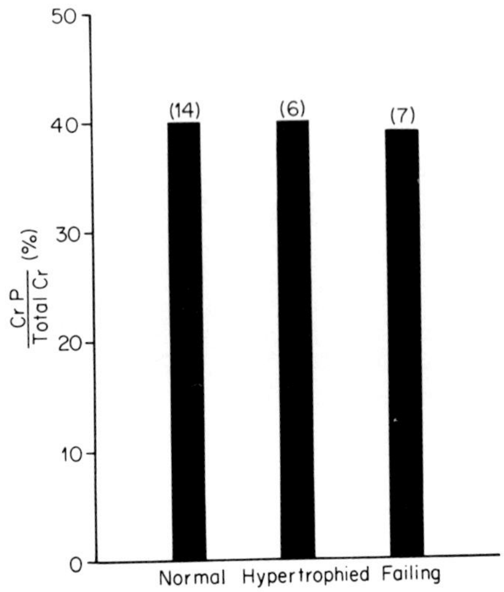

FIG. 1. Percentage of total creatine present as creatine phosphate in normal, hypertrophied, and failing right ventricles.

No changes in these compounds were found in hearts from three dogs with marked ascites and edema produced by partial ligation of the inferior vena cava, and there were no changes in CrP levels in skeletal muscle from animals with heart failure. It was therefore unlikely that a change in extracardiac Cr metabolism was responsible for the alterations found in the failing myocardium.

The dynamics of the decreases in ATP and CrP during failure were next explored by examining the rates at which radioactive inorganic phosphate ($^{32}P_i$) was incorporated into the phosphate groups of ATP. As indicated in Fig. 2, labeling of the terminal (γ) phosphate depends largely on mitochondrial oxidative phosphorylation which, in turn, is regulated by the production of ADP by myofibrillar ATPase. The rate of oxidative phosphoryla-

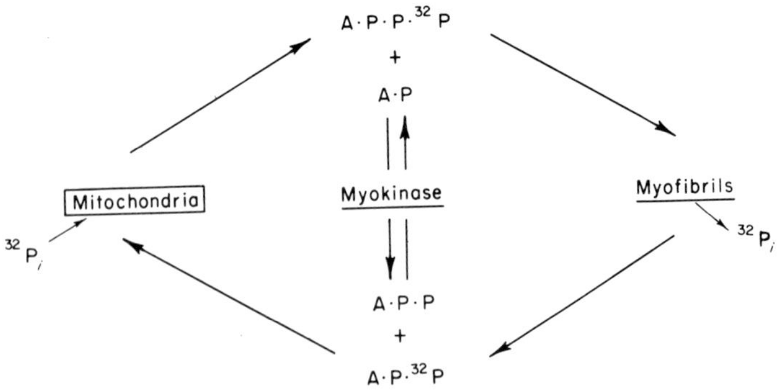

FIG. 2. Principal pathways within the myocardial cell for labeling of ATP phosphates.

tion can be only crudely estimated from the labeling of the γ phosphate of ATP, since "partial" reactions of oxidative phosphorylation such as the P_i–ATP exchange reaction also cause such labeling.

It seemed possible that a more specific, though indirect reflection of the relative rates of ADP production and oxidative phosphorylation might be provided by studying the rate at which the β phosphate of ATP is labeled via the myokinase reaction. This reaction maintains proper ratios of ATP/ADP at the mitochondria. A shift of the myokinase equilibrium towards the production of APP^{32}P would suggest a decreased production of ADP by myofibrillar ATPase; a shift away from the production of APP^{32}P would suggest increased production of ADP at the myofibrils (Fig. 2).

In preliminary studies, the labeling of ATP was examined in the right and left ventricles of normal hearts at varying intervals after injection of $^{32}P_i$ into the inferior vena cava. Comparable degrees of labeling were found in five normal hearts, 5 min after the injection, and labeling did not reach its maximum plateau before 15 min. This suggested that although differences in the permeability of various cell compartments to $^{32}P_i$ might variably retard delivery to the sites of oxidative phosphorylation, rough comparisons could be made between groups of hearts removed after 5 min. There were no differences between the five normal hearts and five failing hearts removed after 5 min. It was also found that labeling of the phosphates of ATP had reached equilibration after 5 min, making it impossible to estimate the direction of the myokinase equilibrium.

To obtain samples before labeling of the γ and β phosphates had reached equilibrium, we injected $^{32}P_i$ into the cross-clamped aorta together with a solution of K citrate, so that only a few contractions occurred before cardiac arrest, extirpation, and freezing. Figure 3 indicates that there were no sig-

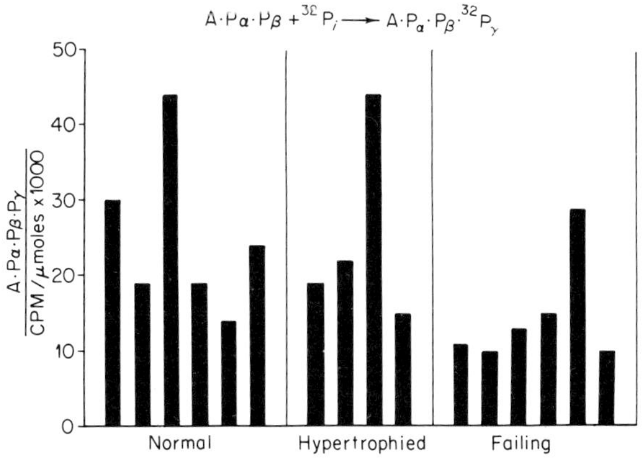

FIG. 3. Specific activity of ATP in normal, hypertrophied, and failing right ventricles immediately after intraaortic injection of $^{32}P_i$.

nificant differences in overall labeling of ATP in normal, hypertrophied, and failing hearts studied in this manner. Total labeling of ATP (largely in the γ phosphate) varied linearly with the amount of $^{32}P_i$ present in the whole tissue extracts, except for a group of hearts studied after injection of dinitrophenol (DNP), which markedly decreased labeling of ATP. This suggested that if a very marked change in oxidative phosphorylation had occurred in the hypertrophied or failing hearts (as in the DNP-treated hearts), our methods could have detected it.

Figure 4 shows that in normal hearts removed after intraaortic injection of $^{32}P_i$, labeling of the γ and β phosphates of ATP had not yet reached the equilibrium found after intravenous injection of $^{32}P_i$. This indicated that such hearts might be used for estimation of the instantaneous mean direction of the myokinase reaction (Fig. 2). Figure 4 also shows that in a small group of hypertrophied failing hearts there were no significant differences from the normal ratio of labeling in the γ and β phosphates of ATP, although the values are scattered.

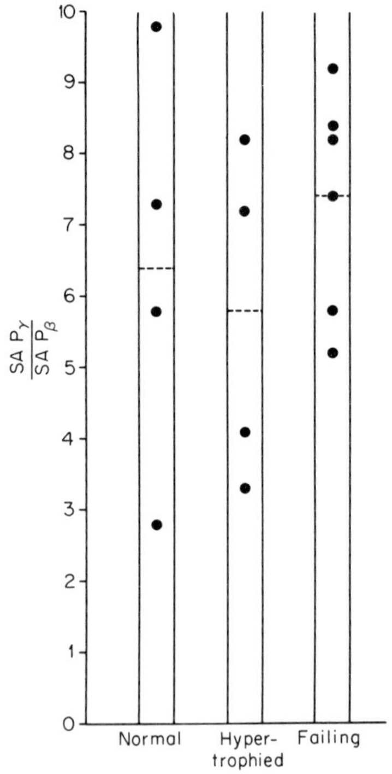

FIG. 4. Ratios between specific activities of the γ and β phosphates of $A \cdot P_\alpha \cdot P_\beta \cdot P_\gamma$ in normal, hypertrophied, and failing right ventricles immediately after intraaortic injection of $^{32}P_i$.

Since ATP and CrP were normal in the hypertrophied right ventricles, the results of the studies with $^{32}P_i$ suggest that with hypertrophy there were no changes in oxidative phosphorylation, in myofibrillar ATPase, or in the steady-state equilibrium between these two processes. With the appearance of right ventricular failure, levels of ATP and CrP fell, and the findings with $^{32}P_i$ seemed most compatible with a shift to a moderate decrease in both oxidative phosphorylation and myofibrillar ATPase activity. The limitations imposed on this conclusion by the techniques we used are detailed elsewhere (Fox and Reed, 1966).

LDH Isoenzymes

In associated studies, we examined the LDH composition of a similar group of canine hearts with marked right ventricular hypertrophy produced by pulmonary artery ligatures. The purpose was to use the isoenzyme patterns as a reflection of the *in vitro* metabolic state, and to help determine whether there is hypoxia in the myocardium that is undergoing hypertrophy in response to an increased pressure load (Fox and Reed, 1969).

LDH is an inducible enzyme that interconverts lactate and pyruvate. There are five isoenzymes which are formed as the two different subunits, *H* and *M*, combine as tetramers (Fig. 5). Early studies suggested that isoenzymes high in *H* subunits predominated in aerobic tissues and favor the conversion of lactate to pyruvate, whereas *M* units predominate in anaerobic tissues and favor the reverse reaction. Although the relevance of the differences in LDH isoenzymes to *in vivo* metabolism has been challenged, there appeared to be an adequate basis for exploring the possibility that if changes were found in

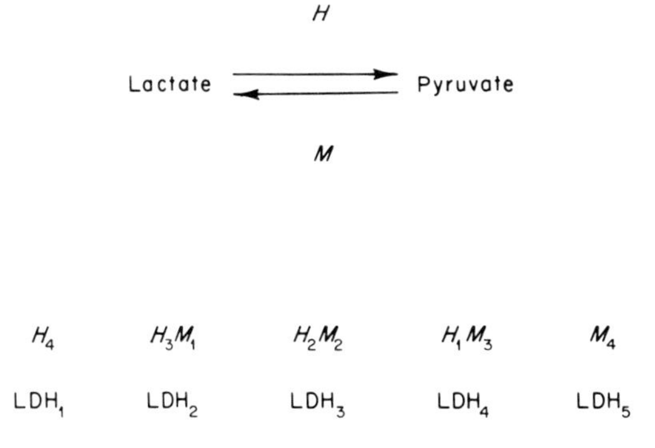

FIG. 5. Action and subunit composition of LDH isoenzymes.

hypertrophied hearts they might reflect hypoxia, growth, or both conditions.

Samples from multiple areas of 13 hypertrophied hearts were trimmed clean of visible vessels, endocardium, and pericardium, homogenized and analyzed for LDH composition by electrophoresis in tubes of 5% polyacrylamide. We determined subunit composition from the proportions found for each isoenzyme by microdensitometry of gels stained with tetrazolium. LDH activity was determined catalytically at low ($3 \times 10^{-4} M$) and high ($1 \times 10^{-2} M$) concentrations of pyruvate. The ratio of activities at low/high pyruvate was shown to vary directly with the concentration of H subunits; with more M subunits the "activity ratios" became lower.

In eight sham-operated hearts, in which ligatures were emplaced but not tightened, there were no significant differences between the LDH composition of the RV and LV (Table III). LDH composition was the same in the outer,

TABLE III

LDH COMPOSITION OF SHAM-OPERATED AND HYPERTROPHIED CANINE HEARTS

Sample		LDH isoenzymes (%) 1	2	3	4	5	H subunits (%)	Activity ratio	Total LDH activity μ/mg sol. protein
Sham-operated (8)	RV	45	48	7	tr.		85	2.73	6,886
	LV	44	47	8	tr.		84	2.76	7,319
RV hypertrophy (13)	RV	31[a]	47	20[a]	2	tr.	76[a]	2.44[a]	7,292
	LV	42	47	10	1	tr.	83	2.66	7,118
Connective tissue from Ivalon implants (8)		1	9	26	29	35	28	1.49	1,400

[a] Significant difference ($P < 0.001$).

inner, and middle thirds of the walls of both ventricles, despite the differences in pO_2 which reportedly exist between subepicardial and subendocardial myocardium in the beating heart (Kirk and Honig, 1964). In the hypertrophied RV's from 13 hearts with tightened pulmonary artery ligatures, there were significant decreases in LDH_1, with corresponding increases in LDH_3 and appropriate changes in the "activity ratios" of the myocardial extracts (Table III). There were no changes in total LDH activity. The differences were significant when compared with the paired LV's of each hypertrophied heart, or with RV's from sham-operated controls.

Additional studies were performed to help determine whether these changes in LDH composition truly occurred within myocardial cells, or simply reflected proliferation of connective tissue cells during hypertrophy. Connective tissue from Ivalon sponges used in the pulmonary artery ligatures showed large amounts of LDH_4 and LDH_5, isoenzymes which were not increased in the hypertrophied hearts (Table III). Furthermore, the LDH content of connective tissue was low, minimizing its potential significance as a contaminant. Proliferation of connective tissue nuclei alone should not have significantly altered the isoenzyme pattern, since we found that 98% of LDH activity was cytoplasmic. The content of collagen was not increased in the two hypertrophied RV's examined (Table IV). Finally, each muscle sample was examined

TABLE IV

COLLAGEN CONTENT OF NORMAL HEARTS AND HEARTS WITH RIGHT VENTRICULAR HYPERTROPHY

	Collagen (mg/100 mg muscle)		
Sample	RV	LV	Septum
Normal	0.66	0.47	0.44
	0.52	0.46	0.45
	0.55	0.37	0.35
Hypertrophied	0.41	0.34	0.32
	0.39	0.33	0.33

histologically and although there was some increase in connective tissue cells in the hypertrophied RV's, the degree of infiltration did not at all correlate with the degree of change in isoenzyme patterns. All of these observations suggested that in the hypertrophied myocardium the changes in LDH isoenzymes had occurred within the muscle cells proper.

Next, we tried to produce regional ischemia in canine hearts to see if this could cause changes in isoenzymes like those we found with hypertrophy. In seven animals, myocardial infarctions were produced by ligation of the anterior descending branch of the left coronary artery and the hearts were examined 3 days to 5 weeks later. Changes in LDH isoenzymes were found only in areas of necrosis or cellular infiltration. In adjacent areas, which were presumed to be relatively hypoxic and histologically normal, the LDH patterns were unchanged. In eight dogs, we produced regional ischemia by constricting the anterior descending and circumflex branches of the left coronary arteries to less than 25% of their normal size. The hearts were examined after 2–12 days and, again, there were no changes in areas that were presumably ischemic and yet histologically normal.

The mechanism of the change we found in isoenzyme patterns is therefore unclear. The changes did not seem related to proliferation of connective tissue cells. If the studies with induced ischemia were valid, the changes did not seem to be related to severe ischemic hypoxia. Similar shifts to a greater proportion of *M* subunits have been noted during growth and during cellular multiplication, particularly under conditions of mild hypoxia (Hellung-Larsen and Andersen, 1968). It therefore seems reasonable to suggest that the shift in LDH patterns during cardiac hypertrophy somehow reflected altered control of protein synthesis during growth, perhaps coincident with very mild hypoxia.

References

Blain, J. M., Schafer, H., Siegel, A. L., and Bing, R. J. (1956) *Amer. J. Med.* **20,** 820.
Fox, A. C., Wikler, N. S., and Reed, G. E. (1965) *J. Clin. Invest.* **44,** 202.
Fox, A. C., and Reed, G. E. (1966) *Am. J. Physiol.* **210,** 1383.
Fox, A. C., and Reed, G. E. (1969) *Am. J. Physiol.* **216,** 1026.
Geha, A. S., Duffy, J. P., and Swan, H. J. C. (1966) *Circ. Res.* **19,** 255.
Kirk, E. S., and Honig, C. R. (1964) *Am. J. Physiol.* **207,** 661.
Hellung-Larsen, P., and Andersen, V. (1968) *Exptl. Cell Res.* **50,** 286.
Spann, J. F., Buccino, R. A., Sonnenblick, E. H., and Braunwald, E. (1967) *Circ. Res.* **21,** 341.

Part IV
The Initiation, Maintenance, and Characteristics of Increased Protein Synthesis in Cardiac Hypertrophy

INITIATION OF PROTEIN SYNTHESIS IN THE ACUTELY OVERLOADED PERFUSED HEART

Sidney S. Schreiber, M. Oratz, and M. A. Rothschild

Prolonged increase in cardiac contractile action is associated with hypertrophy and increased protein synthesis. The factors initiating and maintaining the increased protein synthesis have recently been investigated in *in vivo* preparations with experimental aortic stenosis (Meerson, 1962; Gudbjarnason *et al.*, 1964) and insufficiency (Tomita, 1966) with endocrine-induced hypertension (Wannemacher and McCoy, 1969), and *in vitro* perfusions (Schreiber *et al.*, 1966). The latter methods have allowed the detailed investigation of the early changes resulting in augmented protein synthesis in acute overload under carefully controlled conditions unaffected by homeostatic defenses of the body. The present chapter presents the data obtained and traces the events between the onset of acute hemodynamic overload and the appearance of increased protein synthesis.

General Methods and Results

Guinea pigs, weighing 250–350 gm were used in these experiments. The operative preparation for perfusion and the perfusion apparatus have been described previously (Schreiber *et al.*, 1966). After nembutal anesthesia, the hearts were prepared with perfusion directed into the left ventricle through a cannula secured at the auricular–ventricular ring. The aorta was then cannulated, and fluid presented to the left ventricle was pumped out through the aortic cannula in systole. Aortic flow was measured by a flowmeter attached in line with the aortic cannula; aortic pressure was controlled by varying the flowmeter aperture. Aortic outflow, not directed toward the coronary arteries, emptied into the surrounding bath. Aortic pressures and cardiac rate were measured by a pressure transducer attached in parallel to the aortic outflow and were recorded throughout the studies. The coronary perfusion emptied into the right heart and then out into the surrounding bath through the opened pulmonary artery. The hearts were allowed to beat spontaneously, and were submerged in 500 ml of perfusate which was recirculated to the left ventricle by a polystaltic pump. The perfusate was an amino acid-fortified Krebs–Henseleit solution (Schreiber *et al.*, 1966) oxygenated with 95% O_2–5% CO_2 which maintained the pH at 7.4. The perfusion chamber, a modified glass reaction flask (Ace Glass Co.), capable of withstanding 45 pounds per square inch (psig) gauge pressure (Schreiber *et al.*, 1967a), was used in experiments at normal and hyperbaric pressures (Fig. 1).

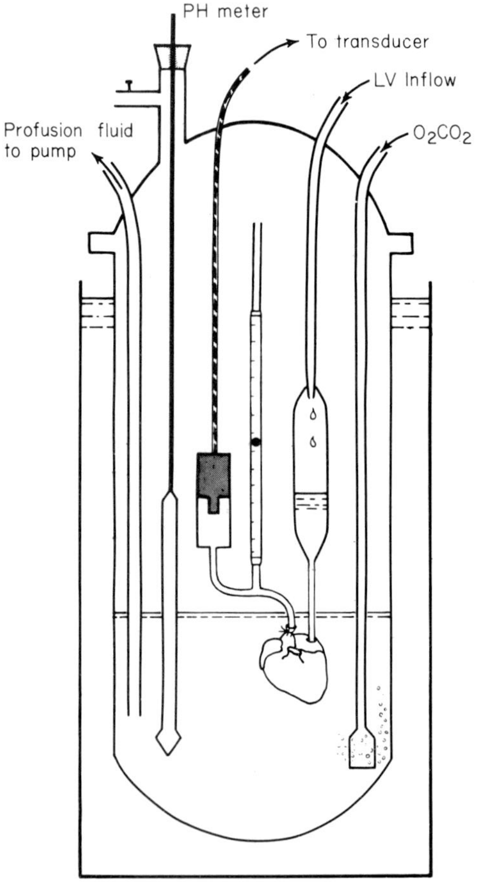

FIG. 1. Perfusion chamber used in normal and hyperbaric experiments. The chamber was a modified glass reaction flask (Ace Glass Co., N.J.) capable of withstanding 45 psig (pounds per square inch gauge pressure). The removable steel top contained ports for entrance and exit of recirculating perfusate, cables for transducer, pH meter probe, and gas tubes for O_2–CO_2.

Coronary perfusion was determined from the difference between ventricular inflow and aortic outflow. Left ventricle "work" was estimated according to the methods of Opie (1965) from the product of the peak systolic pressure and cardiac rate; correction was also made for the apparent cardiac amplitude (measured systolic pressure–diastolic pressure). The hearts (weight 0.9–1.3 gm) could be perfused for 3–4 hr with a left ventricle flow of 7 ml/min and aortic pressure of 25/30 mm Hg without failure. These conditions were considered the control. Failure was considered present if the "amplitude" of ventricle contraction, i.e., the difference between systolic and diastolic pressures, fell to less than $\frac{1}{2}$ of the values seen during the first 30 min. Overload was produced in two ways. First, the aortic outflow was narrowed until the aortic pressure reached 60–70 mm Hg, while the left ventricle perfusion was maintained at control levels of 7 ml/min, and second, by maintaining the aortic pressure at control levels and increasing left ventricle perfusion to 15–20 ml/min. All hearts, both experimental and control, were prepared identically and perfusion initiated at a control level. After 1 min, the overload was induced in the overload group.

Measurement of Left Ventricle Protein Synthesis

In our earlier studies, we were concerned with the time of onset of increased protein synthesis in acute overload, as well as factors relating to this increase. Protein synthesis was measured by determining the incorporation of ^{14}C-lysine into left ventricle protein. Each heart was perfused with the labeled amino acid in 500 ml of the perfusate. Because of the small size of the heart used and the large volume of the perfusate, no change in the lysine specific activity was detectable even after 3 hr of perfusion. The incorporation of lysine into ventricular protein (μmoles lysine/gm Protein N) was determined from the ratio

$$\frac{\mu\text{Ci } ^{14}\text{C/gm protein N}}{^{14}\text{C-lysine sp. act. in perfusate } (\mu\text{Ci}/\mu\text{mole})}$$

The methods of isolation of protein and measurement of the radioactivity were as described (Schreiber *et al.*, 1966).

In the first group, hearts were perfused under control conditions, and the total protein N and incorporation of the labeled lysine into cardiac protein was measured after perfusion for 30–180 min. Failing hearts were not included. The two ventricles differed in protein content and synthesis. Protein N (per 100 gm of wet heart weight) was consistently lower in the right ventricle, but the incorporation of ^{14}C-lysine was significantly greater (Fig. 2), despite the absence of work by the right ventricle in this in vitro system.

The effect of overload on protein synthesis was measured in the left ventricle only. The protein content of left ventricles from overloaded hearts was not significantly changed from the control value after 3 hr of overload perfusion (Fig. 3). Incorporation of the labeled amino acid into left ventricle protein was also unchanged from control levels for 2 hr, but by the third hour there was a marked increase in protein synthesis associated with the increased contractile action (Table I, Fig. 4). In view of the lower or unchanged protein N, there

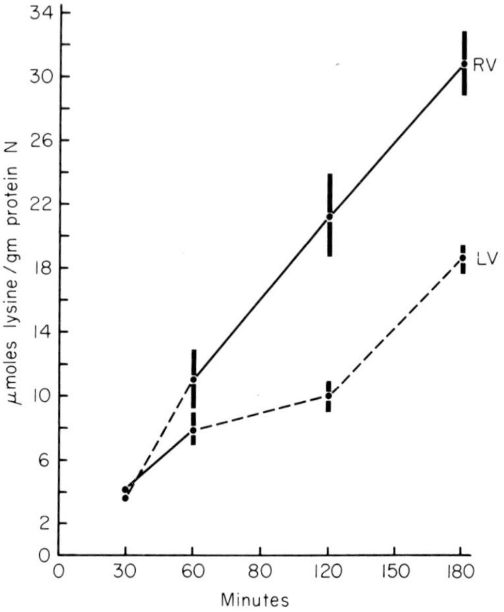

FIG. 2. Time-course study of protein synthesis (Schreiber *et al.*, 1966) in control hearts perfused at 7 ml/min with aortic pressure of 30 mm Hg. Points are means of three or more studies and bars are the SE of the means. The incorporation of the labeled amino acid into protein is plotted as a function of time of perfusion. (RV), Right ventricle; (LV), left ventricle.

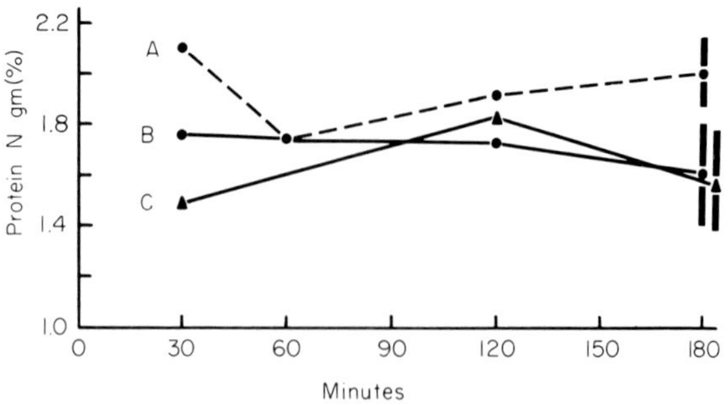

FIG. 3. Protein N/gm ventricle weight plotted as a function of time of perfusion. The points are means of three or more values and the SE are shown for the hearts perfused for 180 min (Schreiber *et al.*, 1966). (A) control; (B) overload resulting from increased perfusion flow; (C) overload resulting from aortic constriction.

TABLE I

^{14}C-LYSINE INCORPORATION INTO LEFT VENTRICLE PROTEIN WITH SYSTOLIC PRESSURE OVERLOAD FOR 3 HR[a]

Sample	^{14}C-lysine incorporated[b]	Protein N gm%	Systolic P ×rate[c]
Control (30)	19.8 ± 2	1.7 ± 0.2	5500 ± 500
Overload (25)	32.5 ± 2	1.5 ± 0.2	12000 ± 600

[a] Numbers in parentheses are the number of separate studies.

[b] μmoles/gm protein N.

[c] Approximation of work (Opie, 1965).

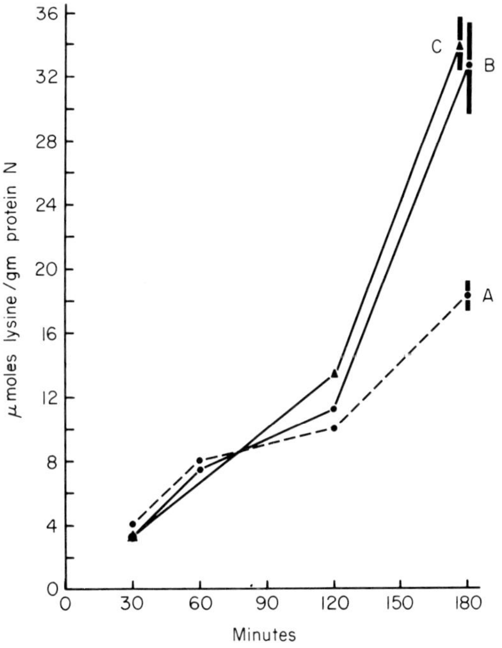

FIG. 4. Protein synthesis in overload left ventricles is plotted as a function of time of perfusion (30–180 min). (A) Controls; (B) overload caused by increased perfusion flow; (C) overload caused by increased systolic pressure. Protein synthesis is expressed as μmoles labeled lysine incorporated into left ventricle protein. The points are means with the range bars representing SE of the mean (Schreiber *et al.*, 1966). Additional experiments for 3 hr are presented in Table I.

must have been marked protein degradation as well as synthesis during the first 3 hr of perfusion. Water content of control and overloaded left ventricles did not differ significantly.

INTRACELLULAR ^{14}C-LYSINE

Since the calculations of protein incorporation of ^{14}C-lysine in our earlier studies were based on the perfusate specific activity, the values were only approximations, even though the specific activity remained constant during perfusion and was the same in all studies. The measurements of intracellular radioactivity in perfused hearts, washed free of ^{14}C-lysine, with a split-stream amino acid analyzer demonstrated that a specific activity was reached after 30–60 min of perfusions that remained constant thereafter (Table II). Furthermore, there was no significant or consistent difference between the intracellular ^{14}C-lysine specific activity of control or overloaded left ventricles,

TABLE II

^{14}C-LYSINE–INTRACELLULAR SPECIFIC ACTIVITY IN THE PERFUSED HEART[a]

	Time of Perfusion (hr)			
Sample	1	2	3	4
	(4)	(6)	(13)	(3)
Control	69[b]	79	70	73
Overload	71	81	68	78

[a] Numbers in parentheses indicate number of studies in each group. The values represent the means for each group.
[b] Specific activity: CPM/μmole lysine $\times 10^3$.

and the increase in protein incorporation of labeled amino acid in overload could not be explained on the basis of increased transport or higher specific activity within the overloaded ventricle. The incorporation data based on perfusate specific activity may be too low by 50% since in the intracellular specific activity never reached more than 50% of that in the perfusate (150,000 cpm/μmole). The latter data are similar to those seen in the perfused liver where ^{14}C-lysine specific activity does not exceed 35% of the perfusate in 3 hr, but this level is reached in 20 min and does not increase thereafter (Schreiber *et al.*, 1966). Similarly, Raacke (1961) has stated that some of the amino acid pool may be relatively inexchangeable during the time of tracer studies, so that the specific activity in the cell may be much lower than that of the perfusate. Of course, it is entirely possible that the specific activity of the exchangeable lysine is equal to that of the perfusate, but at this time it is not feasible to separate the inexchangeable and exchangeable intracellular lysine pools. Of importance is the fact that control and overload ventricles had the same intracellular ^{14}C-lysine specific activity.

Correlation between Work and Protein Synthesis

It was evident that overload was a complex picture with increased contractile action associated with increased systolic pressure or increased ventricular perfusion. In both, the measured coronary flow increased above control levels, and resulted in increased oxygen availability to the myocardium. In an attempt to correlate the measured parameters after 3 hr of perfusion, it was found that the heart rate was not related to protein synthesis (Fig. 5), but by using an approximation of work, the product of systolic pressure and rate (Opie, 1965), a correlation was found. When the latter was corrected by the "net pressure" elaborated by the left ventricle (difference between systolic and diastolic pressure), the correlation was almost a straight line (Fig. 5).

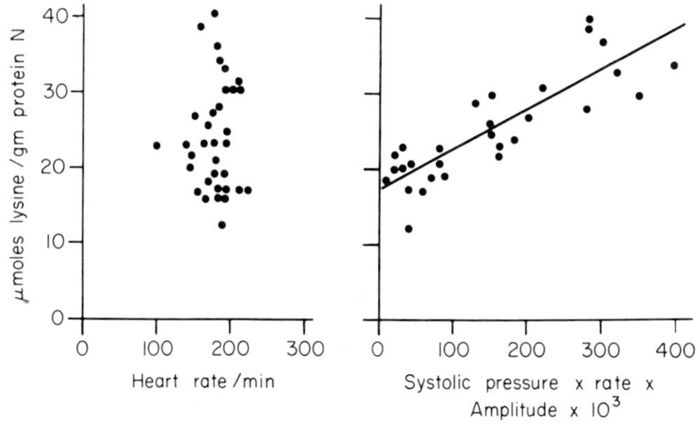

FIG. 5. Correlation between two aspects of cardiac function and protein synthesis after 3 hr of perfusion. Protein synthesis is expressed as micromoles of ^{14}C-lysine incorporated into left ventricle protein (see text).

Effect of Increased Coronary Flow

Since coronary flow increased in overload, this change was tested without ventricular work. Direct back perfusion of the aorta in the presence of intact aortic valves was studied. As the coronary flow increased, there was a concomitant increase in incorporation of the labeled lysine into left ventricle protein (Table III).

TABLE III

DIRECT CORONARY PERFUSION IN THE ABSENCE OF WORK

Coronary flow ml/min	μmoles lysine /gm protein N
3	23.1
4	30.4
7	51.2

EFFECT OF INCREASED OXYGEN TENSION

Since increased coronary flow per se increased protein synthesis in the absence of any measurable ventricular work, the possibility that available oxygen supply controlled protein synthesis was considered. Control perfusion was carried out as above with oxygenated perfusate at atmospheric pressure. In the second group, the hearts were perfused under identical conditions of ventricular flow, aortic pressure, heart rate, and coronary flow, but the oxygen tension was raised to 3 atm (45 psig) during the perfusion using the chamber described (Fig. 1) (Schreiber *et al.*, 1967a). After 3 hr of perfusion in hyperbaric oxygen, there were significant increases in incorporation of the labeled amino acid (34 μmoles lysine compared to 18 in the control) (Table IV) in the absence of any significant difference in lysine intracellular specific activity.

There was also a decrease in protein content under these conditions. Thus, protein degradation and synthesis were markedly increased with increased oxygen tension. Overload produced by aortic constriction in the presence of increased O_2 did not result in a further increase of protein synthesis (Table IV), suggesting that maximum synthesis had been reached for the perfusion conditions.

INCREASED AORTIC PRESSURE WITH CONTROL CORONARY FLOW

The data thus far implied that overload caused increased protein synthesis by increasing coronary perfusion and oxygen availability. However, when hearts were perfused under conditions of increased aortic pressure, with a ventricular flow of 3–4 ml/min all going into the coronary circulation, there was a marked increase in contractile action; and protein synthesis, reflected by increased incorporation of ^{14}C-lysine, was significantly higher than in controls receiving the same coronary flow perfused at 30 mm Hg (Table V). Here again, this group showed a concomitant decrease in protein content and no change in water content.

TABLE IV

LEFT VENTRICULAR PROTEIN SYNTHESIS IN HYPERBARIC OXYGEN[a,b]

Sample	Time of perfusion (min)	μmoles lysine/gm protein N	% Protein N
Controls, atm p.	60	7.1 ± 0.15	1.9 ± 0.13
	120	11.1 ± 1.1	1.9 ± 0.02
	180	18.0 ± 0.4	1.9 ± 0.02
Controls, 45 psig	60	9.95	1.67
	120	20.3 ± 3.1	1.38 ± 0.2
	180	34.1 ± 1.8 $P < 0.001$	1.39 ± 0.05 $P < 0.05$
Aortic constriction, atm p.	180	33.4 ± 1.4 $P < 0.001$	1.5 ± 0.2 $P < 0.2$
Aortic constriction, 45 psig	180	35.1 ± 4.1 $P < 0.01$	1.29 ± 0.09 $P < 0.01$

[a] Data previously reported (Schreiber, *et al.*, 1967a) psig = pounds per square inch gauge pressure; means ± SE.

[b] *P* values refer to comparison with control at 180 min.

TABLE V

^{14}C-LYSINE INCORPORATION INTO LEFT VENTRICLE PROTEIN AFTER 3 hr OF PERFUSION WITH IDENTICAL CORONARY FLOWS[a]

Group	L. Ventricle load (ml/min)	Aortic p. mm Hg	Coronary flow ml/min	gm % Protein N	μmoles lysine/gm protein N
Control (5)	7–8	30	3–4	2.1 ± 0.1 (SE)	18.6 ± 0.3
Elevated systolic pressure (5)	3–4	70–80	3–4	1.5 ± 0.2	38.8 ± 6.0 $P < 0.05$

[a] Number in parentheses represent separate studies.

Thus, increased contractile action in the presence of coronary flow identical to that in control hearts produced augmented protein synthesis and degradation, but an effect of increased coronary pressure could not be excluded.

MICROSOMES OF OVERLOADED LEFT VENTRICLES AND PROTEIN SYNTHESIS

In order to trace the factors initiating protein synthesis in acute overload, studies of subcellular systems were undertaken. It was evident from the experiments with total left ventricle protein that increased synthesis in overload was not apparent until after 2 or 3 hr of stress. Thus, the synthetic factory must have been in operation before that time, and experiments were carried out with microsomes obtained from left ventricles 1, 2, and 3 hr after overload or control perfusion.

The methods of perfusion were as described above. After the perfusion was completed, the left ventricular microsomes were isolated (Schreiber *et al.*, 1967b) and suspended in an incubation medium containing ^{14}C-lysine and also containing their own cell sap as a supply of the pH 5 enzymes and tRNA. After incubation at 37°C for 30 min, microsomes were isolated from the mixture by centrifugation, washed to remove free ^{14}C-amino acids, treated with ice cold trichloroacetic acid to precipitate the protein; the precipitate was repeatedly washed with stable lysine to remove free nonincorporated radioactive amino acid, the resultant protein extracted for lipids and RNA, and finally analyzed for total protein and for radioactivity (Schreiber *et al.*, 1967b). The results of the incubation studies (Table VI) demonstrated

TABLE VI

INCORPORATION OF ^{14}C-LYSINE INTO MICROSOMAL PROTEIN[a,b,c]

Experiment	SP mm Hg	VF ml/min	SP × rate	cpm per mg protein N	Protein N, gm/100 gm ventricle wt
Group A					
Control (4)	33 ± 2(SE)	6.4 ± 0.4	5200 ± 100	213 ± 10	0.13 ± 0.02
Overload (4)	55 ± 5	7.2 ± 0.5	9000 ± 200	515 ± 30	0.12 ± 0.01
				$P < 0.001$	
Group B					
Control (7)	30 ± 3	7.1 ± 0.4	4830 ± 150	1045 ± 120	0.15 ± 0.03
Overload (8)	63 ± 4	8.2 ± 0.5	10640 ± 300	2965 ± 600	0.12 ± 0.02
				$P < 0.01$	

[a] Numbers in parentheses indicate no. of studies.

[b] Microsomes in all experiments were obtained from hearts perfused for 2–3 hr. SP is systolic pressure; VF, ventricular perfusion flow; SP × rate—systolic pressure × rate.

[c] Groups A and B were run identically except for the difference in specific activity of ^{14}C-lysine in the incubation mixture.

that microsomes from ventricles subjected to overload for 2–3 hr had increased protein synthetic capacity. Studies repeated with microsomes from ventricles perfused for shorter periods gave similar results, and it was evident that the increase in the synthetic machinery was in operation 1 hr after the onset of overload. At this point it was uncertain whether the stimulus had been operative through the cytoplasm or the microsomes themselves.

Cross-incubation studies were then set up in order to separate cytoplasmic from microsomal factors. The microsomes were isolated from overloaded and control left ventricles perfused for 1 or more hr on the same day. Microsomes from an overloaded ventricle were tested both in experimental and control cell sap, and similarly, microsomes from the control ventricle were tested in cell sap from control and overloaded ventricles. The results (Table VII) indicated that the microsomes from overloaded ventricles were

TABLE VII

PROTEIN SYNTHESIS IN CROSS-INCUBATION STUDIES WITH MICROSOMES

Expt.	Amino acid ^{14}C-	Time of perfusion (hr)	Microsome–cell sap[a]					
			C-C	C-E	E-C	E-E	C-NP	E-NP
1	lysine	1	100	117	190	270		
2	lysine	1	100	130	105	220		
3	leucine	1	100	99	280	275		
4	leucine	1.5	100	130	180	190		
5	lysine	3	100	110	560	450		
6	leucine	2					100	280
7	leucine	2					100	270
8	phenylalanine	1					100	220
9	phenylalanine	1					100	135
10	phenylalanine	1					100	138
11	phenylalanine	1					100	125

[a] The first letter of each microsome–cell sap pair represents the microsomes, and the second letter of pair represents the cell sap. C is control; E, overloaded; NP, cell sap from nonperfused ventricles. Experiments 1–5 were reported previously (Schreiber *et al.*, 1967b). All figures were compared to controls (C-C) or (C-NP) set at 100.

able to incorporate more amino acid into protein than the controls, whether incubated in their own, in control, or in nonperfused ventricle cell sap. On the other hand, there was only slight increase in control microsome protein synthesis when incubated in cell sap from overloaded ventricles. It is of interest that incorporation of ^{14}C-phenylalanine into microsomal protein has usually been less than the incorporation of leucine or lysine, but the increase in overload has also been significant (Schreiber *et al.*, 1967b).

The above data showed that acute overload in the young guinea pig heart may stimulate augmented protein synthesis independent of the source of cell sap or substrate as early as 1 hr after onset of overload stress, but the specific quality or fraction of the microsome affected was as yet unclear.

Effect of Actinomycin D on Microsomes from Overloaded Ventricles

The specific alteration in the microsome was first studied with actinomycin, whose major action is inhibition of RNA polymerization on the DNA template. In paired experiments, microsomes from ventricles overloaded for 1 hr were studied simultaneously with microsomes from overloaded but actinomycin-treated ventricles. Seven pairs of hearts were used with ^{14}C-leucine or -phenylalanine incorporation taken as an index of protein synthesis.

The perfusion methods were as above. Actinomycin treatment consisted of pretreatment of the guinea pigs with injection of actinomycin in propylene glycol 13 hr prior to perfusion (125 μg/100 gm body weight) and the hearts from these animals were perfused with actinomycin (400 mg/liter) during the study. Control animals were preinjected with identical quantities of propylene glycol and hearts from these animals were overloaded using perfusate containing the same quantity of the solvent as in the actinomycin group.

The hearts subjected to actinomycin treatment were able to withstand the acute overload remarkably well and there was no evidence of failure in any preparation. Approximations of work (systolic pressure × rate) performed by each group were similar (Table VIII). However, there was a significant

TABLE VIII

Effect of Actinomycin-D on Protein Synthesis by Microsomes from Overloaded Left Ventricles[a, b]

Experiment	Microsome protein synthesis[c]	Systolic p. mm Hg	Heart rate	Systolic p. × rate
Without actinomycin (7)	100	73 ± 4	172 ± 6	12600 ± 810
With actinomycin (7)	63 ± 4 $P < 0.001$	67 ± 4	175 ± 9	11850 ± 900

[a] Numbers in parentheses represent separate studies.

[b] The values represent the means of seven hearts in each group (Schreiber *et al.*, 1968).

[c] Cpm of incorporated ^{14}C-leucine/mg microsome RNA expressed as change from overloaded ventricles without actinomycin treatment.

drop in protein synthesis by microsomes derived from actinomycin-treated ventricles to 63% of that of microsomes derived from untreated overloaded ventricles.

A major question to be answered was whether the actinomycin pretreatment and perfusion damaged preexisting or available ribosomes, thus causing an inhibition of the overload effect on protein synthesis. In the next series of studies, control and overloaded hearts with and without actinomycin treatment were perfused for 1 hr on the same day, and microsomes from the left ventricles of each were incubated with ^{14}C-leucine or -phenylalanine (Table IX). The incorporation of labeled amino acids by control microsomes was set at 100 in order to equalize the experiments done on different days. Overload increased phenylalanine incorporation by 138% and leucine incorporation to 219%. Actinomycin did not decrease or interfere with control microsome protein synthesis but reduced the synthetic capacity of microsomes from overloaded ventricles to the same levels as untreated controls. Hence, there was no evidence that actinomycin interfered with or damaged the preexisting ribosomes. The suggestion at this time was that we were seeing the predominant action of actinomycin at work, i.e., an interference with either mRNA or possibly ribosomal RNA formation, which had been stimulated in overload.

Polyuridylic Acid and Microsome Protein Synthesis

To explore this point further, experiments with the artificial messenger, poly U, were performed. If overload initiated increased protein synthesis because of an increased number of functioning ribosomes, poly U should further stimulate synthesis in microsomes from overloaded ventricles. On the other hand, if the very early response to overload stress was release or formation of new mRNA, as had been suggested by the actinomycin experiments, the new mRNA would bind to the ribosomes, and the addition of poly U would not result in a further stimulation of the same ribosome population to manufacture more protein.

Microsomes were isolated from control and overloaded left ventricles obtained from actinomycin-treated and untreated guinea pig hearts perfused for 1 hr. The incubation time and the amount of poly U added were identical in all incubation tubes (Schreiber *et al.*, 1968). The data obtained for the group are summarized in Table X. Each group without poly U is set at 100 and the effect of poly U related to this standard. Control microsomes showed increased incorporation of labeled phenylalanine with poly U, indicating available functioning ribosomes unbound to mRNA. Although microsomes from overloaded ventricles incorporated more phenylalanine than did controls (Table IX), the addition of poly U did not stimulate further incorporation of the labeled amino acid (Table X). Therefore, microsomes from overloaded

TABLE IX

EFFECT OF ACTINOMYCIN-D ON PROTEIN SYNTHESIS BY MICROSOMES FROM CONTROL AND OVERLOADED LEFT VENTRICLES[a, b]

Expt. ^{14}C-	Control	Control with actinomycin	Overloaded	Overloaded with actinomycin
phenylalanine (5)	100	110 ± 4 NS	138 ± 4 $P < 0.001$	102 ± 8 NS
leucine (3)	100	99 NS	219 ± 17 $P < 0.001$	115 ± 5 NS

[a] Schreiber *et al.* (1968).

[b] Numbers in parentheses refer to numbers of complete experiments. Values are cpm in microsomal protein/mg RNA in the microsomes compared to controls set at 100. NS, not significant. *P* values refer to untreated controls. Figures are means $\pm$ SE of mean.

TABLE X

POLYURIDYLIC ACID AND MICROSOME PROTEIN SYNTHESIS[a]

Sample	Without poly U	With poly U	
Control, untreated	100	140 ± 10[b]	$P < 0.01$
Overload, untreated	100	83 ± 8	NS
Control + Actinomycin	100	145 ± 5	$P < 0.02$
Overload + Actinomycin	100	139 ± 5	$P < 0.01$

[a] Schreiber *et al.* (1968).

[b] SE.

ventricles contained ribosomes bound to mRNA presumably newly formed or released, rather than an increase in the free ribosome population. Control microsomes from actinomycin-treated ventricles responded to poly U as did untreated controls and protein synthesis increased, again supporting the concept that actinomycin in this situation had not damaged the available ribosomes. Whereas microsomes from overloaded ventricles treated with actinomycin showed no increased ^{14}C-phenylalanine incorporation into protein above the untreated control level, poly U was able to stimulate these microsomes, and protein synthesis rose to levels seen with controls. Thus, both the actions of actinomycin and poly U supported an early formation of mRNA in acute overload. The increased mRNA bound all of the available ribosomes, and the artificial messenger poly U had no free ribosomes available for stimulation. Actinomycin, inhibiting mRNA formation, now allowed the poly U to effectively stimulate the free ribosomes.

Acute Overload and RNA Synthesis

The suggestion of increased mRNA formation very early in overload led to the evaluation of the ribosome and polysome synthesis in left ventricles subjected to acute stress of increased systolic pressure. Ribosomes and polysomes were isolated from perfused control and overloaded ventricles and were examined on sucrose gradients. After perfusion for 1 or 2 hr, the ventricles were homogenized in buffer with deoxycholate, the ribosomes and polysomes separated by 1–2 *M* sucrose zone centrifugation, and the isolated mixture of ribosomes and polysomes suspended on a 10–30% linear sucrose gradient (Schreiber *et al.*, 1968; Earl and Korner, 1965; Munro *et al.*, 1964). Uridine-^{3}H was used in the perfusate as a precursor of RNA, and the synthesis of RNA was estimated from the determinations of the radioactivity incorporated into RNA in samples collected from the sucrose gradient. Ferritin was used as a 70-S marker in a gradient run at the same time under identical conditions. Early data with this method showed a major initial peak consistent with ribosomes, followed by smaller peaks indicating collections of heavier aggregates, or polysomes. Specific activity determinations were hampered by contamination of all of the peaks with free nonincorporated ^{3}H-uridine despite the separation methods (Fig. 6). This necessitated repurification of the ribosome–polysome pellet by an additional zone centrifugation through 1 *M* sucrose (Schreiber *et al.*, 1968). The gradients obtained with the repurified ribosomes and polysomes showed that the incorporation of labeled uridine into the ribosomes from control and overloaded ventricles was essentially the same (Fig. 7), but incorporation of the label was markedly increased in heavier aggregates in the overloaded (fractions 3 and 5, Fig. 7). In the face of apparently unchanged ribosome RNA synthesis, the increase in ^{3}H-uridine activity in the polysome aggregates again supported the earlier suggestion that mRNA synthesis was increased early in acute overload.

If the higher activity of labeled uridine in the heavier aggregates from overloaded ventricles was due to new mRNA, then actinomycin, in dosage levels that had inhibited microsome protein synthesis in the overloaded ventricle, should obliterate the former, and this is precisely what was seen in analyses of ribosomes and polysomes from actinomycin-treated overloaded ventricles (Fig. 8).

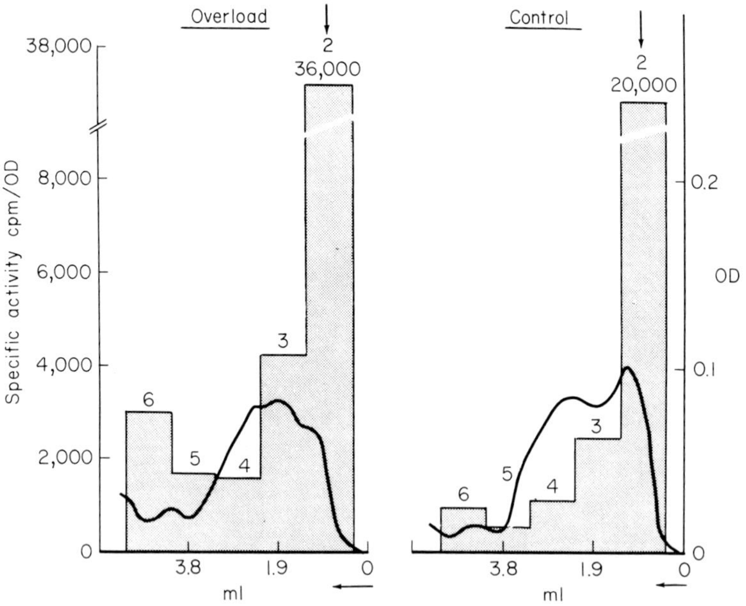

FIG. 6. Analysis of ribosomes and polysomes obtained from perfused control and overloaded left ventricles (Schreiber *et al.*, 1968). The ribosome–polysome mixture was originally separated by centrifugation through a 1–2 *M* zone sucrose gradient after homogenizing the left ventricle of a heart perfused for 2 hr with ^{3}H-uridine. The resultant purified ribosome–polysome mixture was then analyzed on a 10–30% linear sucrose gradient shown here. The smooth line curve represents the continuous readings as the gradient passed through a UV analyzer; the shaded bars represent activity (cpm due to ^{3}H-uridine/OD) of fractions collected. The arrows are the sedimentation of ferritin (70s) run simultaneously. Numbers 2–6 represent the fractions collected and analyzed for activity after the gradient had passed through the analyzer. Decreases in peaks or differences in the shapes of the curves were not consistent. The activity of fraction 2, the ribosomes, was markedly increased due to contamination with ^{3}H-uridine nonspecifically adsorbed to the ribosomes. This contamination was eliminated by repeated centrifugation through a 1 *M* sucrose zone gradient prior to further analysis on a linear gradient (Schreiber *et al.*, 1968). Figure 7 shows the analysis of repurified ribosomes and polysomes.

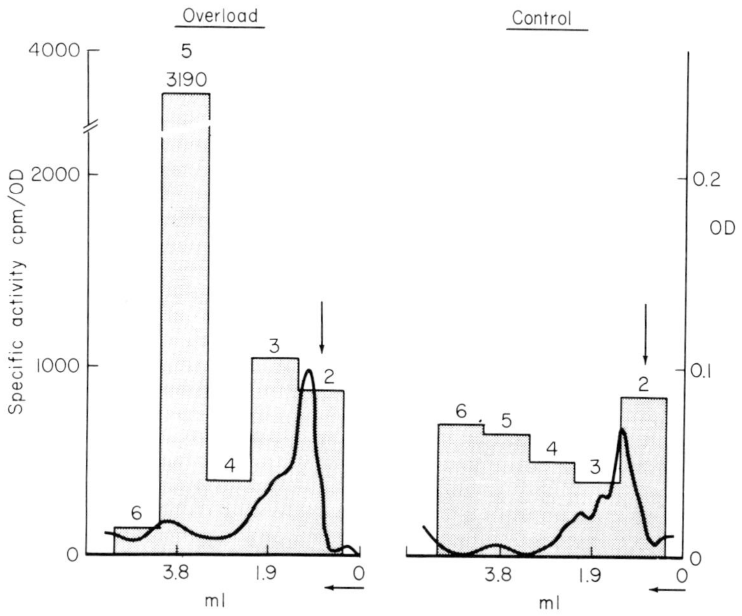

FIG. 7. Analysis of ribosomes and polysomes from ventricles taken from hearts perfused with ^{3}H-uridine and reported previously (Schreiber *et al.*, 1968). The polysomes and ribosomes were centrifuged twice through a zone of 1–2 *M* sucrose to remove contaminating labeled uridine. The difference in ribosome peak size between control and overloaded ventricles is a result of the quantity of material isolated and is not significant. However, incorporation of the labeled uridine was significantly elevated in fractions 3 and 5 in the overloaded preparations.

MESSENGER ACTIVITY OF RNA REMOVED FROM OVERLOADED LEFT VENTRICLE NUCLEI

Since increased microsome protein synthesis early in acute overload appeared to be a result of increased mRNA available to the ribosomes, studies were

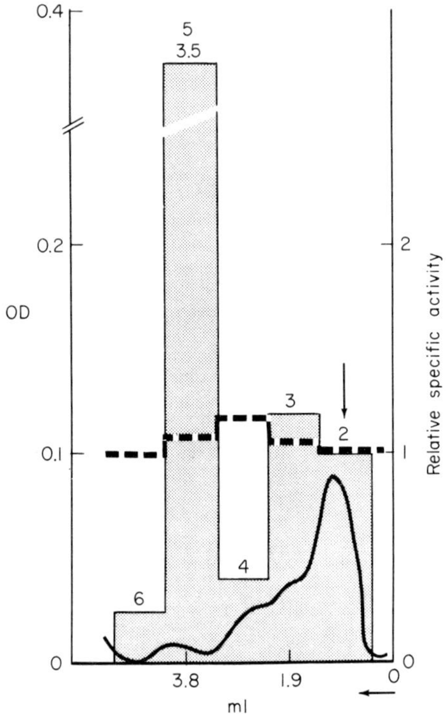

FIG. 8. Analysis of ribosomes and polysomes from overloaded and control ventricles after perfusion with uridine (Schreiber *et al.*, 1968). Smooth line curve represents the OD reading as the gradient passed through the UV analyzer and shows the gradient of an overloaded ventricle. Treatment with actinomycin D gave similar results. The shaded bar graph represents ^{3}H-uridine activity of the overloaded ventricle ribosomes and polysomes (seen in Fig. 7) and the broken line that of the actinomycin D treated and overloaded left ventricle. The ribosome-specific activities have been equalled so that changes in specific activity relative to the ribosomes are shown. Actinomycin D treatment abolished the increased activity seen in the heavier aggregates.

initiated to see if nuclei from overloaded left ventricles contained more mRNA activity. Messenger activity of the RNA isolated from ventricular nuclei was tested by the ability of the RNA to stimulate liver microsomes' incorporation of labeled amino acid into protein. The methods of isolation of nuclei, purification and isolation of the RNA and incubation were as outlined by Bondy and Roberts with an *E. coli* test system (Bondy and Roberts, 1967). After perfusion was completed, the ventricles were homogenized and the nuclei separated by centrifugation, purified by recentrifugation through 2 *M* sucrose, and the RNA isolated. Because of the small yield per heart, the nuclear RNA from four to six identically treated left ventricles were pooled (Schreiber *et al.*, 1969). Hepatic microsomes were isolated and incubated, using standard methods (Rothschild *et al.*, 1968). The system was initially tested with nuclear RNA obtained from nonperfused hearts. Cardiac nuclear RNA did have messenger activity, as indicated by the ability to stimulate incorporation of phenylalanine or leucine into protein by liver microsomes (Table XI).

TABLE XI

EFFECT OF POLYURIDYLIC ACID AND CARDIAC NUCLEAR RNA ON LIVER MICROSOMES' ABILITY TO INCORPORATE AMINO ACIDS INTO PROTEIN[a,b]

	RNA or poly U	Amino acid incorporation (cpm/mg protein)
^{14}C-phenylalanine		
Preincubated microsomes	None	0
Preincubated microsomes	Cardiac nuclear RNA (143 mg)	2560
Preincubated microsomes	Poly U (142 mg)	16,800
^{14}C-leucine		
No preincubation	None	134,000
Preincubated liver microsomes	None	31,400
Preincubated liver microsomes	Cardiac nuclear RNA (300 mg)	43,700

[a] Schreiber *et al.* (1969).

[b] Preincubations were for 15 min, and incubations for 30 min with the cardiac nuclear RNA or with Poly U. The cardiac nuclear RNA was obtained from nonperfused hearts.

Pooled nuclear RNA from left ventricles subjected to control or overload perfusion, were now tested for messenger activity (Table XII). There was no consistent difference in the messenger effect between nuclei from control and overloaded ventricles. The DNA/RNA ratios in both groups were identical. Thus, if acute overload caused increased mRNA formation, the mRNA had been rapidly released from the nuclei, as would be expected from the earlier data with microsomes and polysomes.

TABLE XII

EFFECT OF VENTRICULAR NUCLEAR RNA FROM PERFUSED HEARTS ON PROTEIN SYNTHESIS BY PREINCUBATED LIVER MICROSOMES[a]

	Control	Overload	% change
Perfusion rate (ml/min)	7.1 ± 0.2[b]	7.2 ± 0.2	
Mean donor heart systolic pressure	33 ± 0.6	72 ± 1.7	+118
Incorporation of ^{14}C-leucine cpm/mg microsome protein			
Expt. 1	14,300	15,100	+ 6
2	7,210	6,910	− 4
3	15,000	11,090	− 26
4	7,500	8,250	+ 10
DNA/RNA ratio in donor nuclei	11.7 ± 1.1	11.5 ± 1.0	
Number of donor ventricles	33	25	

[a] Schreiber *et al.* (1969).
[b] Mean ± SE.

NUCLEAR RNA POLYMERASE ACTIVITY IN ACUTELY OVERLOADED LEFT VENTRICLES

In order to study the mRNA synthetic capacity of cardiac nuclei, RNA polymerase activity of isolated nuclei was studied as outlined by Nair *et al.*, (1967). After perfusion under control or overload conditions, the left ventricular nuclei were isolated and purified. Nuclear suspensions in sucrose and $MgCl_2$ containing the same amounts of DNA were incubated in media with Mn^{2+}–$(NH_4)_2SO_4$ or with Mg^{2+} (Nair *et al.*, 1967). RNA polymerase activity was determined by using ^{32}P-labeled UTP in the incubation media and by measuring the activity of ^{32}P/mg isolated RNA corrected for DNA content (Schreiber *et al.*, 1969). The results were expressed as percent change from controls (Nair *et al.*, 1967).

The data obtained from 12 hearts perfused from 20–120 min indicated that there was an initial increase in Mn^{2+}-stimulated polymerase activity which rapidly dropped. On the other hand, the initially low Mg^{2+} stimulation activity appeared to increase with perfusion time (Fig. 9). The early difference in RNA polymerase activity of nuclei from overloaded ventricles incubated in Mn^{2+} or Mg^{2+} was found to be significant at 20 min (Table XIII).

Since Mn^{2+}-stimulated polymerase activity favors the formation of DNA like RNA or mRNA (Nair *et al.*, 1967), the data implied that early in acute overload there was a rapid and brief increase in mRNA synthesis, which supports the data obtained with actinomycin and poly U experiments performed above. This was then followed by an increase in ribosome-like RNA

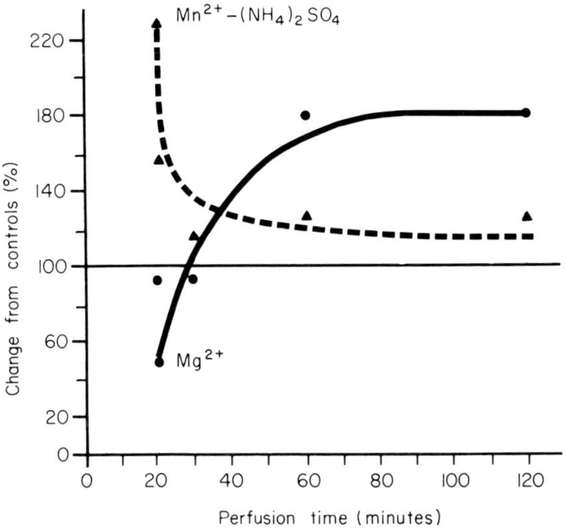

FIG. 9. RNA polymerase activity of nuclei obtained from acutely overloaded left ventricles in hearts perfused from 20–120 min. Each point represents a comparison of the ^{32}P specific activity of the RNA obtained from nuclei from an overloaded left ventricle after incubation with UTP-^{32}P compared with a simultaneously run control. The control value was set at 100. (---) Polymerase activity with $Mn^{2+}-(NH_4)_2SO_4$; (—) activity in Mg^{2+} media. Values have been corrected for the DNA content per incubation tube; each experiment was run in duplicate or triplicate (Schreiber *et al.*, 1969).

TABLE XIII

NUCLEAR POLYMERASE STUDIES OF NUCLEI OBTAINED FROM PERFUSED OVERLOADED HEARTS[a,b]

	Mn^{2+}	Mg^{2+}
Perfusion for 20 min	136 ± 9[c]	80 ± 9 $P < 0.001$
Perfusion for 30 min	93 ± 4	98 ± 10 NS

[a] Schreiber *et al.* (1969).

[b] Total number of experiments included 16 pairs of hearts. An overload and control were perfused on the same day and the polymerase studies of the nuclei from both run simultaneously.

[c] Expressed as percent change from values obtained with control Nonoverloaded hearts $\pm$ SE of the mean.

formation (Mg^{2+} stimulation). A later increase in ribosomal RNA has been reported (Nair *et al.*, 1967).

Thus, in tracing the increased cardiac protein synthesis in acute overload from its inception, the data suggest that acute overload rapidly produces an effect on the ventricular nuclei that results in increased mRNA formation leading to increased protein synthesis. As the overload persists, augmented ribosomal RNA formation allows further increase in protein synthesis (Nair *et al.*, 1967; Moroz, 1967; Posner and Fanburg, 1968).

Types of Protein Synthesized in Acute Cardiac Overload

The question now arose as to just what kind of protein was so rapidly synthesized. Earlier data with crude fractionation by centrifugation showed that the ^{14}C-lysine specific activity of protein obtained from the myofibrillar and nuclear fraction and soluble protein fraction were the highest; that of mitochondria was the lowest (Fig. 10).

A more detailed and careful analysis of synthesis of myosin, myoglobin, and of connective tissues was undertaken.

Connective Tissue

To measure connective tissue synthesis, the hearts were perfused with ^{14}C-proline in perfusate which was otherwise identical to that used in the experiments above. After 1–3 hr of systolic pressure overload, the hearts were washed free of radioactivity and the left ventricles hydrolyzed in 6 N HCL for 24 hr. The mixture was freeze-dried, resuspended in buffer, and analyzed for proline and hydroxyproline in an amino acid analyzer or by isolation methods described by Buccino *et al.* (1969). Preliminary data obtained thus far with the analyzer have indicated that connective tissue synthesis, measured by hydroxyproline specific activity, is very low, and there was no significant difference after 3 hr of perfusion between control and overloaded ventricles. With the toluene method (Buccino *et al.*, 1969), using the ^{14}C-proline as precursor, hydroxyproline synthesis after 3 hr of overload perfusion appeared to be greater than controls. However, the increased synthesis was open to question in view of the contamination of the ^{14}C-hydroxyproline by non-specific adsorption of ^{14}C-proline, and further studies are needed.

Myoglobin

Myoglobin synthesis was determined by measuring the incorporation of ^{14}C-lysine into isolated and purified myoglobin (Theorell and deDuve, 1947). Standard procedures for carrier dilution were used in view of the small yield of myoglobin. Following perfusion, the left ventricles were homogenized in buffer (Theorell and deDuve, 1947) in the presence of a known and exactly measured quantity of whale myoglobin. The addition of a known quantity

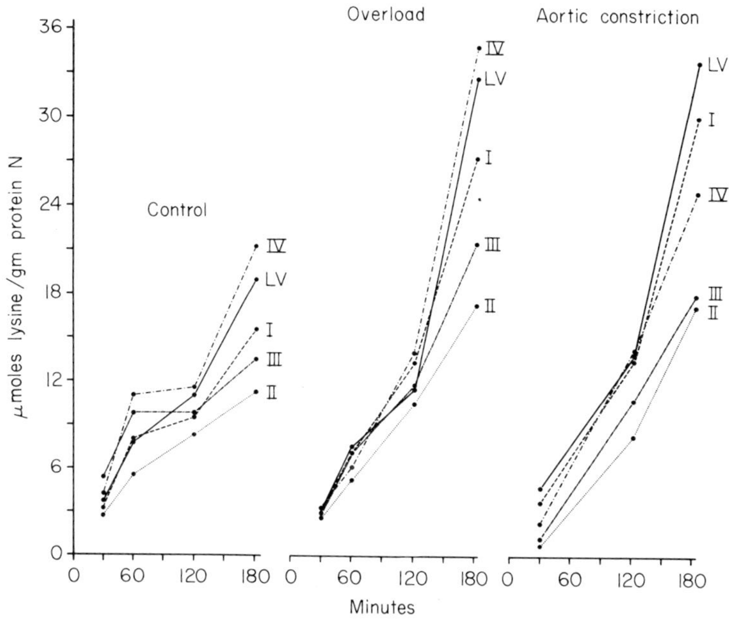

FIG. 10. Protein synthesis in control and overloaded ventricles plotted as a function of time of perfusion; overload represents increased ventricular perfusion (15 ml/min compared to control of 7 ml/min) and aortic constriction represents overload with elevation of systolic pressure above 60 mm Hg (controls were at 30 mm Hg). Protein synthesis is measured by incorporation of ^{14}C-lysine into protein isolated from the left ventricle or from the protein isolated from different fractions. Crude fractions were obtained by centrifugation. LV, total left ventricle represents (I) Myofibrillar and nuclear obtained with 600–1,000 × g; (II) mitochondrial protein obtained from mitochondria precipitated at 20–30,000 × g; (III) microsomal protein from microsomes precipitated at 105,000 × g; and (IV) protein from the supernatant obtained after centrifugation of the microsomes. Each point represents the mean of three or more studies.

of myoglobin permitted the careful isolation and purification of myoglobin by repeated precipitations at increasing salt concentrations, isolation in 100% ammonium sulfate, and dialysis and removal of salt (Theorell and deDuve, 1947). The isolated and dialyzed myoglobin was tested for purity by an acrylamide gel electrophoresis method (Miyoshi *et al.*, 1968). Skeletal muscle myoglobin forms a main electrophoretic band preceded by three smaller bands (Miyoshi *et al.*, 1968). Our studies with whale myoglobin used as a carrier gave identical patterns. Pooled guinea pig ventricular myoglobin demonstrated the main band 1 and band 3 when run on the acrylamide gel alone, but gel electrophoresis of the mixture of carrier myoglobin and guinea pig ventricle gave patterns identical to those seen by purified carrier myoglobin alone. The method is exquisitely sensitive in isolating contaminants since fractions of micrograms will give distinct electrophoretic bands (Miyoshi *et al.*,

1968). Thus, the isolation of pure cardiac ventricle myoglobin in the presence of carrier myoglobin was assured by the identical gel electrophoresis pattern. The specific activity of the ^{14}C-lysine in the isolated and purified myoglobin was determined and μmoles of protein synthesized, calculated by standard isotope-carrier dilution methods.

Data obtained so far indicate that after 3 hr of perfusion there was no significant difference in myoglobin synthesis between control and overloaded left ventricles despite the marked increase in synthesis of the "total" left ventricle protein (Table XIV).

TABLE XIV

SYNTHESIS OF CARDIAC MYOGLOBIN

Time of perfusion	2 hr: cpm/μmole myoglobin	2 hr: μmoles[a] myoglobin synthesized	3 hr: cpm/μmole myoglobin	3 hr: μmoles[a] myoglobin synthesized
Control	682	298	1010	449
	668	280	1045	466
	564	246	720	312
	615	270		
Overload	565	244	1025	445
	615	270	974	440
			975	423

[a] All synthesis figures are $\times 10^{-6}$.

MYOSIN

Myosin was isolated from the left ventricles of overloaded and control hearts perfused for 1–4 hr with ^{14}C-lysine. The methods of isolation and purification of myosin were described by Davis *et al.* for cardiac muscle myosin (Davis *et al.*, 1960). The presence of a pure protein was verified by acrylamide gel electrophoresis according to the methods of Small *et al.* (1961), where myosin subunits move as a single band.

For convenience, left ventricle protein synthesis is expressed in the same terms used in earlier studies (Table XV), and shows increased incorporation of ^{14}C-lysine into protein with systolic pressure overload. The intracellular ^{14}C-lysine specific activity in control and overload was not significantly different (Table II). Myosin synthesis (cpm resulting from ^{14}C-lysine/mg isolated and purified myosin) showed no increase with overload until 3 hr when there was a significant increase thereafter. The percentage increase appeared to lag behind that of the total left ventricle protein (Table XV).

TABLE XV

^{14}C-LYSINE INCORPORATION IN LEFT VENTRICULAR MYOSIN OF PERFUSED HEARTS[a]

	1 hr (4)		2 hr (9)		3 hr (12)		4 hr (3)	
	LV	Myosin	LV	Myosin	LV	Myosin	LV	Myosin
Control	7.2	370	15.0	455	22.0 ± 2	570 ± 20	26.1	570
Overload	8.1	310	14.6	500	36.2 ± 2	735 ± 25	44.0 ± 4	810 ± 10
% change from control	110	84	97	110	165	130	170	142
					$p < 0.001$	$p < 0.005$	$p < 0.001$	$p < 0.001$

[a] Numbers in parenthesis indicate number of hearts for each group.
[b] Means expressed as mean ±SE.
[c] LV, Total Protein Incorporation: μmoles lysine/gm protein N. Myosin incorporation: cpm ^{14}C-lysine/mg purified myosin.

Thus, of the three proteins, connective tissues, myoglobin, and myosin, the myosin appeared to be the protein synthesized more rapidly in the overloaded ventricle after 3 hr of stress.

Discussion

The heart that is subjected to acute or chronic hemodynamic overload responds to the stress with many intracellular alterations, some of which are involved with glucose utilization and fat metabolism (Crass *et al.*, 1969; Opie *et al.*, 1962), energy availability (Meerson *et al.*, 1964; Cohen *et al.*, 1969), and increased protein synthesis (Meerson, 1962; Gudbjarnason *et al.*, 1964; Tomita, 1966; Wannemacher and McCoy, 1969; Schreiber *et al.*, 1966). Although it is not possible at this time to review all of the changes, and cite the many references concerned with metabolic alterations, this chapter attempts to trace the sequence of events from the onset of acute overload stress applied to the left ventricle, to the increased protein synthesis that ultimately results.

Following the exposure of the heart to increased work load, and using a variety of techniques in rats and rabbits, changes have been reported as late as the first day after *in vivo* aortic constriction (Meerson, 1962; Gudbjarnason *et al.*, 1964; Hatt *et al.*, 1965; Zuhlke *et al.*, 1966), or insufficiency (Tomita, 1966), or as early as 4 hr (Posner and Fanburg, 1968). The use of the isolated guinea pig heart permitted examination of very early changes, with noticeable increase in protein synthesis seen in overloaded ventricles as early as 2–3 hr (Schreiber *et al.*, 1966). Short-term measurements following major operative procedure in the *in vivo* methods involving all the body's homeostatic mechanisms, neurogenic and endocrine, may be difficult. It is not implied that preparation of the heart for *in vitro* perfusion does not subject the heart to stress, but the overload enforced on an excised heart produces its effect from a recognizable and, what is most important, a reproducible baseline level which is equal and standardized in all preparations.

The measurement of protein synthesis *in vivo* has usually involved single injection of the radioactive labeled amino acid and the determination of the amount of label incorporated into protein. Although sham-operated animals have served as controls, it is possible that the plasma levels, rates of removal, excretion, and distribution of the labeled and unlabeled amino acid in the sham-operated control are different than that in the overloaded (and sometimes failing preparation). Thus, measurements of cardiac protein synthesis after a single injection of the label may be questioned, especially if the intracellular specific activity is not known. Using skeletal muscle, it has also been reported that entry of a nonutilizable amino acid is increased during hypertrophy, and the suggestion has been made that augmented protein synthesis may depend on this increase in amino acid transport (Goldberg and Goodman, 1969). In the present studies using the *in vitro* perfusion, the amino acid specific activity both in the perfusate and intracellularly, has been constant and the same in controls and overloaded ventricles after the first 30 min to 1 hr. Thus, the increase in protein synthesis in the perfused heart was not a result of altered intracellular amino acid specific activity and the variations described above were not active.

Variations in RNA synthesis have also been reported (Schreiber *et al.*, 1969; Fanburg and Posner, 1968), with the differences in part explained by the items described above. An additional note should be added concerning centrifugation of labeled particles as RNA and determination of synthesis by measuring the incorporation of labeled presursors. The finding that non-specific adsorption of the labeled precursors occurs in sucrose gradient analysis of RNA (Schreiber *et al.*, 1968) raises the question as to measurement of the particle specific activity with these methods without some method of eliminating the precursor not involved in synthesis.

The discovery of increased cardiac muscle protein synthesis with overload led to studies of cardiac RNA, ribosomes, and polysomes. Increased total RNA synthesis was not seen after 2–3 hr (Schreiber *et al.*, 1968), but was reported as early as 4 hr in *in vivo* heart preparation (Fanburg and Posner, 1968) and after 24 hr in heart and skeletal muscle stress (Moroz, 1967; Hamosh *et al.*, 1967). Recent studies (Nair *et al.*, 1967, 1968), have shown that one of the early responses (12 hr) in hearts, subjected to *in vivo* aortic constriction is increased nuclear Mg^{2+}-stimulated RNA polymerase activity, indicating increased formation of ribosome-like RNA at that time. Tracing the stimulus back toward the onset of overload, with the *in vitro* preparation, demonstrated that after 1 hr of overload, microsomes from stressed ventricles were programmed to increase protein synthesis (incorporation of labeled amino acid into protein). The early change in the microsomes from loaded ventricles (after 1 hr) did not appear to result from an increase in free ribosomes, since the addition of poly U did not further stimulate ^{14}C-phenylalanine incorporation into protein. These results also suggest that the ribosome population was now bound to newly available mRNA (Schreiber *et al.*, 1968). Actinomycin inhibited the expected increase in protein synthesis by microsomes obtained from overloaded hearts, supporting the suggestion that mRNA was rapidly synthesized very early in overload stress. Further, stimulation of nuclear RNA polymerase activity in Mn^{2+} carried out 20–30 min after onset of stress (Schreiber *et al.*, 1969) also indicated that an early effect of stress was an increase in mRNA synthesis. Finally, studies with ^{3}H-uridine, as a precursor of RNA synthesis, pointed to a rapid mRNA synthesis, since incorporation of the label into ribosomal RNA was not increased in overload, whereas incorporation was increased in the polysome aggregates, and the latter increase was abolished by actinomycin.

Selective incorporation of precursor by any one species of RNA, measured after separation on sucrose gradients, was not found in the *in vivo* preparation 4–8 hr after aortic constriction, although total RNA synthesis was increased (Fanburg and Posner, 1968). The difference between the *in vitro* and *in vivo* data could be due to the difficulties in methods described above, and could also be one of time, since the increase in mRNA was of brief duration (Schreiber *et al.*, 1969), and subsequently, an increase in the total RNA synthetic machinery (4–8 hr) could occur. In the *in vitro* preparation, this overall increase in RNA synthesis had not occurred by 2 hr after the stress (Schreiber *et al.*, 1969).

The type of cardiac protein involved in the early response to acute overload has not been clearly defined. Our earlier studies, employing crude fractionation techniques, showed that both the soluble protein, not located in intracellular organelles, and the myofibrillar fraction, paralleled the increase in total ventricular synthesis most closely in the response to overload. Recently, radioautography studies with ^{3}H-thymidine, 1–10 days after aortic constriction *in vivo*, revealed that 99% of the labeling occurred in the connective tissue and endothelial nuclei, suggesting an increase in number of the cells in these areas (Morkin and Ashford, 1968). The higher proliferative activity of nuclei of cardiac connective tissues in hypertrophy was also suggested by Meerson *et al.* (1968), and an increase in cardiac connective tissues, measured by hydroxyproline content, was reported in cats 3–90 days after experimental right ventricle hypertrophy (Buccino *et al.*, 1969).

However, studies with the perfused hearts have not provided conclusive evidence of the role of cardiac connective tissue during acute cardiac stress. The content of stable hydroxyproline is not altered during overload, and there is little evidence of increase in ^{14}C-hydroxyproline incorporation. A major problem in the analysis is the contamination of the newly made ^{14}C-hydroxyproline with the ^{14}C-proline precursor; this remains to be settled before any definite statement can be made concerning early connective tissues synthesis.

The isolation and purification of myoglobin has permitted the study of the synthesis of new myoglobin, using ^{14}C-lysine as the label. In rats, synthesis of this respiratory protein has been studied in cardiac hypertrophy due to hypoxia of high altitude. There is an increase in cardiac but not skeletal muscle, myoglobin concentration 3–10 days after the onset of hypoxia (Anthony *et al.*, 1969). In contrast, the present report indicates that measurements of specific activity of incorporated labeled lysine in purified myoglobin are the same in control and acutely overloaded left ventricles up to 3 hr after onset of the stress. Although these data do not imply that there is no later increase, they show that myoglobin synthesis apparently is not an early response to overload stress.

A significant increase in myosin synthesis was seen early in the response to acute overload, and although the percentage increase was less than that of the protein in the total left ventricle, the time of increase was the same. No data were obtained concerned with myosin degradation, but studies by Hatt *et al.* (1965) indicate myofibrillar lysis (and presumably myosin degradation) following experimental aortic stenosis *in vivo*, followed by the appearance of new fibrils with the presumptive synthesis of myosin. Although these events occurred much later than the data obtained with the perfused heart would indicate, they fit the concept that overload to the left ventricle produces a significant early effect in the contractile proteins.

Thus, increased protein synthesis in acute left ventricular load has been traced back to a rapid response of cardiac nuclei to make a DNA-like RNA, or mRNA; the mRNA is released to the ribosomes, which increase protein synthesis in the left ventricle, with a major response seen in myosin by the third hour of stress. As the overload continues, ribosomes are increased, which further augment synthesis. What triggers the train of events is still unknown. There is little doubt that metabolic and enzymatic alterations are widespread in overload, but is is uncertain as to whether these set off increased protein synthesis or whether they are the result of an overall increase in metabolism that accompanies the stress. Furthermore, in view of the increase in protein synthesis following many external alterations (Schreiber *et al.*, 1966, 1967a), it is unlikely that the stimulus is the same for all conditions. There are data indicating early responses of nuclei to overload (Schreiber *et al.*, 1969; Nair *et al.*, 1967, 1968), and it is entirely possible that cytoplasmic, metabolic, or enzymatic changes initiate the nuclear response. There is, however, at least one other alternative, and that is the direct effect of overload and increased contractility on the nucleus itself. Myocardial nuclei have been found to undergo drastic changes in conformation with contraction of the muscle (Bloom and Cancello, 1969). With increased contractile action seen in overload, these changes in nuclear shape may be even more drastic. It is not impossible to assume that this physical nuclear change is translated to a DNA effect, e.g., release of an inhibitor, which now allows mRNA formation. As the stress continues, new stimuli as myosin breakdown, increase in amino acid pool, alterations in mitochondria, lysosomes, among others, may further stimulate production of ribosomes to allow the continued synthesis of new protein leading to hypertrophy. The exact place of all of the intracellular changes in this picture of increased protein synthesis in acute overload awaits further investigation.

ACKNOWLEDGMENT

Supported in part by a grant from the National Institutes of Health No. 09562.

REFERENCES

Anthony, A., Ackerman, E., and Strother, G. (1969). *Amer. J. Physiol.* **196**, 512.
Bloom, S., and Cancello, P. A., (1969). *Circ. Res.* **24**, 189.
Bondy, S. C., and Roberts, S. (1967). *Biochem. J.* **105**, 1111.
Buccino, R. A., Harris, E., Spann, J. F., Jr., and Sonnenblick, E. H. (1969). *Amer. J. Physiol.* **216**, 425.
Cohen, J., Feldman, R. E., and Whitbeck, A. A. (1969), *Amer. J. Physiol.* **216**, 76.
Crass, M. F. III, McCaskill, E. S., and Shipp, J. C. (1969). *Amer. J. Physiol.* **216**, 1569.
Davis, J. O., Carroll, W. R., Trapasso, M., Yankopoulos, N. A., and Casper, A. (1960). *J. Clin. Invest.* **39**, 1463.
Earl, D. C. N., and Korner, A. (1965). *Biochem. J.* **94**, 721.
Fanburg, B. L., and Posner, B. I. (1968). *Circ. Res.* **23**, 123.
Goldberg, A. L., and Goodman, H. M. (1969). *Amer. J. Physiol.* **216**, 1111.
Gudbjarnason, S., Telerman, M., and Bing, R. J. (1964). *Amer. J. Physiol.* **206**, 294.
Hamosh, M., Lesch, M., Baron, J., and Kaufman, S. (1967). *Science* **157**, 935.
Hatt, P. V., Ledoux, C., Bonvalet, J. P., and Guillemat, H. (1965). *Arch. Malad. Coeur Vaisseaux* **58**, 1703.
Meerson, F. Z. (1962). *Circ. Res.* **10**, 250.
Meerson, F. Z., Zaletayeva, T. A., Lagutchev, S. S., and Pshennikova, M. G. (1964). *Exp. Cell. Res.* **36**, 568.
Meerson, F. Z., Alekhina, G. M., Aleksandrov, P. N., and Bazardjan, A. G. (1968). *Amer. J. Cardiol.* **22**, 337.
Miyoshi, K., Saijo, K., Kuryu, Y., Oshima, Y., Nakano, M., and Kawai, H. (1968). *Science* **159**, 736.
Morkin, E., and Ashford, T. P. *Amer. J. Physiol.* **215**, 1409.
Moroz, L. A. (1967). *Circ. Res.* **21**, 449.
Munro, A. J., Jackson, R. J., and Korner, A. (1964). *Biochem. J.* **92**, 289.
Nair, K. G., Rabinowitz, M., and Chen-Tu, M. (1967). *Biochemistry* **6**, 1898.
Nair, K. G., Cutilletta, A. F., Zak, R., Korde, T., and Rabinowitz, M. (1968). *Circ. Res.* **23**, 451.
Opie, L. H., (1965). *J. Physiol.* (*London*) **180**, 539.
Opie, L. H., Shipp, J. C., Evans, J. R., and LeBoeuf, B. (1962). *Amer. J. Physiol.* **203**, 839.
Posner, B. I., and Fanburg, B. L. (1968). *Circ. Res.* **23**, 137.
Raacke, I. D. (1961). "Metabolic Pathways," 2nd Ed., Vol. II, pp. 263–388. Academic Press, New York.
Rothschild, M. A., Oratz, M., Mongelli, J., and Schreiber, S. S. (1968). *J. Clin. Invest.* **47**, 2591.
Schreiber, S. S., Oratz, M., and Rothschild, M. A. (1966). *Amer. J. Physiol.* **211**, 314.
Schreiber, S. S., Evans, C., Oratz, M., and Rothschild, M. A. (1967a). *Amer. J. Physiol.* **212**, 35.
Schreiber, S. S., Oratz, M., and Rothschild, M. A. (1967b). *Amer. J. Physiol.* **213**, 1552.
Schreiber, S. S., Oratz, M., Evans, C., Silver, E., and Rothschild, M. A. (1968). *Amer. J. Physiol.* **215**, 1250.

Schreiber, S. S., Oratz, M., and Rothschild, M. A. (1969). *Amer. J. Physiol.* **217**, 1305.
Small, P. A., Harrington, W. E., and Kielley, W. W. (1961). *Biochim. Biophys. Acta* **49**, 462.
Theorell, H., and deDuve, C. (1947). *Arch. Biochem.* **12**, 113.
Tomita, K. (1966). *Jap. Heart J.* **7**, 566.
Tristram, G. R. (1949). Advan. Protein Chem. **5**, 83.
Wannemacher, R. W., and McCoy, J. R. (1969). *Amer. J. Physiol.* **216**, 781.
Zuhlke, V., de Rochemont, W. du M., Gudbjarnason, S., and Bing, R. (1966) *Circ. Res.* **18**, 558.

STUDIES ON PROTEIN SYNTHESIS IN HEART MUSCLES DURING DEVELOPMENT AND IN EXPERIMENTALLY PRODUCED HYPERTROPHY

Radovan Zak and Donald A. Fischman

In 1941, both Brachet (1941) and Caspersson (1941) published their classical experiments independently showing that the protein synthetic activity of a given tissue is directly proportional to the RNA concentration in that tissue. This basic correlation can also be demonstrated in various types of muscle (Zak, 1962). Rabbit heart, diaphragm, and gastrocnemius are all muscles that differ in their respective contraction rates. The heart, which is the most active of these muscles, has the highest RNA concentration and the highest incorporation of ^{14}C-lysine into its myofibrils, followed by the less active diaphragm and gastrocnemius muscles (Table I).

These observations were later refined, mainly in two aspects. First, it was established that ribosomes comprise 85% of RNA, ~15% is made up of

TABLE I

RNA CONCENTRATION AND PROTEIN LABELING IN DIFFERENT TYPES OF RABBIT MUSCLE[a]

Muscle	RNA (mg RNA·P/mg PN)[b]	^{14}C-Lysine incorporation into myofibrils (cmp/mg protein)	
		90 min	120 min
Heart	9.9 ± 0.5	450	540
Diaphragm	7.0 ± 0.5	350	450
Gastrocnemius	4.6 ± 0.6	220	260

[a] 100 μCi/kg of uniformly labeled ^{14}C-lysine was injected I.P./kg of body weight.
[b] RNA concentrations expressed as mg of RNA phosphorus per mg of protein nitrogen.

transfer RNA, and less than 1% consists of messenger RNA (Gilbert, 1963). Second, it was demonstrated that only a fraction of the ribosomes is actively involved in protein synthesis at any given time. These are the ribosomes held together by messenger RNA in the form of polysomes. The tissues that have a higher rate of protein synthesis contain a higher ratio of polysomes to single ribosomes (Villa-Trevino *et al.*, 1964; Fleck *et al.*, 1965). Polysomes are rather fragile structures, easily disrupted by mechanical forces. Since homogenization of adult muscle is very difficult to achieve, it must be realized that polysomes visualized as optical density profiles on sucrose density gradients may not be true images of living cells. Polysomes, however, can be readily isolated from embryonic muscle cells (Heywood *et al.*, 1967; Zak *et al.*, 1967), which are comparatively easy to disrupt by homogenization.

What interests us in a study of cardiac hypertrophy is how these basic relationships hold when the differentiated mature heart in a balanced state of metabolism is induced to markedly increase its rate of protein synthesis. After aortic constriction, the rat heart increases its protein mass by 40% in 2 days (Nair *et al.*, 1968). This represents the synthesis of approximately 1 mg of protein per gram of heart per hour, as compared for example with the 6 mg hemoglobin made by 1 gm of reticulocytes (Borsook, 1955).

Correlation of RNA Concentration and Amino Acid Incorporation into the Heart Muscle

The RNA concentration in the heart is elevated as early as 24–48 hr after aortic constriction. During the first postoperative week, the percent increase of the RNA concentration is proportional to the degree of heart enlargement (Nair *et al.*, 1968). The synthesis of both ribosomal and transfer RNA as measured by ^{32}P- and ^{3}H-uridine incorporation also increases proportionately (Fanburg and Posner, 1968; Koide and Rabinowitz, 1969).

The correlation between cardiac enlargement after aortic constriction and the RNA concentration and amino acid incorporation into protein is shown in Fig. 1. The percent heart enlargement is calculated from the ratio of heart–body weight of sham-operated rats. It can be seen that 72 hr after aortic constriction, both the RNA concentration and the incorporation of ^{14}C-amino acids in protein during a 15-min pulse are positively correlated with heart enlargement.

A similar relationship between RNA concentration and the amino acid incorporating activity was also found in embryonic chick hearts. As seen in Fig. 2, the RNA concentration of the embryonic heart peaks at approximately the 10th day of incubation. The incorporation of a ^{14}C-labeled mixture of amino acids into beating hearts incubated in Eagle's basic medium was also found to be higher in 10-day than in 15-day hearts.

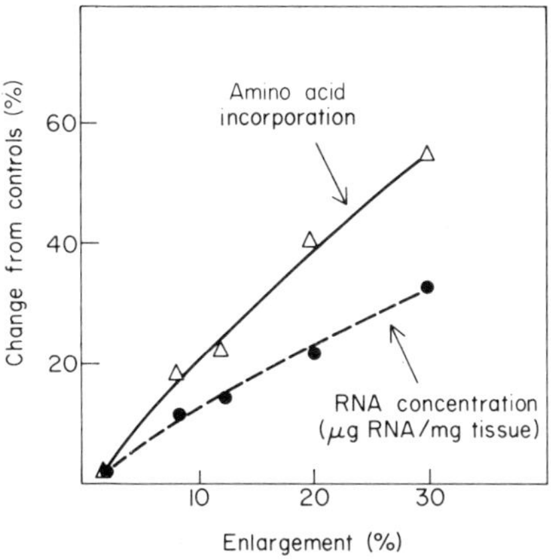

FIG. 1. Relationship of RNA concentration and amino acid incorporation into protein is demonstrated.

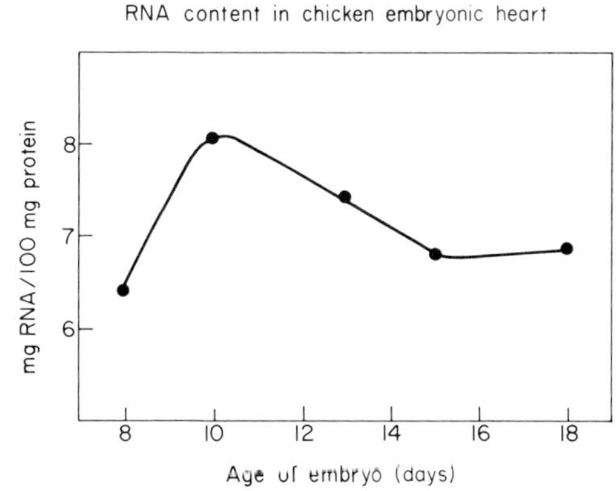

FIG. 2. RNA content in chick embryonic heart. See text for further explanation.

Therefore, the protein synthetic activity of a muscle indicates a positive correlation with RNA concentration not only in different types of muscle, but also in individual muscles growing at different rates, and at different stages of development.

Proportion of Polysomes to Monosomes in the Enlarging Heart

Moroz (1967) demonstrated that microsomes isolated from hypertrophic rat hearts are more active in protein synthesis when measured in an *in vitro* amino acid-incorporating system. This difference, however, is entirely explained by the higher content of ribosomes in microsomal preparations

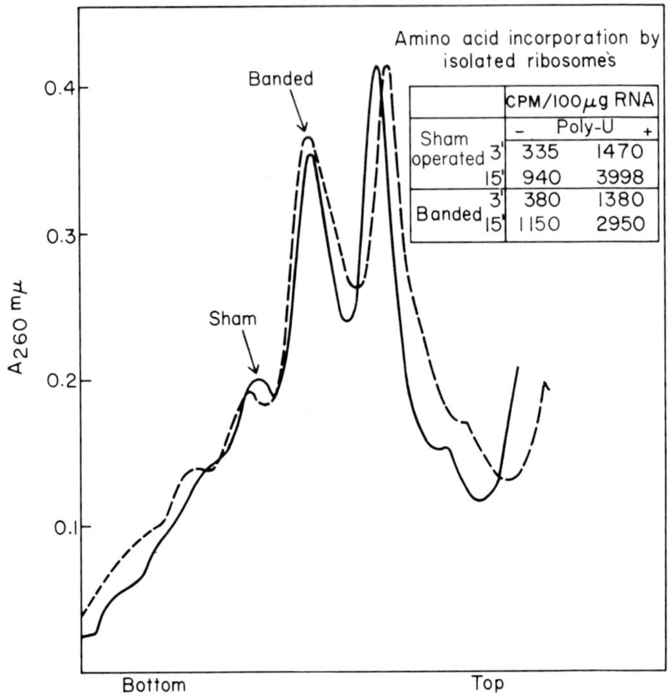

FIG. 3. Five O.D.$_{260\,m\mu}$ units of ribosomes were loaded on the top of 15–30% sucrose density gradient and centrifuged for 90 min at 39,000 rpm in Spinco SW 39 rotor. Ribosomal profiles and amino acid incorporation in banded and sham-operated rats are demonstrated.

isolated from hypertrophied hearts. No evidence was found for more active ribosomal fractions or for larger proportion of ribosomal aggregates in hypertrophy. Our observations are similar (Fig. 3). We found no substantial difference in incorporation of ^{14}C-phenylalanyl-rRNA into trichloroacetic acid insoluble material by heart ribosomes with or without polyuridylic acid between sham-operated and banded animals. A sucrose density gradient analysis of the total ribosomal population did not reveal any substantial shift to larger polysomes during hypertrophy.

A similar situation is apparently true in chick embryonic hearts at different stages of development. The 10-day embryonic heart incubated in Eagle's medium incorporates ^{14}C-amino acids into proteins more rapidly than a 15-day-old heart, but the protein synthetic activity of ribosomes isolated from hearts of both ages are comparable (Table II). The only difference is that the 10-day heart has a higher concentration of RNA, and presumably more ribosomes.

Since the enlarging heart contains more total ribosomes and more t-RNA,

TABLE II

AMINO ACID INCORPORATION INTO MYOFIBRILLAR AND RIBOSOMAL PROTEINS OF CHICK EMBRYONIC HEARTS INCUBATED *In Vitro*[a]

Age of embryo	Amino acid incorporation into protein (cpm/mg protein) (Time of incubation) 12 min	20 min
Myofibrils		
10 days	410	1050
15 days	200	580
Ribosomes		
10 days	500	900
15 days	540	850

[a] Ten whole hearts in each age group were incubated at 37° in 10 ml of Eagle's basic medium containing 1 μCi of ^{14}C-labeled amino acid mixture/ml.

but shows no increase in the ratio of monosomes to polysomes, it must be concluded that synthesis of messenger RNA proceeds at a similar rate to bulk RNA synthesis. That there is no preferential synthesis of messenger RNA is also indicated by the incorporation of ^{32}P- and ^{3}H-uridine into RNA. Although RNA synthesis is increased several times after aortic constriction, no elevation in the rate of messenger RNA synthesis is detectable (Fanburg and Posner, 1969; Koide and Rabinowitz, 1969).

Proportionality of Amino Acid Incorporation into Subcellular Fractions of Heart

Hearts were fractionated as outlined in Fig. 4. The adult rat hearts were homogenized for 20 sec in a blade-type MSE homogenizer (14,000 rpm); the chick embryonic hearts were disrupted by ten strokes in a tightly fitting Dounce homogenizer. The following solutions were used: buffer I: 0.3 *M* sucrose, 0.05 *M* tris/HCl pH 7.5, 0.001 *M* $MgCl_2$; buffer II: 0.25 *M* sucrose, 0.01 *M* tris/HCl; pH 7.5, 0.01 *M* KCl, 0.001 *M* EDTA; buffer III: 0.25 *M* sucrose, 0.05 *M* tris/HCl pH 7.8, 0.15 *M* KCl, 0.005 *M* $MgCl_2$; buffer IV: 0.5 *M* sucrose, 0.001 *M* $MgCl_2$; buffer V: 0.05 *M* tris/HCl pH 7.5, 0.1 *M* KCl, 0.001 *M* EDTA.

The purity of individual fractions was checked by electron microscopy (Fig. 5) and by quantitation of biochemical markers selected on the basis of possible contamination indicated by electron microscopic examination (Table III). The highest degree of purification was obtained in the preparations of

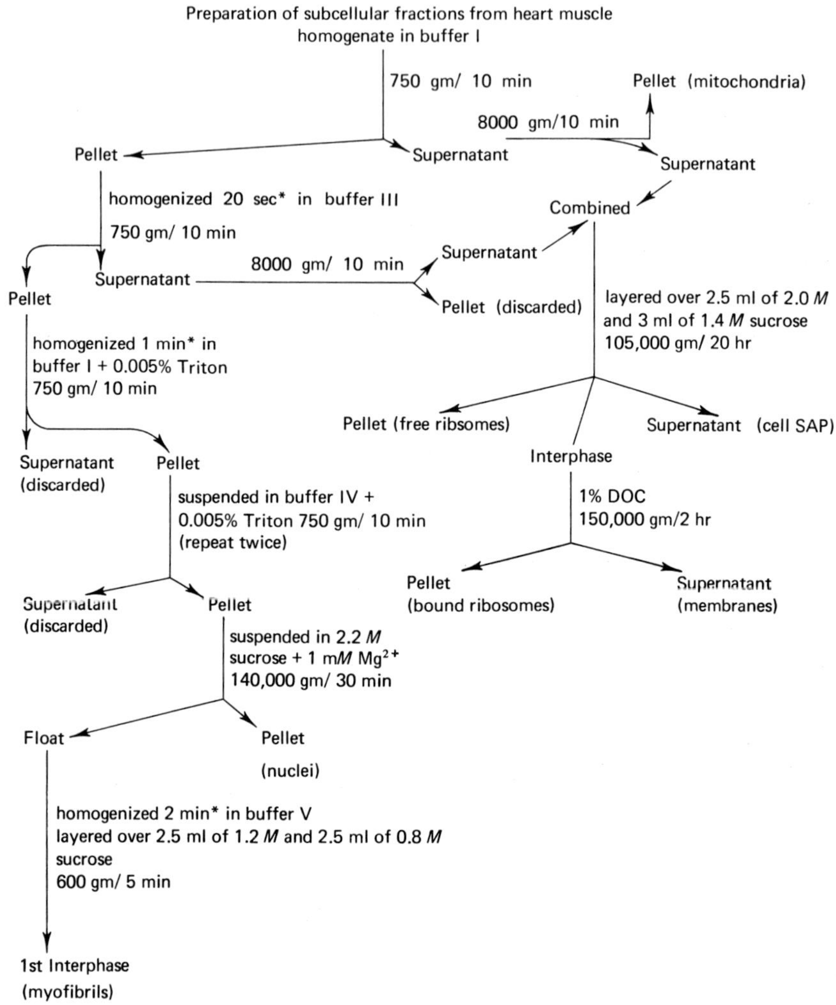

FIG. 4. Preparation of subcellular fractions from heart muscle homogenate in buffer I: Note that asterisk (*) applies only to rat heart; chick embryo hearts were resuspended at each step by ten strokes in Dounce homogenizer. Mitochondria were further purified in buffer II by two cycles of suspension and centrifugation at 750 gm/10 min and five cycles of suspension and pelleting at 8000 gm/10 min. Nuclei were suspended in 2.2 *M* sucrose (+1 m*M* $MgCl_2$), layered over 1 ml of the same sucrose and pelleted by 30 min centrifugation at 140,000 gm. Myofibrils were washed three more times in buffer V containing 0.005% Triton X-100 and were finally suspended in 2.2 *M* sucrose and floated by 30-min centrifugation at 140,000 gm.

TABLE III

RELATIVE PURITY OF HEART CELL FRACTIONS[a]

Marker	Unit: 100 mg protein	Homogenate	Myofibrils	Mitochondria	Nuclei	Membranes	Ribosomes
RNA	mg	7.35	0.23	–	6.8	8.2	112
DNA	mg	5.40	0.51	–	58.5	–	–
phospholipids	μg P_i	730	8	–	–	950	–
cytochrome oxidase	sec^{-1}	2900	negative	540	–	500	–
Ca^{2+} uptake	μmoles	–	negative	negative	–	150	–

[a] The following analytical methods were used: RNA and DNA, Nair *et al.* (1968); phospholipids, Manganiello and Phillips (1965); cytochrome oxidase, Cooperstein and Lazarow (1951); Ca^{2+} uptake, Martonosi and Feretos (1964).

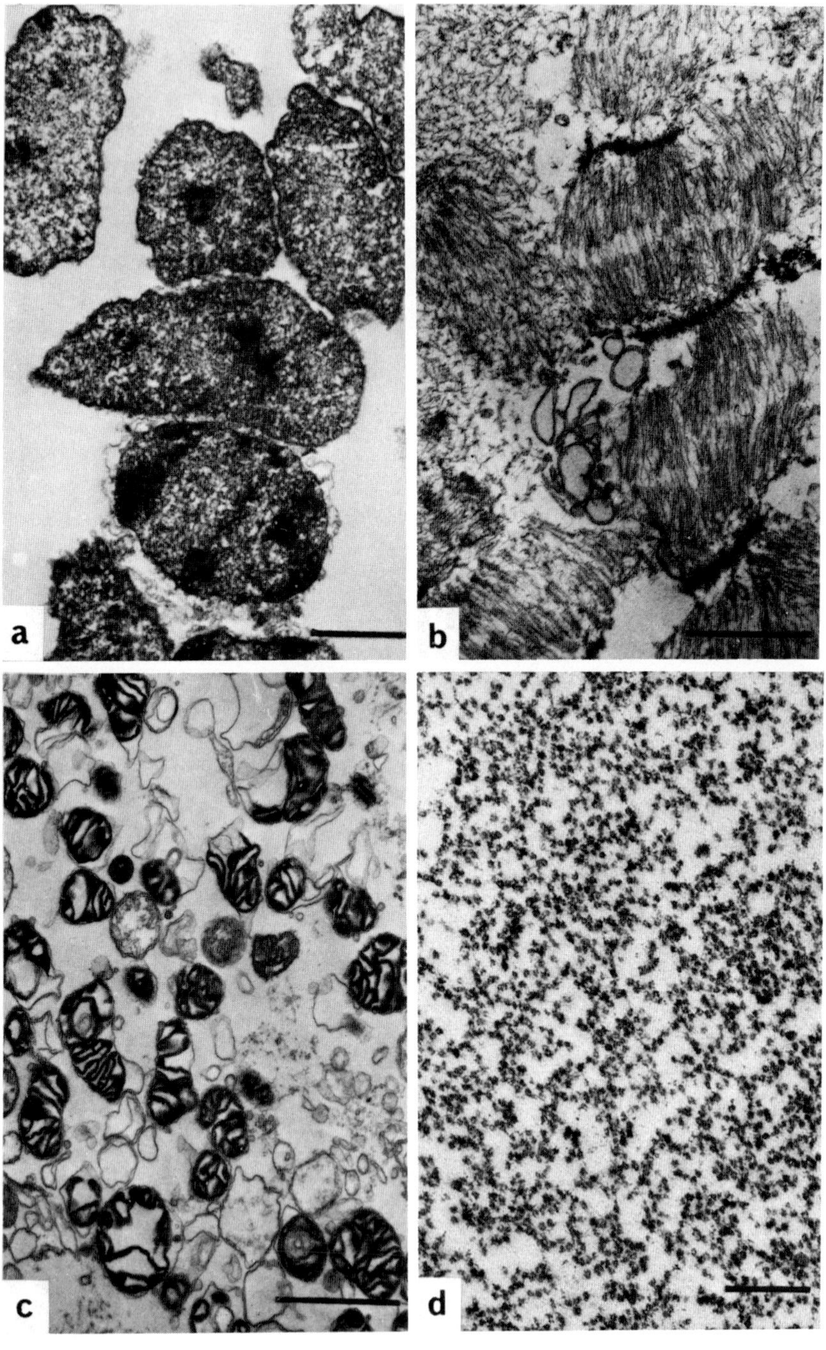
a
b
c
d

nuclei, mitochondra, and ribosomes. Myofibrils contained some fragments of smooth membranes on electron microscopy, but only traces of phospholipids could be detected biochemically and Ca^{2+} uptake was not measurable. Contamination of myofibrils with nuclei and ribosomes was also very low as judged from DNA and RNA analysis. The preparation of membranes contained less than 10% mitochondrial fragments as calculated from their cytochrome oxidase activity before and after Lubrol activation.

The incorporation of ^{14}C-labeled mixture of amino acids into subcellular muscle fractions prepared from hearts of sham-operated and banded animals may be seen in Fig. 6. The specific activity of the total homogenate from each group of sham and banded rates was chosen as unity. The graph thus compares the specific activity of subcellular fractions of hearts with that of the homogenate in sham-operated and banded animals. The nuclei of sham-operated hearts show the lowest incorporation during the first 15 min of labeling, and the ribosomes show the highest. When the same comparison is made in hearts 60 hr after aortic constriction, it is apparent that the general cell proportionality is maintained. Nuclei, mitochondria, and ribosomes are

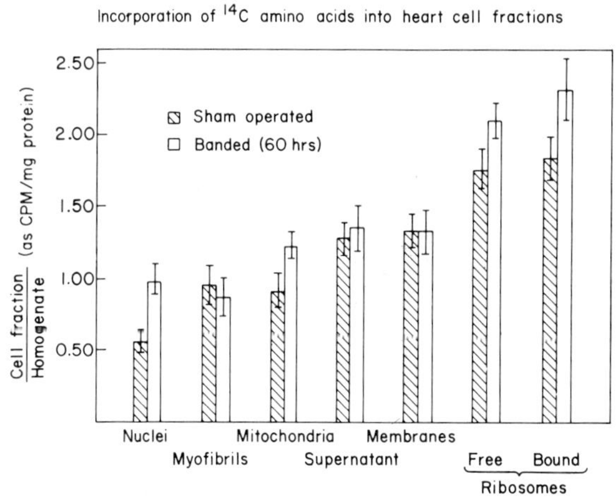

FIG. 6. Results are expressed as means ± S.E.M. incorporation of ^{14}C-amino acids into heart cell fractions.

FIG. 5. Electron micrographs of thin-sectioned pellets from adult rat myocardium fractioned as outlined in Fig. 4. All pellets were fixed in 2.5% gluteraldehyde, 0.1 *M* cacodylate buffer, pH 7.4, subsequently postfixed in OsO_4, and embedded in Araldite. Thin sections were stained with uranyl acetate and lead citrate and examined in an AEI EM 6B electron microscope. (a) Nuclear pellets, magnification, 13,000×; calibration bar, 1 μm. (b) Myofibrils with a small contamination of smooth membranes; magnification, 17,000×; calibration bar, 1 μm. (c) Mitochondrial pellet; magnification, 17,000×; calibration bar, 1 μm. (d) Free ribosomes; magnification, 48,000×; calibration bar, 0.25 μm.

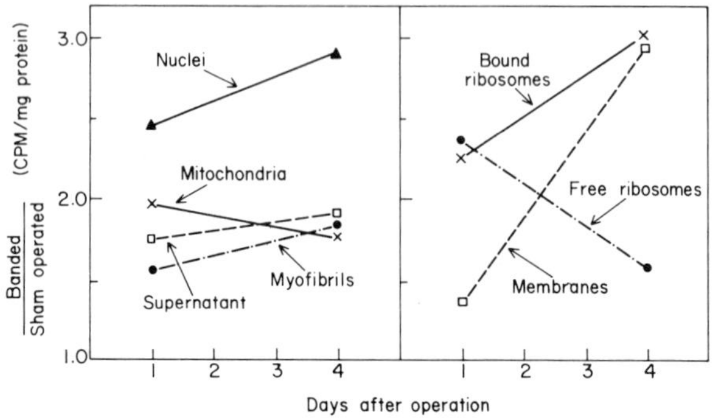

FIG. 7. Change in amino acid incorporation into heart cell fractions is shown after aortic constriction.

synthesized, however, at relatively higher rates than the other cell components during hypertrophy.

Figure 7 shows the changes in amino acid incorporation into heart subcellular fractions 24 and 96 hr after aortic constriction. The striking feature of this comparison of early and later response to aortic banding is the decline in the amino acid incorporation into free ribosomes, and the sharp increase in labeling of the membrane-bound ribosomes and of the membranes themselves.

Free and Membrane-Bound Ribosomes in Enlarging Heart

Two examples of heart enlargement were selected for the study of distribution of free and membrane-bound ribosomes: Rat hearts 72 hr after aortic constriction were compared with sham-operated hearts, and 12-day-old chick embryo hearts were compared with hearts from 16-day-old embryos. In both cases of elevated rate of protein synthesis, the proportion of membrane bound ribosomes to free ribosomes was increased (Table IV).

The role of membrane-bound ribosomes in synthetic activities of heart muscle is not clear. Porter and Palade (1957) noted that their electron-microscopic preparations of the sarcoplasmic reticulum in skeletal muscle showed a striking scarcity of rough-surfaced membranes compared with preparations of cells manufacturing proteins for export, such as the liver or pancreas. During recent years, however, evidence has accumulated for the existence of a small but significant amount of rough membrane both in skeletal muscle (Schiaffino and Margreth, 1969) and in the heart (Fawcett and McNutt, 1969). The population of membrane bound ribosomes isolated from whole heart also includes ribosomes from nonmuscle cells (fibroblasts, endothelium, etc.), which could make up as much as 75% of the total cell number, but only

TABLE IV

RELATIVE PROPORTIONS OF FREE AND MEMBRANE-BOUND RIBOSOMES

Experiment	Free (%)	Bound (%)	No. of experiments
Rat heart			
sham-operated	86 ± 8	14 ± 1	6
banded	65 ± 7	35 ± 4	6
Chicken embryonic heart			
12 days old	74	26	2
16 days old	84	16	2

a small percentage of the myocardial volume (Grove *et al.*, 1969). Membrane-bound ribosomes are clearly visible both in fibroblasts (Goldberg and Greene, 1967) and in endothelial cells of blood vessels (Bruns and Palade, 1968). Thus, the increased proportion of membrane-bound ribosomes in hypertrophic hearts could be explained by either an increased population of connective tissue cells (Grove *et al.*, 1969) or an increased amount of rough endoplasmic reticulum within the muscle cells themselves. These alternatives can be resolved by electron-microscopic examination of the hypertrophic myocardium.

ACKNOWLEDGMENTS

Supported by Grants HE 09172 and HE 05447 from the U.S.P.H.S., and by Chicago Heart Association Research Grant N 69-32 and National Science Foundation Grant GH-7591. We wish to thank Dr. Murray Rabinowitz for his discussions, interest, and support of this work.

REFERENCES

Borsook, H. (1955). *Proc. 3rd Int. Congr. Biochem.*, Academic Press, N.Y., 54.
Brachet, J. (1941). *Arch. Biol.* **53,** 207.
Bruns, R. R., and Palade, G. E. (1968). *J. Cell Biol.* **37,** 244.
Caspersson, T. (1941). *Naturwissenschaften* **29,** 33.
Cooperstein, S. J., and Lazarow, A. (1951). *J. Biol. Chem.* **189,** 665.
Fanburg, B. L., and Posner, B. I. (1968). *Circ. Res.* **23,** 137.
Fawcett, D. V., and McNutt, N. S. (1969). *J. Cell Biol.* **42,** 1.
Fleck, A., Shepherd, J., and Munro, H. N. (1965). *Science* **150,** 628.
Gilbert, W. (1963). *J. Mol. Biol.* **6,** 389.
Goldberg, B., and Green, H. (1967). *J. Mol. Biol.* **26,** 1.
Grove, D., Zak, R., Nair, K. G., and Aschenbrenner, V. (1969). *Circ. Res.* **25,** 473.
Heywood, S. M., Dowben, R. M., and Rich, A. (1967). *Proc. Nat. Acad. Sci. U.S.* **57,** 1002.
Koide, T., and Rabinowitz, M. (1969). *Circ. Res.* **24,** 9.

Manganiello, V. C., and Phillips, A. H. (1965). *J. Biol. Chem.* **240,** 3951.
Martonosi, A., and Feretos, R. (1964). *J. Biol. Chem.* **239,** 648.
Moroz, L. A. (1967). *Circ. Res.* **21,** 449.
Nair, K. G., Cutilletta, A. F., Zak, R., Koide, T., and Rabinowitz, M. (1968). *Circ. Res.* **23,** 451.
Porter, K. R., and Palade, G. E. (1957). *J. Biophys. Biochem. Cytol.* **3,** 269.
Schiaffino, S., and Margreth, A. (1969). *J. Cell Biol.* **41,** 855.
Villa-Trevino, S., Farber, E., Staehelin, T., Wettstein, F. O., and Noll, H. (1964). *J. Biol. Chem.* **239,** 3826.
Zak, R. (1962). *Fed. Proc. Fed. Amer. Soc. Exp. Biol.* **21,** 2.
Zak, R., Rabinowitz, M., and Platt, C. (1967). *Biochemistry* **6,** 2493.

MYOCARDIAL NUCLEIC ACID METABOLISM IN EXPERIMENTAL CARDIAC HYPERTROPHY

Eugene Morkin

Because of the importance of nucleic acids in growth and differentiation, there has been much recent interest in myocardial nucleic acid metabolism during development of cardiac hypertrophy. In this chapter, I discuss certain problems associated with obtaining the precise kind of information about nucleic acid metabolism in the myocardium that has been possible with other tissues. First, the interstitial cells within the heart are nearly three times more numerous than muscle cells; they dominate nucleic acid metabolism in the organ. Second, a variety of factors influence the nucleic acid content of the myocardium, including changes in the rate of nucleic acid synthesis, alterations in content and turnover rate of nucleic acid precursors, and possibly alterations in the rate of nucleic acid degradation as well. These factors make accurate assessment of changes in myocardial nucleic acid metabolism induced by increased work load particularly difficult. I would like to discuss these problems in some detail as it would appear that their importance has not been generally recognized.

Dominance of Interstitial Cells in Myocardial Nucleic Acid Metabolism

Since the increased muscle mass in cardiac hypertrophy is thought to represent primarily an enlargement of individual cardiac cells without an accompanying increase in nuclei (Grove *et al.*, 1969b; Karnser, 1925), the increased DNA content reported for hypertrophied hearts by several investigators (Gluck *et al.*, 1964; Grimm *et al.*, 1966; Summer and McIntosh, 1963) seemed puzzling and prompted us to measure and localize myocardial DNA synthesis during development of cardiac hypertrophy (Morkin and Ashford, 1968).

Rats (200–220 gm) were injected with thymidine-methyl-^{3}H (15.6 Ci/mM) on the first, second, third, seventh, and tenth days following either aortic coarctation (19 animals) or sham operation (9 animals). Blocks of tissue were taken from the heart for histological study and the remainder used for analysis of nucleic acids by a modification of the Schmidt-Thannhauser technic (Schmidt and Thannhauser, 1945). Radioactivity in the DNA fraction was measured by liquid scintillation counting in Bray's solution (Bray, 1960) with appropriate corrections for background radioactivity and quenching.

For microscopic examination and autoradiography, tissue was fixed in phosphate-buffered 4% glutaraldehyde (pH 7.4) and embedded in epoxy resin, "Epon," from which 0.5 μm sections were cut with a Sorvall microtome. Autoradiography was performed as described by Caro (1964) using Ilford K-5 emulsion. After developing, the sections were stained with freshly filtered methylene blue. The relative frequency of nuclei of different cell types and the distribution of radioactivity between them was determined in each animal by examining the nuclei contained in 100 high-power fields.

Changes in ventricular weight, nucleic acid concentration, and thymidine-^{3}H incorporation following aortic coarctation and sham operation are shown in Fig. 1. Sham-operated rats sacrificed during the first week after operation showed no systematic difference in ventricular weight, nucleic acid concentration, or thymidine-^{3}H incorporation, and have been summarized as a single control group. As shown in the upper graph in Fig. 1(a), there was a rapid increase in left ventricular (LV) weight following coarctation; by the third

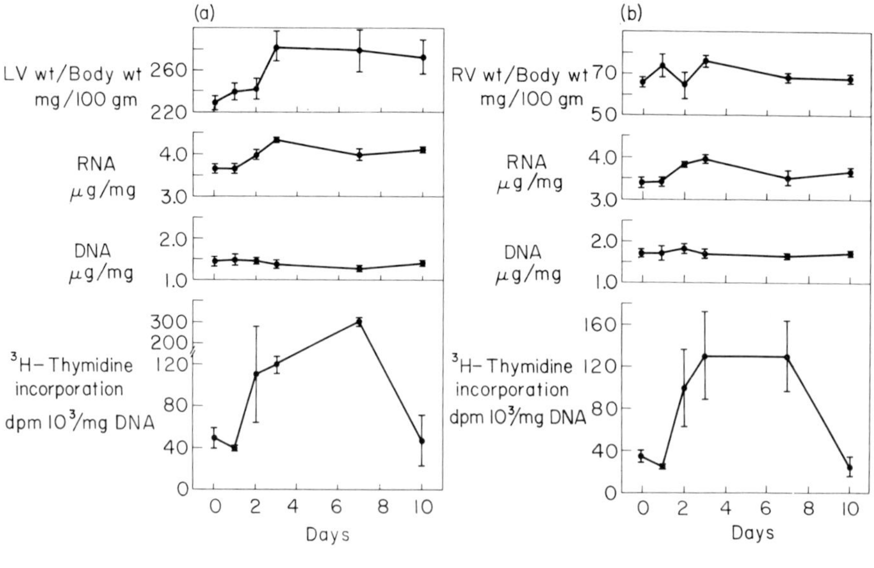

FIG. 1. Changes in left (a) and right (b) ventricular weight, RNA concentration, DNA concentration and thymidine-^{3}H incorporation following aortic coarctation. Values are mean $\pm$ S.E. (By permission of the American Physiological Society.)

postoperative day, LV weight was increased by 23%, as compared with controls ($P < 0.01$).

Concomitant with the increase in LV weight, LV RNA concentration increased 17% ($P < 0.1$), remaining approximately at this level for the remainder of the period of observation. On the contrary, LV DNA concentration decreased about 10% during the phase of rapid increase in ventricular weight. However, by the 10th day after operation, continuing DNA synthesis returned the DNA concentration nearly to normal level.

As shown in the lowermost graph in Fig. 1(a), there was little change in LV DNA synthesis, as measured by the rate of thymidine-^{3}H incorporation into DNA, until the second postoperative day. The rate of DNA synthesis was markedly increased between the second and seventh postoperative days, averaging three to five times control ($P < 0.01$). By the 10th postoperative day, DNA synthesis had returned toward control level.

Interestingly, RV nucleic acid concentration and thymidine-^{3}H incorporation underwent similar, but smaller changes than those observed in LV [Fig. 1(b)]. Increased RV weight and RNA concentration have been reported previously following left ventricular overload (Gluck *et al.*, 1964), apparently because of elevation of LV filling pressure and pulmonary arterial and RV pressures (Zuhlke *et al.*, 1966).

Autoradiographs from hypertrophied and control ventricles revealed that labeling is confined almost entirely to the nuclei of endothelial and connective tissue cells [Fig. 2(a) and (b)]. There was no increase over background in

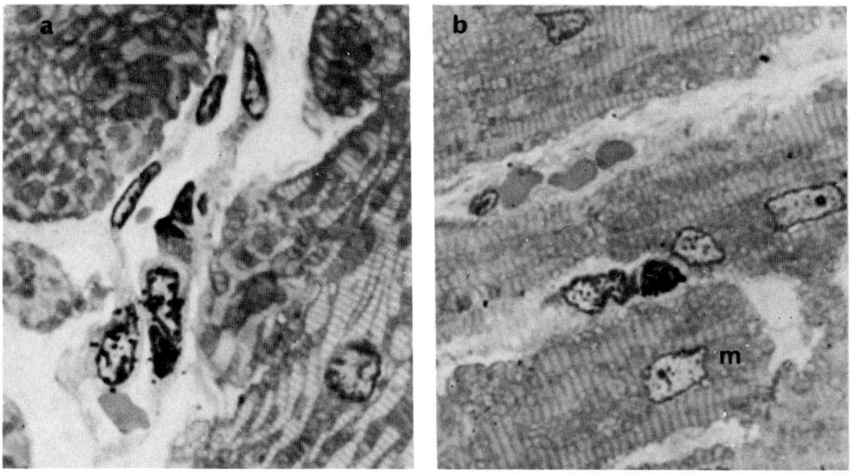

FIG. 2. Autoradiographic localization of thymidine-^{3}H incorporation in hypertrophied rat heart. (a), Labeled capillary endothelial nuclei; (b), labeled connective tissue nucleus. Muscle nuclei (*m*) are not labeled. (×1,600).

labeling of possible extranuclear sites (mitochondria) of DNA synthesis. An analysis of autoradiographed sections of myocardium from sham-operated and stenosed rats is shown in Fig. 3. The upper bar graphs represent the composition of myocardial nuclei in sham-operated and stenosed animals at various times after coarctation: 1–2 days, 3–7 days, and 10 days. In the sham-operated group (day 0), about 27% of the total myocardial nuclei are muscle nuclei, about 35% are connective tissue nuclei, and about 38% are endothelial nuclei. After coarctation, there is a slight increase in the proportion of blood vessel endothelial nuclei. Although there are some binucleate cells in the heart, these data can be taken to approximate an analysis of myocardial cell types.

The distribution of label among these nuclear types is shown in the lower part of Fig. 3. A small fraction of a percent of labeled muscle nuclei were found in sham-operated animals, whereas about 2% of the interstitial nuclei were labeled. Following operation there is a marked increase in labeling of interstitial cells which is greatest during the 3rd–7th days after coarctation. No labeled muscle nuclei were observed in ventricular tissue of stenosed rats.

This analysis revealed two striking facts: First, there is a nearly 3:1 predominance of interstitial cells as compared to muscle cells in the heart. Second, during development of cardiac hypertrophy, there is an increase in labeling of connective tissue and blood vessel endothelium without any evidence of thymidine-^{3}H incorporation by muscle nuclei. Since the nucleus of each somatic cell contains approximately the same diploid complement

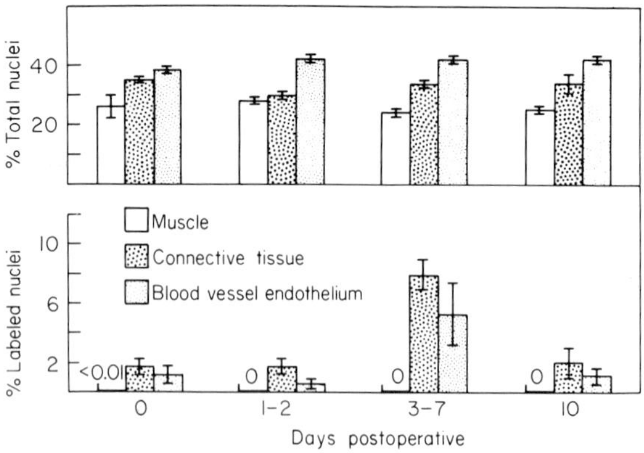

FIG. 3. Distribution of thymidine-^{3}H labeling of myocardial cell types. Percent of total nuclei represented by cardiac muscle, connective tissue cells, and blood vessel endothelium is shown above. The percent of labeled nuclei of each type is represented below. The values are mean ± S.E.

of DNA (Boivin *et al.*, 1948), it would appear that three-fourths of myocardial DNA is of connective tissue and endothelial origin. Hence, changes in the DNA content of the heart can be readily ascribed to alterations in the rate of DNA synthesis by interstitial cells. Similar results and conclusions have been obtained by Rumyantsev *et al.*, (1967) and by Grove and co-workers (1969a, b).

Since RNA is synthesized primarily within the nucleus these data suggested the need for localizing RNA synthesis within the heart. For these studies it proved convenient to use an *in vitro* labeling system. Heart slices (0.3-mm thickness) were incubated in Eagle's medium containing penicillin (100 units/ml) and streptomycin (100 μg/ml). For measurement of RNA synthesis, uridine-5-^{3}H (26.3 Ci/m*M*) was added at a concentration of 25 μCi/ml. In some experiments, protein synthesis also was determined by replacing unlabeled leucine in the medium with L-leucine-1-^{14}C (30.3 mCi/m*M*) at a concentration of 0.5 μCi/ml. Two or three slices weighing ~250 mg were incubated in 4 ml medium at 37°C with gentle shaking in a Dubnoff metabolic incubator through which 95% O_2–5% CO_2 was bubbled. Experiments were terminated by placing the flasks in an ice bath and by adding uridine or leucine in unlabeled form. After removing blocks of tissue for microscopic study, the remaining tissue was analyzed for RNA (Schmidt and Thannhauser, 1945) and protein.

As shown in Fig. 4, RNA and protein synthesis were nearly constant in

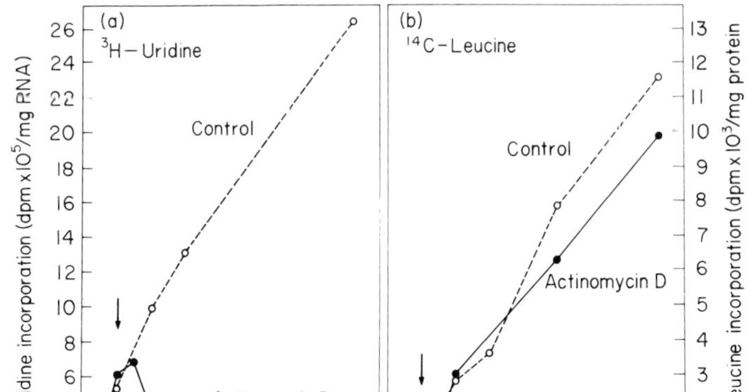

FIG. 4. Incorporation of uridine-5-^{3}H and L-leucine-1-^{14}C into RNA and protein in heart slices. After addition of 12.5 μg actinomycin-D (indicated by arrow) there was a prompt cessation of RNA synthesis while protein synthesis continued at nearly 80% of the control rate.

these slices for at least 8 hr, and continued at a diminished rate for several more hours. RNA synthesis was completely inhibited within 30 min of addition of actinomycin D to the flasks, whereas protein synthesis continued at almost 80% of the control rate for many hours, suggesting that most myocardial proteins are made on long-lived RNA templates. The diminution in RNA specific activity after addition of actinomycin D presumably reflects continuing degradation of RNA unopposed by further synthesis.

Figure 5 shows autoradiographs prepared from a slice incubated for 2 hr in uridine-^{3}H. Almost all the interstitial cells appear heavily labeled; lightly labeled muscle nuclei (1–2 grains/nucleus) also are identified. Slices from hypertrophied hearts show a similar predominance of interstitial labeling so that careful quantitative analysis of grain density and distribution will be necessary to determine the exact extent of change in RNA synthesis. Nevertheless, the 3 : 1 predominance of interstitial cells in conjunction with their apparently greater RNA synthetic activity clearly indicates that studies of RNA synthesis in whole heart homogenates (Fanburg and Posner, 1968; Koide and Rabinowitz, 1969), or using nuclear enzymes (Nair *et al.*, 1968) from whole heart homogenates, primarily reflect alterations in the RNA metabolism of interstitial cells and cannot be expected to shed much light upon changes in muscle cells.

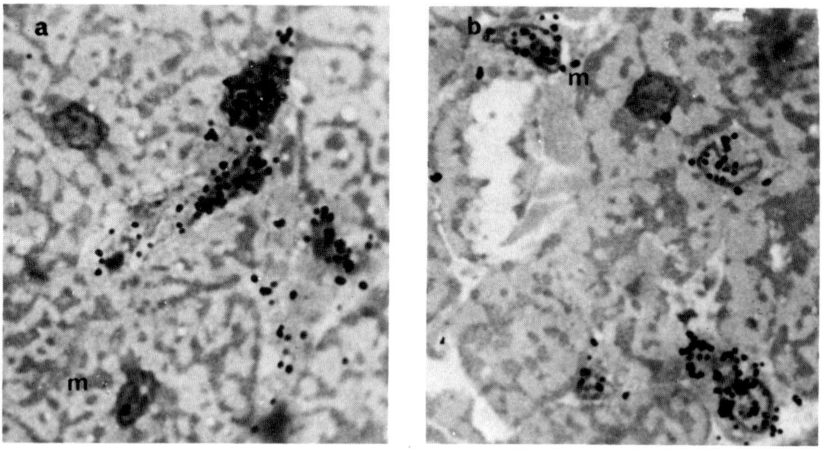

FIG. 5. Autoradiographs prepared from heart slice labeled *in vitro* with uridine-5-^{3}H. Muscle fibers are shown in cross section. In both (a) and (b) nearly all blood vessel and connective tissue nuclei are heavily labeled; occasional muscle nuclei (m) are lightly labeled (×2,000).

Factors Influencing Measurement of RNA Synthesis

Let us now turn our attention to an analysis of factors influencing the measurement of nucleic acid synthesis during development of cardiac hypertrophy. A summary of data from three laboratories (Fanburg and Posner, 1968; Koide and Rabinowitz, 1969; Morkin and Ashford, 1968) (Fig. 6) shows the percent changes in left ventricular (LV) weight, RNA content, and rate of RNA synthesis measured by RNA specific activity that occurs during the first week following aortic coarctation. Left ventricular weight does not increase significantly until the second or third day. An increase in total RNA content occurs simultaneously because of an increase in RNA concentration and ventricular weight. The lower part of Fig. 6 shows the specific activity of RNA following a pulse label on successive days after operation. The peak increase in specific activity occurs at about 12 hr in the study of Fanburg and Posner (1968) in which ^{32}P was used for RNA labeling, but does not reach a peak until 48 hr in the experiments of Koide and Rabin-

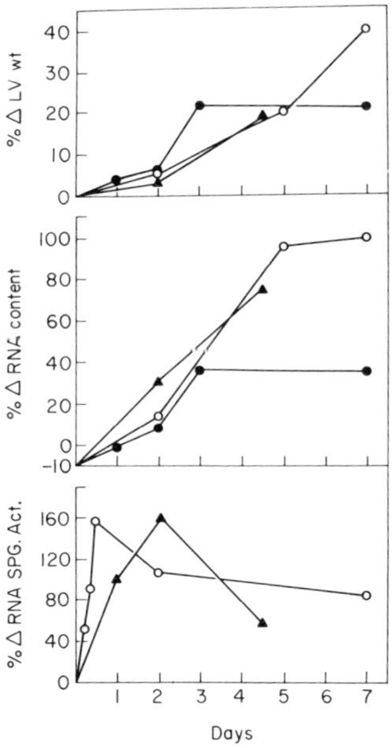

FIG. 6. Changes in left ventricular weight, RNA content, and RNA specific activity following aortic coarctation. Represented are average results from three groups of investigators: (●—●) Morkin and Ashford (1968); (○—○) Fanburg and Posner (1968); (Δ—Δ) Koide and Rabinowitz (1969).

witz (1969) in which uridine-^3H was employed. However, there is fair agreement as to the magnitude of the increase in RNA specific activity–$\sim$120–160%.

Before an estimate of the actual rate of RNA synthesis can be made, corrections must be made for the effects of changes in metabolism of nucleotide precursors and for dilution of newly formed RNA by the increased RNA content of the heart. Koide and Rabinowitz (1969) have included these corrections in what they term the "Index of RNA Synthesis" [Eq. (1)]:

$$\varepsilon = \frac{a \times S}{I_U} \times \frac{1}{fr_U} k \tag{1}$$

$$\% \, \Delta\text{RNA synthesis} = \frac{\varepsilon_c - \varepsilon_s}{\varepsilon_s} \tag{2}$$

where ε is the index of RNA synthesis, units/hr; c, s, coarctation and sham operation; a, specific activity of RNA, (mμCi/mg); S, RNA content of heart (mg); I_U, integrated specific activity–time curve (0–24 hr) for uridine monophosphate (mμCi/hr/μgUMP); fr_U, uridine monophosphate fraction of RNA by weight; and k, constant for uncontrolled variables.

The important points are, first, that the effect of changes in radioactivity of the precursor is incorporated into (I) the specific activity–time factor, and second, that the specific activity of RNA (a) is multiplied by the total amount of RNA (S). This corrects for dilution of radioactivity by the increased RNA content of the heart.

As indicated in Eq. (2), the percent change in RNA synthesis can be computed from the Indices of RNA Synthesis of animals with coarctation (ε_c) as opposed to sham operation (ε_s).

The influence of these corrections on the apparent rate of RNA synthesis and the resultant increase in ventricular RNA content as determined by Koide and Rabinowitz (1969) is illustrated in Fig. 7. After correction of the observed RNA specific activity for changes in uridine precursor pool, the maximum apparent rate of synthesis is increased from 169% to over 200%.* Further correction for the increased RNA content observed on the second day increases the peak rate of RNA synthesis to 300% of control. From days 2 to 5, there is a rapid decline in the rate of RNA synthesis.

Let us now ask whether these changes in labeling of RNA can account for

* Measurement of UMP or AMP specific activity is not an entirely satisfactory measure of RNA precursor labeling. Since RNA polymerase reacts only with nucleotide triphosphates, when radioactive uridine or adenine are injected determination of labeling of UTP or ATP would seem to be a more valid approach. When ^{32}P is injected, only the radioactivity associated with the α-phosphate of the nucleotide triphosphates is an accurate indicator of RNA precursor labeling.

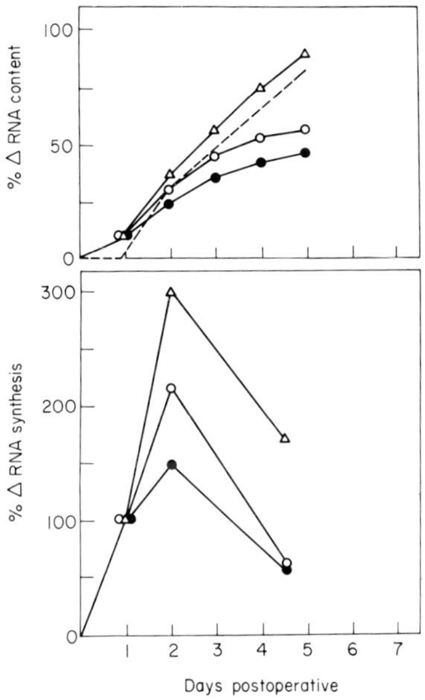

FIG. 7. Changes in myocardial RNA content and rate of RNA synthesis during development of cardiac hypertrophy using data of Koide and Rabinowitz (1969). (*Above*), LV RNA content predicted from changes in RNA specific activity (●—●) as measure of rate of synthesis; after correction of apparent synthetic rate for changes in RNA precursor pool size and turnover rate (○—○) after further correction of apparent synthetic rate for dilution by increased RNA content (Δ—Δ). Measured change in RNA content (---). (*Below*), Apparent rate of RNA synthesis as indicated by RNA specific activity following injection with uridine-^{3}H (●—●); after correction for UMP pool size and turnover rate (○—○); and after additional correction for increased RNA content (Δ Δ).

the increase in RNA content observed by the investigators. The calculations of RNA contents shown in the upper part of Fig. 7 were made from the data on RNA synthesis by assuming a turnover time of 5½ days for cardiac RNA as measured in the adult mouse heart by Baserga and co-workers (1966). The increase in RNA content predicted from the change in RNA specific activity is substantially less than that actually observed. After correction for changes in labeling of nucleotide precursor there is an increase in the amount of RNA synthesized, which still falls appreciably short of that observed. After further correction of the apparent rate of synthesis for dilution by the increased amount of RNA, there is better agreement between observed and computed values.

When a similar sequence of corrections is applied to the data of Fanburg and Posner, the results are less favorable (Fig. 8). The specific activity of

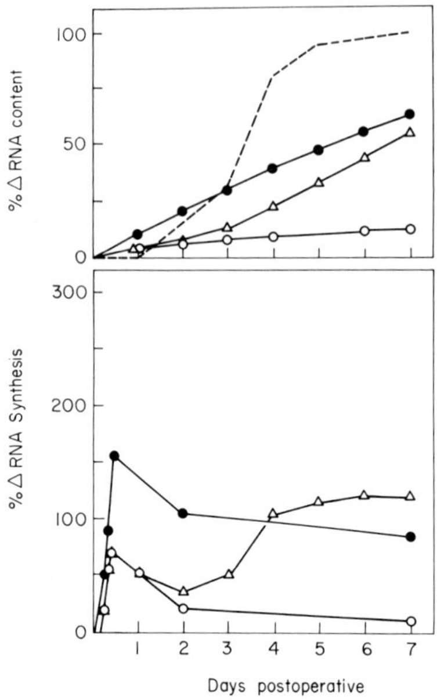

FIG. 8. Changes in myocardial RNA content and rate of RNA synthesis during development of cardiac hypertrophy using data of Fanburg and Posner (1968). (*Above*) LV RNA content calculated from changes in RNA specific activity (●—●); after correction of apparent synthetic rate for changes in labeling of RNA precursor pool (○—○); after further correction of apparent synthetic rate for dilution by increased RNA content (Δ—Δ). Measured change in RNA content (---). (*Below*) Apparent rate of RNA synthesis as indicated by RNA specific activity following injection with ^{32}P (●—●); after correction for AMP specific activity (○—○); and after additional correction for increased RNA content (Δ—Δ).

AMP following labeling with ^{32}P was markedly increased in hearts from stenosed rats so that the RNA specific activity is diminished by this correction. Equally interesting is the influence of the increasing RNA content, which in combination with a persistently elevated RNA specific activity, produces a biphasic curve of RNA synthesis. Before attempting any interpretation of this result, discrepancies between these data and those of Koide and Rabinowitz must be resolved.

The foregoing comments on factors influencing calculation of myocardial RNA synthesis also apply to synthesis of DNA. However, the ventricular thymidine-^{3}H pool is similar in normal and hypertrophied hearts (Grove *et al.*, 1969b), and the increase in DNA content during hypertrophy is small as compared to the increase in RNA content (Morkin and Ashford, 1968).

Myocardial RNA Turnover during Cardiac Hypertrophy

Finally, I would like to make a few comments about degradation of myocardial RNA. Figure 9 shows the data of Baserga and co-workers (1966) on the turnover of RNA in the mouse heart which have been replotted on semilog coordinates. In the adult heart, the decrease in radioactivity of RNA is rapid at first, then quite slow. This might be the result of RNA species turning over with markedly different half-lives, or possibly, the result of reutilization of label. Curiously, in the newborn mouse RNA turnover seems to be slower and to obey simple first-order kinetics.

Using the initial downslope of the curve of RNA radioactivity, the half-life of cardiac RNA in the adult mouse heart is $5\frac{1}{2}$ days. This value is similar to the half-life reported for rat liver RNA (Hirsch and Hiatt, 1966).

Although in calculating the amount of RNA synthesized, I have assumed that RNA degradation is unchanged during development of cardiac hypertrophy, there is, in fact, no reason for believing that changes in degradation may not occur. As an example, Hirsch and Hiatt (1966) have demonstrated decreased RNA synthesis and increased degradation to be responsible for depletion of ribosomes from the liver during starvation.

We have recently attempted to assess degradation of RNA during development of cardiac hypertrophy (Table I). For these experiments, rats were injected with 0.5 mCi/100 gm body weight uridine-5-^{3}H (26.3 Ci/mM). The following day, three were sacrificed and the remaining six subjected to sham operation or aortic coarctation. At the end of 5 days, total LV RNA

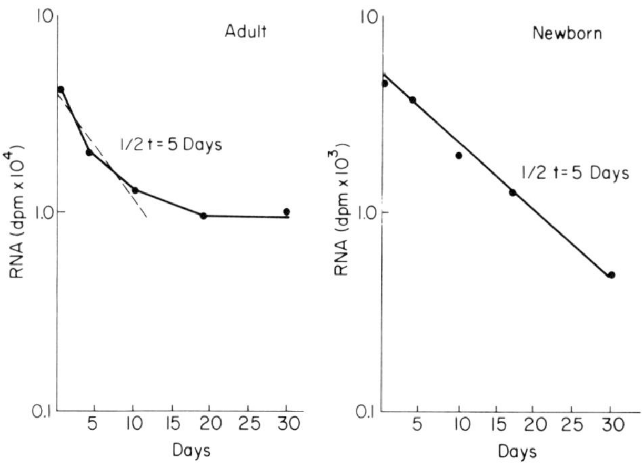

FIG. 9. Turnover of a cardiac RNA in the adult (left) and newborn (right) mouse heart. Data from Baserga and co-workers (1966).

TABLE I

RNA TURNOVER DURING DEVELOPMENT OF CARDIAC HYPERTROPHY

Postoperative day[a]	Type	LV wt (100 gm body wt)	LV RNA (dpm × 10^4)
0 (3)	Unoperated	218.3 ± 3.3	19.6 ± 4.5
5 (3)	Sham	217.5 ± 1.5	9.1 ± 0.1
5 (3)	Stenosed	320.7 ± 11.0	16.8 ± 1.3
5 (1)	Stenosed + uridine infusion	303	19.9

[a] Mean value ± S.E. Numbers in parentheses are numbers of animals.

radioactivity in sham-operated animals decreased to less than one-half the initial value, but radioactivity in the RNA fraction of stenosed rats showed little change. This result might arise either by decreased RNA degradation and/or increased reutilization of label. In an attempt to assess the role of nucleoside reutilization, a continuous intravenous infusion of unlabeled uridine (10 mg/day) was given to an additional rat for 5 days after coarctation. In this animal, the total counts in the LV RNA fraction after five days was not significantly reduced as compared to stenosed animals not receiving an infusion, suggesting that reutilization at the nucleoside level is not primarily responsible for the slower RNA turnover observed. Although these results are only preliminary, they illustrate the difficulty of accurately determining RNA turnover and suggest the need for careful appraisal of myocardial RNA degradation, as well as synthesis, during development of cardiac hypertrophy.

Summary

In summary, I have tried to review recent advances in myocardial nucleic acid metabolism with particular emphasis upon three points: (1) the dominant role of interstitial cells in measurements of total nucleic acid synthesis in the heart; (2) the influence of both changes in precursor radioactivity and increasing RNA content on measurements of ventricular RNA synthesis during development of cardiac hypertrophy; and (3) the possible role of decreased degradation and/or nucleoside reutilization in measurements of RNA turnover.

ACKNOWLEDGMENTS

This research was supported by grants from the Life Insurance Medical Research Fund, the Greater Boston Chapter of the Massachusetts Heart Association, and the National Institutes of Health (HE-13317 and HE-11414). The author is a recipient of a Research Career Development Award (HE-13639).

References

Baserga, R., Petersen, R. O., and Estensen, R. D. (1966). *Biochim. Biophys. Acta* **129,** 259.

Boivin, A., Vendrely, R., and Vendrely, C. (1948). *Compt. Rend. Acad. Sci.* **226,** 1061.

Bray, G. A. (1960). *Anal. Biochem.* **1,** 279.

Caro, L. G. (1964). "In Methods in Cell Physiology" (D. M. Prescott, ed.), Vol. 1, p. 327. Academic, New York.

Fanburg, B. L., and Posner, B. I. (1968). *Circ. Res.* **23,** 123.

Gluck, L., Talner, N. S., Stein, H., Gardner, T. H., and Kulovich, M. V. (1964). *Science* **144,** 1244.

Grimm, A. F., Kubota, R., and Whitehorn, W. V. (1966). *Circ. Res.* **19,** 552.

Grove, D., Nair, K. G., and Zak, R. (1969a). *Circ. Res.* **25,** 463.

Grove, D., Zak, R., Nair, K. G., and Aschenbrenner, V. (1969b). *Circ. Res.* **25,** 473.

Hirsch, C., and Hiatt, H. (1966). *J. Biol. Chem.* **241,** 5936.

Karnser, H., Saphir, O., and Todd, T. W. (1925). *Amer. J. Pathol.* **1,** 351.

Koide, T., and Rabinowitz, M. (1969). *Circ. Res.* **24,** 9.

Morkin, E., and Ashford, T. P. (1968). *Amer. J. Physiol.* **215,** 1409.

Nair, K. G., Cutilletto, A. F., Zak, R., Koide, T., and Rabinowitz, M. (1968). *Circ. Res.* **23,** 451.

Rumyantsev, P. P., Aljekhina, G. A., and Meerson, F. S. (1967). *Tsitologiia* **9,** 311.

Schmidt, G., and Thannhauser, S. J. (1945). *J. Biol. Chem.* **161,** 83.

Summer, R. G., and McIntosh, D. H. (1963). *Circ. Res.* **12,** 170.

Zuhlke, V., de Rochemont, W. du M., Gudbjarnson, S., and Bing, R. J. (1966). *Circ. Res.* **18,** 558.

RIBONUCLEIC ACID SYNTHESIS IN EXPERIMENTAL CARDIAC HYPERTROPHY

Barry L. Fanburg, Barry I. Posner, and Satoru Matsushita

Changes in nucleic acid metabolism play an early and central role in several examples of rapid tissue growth (Gorski and Nicolette, 1963; Korner, 1964; Wicks *et al.*, 1965; Greenman *et al.*, 1965; Benjamin and Gelhorn, 1966; Malt and Stoddard, 1966; Hamilton *et al.*, 1967). A study of these changes in experimental cardiac hypertrophy provides a focus for assessing the mechanism that translates increased mechanical activity into heart muscle growth. The present report is concerned with some of the investigations that have been carried out in this laboratory into the stimulation of RNA synthesis resulting from the imposition of a work load on the rat heart *in vivo*.

Cardiac hypertrophy was produced, as previously described (Fanburg and Posner, 1968), in anesthetized Charles River male rats weighing 180–220 gm. The mediastinum was entered through a midsternal incision, and a constriction was placed around the ascending aorta between the right innominate and left internal carotid arteries. The constriction was imposed by making a tight ligature around the aorta and an adjacent 1.17-mm-diameter stainless steel needle, and subsequently removing the needle. This procedure resulted in ~30% increase in heart weight and ~40% increase in the heart weight/body weight ratio of animals with aortic constriction, as compared with sham-operated controls at 7 days after operation (Fig. 1). These values remained relatively constant over the next 3 weeks of the study. In some experiments the left ventricular pressure was recorded through a transdiaphragmatic puncture (Posner and Fanburg, 1968), and the peak systolic pressure was found to be elevated ~30% above that of controls at 1–2 hr after constriction. The increase in pressure was even more marked at 7 days after operation, a time at which the growth process had reached a plateau.

RNA and DNA determinations (Fig. 2) were carried out on the hearts from a group of these animals. The RNA concentration in hearts from animals with aortic constriction showed little, if any, difference from that of control animals at 1 day after operation. At 2 days after operation, there was a 30%

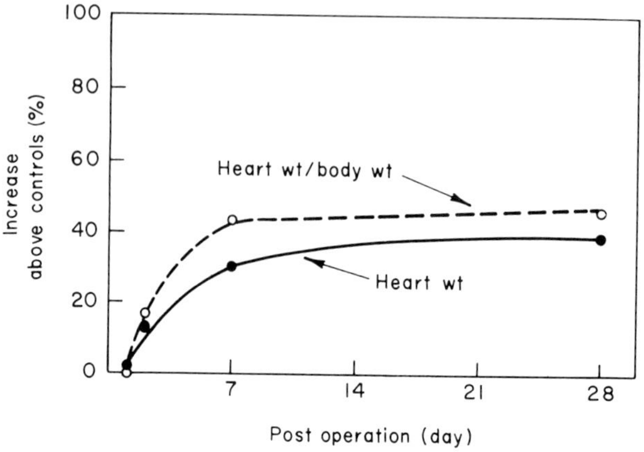

FIG. 1. Changes in heart weight and heart weight/body weight ratio after aortic constriction. Average weights were determined on at least eight animals at each time.

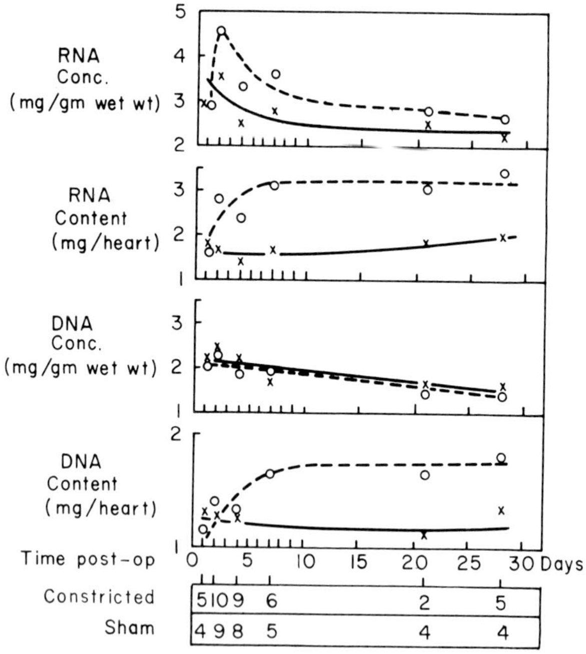

FIG. 2. Changes in total and concentration of heart RNA and DNA in rats with aortic constriction. RNA was determined by the orcinol procedure (Schneider, 1957). DNA was determined by the diphenylamine procedure of Burton (1956). The number of animals used at each time is noted at the bottom of the figure. (0- - -0) Hearts from animals with constricted aortas; (x—x) hearts from sham-operated animals.

increase above controls in the RNA concentration of the animals with aortic constriction. Thereafter, the concentration gradually returned toward the control level. The total heart RNA content also increased by the second day after operation and remained elevated above that for control animals throughout the period of the study. However, the DNA concentration of the animals with aortic constriction remained unchanged from that of the controls. There was a gradual decrease in this value as the animals grew. The total DNA content per heart of animals with aortic constriction increased proportionately to the increase in heart weight.

The pattern and extent of labeling of heart RNA was determined with a radioactive precursor of RNA at various times after operation. RNA was isolated by extraction with phenol, purification, and fractionation on a sucrose density gradient as has been previously described in detail (Fanburg and Posner, 1968; Posner and Fanburg, 1966).

When a 4-hr period of labeling with $^{32}P\text{-}H_3PO_4$ was carried out at 20 hr after operation, the pattern of labeling of RNA corresponded closely to that of the optical density profile (Fig. 3). The specific activity of RNA from hearts of animals with aortic constriction was increased throughout the gradient. A shorter period of labeling, for 1 hr at 7 hr after operation, resulted in less correspondence of the labeling pattern to the optical density profile. However, there was still a general increase in RNA labeling throughout the gradient for hearts from animals with aortic constriction. At no time did we see any

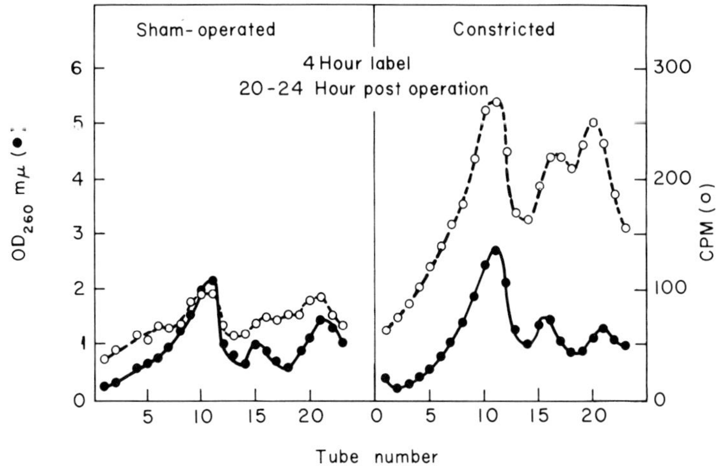

FIG. 3. Pattern of labeling of heart RNA between 20 and 24 hours after aortic constriction. Each animal was injected intravenously with 2 μCi/gm body weight of $^{32}P\text{-}H_3PO_4$. RNA was extracted from pooled hearts of four animals for each group.

selective increase in labeling of any one area of the gradient. This indicated that all species of RNA were being stimulated to about the same extent.

The specific activity of RNA was determined at various times after aortic constriction. In addition to the total RNA, the specific activity of 28 S ribosomal RNA was analyzed. The specific activities of both total and 28 S RNA from hearts of animals with aortic constriction were increased above sham values at 4 hr after operation. These reached a peak at about 8 hr after operation, and, thereafter, gradually decreased (Fig. 4).

The specific activity of the α-phosphate of tissue ATP was determined after enzymatic hydrolysis of ATP with apyrase and separation of the resulting AMP by Dowex-1 formate column chromatography according to the technique of Bergkvist and Deutsch (1954). The labeling of RNA was then corrected for the labeling of precursor ATP as has been described (Fanburg and Posner, 1968). The validity of this type of correction for precursor specific activity depends upon an assumption of the absence of compartmentalization of precursor in the tissue and similar rates for the incorporation of other

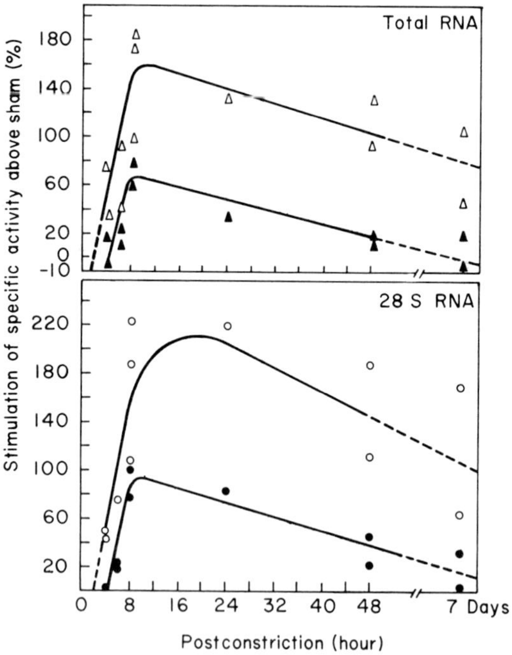

FIG. 4. Time course of labeling of RNA. Open circles and triangles represent the percent increase in specific activity of RNA above sham values without correction for AMP labeling. Closed circles and triangles represent the percent increase with correction for AMP labeling.

nucleotides into RNA as that for the adenosine nucleotide. With this correction for precursor, it was found that there was about a 4-hr lag period before the occurrence of any demonstrable increase in labeling of RNA in hearts from animals with aortic constriction (Fig. 4). Again, the peak increase in labeling occurred at about 8 hr after operation and, thereafter, gradually decreased. From this analysis, it could be seen that part of the increase in labeling of RNA with aortic constriction could be accounted for by an increase in the labeling of precursor. The increase in labeling of the immediate precursor may be accounted for, in turn, by an increase in the specific activity of inorganic phosphorus in the acid-soluble pool of hearts from animals with aortic constriction (Fanburg and Posner, 1968).

The base composition of heart RNA was determined by a nearest neighbor frequency analysis. Heart RNA was labeled by injecting animals with ^{32}P-H_3PO_4 and was fractionated on a sucrose density gradient. The fractions from various areas of the gradient were pooled, and the RNA was recovered and hydrolyzed in 0.3 *N* KOH for approximately 16 hr at 20°C. The four component nucleotides of RNA were separated as described by Blattner and Erickson (1967) on an AG 50W-X4 column chromatography. The results from this analysis are recorded in Table I. No appreciable difference was found between control animals and those with aortic constriction in the distribution of labeling in RNA. This provides further support that there was no alteration in the type of RNA produced during hypertrophy.

Actinomycin D and puromycin are known inhibitors of RNA and protein

TABLE I.
Comparison of Base Composition of Heart RNA from Normal Animals and Animals with Aortic Constriction

RNA fraction	Type of animal	% ^{32}P in CMP	AMP	GMP	UMP	$\frac{A + U}{G + C}$
> 28 S	N	21.8 ± 2.7	19.3 ± 1.6	29.4 ± 0.5	29.4 ± 1.2	0.96 ± 0.11
	C	25.2 ± 2.9	14.6 ± 1.8	28.1 ± 1.3	32.0 ± 1.7	0.88 ± 0.08
28 S	N	22.6 ± 2.5	15.5 ± 0.5	31.2 ± 1.4	30.7 ± 1.2	0.86 ± 0.05
	C	25.9 ± 3.2	13.4 ± 0.9	30.9 ± 0.6	31.0 ± 1.9	0.77 ± 0.08
18 S	N	18.2 ± 2.4	21.8 ± 2.6	25.5 ± 2.8	34.2 ± 2.4	1.32 ± 0.25
	C	21.9 ± 3.05	18.1 ± 2.4	26.1 ± 0.4	33.7 ± 3.4	1.09 ± 0.13
4-18 S	N	17.2 ± 1.9	19.8 ± 0.7	26.9 ± 1.5	36.0 ± 0.5	1.26 ± 0.02
	C	19.7 ± 2.2	20.3 ± 3.1	22.5 ± 1.0	37.4 ± 3.9	1.39 ± 0.2
4 S	N	17.5 ± 1.7	19.0 ± 0.1	23.3 ± 1.5	38.3 ± 2.1	1.46 ± 0.05
	C	21.2 ± 2.5	20.2 ± 0.7	22.0 ± 2.6	36.3 ± 4.8	1.38 ± 0.3
sRNA	N	24.5	13.8	24.4	37.5	1.05
	C	20.5	17.9	27.0	34.6	1.1

synthesis, respectively. The effects of these antibiotics on heart RNA synthesis were studied in animals with aortic constriction.

In experiments with actinomycin D, 2 μCi/gm body weight of $^{32}P\text{-}H_3PO_4$ was injected at 4 hr after aortic constriction, and animals were sacrificed 4 hr later. Actinomycin D was injected in divided doses over the entire 8-hr period. Inhibition of RNA synthesis in sham-operated animals occurred only when the total intravenous dosage of actinomycin was 10 μg or more per animal. At 5 μg per animal, there was essentially no inhibition of labeling of heart RNA from sham-operated animals, whereas labeling of 28 S heart RNA from animals with aortic constriction was inhibited 46% (Fig. 5). The same pattern of inhibition, though less in magnitude, was obtained when total RNA labeling was evaluated. Although it is tempting to postulate that there was an increased sensitivity of the DNA template to actinomycin, possibly representing new sites for RNA transcription, it is necessary to be cautious in the interpretation of the mechanism of the inhibition of labeling in the hypertrophying heart. An increase in the concentration of actinomycin in the hearts of animals with aortic constriction was excluded by measurements of the uptake of radioactive actinomycin (Posner and Fanburg, 1968).

The effect of puromycin on heart muscle protein synthesis was determined. Hourly intravenous administration of puromycin in 10 mg aliquots during a

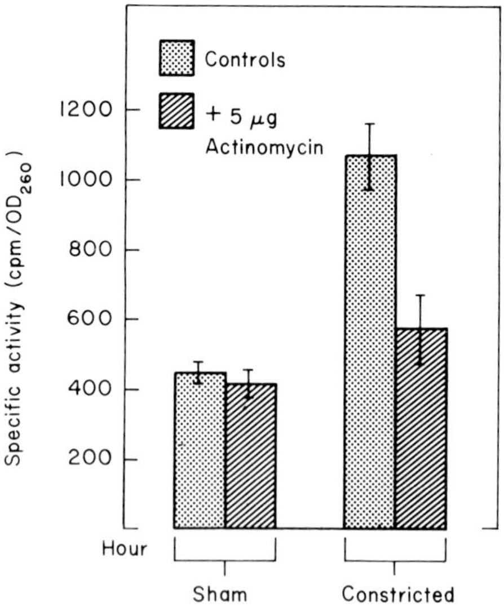

FIG. 5. Effect of actinomycin on labeling of heart RNA. The average specific activity of 28 S RNA was determined from 3–4 animals in each group, and the standard error is recorded with brackets. Actinomycin (total of 5 μg) was given intravenously in divided doses every 2 hr during the 8-hr interval.

4-hr labeling period resulted in a 70% inhibition of the labeling of heart muscle protein with ^{3}H-leucine. This was similar to the results obtained for the heart in studies by Gorski *et al.* (1961).

In experiments in which the effect of puromycin on RNA synthesis was studied, animals received $^{32}P\text{-}H_3PO_4$ 4 hr after operation and were sacrificed 4 hr later. Puromycin was given in hourly intravenous injections of 10 mg. Figure 6 demonstrates the inhibition of labeling of 28 S RNA by puromycin. A similar but less pronounced effect was seen when total RNA labeling was determined. When puromycin was given every hour from the time of operation throughout the entire 8 hr of the study, the stimulation of RNA labeling that occurred in animals with aortic constriction was abolished. When puromycin was administered hourly starting from the time of labeling with $^{32}P\text{—}H_3PO_4$ (4 hr after constriction), the labeling of 28 S RNA was inhibited by only 19%. Puromycin, given only during the first 4 hr after constriction, produced the same inhibition as when it was given for the entire 8 hr. This experiment raises the question of whether puromycin might have inhibited the formation of a protein synthesized during the first 4 hr after constriction, which is critical for the increase in RNA labeling.

It is possible that the effects of both actinomycin and puromycin could have occurred through alterations in myocardial mechanics resulting from these drugs. We have no evidence for or against this consideration.

Recently, we have been interested in the effects of aortic constriction on

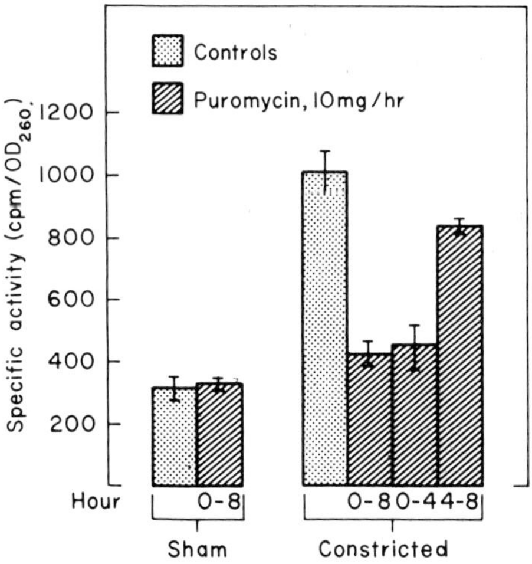

FIG. 6. Effect of puromycin on labeling of heart RNA. The average specific activity of 28 S RNA was determined from 3–4 animals in each group, and the standard error is recorded with brackets. Puromycin was given intravenously over the time periods noted on the abscissa.

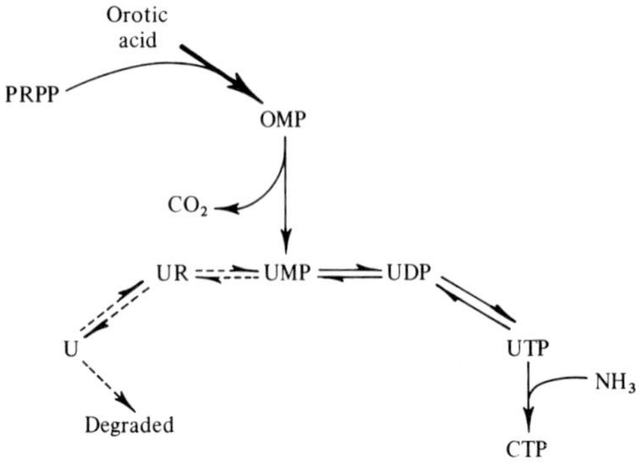

FIG. 7. Pathways of pyrimidine metabolism.

the intermediary steps in nucleic acid metabolism and, in particular, on pyrimidine metabolism. Most tissues have the option of using one of two pathways for the formation of pyrimidines (Fig. 7). The predominant *de novo* pathway in tissues—such as the liver—where this has been studied extensively, involves the utilization of orotic acid. In this pathway, orotic acid, formed from smaller precursors, is converted to OMP* in the presence of PRPP. The OMP is then decarboxylated to UMP. The UMP is subsequently phosphorylated to UDP and UTP prior to entry into RNA.

The other pathway, the so-called "salvage pathway," involves the conversion of uracil to uridine and subsequent phosphorylation to UMP, UDP, and UTP. Conversion of uracil to uridine requires ribose-1-phosphate and the enzyme, uridine phosphorylase. The subsequent phosphorylation of uridine requires the enzyme uridine kinase and the presence of ATP and Mg.

We have studied the incorporation of various radioactive substrates of these pathways into heart RNA. There was considerably less incorporation of ^{3}H-5-orotic acid into RNA in incubated heart tissue slices than there was of ^{3}H-5-uridine or ^{3}H-5-UMP. Transport of orotic acid into the cell did not appear to be rate limiting.

We have assayed several enzymes involved in these pathways from a particle-free extract from rat heart after centrifugation of the heart homogenate at 100,000 × gm for 90 min. The assay systems contained labeled substrates and substrates and products were separated after incubation on paper or thin-layer chromatography. The assays were carried out under what we found to be optimal conditions during a time period of linear enzymatic activity and within a range of concentration-dependent enzymatic activity.

* The abbreviations used are as follows: OMP, Orotidine monophosphate; PRPP, 5-phosphorylribose-1-pyrophosphate; UMP, uridine monophosphate; UDP, uridine diphosphate; UTP, uridine triphosphate.

We found no measurable conversion of orotic acid to UMP by heart extract from either the control animals or from those with aortic constriction, under conditions in which there was good activity from extracts of other organs. For these studies, the assay medium contained 5 mM ribose-5-phosphate, 5 mM ATP, 15 mM phosphoglyceric acid, 10 mM $MgCl_2$, 10 mM tris pH 7.4, 5 μCi/ml of ^{3}H-5-orotic acid (sp. act. = 940 mCi/mM), and 0.5 ml tissue extract/1 ml assay volume. In some additional studies, the inclusion of PRPP in the assay system appeared to enhance the activity of the heart extract and the significance of this is being investigated. Uridine kinase, uridylate kinase, and uridine phosphorylase activities were high in the heart extract. These data suggested that the "salvage" pathway might play an important role in the synthesis of pyrimidine nucleotides in the heart.

We, therefore, measured uridine kinase activity in the heart after aortic constriction (Fig. 8). An increase in this activity occurred about 4–8 hr following constriction, and reached a peak level of ~70% increase above sham-operated values at 1–2 days after operation. If uridine kinase is a rate-

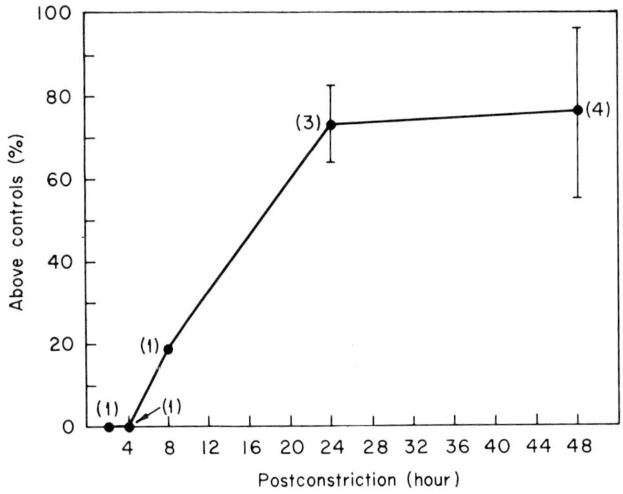

FIG. 8. Uridine kinase activity in heart extract at various times after aortic constriction. The assay medium contained 50 mM tris, pH 7.8, 50 mM $MgCl_2$, 5 mM ATP, 0.005 mM uridine, and 5 μCi/ml of ^{3}H-5-uridine (sp. act. = 28 Ci/mM). The reaction was carried out with 0.05 ml heart extract (25% homogenate in 0.05 M Na acetate) in a total assay volume of 0.7 ml for 30 min at 37°C. Descending chromatography was done on DEAE cellulose paper with a solvent containing 4 N formic acid and 0.1 N NH_4 formate. Areas of the chromatogram were counted in a scintillation counter, and the conversion of uridine to total uridine nucleotides determined. In each experiment, heart extracts from 3–4 animals with aortic constriction were compared with those from the same number of sham-operated animals. The number of experiments at each time is indicated in parentheses. The average percent increase in activity above controls ± 1 S.E. is recorded.

limiting enzyme, an increase in its activity may be important in increasing the supply of pyrimidine nucleotides for RNA synthesis. Further studies are now being carried out on the activity of the enzymes for pyrimidine synthesis in the hypertrophying heart.

In conclusion, it appears from these experiments that a generalized increase in ribonucleic acid synthesis begins very shortly after the imposition of an acute work load on the heart and represents one of the earliest biochemical events in experimental cardiac hypertrophy. An increase in RNA polymerase which reportedly follows aortic constriction (Nair *et al.*, 1968) appears to occur later than the increase in RNA labeling. The reason for this is not clear. An increase in labeling of DNA follows that of RNA, and the incorporation of label is predominantly into the DNA of interstitial cells (Morkin and Ashford, 1968; Grove *et al.*, 1968; Kako *et al.*, 1969).

Acknowledgments

This investigation was supported by Grant No. 5R01 HE06924 from the National Institutes of Health, U.S. Public Health Service. We would like to express our appreciation to Dr. Maurice S. Raben for his support and encouragement in carrying out this work.

References

Benjamin, W., and Gelhorn, A. (1966). *J. Lipid Res.* **7,** 285.
Bergkvist, R., and Deutsch, A. (1954). *Acta Chem. Scand.* **8,** 1877.
Blattner, F. R., and Erickson, H. P. (1967). *Anal. Biochem.* **18,** 220.
Burton, K. (1956). *Biochem. J.* **62,** 315.
Fanburg, B. L., and Posner, B. I. (1968). *Circ. Res.* **23,** 123.
Gorski, J., and Nicolette, J. (1963). *Arch. Biochem. Biophys.* **103,** 418.
Gorski, J., Aizawa, Y., and Mueller, G. C. (1961). *Arch. Biochem. Biophys.* **95,** 508.
Greenman, D. L., Wicks, W. D., and Kenny, F. T. (1965). *J. Biol. Chem.* **240,** 4420.
Grove, D., Zak, R., and Nair, K. G. (1968). *Clin. Res.* **16,** 231.
Hamilton, T. H., Widnell, C. C., and Tata, J. R. (1967). *Nature* (*London*) **213,** 992.
Kako, K., French, I., Garg, V., Rajhathy, J., and Beznak, M. (1969). *First Winter Mtg. Can. Physiol. Soc.* 1969.
Korner, A. (1964). *Biochem. J.* **92,** 449.
Malt, R. A., and Stoddard, S. K. (1966). *Biochim. Biophys. Acta* **119,** 207.
Morkin, E., and Ashford, T. P. (1968). *Amer. J. Physiol.* **215,** 1409.
Nair, K. G., Cutilletta, A. F., Zak, R., Koide, T., and Rabinowitz, M. (1968). *Circ. Res.* **23,** 451.
Posner, B. I., and Fanburg, B. L. (1966). *Circ. Res.* **19,** 805.
Posner, B. I., and Fanburg, B. L. (1968). *Circ. Res.* **23,** 137.
Schneider, W. C. (1957). *Methods Enzymol.* **3,** 680.
Wicks, W. D., Greenman, D. L., and Kenney, F. T. (1965). *J. Biol. Chem.* **240,** 4414.

SYNTHESIS AND TURNOVER OF HEART MITOCHONDRIA IN NORMAL, HYPERTROPHIED, AND HYPOXIC RAT

Murray Rabinowitz, V. Aschenbrenner, R. Albin, N. J. Gross, R. Zak, and K. G. Nair

The energy requirements of normal heart muscle are supplied almost exclusively from aerobic metabolism. Heart muscle contains only a very limited reserve of high-energy phosphates so that mitochondrial synthesis of ATP must be very finely adjusted to needs. The principal mechanism by which the oxidative metabolism and ATP synthesis are altered according to changes in energy requirements is by the process of respiratory control based primarily on the availability of ADP as phosphate acceptor. Mitochondrial functional mass is maintained at a level adequate to provide ATP during periods of extreme activity during which ATP requirement may increase severalfold. An important adjustment, which maintains adequate levels of mitochondrial functional mass, is the regulation of the synthesis and degradation of mitochondria. Mitochondrial mass increases during periods of prolonged increase in work load, accompanying the general hypertrophic process.

For some time we have been studying the general problem of the mechanism of mitochondrial biogenesis, and more recently, we have begun to look into the question of control of mitochondrial synthesis and breakdown in heart muscle in response to increase work load, hypoxia, and deprivation and overdosage of thyroid hormone. Our studies have led to the concept that mitochondria are normally in a very active state of flux; they are rapidly synthesized and destroyed within cells. Accumulation of mitochondria in cardiac hypertrophy may be accomplished by enhancing the rate of synthesis or by decreasing the rate of breakdown.

During the past few years it has been established that mitochondria are semi-independent organelles having their own genetic material (Granick and Gibor, 1967; Rabinowitz, 1968; Rabinowitz and Swift, 1970; Roodyn and Wilkie, 1968) and their own systems for synthesis of DNA (Iwashima and Rabinowitz, 1969; Kalf and Ch'Ih, 1968; Parson and Simpson, 1967), RNA (Luck and Reich, 1964), and protein (McClean *et al.*, 1958; Roodyn *et al.*, 1961; Webster, 1954). Mitochondria exist in cells as symbionts since they are dependent in part for their formation upon the information and synthetic capacity of the remainder of the cell. On the other hand, mitochondrial synthesis of ATP is essential to the life of all but the most primitive of eukaryote cells.

At about the same time that Luck and Reich showed that *Neurospora* mitochondria contained DNA with a lower guanine–cytosine content than that of nuclear DNA (Luck and Reich, 1964), our laboratory showed that mitochondria in higher organisms also contained DNA with a different base composition from that of the nuclear DNA (Rabinowitz *et al.*, 1965). Figure 1 demonstrates the determination of the buoyant density of chick heart mitochondrial and nuclear DNA by isopyknic CsCl density gradient centrifugation. Mitochondrial DNA has a buoyant density considerably heavier than that of nuclear DNA. Since the buoyant density of DNA is linearly related to its guanine–cytosine content, the result shows that chick mitochondrial DNA has a guanine–cytosine content of ~8% higher than that of chick nuclear DNA.

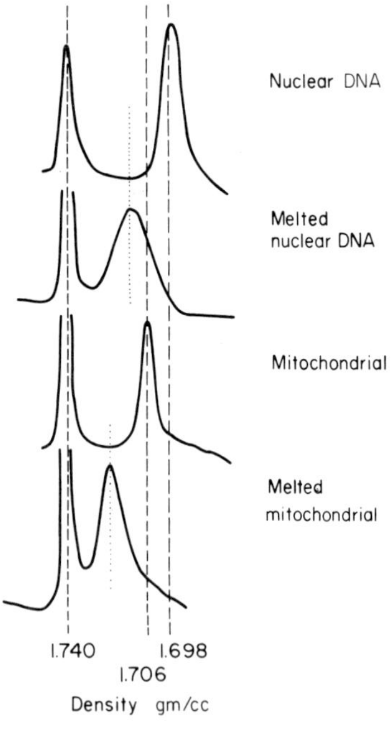

FIG. 1. Buoyant density of native and denatured chick mitochondrial and nuclear DNA. (From Rabinowitz *et al.*, 1965.)

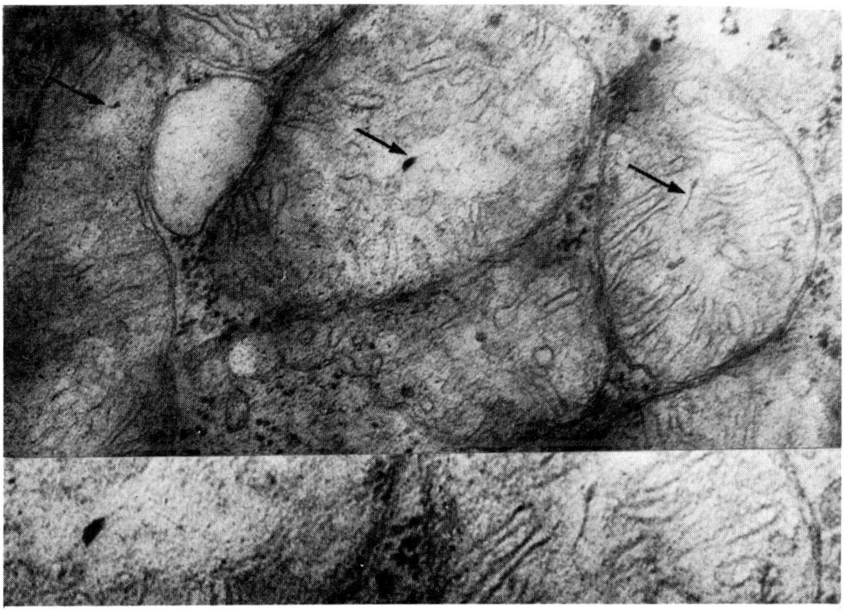

Fig. 2. Chick heart (18-day embryo) fixed in osmium tetroxide, showing mitochondria with filament (arrows) plate 1 (× 20,000). Detail showing typical filamentous inclusion, plate 2 (× 48,000). Electron micrographs by H. Swift. (From Rabinowitz *et al.*, 1965.)

Figure 2 illustrates DNA filaments in heart mitochondria. DNAse specifically removes these filaments. Subsequent investigations have shown that mitochondria are capable of replicating mitochondrial DNA by a semi-conservative process, independent of DNA replication in the nucleus (Gross and Rabinowitz, 1969a; Reich and Luck, 1966; Smith *et al.*, 1968). A mitochondrial DNA polymerase that differs from nuclear DNA polymerase is responsible for mitochondrial DNA replication (Iwashima and Rabinowitz, 1969; Kalf and Ch'Ih, 1968; Parson and Simpson, 1967).

Mitochondrial DNA is unique in that it has a circular form in higher organisms (Kroon *et al.*, 1966; Nass, 1966; Sinclair and Stevens, 1966; Van Bruggen *et al.*, 1966). An electron micrograph of mitochondrial DNA is seen in Fig. 3. The circular forms are similar to those of viruses such as polyoma virus, and are present in highly twisted or open configurations. The property of circularity alows specific separation and identification of mitochondrial DNA in species such as the rat, where base composition and buoyant density are similar. Mitochondria also contain RNA polymerase (Luck and Reich, 1964), which uses the information in mitochondrial DNA to synthesize mitochondrial ribosomal (Fauman *et al.*, 1969; Rifkin *et al.*, 1968; Rogers *et al.*, 1967; Wintersberger, 1967; Wood and Luck, 1969), transfer, and messenger RNA (Barnett and Brown, 1967; Buck and Nass, 1969; Casey

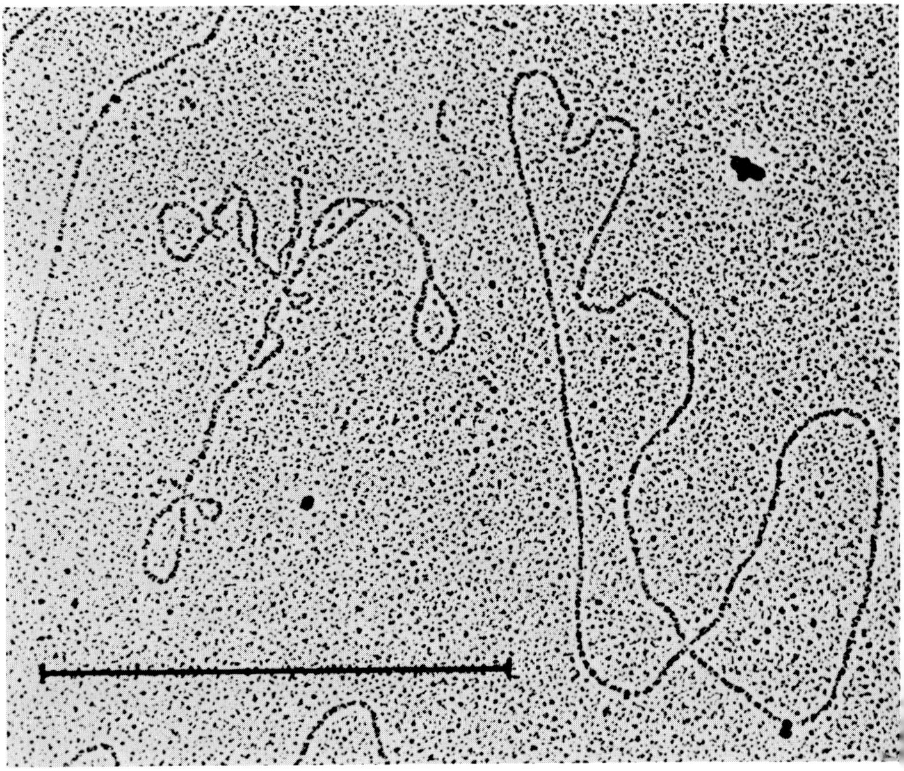

FIG. 3. Electron micrographs of shadowed preparations of mitochondrial DNA showing supercoiled configuration on the left and an "open circle" on the right. (From Rabinowitz, 1969.) Courtesy of B. J. Stevens and J. Sinclair.

et al., 1969; Nass and Buck, 1969; Suyama and Eyer, 1967). Mitochondria also contain their own systems for protein synthesis, mitochondrial ribosomes that resemble bacterial ribosomes (Rifkin *et al.*, 1968). Thus, mitochondria are almost cells within cells. In higher organisms, however, the mitochondrial DNA is only 5 μ (10^7 daltons), a size that can provide sufficient information to code only a few of the components of mitochondria (Sinclair and Stevens, 1966; Sinclair *et al.*, 1967; Van Bruggen *et al.*, 1966). It is probable that the entire outer mitochondrial membrane, the matrix enzymes, and many of the inner membrane enzymes are synthesized by extramitochondrial ribosomes using information derived from the nucleus. It is apparent from this discussion that the process of mitochondrial accumulation during cardiac enlargement involves stimulation of mitochondrial nucleic acid and protein synthesis, in addition to the integrated stimulation of nuclear and cytoplasmic synthesis of those mitochondrial components that are formed outside the organelle.

As a preliminary to the study of changes in cardiac mitochondria following a growth stimulus, our laboratory investigated the turnover of various mitochondrial components in normal rat heart and liver. Several years ago, Fletcher and Sanadi (1961) postulated from their observation that total mitochondrial proteins, cytochrome c, and total mitochondrial lipids in rat liver turnover with very similar half-lives, ~8–10 days, that mitochondria are synthesized and degraded as a unit. We reinvestigated this problem using a variety of specific mitochondrial components and a variety of labeled precursors, first comparing the apparent half-lives of mitochondrial DNA and the phospholipid cardiolipin, which is specifically localized in the inner mitochondrial membrane (Gross *et al.*, 1969).

The observed half-lives of rat liver mitochondrial DNA labeled with ^{3}H-thymidine, and cardiolipin and other mitochondrial phospholipids labeled with ^{32}P were found to be very similar, ~8 days (Fig. 4). The turnover of liver nuclear DNA however, was very slow, perhaps several years, as would be expected from the long life of hepatocytes. Incorporation of ^{3}H-thymidine into mitochondrial DNA was 30–50 times greater than nuclear DNA. These data tend to confirm the hypothesis of synchronous turnover of mitochondria.

In heart, however, the situation was more complex. Mitochondrial DNA turned over more rapidly than in liver, with a half-life of ~5.5 days (Fig. 5). Nuclear DNA also showed significantly accelerated turnover, ~29 days,

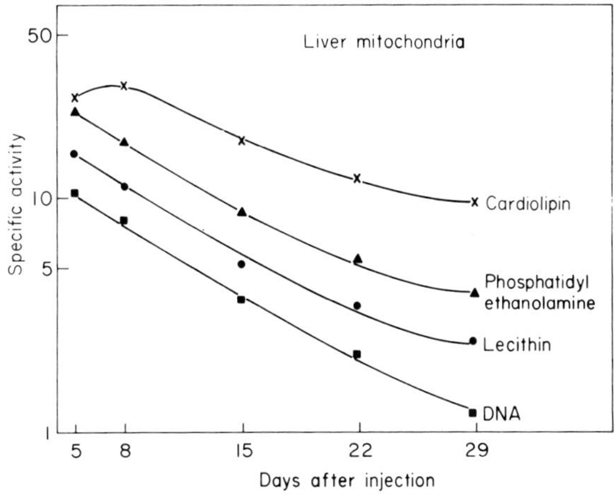

FIG. 4. Turnover of phospholipids and DNA in rat liver mitochondria. Specific activity is expressed in arbitrary units on a logarithmic scale on the ordinate. (From Gross *et al.*, 1969.)

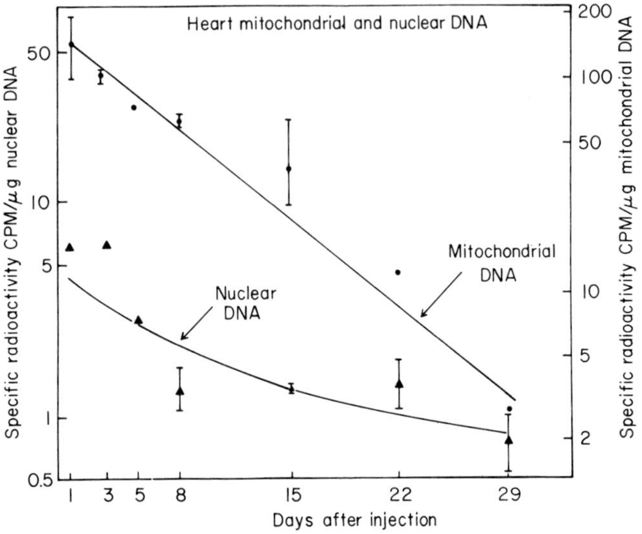

FIG. 5. Turnover of nuclear and mitochondrial DNA from rat heart. Specific activities ± 1 sd are given. (From Gross *et al.*, 1969.)

perhaps reflecting the turnover of connective tissue cells in the heart, as has been shown to occur in acutely induced hypertrophy.

Cardiolipin and other mitochondrial phospholipids showed variable but slower turnover rates than mitochondrial DNA (Fig. 6). The data therefore tend to negate the original hypothesis. It is now apparent, however, that in the cases illustrated, reutilization of labeled precursor after degradation of the product may be very efficient, and may greatly alter the calculated half-life. Furthermore, reutilization may differ markedly in organs such as heart and liver. Liver cells are specialized for the function of protein synthesis, and an efficient pathway for reutilization of breakdown products might be anticipated. In heart, however, protein synthesis is largely reparative, or adaptive to increased work load, so that such an efficient mechanism might not be expected, at least in the normal state.

This question was studied using a precursor such as ^{3}H-leucine which may be reutilized, and a nonreutilizable precursor such as ^{14}C-guanido-labeled arginine, in comparing the turnover of mitochondrial proteins of heart and liver. In the latter case, liver arginase rapidly converts the guanido group of arginine to urea, which is excreted and not available for the further synthesis of proteins.

The observed half-life of liver mitochondrial proteins labeled with ^{3}H-leucine is $\sim$8 days, but with arginine it is only about $5\frac{1}{2}$ days. Thus, a very efficient pathway for reutilization of leucine is present in liver.

In contrast, the results in heart show that the half-lives of mitochondrial proteins labeled with ^{3}H-leucine (Fig. 7) and ^{14}C-guanido-labeled arginine are very similar, ~5.0–6.0 days. The data suggest that reutilization of amino acids is not very important in heart in the normal steady state. Whether the pathway becomes more significant when growth is stimulated, still remains to be tested.

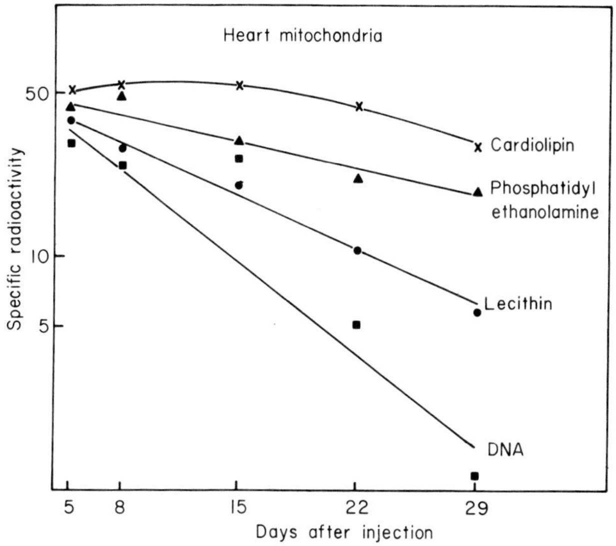

FIG. 6. Turnover of phospholipids and DNA in rat heart mitochondria. (From Gross *et al.*, 1969.)

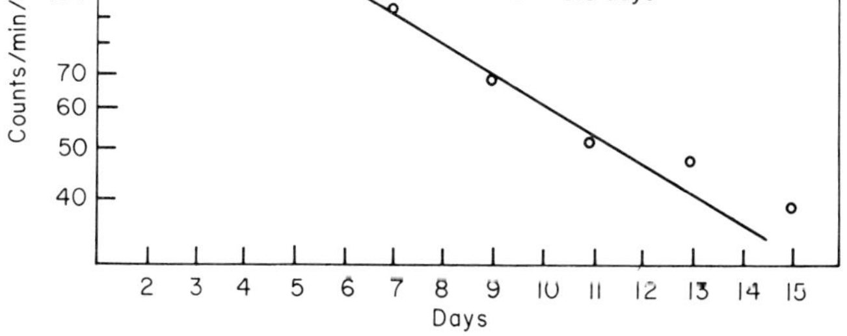

FIG. 7. Turnover of rat heart mitochondrial proteins labeled with ^{3}H-leucine.

It is possible that arginase may be lacking in heart, and that the true turnover of mitochondrial proteins would be still more rapid if a truly nonreutilized precursor were used.

To test this hypothesis, ^{3}H-δ-aminovulinic acid (ALA) was used to label the heme group of cytochromes a, b, and c, which are located on the inner mitochondrial membrane. ALA is truly a nonreutilizable precursor, since hemes are degraded to bilirubin, which is excreted in the bile and is not available for synthesis of new hemes.

The turnover of heart and liver cytochrome c labeled with tritiated ALA is shown in Fig. 8. The half-lives are essentially identical, ~5.5 days, which is

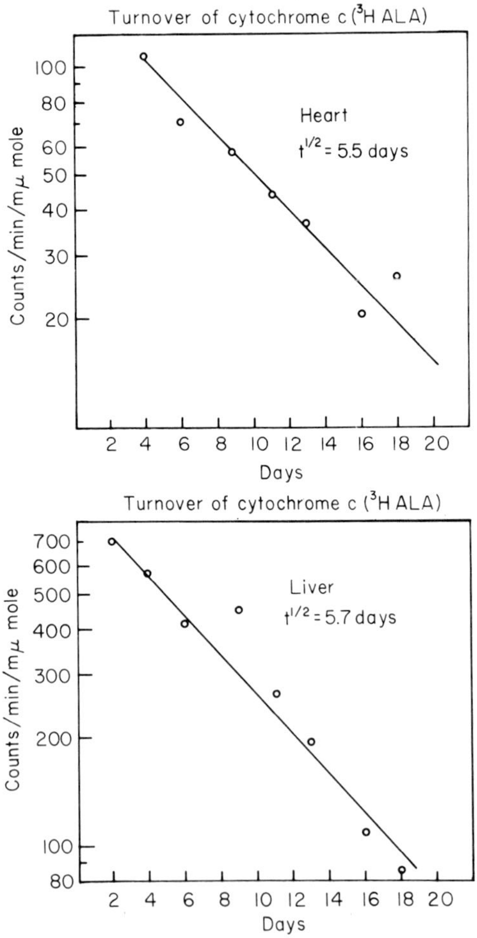

FIG. 8. Turnover of cytochrome c from rat heart and liver labeled with ^{3}H-δ-aminolevulinic acid.

similar to the turnover of total liver proteins labeled with arginine, and heart proteins labeled with either arginine or leucine.

The turnover rate of heme a of rat heart is also very similar to that of cytochrome c, and to total mitochondrial proteins (Aschenbrenner *et al.*, 1970). The results provide further evidence that reutilization of amino acids is not significant in heart as compared with liver.

Similarly, the turnover of cytochromes c and hemes a and b in liver are essentially identical (Aschenbrenner *et al.*, 1970); Druyan *et al.*, 1969). However, both cytochrome b_5 located in the outer mitochondrial membrane, and cytochrome b_5 located in the microsomes, have significantly faster half-lives than inner membrane components and different from each other (Druyan *et al.*, 1969). These and other data (DeBarnard *et al.*, 1969) lead us to conclude that the inner mitochondrial membrane, or a large unit of it, turns over as a unit in $\sim$5 days, whereas the outer mitochondrial membrane turns over more rapidly. Several inducible matrix enzymes such as δ-aminolevulinic acid synthetase (Marver *et al.*, 1966; McKay *et al.*, 1969), and alanine and ornithine aminotransferases (Swick *et al.*, 1968) turn over rapidly, independently of inner membrane enzymes.

Our studies on the control of mitochondrial synthesis and degradation in heart have used three different model systems, viz., banding of the ascending aorta; exposure to periods of severe hypoxia; and administration of thyroxine to thyroidectomized and euthyroid rats. Some of the questions we asked were (1) whether the synthesis of the various cell components in response to a stimulus to cardiac growth is symmetrical, or whether organelles such as mitochondria are preferentially synthesized very early in growth; (2) whether mitochondria may be involved in the mechanism whereby hypertrophy is initiated; and (3) whether mitochondrial accumulation is a result of an increased rate of synthesis, a decreased rate of degradation, or a combination of both.

The effect of banding the ascending aorta of rats (Nair *et al.*, 1968) on the activity of three mitochondrial enzymes, representing different sites on the electron transport system is shown in Fig. 9. The specific activities of the three enzymes with respect to protein are increased in heart homogenates 24 hr after aortic constriction. Total cardiac activities are increased to an even greater extent. Enzyme-specific activity of purified mitochondria did not change; the results therefore reflect synthesis of additional mitochondrial functional mass. The increased enzyme activities relative to homogenate protein content indicate that the mitochondria are synthesized more rapidly than the average myocardial protein. The data also suggest an asymmetrical development of mitochondria. Succinic dehydrogenase, a simple flavoprotein, increases to a greater extent than the more complex cytochrome c reductase and oxidase components.

Incorporation of a 1-hr pulse of labeled amino acid 24 hr after aortic

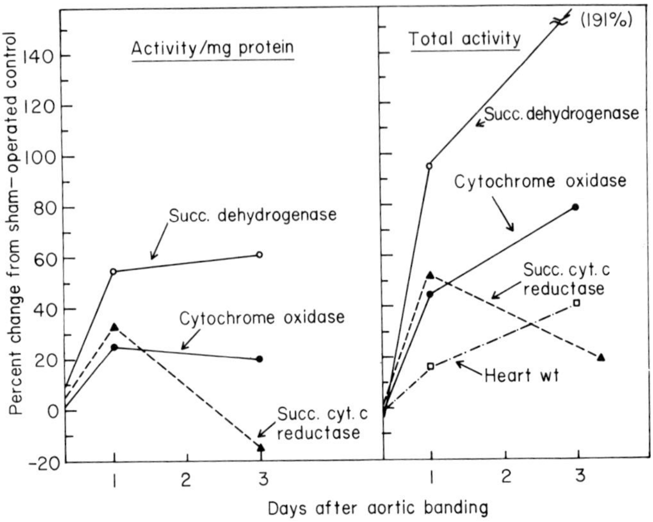

FIG. 9. Effect of banding the ascending aorta in rats on the cardiac mitochondrial respiratory enzyme activities.

banding into various myocardial cell fractions also indicates an asymmetrical accumulation of cell proteins (Fig. 10). The increment in incorporation of ^{3}H-leucine into mitochondria after aortic banding is greater than the increase seen in myofibrils, membranes, or supernatant protein. Ribosomes and nuclear fractions, however, show an even greater increase in amino acid incorporation than do mitochondria. The interpretation of the data assumes that specific radioactivities of mitochondrial and supernatant leucyl-t-RNA's are identical. Thus, two sets of data suggest an asymmetric increase of cardiac muscle components during rapid growth.

We have also investigated the effect of short periods of severe hypoxia on mitochondrial generation. One hypothesis for the mechanism by which increased work load results in cardiac hypertrophy is that local tissue hypoxia is the immediate stimulus for cell growth.

This hypothesis was tested by exposing rats to 6-hr periods of 4% oxygen. Mitochondrial proteins were prelabeled several days before with ^{14}C-arginine. Synthesis of new mitochondrial protein was estimated from the dilution of specific radioactivity of mitochondrial proteins by newly synthesized unlabeled proteins during and after hypoxia. The effect of hypoxia on mitochondrial turnover was also followed. A 15–20% dilution of specific activity of mitochondrial protein ensued after hypoxia (Fig. 11). Mitochondrial turover after return to normal O_2 tension however was not significantly affected. The data are interpreted to indicate that hypoxia leads to a destruction of about

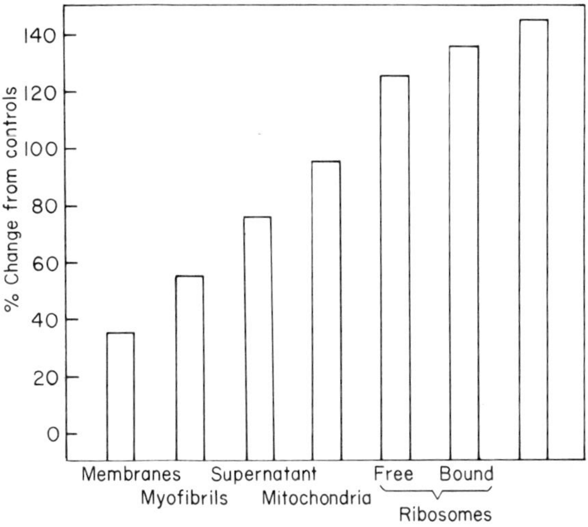

FIG. 10. Relative incorporation of ^{3}H-leucine into proteins of myocardial cell fractions. Results obtained 24 hr after aortic banding are compared to sham-operated controls.

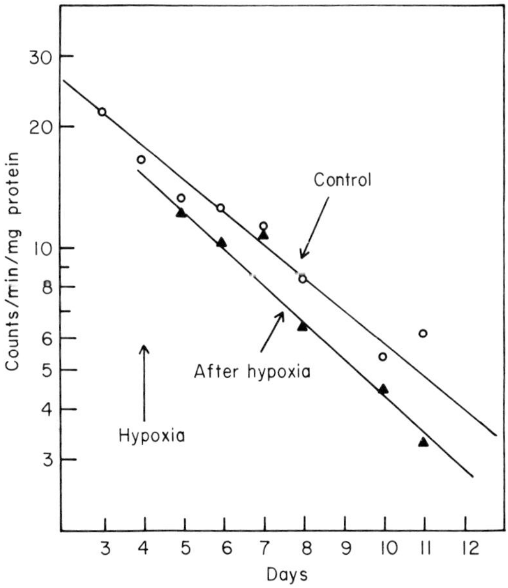

FIG. 11. Effect of hypoxia on specific activities of mitochondrial proteins labeled previously with ^{14}C-guanido-arginine. 6 hr periods of 4–5 % oxygen were given to experimental animals, which were killed at intervals thereafter. The specific radioactivity of purified mitochondria was measured.

15% of cardiac mitochondria, which are resynthesized after return to normal O_2 tension. No increase in the subsequent turnover rate of mitochondria exposed to hypoxia could be demonstrated.

This interpretation was supported by experiments measuring the incorporation of 1-hr pulses of ^{3}H-leucine into mitochondrial protein during and after hypoxia (Fig. 12). It is apparent that there was no increase in leucine incorporation during hypoxia, but that after return to a normal atmosphere, incorporation increased 2- to 3-fold for 5–6 hr, returning to normal in 24 hr. The results are similar to those obtained with yeast (Rabinowitz *et al.*, 1969; Slonimski, 1953), and with mammalian cells in tissue culture (Hakami and Pious, 1967), in which hypoxia inhibits mitochondrial synthesis and oxygen induces mitochondrial development. The data weigh against the hypothesis that hypoxia per se is the immediate stimulus for mitochondrial synthesis in experimental cardiac hypertrophy.

The final system used to study mitochondrial synthesis and breakdown in heart was the administration of thyroid hormone to thyroidectomized and euthyroid rats. Tata has previously shown that thyroxine stimulates mitochondrial protein synthesis and mitochondrial development (Tata, 1964). The system provides reproducible and striking changes in mitochondrial function and mass.

The effects of thyroxine administration on succinate cytochrome c reductase activity in homogenates and purified mitochondria are seen in Fig. 13. Changes were particularly striking in thyroidectomized animals. In heart

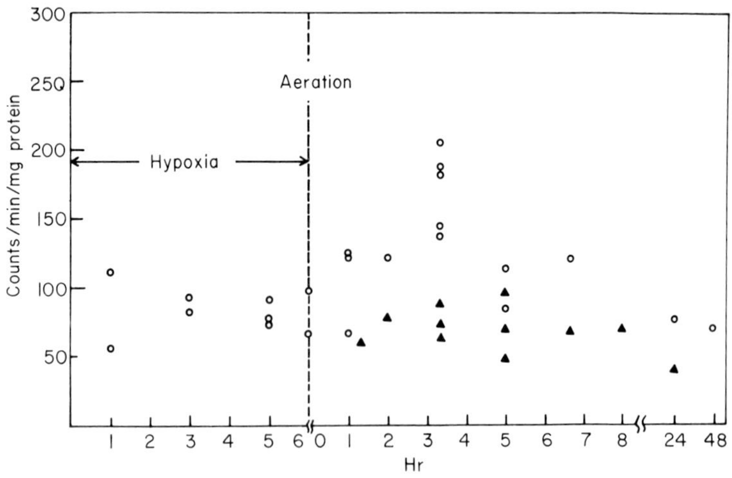

FIG. 12. Incorporation of ^{3}H-leucine into purified rat heart mitochondrial proteins during and after a 6-hr period in 4–5% oxygen. 1-hr pulses of ^{3}H-leucine were given. (▲) Control group; (O) hypoxia.

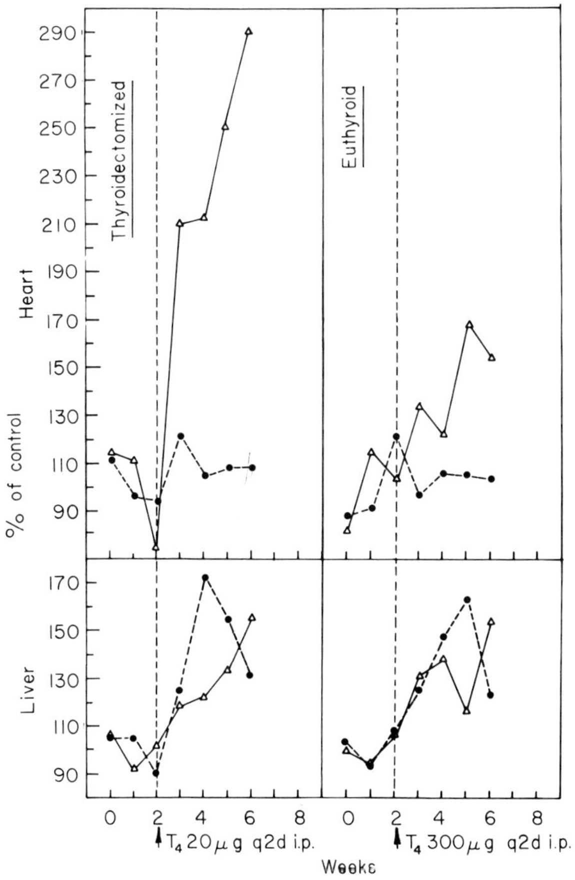

FIG. 13. Effect of thyroxine administration on total homogenate and mitochondrial specific activities of succinate cytochrome c reductase in rat liver and heart. Thyroidectomized animals on the left, euthyroid animals on the right. Results are expressed in percentage change from control. (△) Total activity; (●) mitochondrial sp. act.

there was a marked increase in total homogenate activity whereas mitochondrial specific activity was very little affected. A brisk synthesis of new mitochondria is therefore indicated by the data. In liver however, the response to thyroxine was less striking. The increase in total homogenate activity could be accounted for entirely by an increase in mitochondrial specific activity. In liver, therefore, thyroid hormone seems to increase enzyme activity of existing mitochondria, little synthesis of new mitochondria taking place. Similar but smaller changes occurred after thyroxine administration to euthyroid rats.

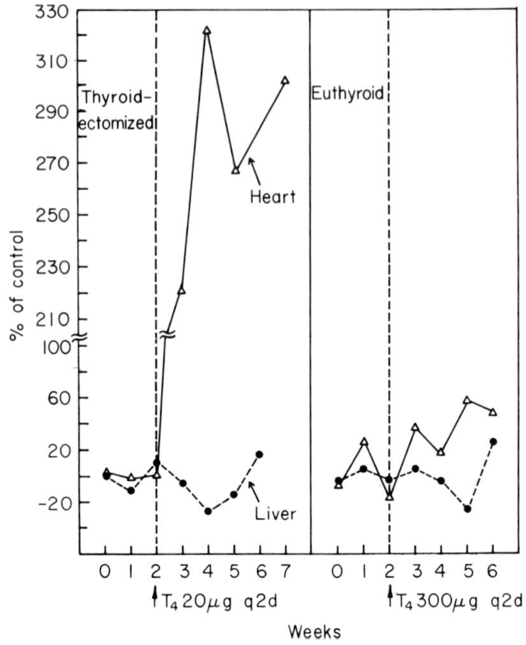

FIG. 14. Changes in calculated mitochondrial mass in rat heart and liver following thyroid administration to thyroidectomized and euthyroid animals.

This interpretation is illustrated in Fig. 14, where changes in mitochondrial mass have been calculated from homogenate and mitochondrial enzyme activities. Thyroxine administration causes a striking increase in calculated cardiac mitochondrial mass but little or no change in liver.

This system of rapid mitochondrial accumulation affords an opportunity for testing the hypothesis that changes in the rate of destruction of mitochondria are equally as important as changes in rate of synthesis during accumulation of mitochondrial mass. (Gross, 1971; Gross and Rabinowitz, 1969b).

Mitochondrial proteins were labeled with ^{14}C-arginine and the decay in specific activity was followed before and after thyroid hormone administration (Fig. 15). A second dose of ^{14}C-arginine was administered at $2\frac{1}{2}$ weeks to account for the new level of the baseline. A normal decay rate was seen in the euthyroid animals. After administration of large doses of thyroxine there was a marked decrease in the rate of decay. It is apparent that the rate of mitochondrial destruction has been substantially reduced. These conclusions are valid even when corrections are made for accumulation of new unlabeled mitochondrial protein secondary to administration of thyroid hormone.

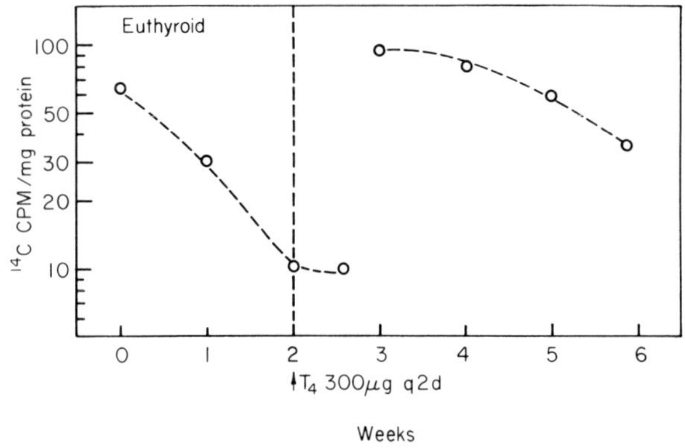

FIG. 15. Changes in turnover of total mitochondrial proteins of rat heart labeled with ^{14}C(guanido)arginine following thyroxine administration to euthyroid animals. From Gross 1971.

Similar results were obtained when thyroid hormone was given to thyroidectomized rats (Fig. 16). In this case a very slow mitochondrial turnover rate was already present in the thyroidectomized animals. After thyroxine administration, despite rapid accumulation of mitochondria and return to the euthyroid state, the slow rate of mitochondrial decay persisted. Thus, both decreased rate of destruction probably contributes to the increase in mitochondrial functional mass after thyroxine administration.

In summary, we have presented some of our recent work, still in progress, showing that cardiac mitochondria turnover rapidly in about 5–6 days; that hypoxia results in destruction, and aeration in resynthesis of mitochondria; and that decreased rate of destruction as well as increased rate of synthesis is an important mechanism in mitochondrial accumulation.

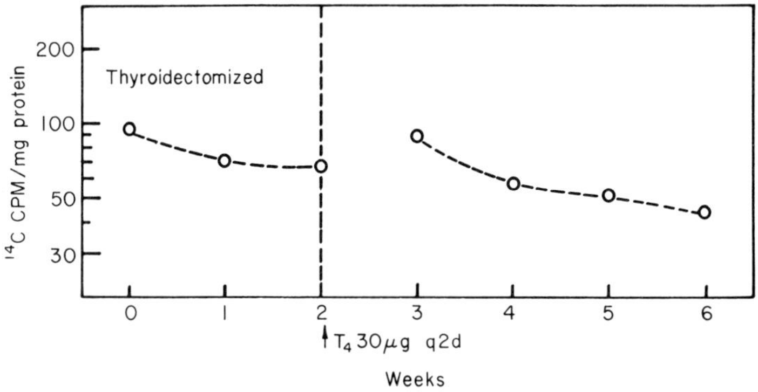

FIG. 16. Turnover of rat heart mitochondrial proteins labeled with ^{14}C(guanido)arginine in thyroidectomized rats before and after thyroxine administration. From Gross 1971.

Much additional work remains to be done to elucidate how changes in mitochondrial nucleic acid and protein synthesis are integrated with the synthetic activities of the rest of the cell.

Acknowledgments

This investigation was supported in part by grants from the National Heart Institute, National Institutes of Health, Bethesda, Maryland, the Chicago and Illinois Heart Association and the Myocardial Infarction Research Unit PH 4368133.

References

Aschenbrenner, V., Druyan, R., Albin R., and Rabinowitz, M. (1970). *Biochem. J.* **119**, 157.
Barnett, W. E., and Brown D. H. (1967). *Proc. Nat. Acad. Sci. U.S.* **57,** 452.
Buck, C. A., and Nass, M. M. K. (1969). *J. Mol. Biol.* **41,** 67.
Casey, J., Fukuhara, H., Getz, G. S., and Rabinowitz, M. (1969). *J. Cell Biol.* **43**, 18A.
DeBernard, B., Getz, G. S., and Rabinowitz, M. (1969). *Biochim. Biophys. Acta* **193,** 58.
Druyan, R., DeBernard, B., Getz, G. S., and Rabinowitz, M. (1969). *J. Biol. Chem.* **193,** 58.
Fauman, M., Rabinowitz, M., and Getz, G. S. (1969). *Biochim. Biophys. Acta* **182,** 355.
Fletcher, M. J., and Sanadi, D. R. (1961). *Biochim. Biophys. Acta* **51,** 356.
Granick, S., and Gibor, A. (1967). *Progr. Nucl. Acid Res. Mol. Biol.* **6,** 143.
Gross, N. J., (1971). *J. Cell. Biol.* **48,** 29.
Gross, N. J., and Rabinowitz, M. (1969a). *J. Biol. Chem.* **244,** 1563.
Gross, N. J. and Rabinowitz, M. (1969b). *Clin. Res.*, **17**, 459.
Gross, N. S., Getz, G. S., and Rabinowitz, M. (1969). *J. Biol. Chem.* **244**, 1552.
Hakami, N., and Pious, D. A. (1967). *Nature* (*London*) **216,** 1087.
Iwashima, A., and Rabinowitz, M. (1969). *Biochim. Biophys. Acta* **178,** 283.
Kalf, G. F., and Ch'Ih, J. J. (1968). *J. Biol. Chem.* **243,** 4904.
Kroon, A. M., Borst, P., Van Bruggen, E. F. J., and Ruttenberg, G. J. C. M. (1966). *Proc. Nat. Acad. Sci. U.S.* **56,** 1836.
Luck, D. J. L., and Reich, E. (1964). *Proc. Nat. Acad. Sci. U.S.* **52,** 931.
McClean, J. R., Cohen, G. L., Brandt, I. K., and Simpson, M. V. (1958). *J. Biol. Chem.* **233,** 657.
McKay, R., Druyan, R., Getz, G. S., and Rabinowitz, M. (1969). *Biochem. J.* **114,** 455.
Marver, H. S., Tschudy, D. P., Periroth, M. G., and Collins, A. (1966). *J. Biol. Chem.* **241,** 2803.
Nair, K. G., Cutilletta, A. F., Zak, R., Koide, T., and Rabinowitz, M. (1968). *Circ. Res.* **23,** 451.
Nass, M. M. K. (1966). *Proc. Nat. Acad. Sci. U.S.* **56,** 1215.
Nass, M. M. K., and Buck, C. A. (1969). *Proc. Nat. Acad. Sci. U.S.* **62,** 506.
Parson, P., and Simpson, M. V. (1967). *Science* **155,** 91.
Rabinowitz, M. (1968). *Bull. Soc. Chim. Biol.* **50,** 311.
Rabinowitz, M., and Swift, H. (1970). *Physiol. Rev.* **50**, 376.
Rabinowitz, M., Sinclair, J., DeSalle, L., Haselkorn, R., and Swift, H. (1965). *Proc. Nat. Acad. Sci. U.S.* **53,** 1126.
Rabinowitz, M., Getz, G. S., Casey, J., and Swift, H. (1969). *J. Mol. Biol.* **41,** 381.
Reich, E., and Luck, D. J. (1966). *Proc. Nat. Acad. Sci. U.S.* **55,** 1600.

Rifkin, M. R., Wood, D. D., and Luck, D. J. L. (1968). *Proc. Nat. Acad. Sci. U.S.* **58,** 1025.
Rogers, P. J., Preston, B. N., Titchener, E. B., and Linnane, A. W. (1967). *Biochem. Biophys. Res. Commun.* **27,** 405.
Roodyn, D. B., and Wilkie, D. (1968). "The Biogenesis of Mitochondria." Methuen, London.
Roodyn, D. B., Reis, P. J., and Work, T. S. (1961). *Biochem. J.* **80,** 9.
Sinclair, J. H., and Stevens, B. J. (1966). *Proc. Nat. Acad. Sci. U.S.* **56,** 508.
Sinclair, J. H., Stevens, B. J., Gross, N., and Rabinowitz, M. (1967). *Biochim. Biophys. Acta* **145,** 528.
Slonimski, P. P. (1953). "Formation des Enzymes Respiratories chez la Levure." Masson, Paris.
Smith, D., Tauro, E., Schweizer, E., and Halvorsen, H. O. (1968). *Proc. Nat. Acad. Sci. U.S.* **60,** 936.
Suyama, Y., and Eyer, J. (1967). *Biochem. Biophys. Res. Commun.* **28,** 746.
Swick, R. N., Rexroth, A. K., and Stange, J. L. (1968). *J. Biol. Chem.* **243,** 3581.
Tata, J. R. (1964). *In* "Actions of Hormones on Molecular Process" (G. Litwack and D. Kritchevsky, eds.), p. 58. Wiley, New York.
Van Bruggen, E. F., Borst, P., Ruttenberg, C. J. C. M., Gruber, M., and Kroon, A. M. (1966). *Biochim. Biophys. Acta* **119,** 437.
Webster, G. C. (1954). *Plant Physiol.* **29,** 202.
Wintesberger, E. (1967). *Z. Physiol. Chem.* **348,** 1701.
Wood, D. D., and Luck, D. J. L. (1969). *J. Mol. Biol.* **41,** 211.

BIOCHEMICAL EVENTS DURING HYPERTROPHY OF SKELETAL MUSCLE

Alfred L. Goldberg

The major goal of research into the mechanisms of work-induced hypertrophy is to determine how increased work initiates muscle growth and how such growth is terminated once the muscle has compensated for the increased demand. An essential first step toward this goal is to obtain detailed biochemical information about the growth process. In other words, before we can identify the signal for hypertrophy, we must understand how the hypertrophying muscle differs from a nongrowing one.

For the past few years, we have been studying work-induced hypertrophy in rat skeletal muscle. As discussed in pages 39–53, a simple technique was developed for inducing rapid hypertrophy of the soleus and plantaris muscles of one hind limb of the rat. If the tendon of the gastrocnemius is cut on one limb, the synergistic soleus and plantaris are forced to support the body weight on that side. Within 1 week, these muscles become 40 and 20% larger than the corresponding muscles of the contralateral limb (Fig. 1).

This experimental system offers many technical advantages for the study of compensatory hypertrophy. The growth is rapid and highly reproducible. The opportunity of comparing a hypertrophying muscle and a non growing control organ within the same animal is especially useful for studying biochemical aspects of the growth process. Such an internal control is clearly impossible in studies of hypertrophy of the heart. Using this experimental system, we were able to demonstrate that work-induced hypertrophy does not require pituitary hormones. Hypophysectomized rats (Goldberg, 1967a) were therefore used in most experiments in order that we might study work-induced hypertrophy independent of total body growth.

The gain in weight of the soleus which results from tenotomy of the gastrocnemius occurs primarily through an increase in muscle protein (Table I). Such growth leads to a larger mean diameter of the muscle fibers (Goldberg, 1967a), without a change in their number. Both sarcoplasmic (soluble) and myofibrillar (contractile) proteins increase in absolute amount

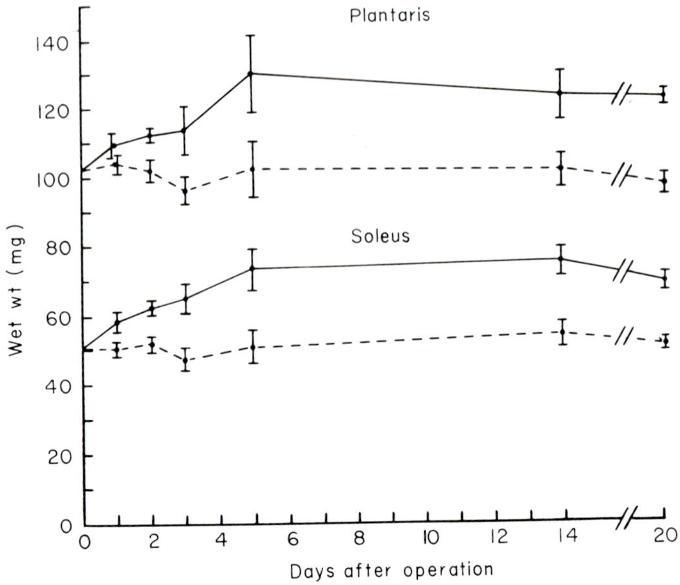

FIG. 1. Sizes of soleus and plantaris after section of the gastrocnemius tendon in hypophysectomized rats. Rapid growth of the muscles of the tenotomized limb is evident. (—), Operated limb; (---), control group.

during hypertrophy, although the proportion of soluble proteins increases differentially (Table I). At present we have no idea of the physiological significance of this interesting and unexpected change in the relative proportions of the two classes of proteins.

In addition to these changes in protein content, the hypertrophied muscle contains greater amounts of DNA than the contralateral control (Hamosh

TABLE I

PROTEIN CONTENT OF HYPERTROPHIED AND CONTROL SOLEUS 6 DAYS AFTER TENOTOMY OF GASTROCNEMIUS

Group	Total protein[a] (mg nitrogen/muscle)	% (Noncollagenous) protein	
		Soluble	Myofibrillar
Control soleus	1.58 ± 0.16	26.4 ± 1.4	73.5 ± 1.4
Hypertrophied soleus	2.22 ± 0.18	33.4 ± 1.9	66.5 ± 1.9
Increment	0.64 ± 0.22 ($p < 0.02$)	7.0 ± 2.2 ($p < 0.02$)	

[a] Mean ± S.E., seven animals.

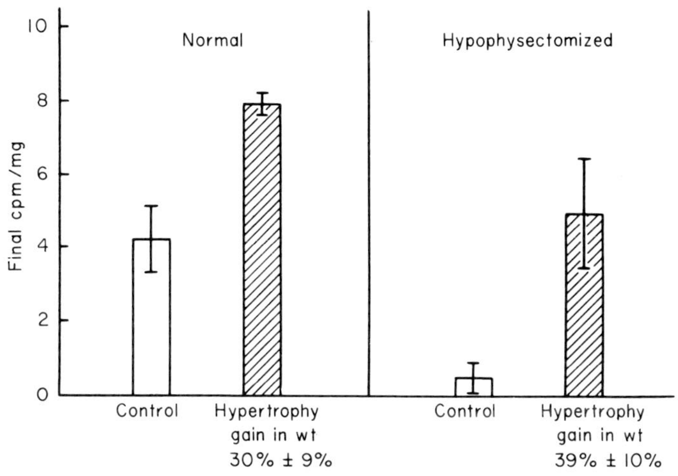

FIG. 2. Incorporation of ^{3}H-thymidine into DNA during muscular hypertrophy. Animals were given daily injections of ^{3}H-thymidine following tenotomy of the gastrocnemius. The rats were sacrificed 6 days later, and the muscles perfused to remove labeled cells from the vascular space of the muscle. The increase in incorporation by the hypertrophying muscle is highly significant ($p < 0.001$) in both normal and hypophysectomized rats. Each point is the average of five animals. At least 90% of the labeled nuclei are of connective tissue origin.

et al., 1967). Measurements of the incorporation of ^{3}H-thymidine further indicate new DNA synthesis within the hypertrophied muscle (Fig. 2) (A. L. Goldberg, and R. L. Sidman, unpublished data). Although the findings at first suggested the somewhat heretical possibility of division of muscle cells, on autoradiography the great majority of the labeled nuclei were found to be of connective tissue origin. Several groups have also found increased DNA synthesis by nonmuscular cells during hypertrophy of the heart (see chapters by Morkin and Nair, this volume). Thus, in both types of muscle, increased work leads to hypertrophy of muscle cells and concomitant hyperplasia of the stromal components.

The physiological significance of the proliferation of connective tissue cells is, however, unclear since we have no idea of function of the nonmuscular components. Of related interest was the finding that the collagen content of the overworked soleus also increased during hypertrophy. Similar observations have been made by Spann and co-workers (see pages 141–145) in the hypertrophied heart. Presumably increased synthesis of collagen represents a compensatory response of the connective tissue cells, permitting the hypertrophied muscle to exert increased force.

Protein and RNA Synthesis during Hypertrophy

A number of experiments have been carried out in our laboratory to investigate protein synthesis during compensatory growth; nevertheless, definitive evidence of altered rates of protein synthesis during hypertrophy was not easy to obtain. Although greater incorporation of a pulse of radioactive amino acids into protein was found consistently in the hypertrophying muscle, these results do not, by themselves, prove greater protein synthesis. Such a result could occur, for example, simply through changes in the sizes, rates of labelling, or specific activities of intracellular precursor pools. In fact, it is known that blood flow and amino acid transport into muscle cells vary with the amount of muscular work, as discussed below.

To minimize such complications (which are most serious for experiments involving a pulse of a radioactive precursor), we administered radioactive leucine chronically during the growth period, i.e., beginning at the time of operation and continuing for the subsequent 5 days. The total amount of label incorporated by the growing and nongrowing muscles were then compared at the time when hypertrophy was complete (Fig. 3). In all 20

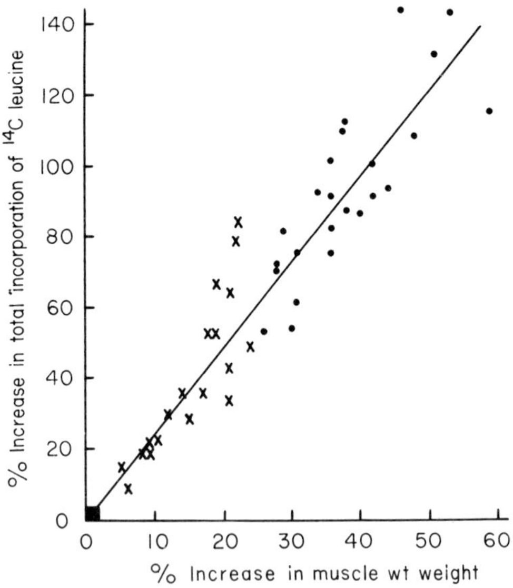

FIG. 3. Relationship of total incorporation of ^{14}C-leucine to gain in weight by hypertrophied muscle. Net growth and amino acid incorporation are both expressed as per cent increase above that found in muscles of contralateral, sham-operated limb. All measurements were made 6 days after tenotomy of the gastrocnemius in animals injected daily with leucine-^{14}C. Control animals received no operations or received sham operations on both limbs. (■) Control group; (X) plantaris; (●) soleus.

animals studied, the hypertrophied muscles had incorporated more leucine-^{14}C than did the contralateral controls. Furthermore, the increase in muscle weight was found to be directly proportional to the increase in amino acid incorporation and thus presumably new protein synthesis. (Goldberg, 1968a.) The conclusion of increased protein synthesis during hypertrophy received further support from Hamosh *et al.* (1967), who observed that cell-free extracts from hypertrophying muscles were more active than controls in incorporating amino acids into protein (see chapter by Lesch, pp. 147–155).

Although anticipated, the finding of a linear relationship between the gain in muscle weight and the increased amino acid incorporation is not completely trivial. First, Fig. 3 provides evidence that incorporation data are not experimental artifacts, but are intimately related to the growth process. Qualitative data relating growth to amino acid incorporation previously have been obtained only in exponentially growing bacteria. The relationship between growth and synthetic events is far more complicated in mammalian tissues than in bacteria, as a result of the greater protein catabolism found in higher organisms (Mandelstam, 1960) and the fact that appreciable synthesis must

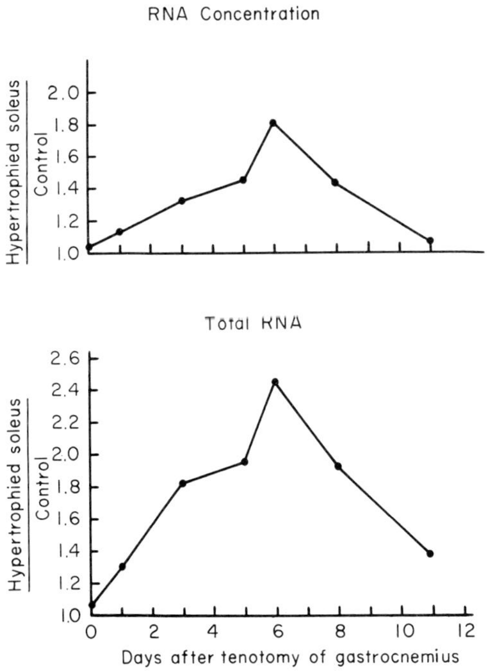

FIG. 4. Changes in RNA content during hypertrophy. RNA content in the hypertrophying muscle is expressed relative to that of the contralateral control. Each point is the average of the ratios in five animals.

occur in mammalian tissues even in the absence of growth. Thus the slope of Fig. 3 is also a function of the average rate of protein turnover in the muscles (see below). Quantitative data, such as those presented in Fig. 3, are difficult to obtain in higher organisms, because of technical problems in quantifying organ growth and the associated biochemical changes without using prohibitively large numbers of animals. In the present experiments this difficulty was circumvented by comparing data on paired growing and nongrowing muscles in the same hypophysectomized animal.

These findings led us to investigate the RNA content of the hypertrophying soleus. (Fig. 4) (A. L. Goldberg, and R. L. Torkelson, unpublished data). During such growth, there occurs a marked increase in the total RNA and in the RNA concentration in the muscle. The RNA concentration within the hypertrophied soleus was maximal 6 days after tenotomy of the gastrocneumius, and declined to control levels following the period of rapid growth.

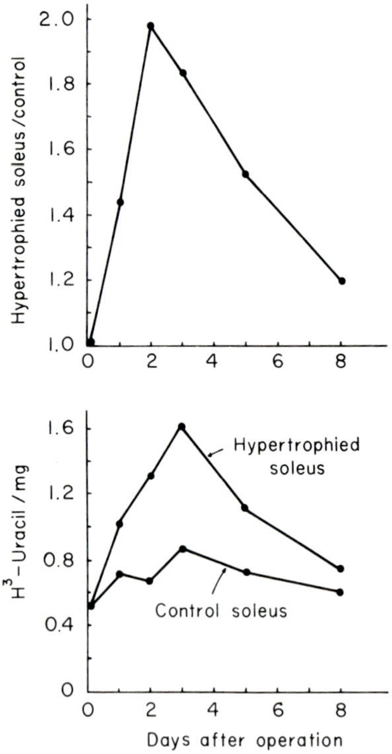

FIG. 5. Total incorporation of ^{3}H-uracil during hypertrophy. Each point represents the average of five animals. In the upper graph, the total incorporation in the hypertrophied muscle is expressed relative to the contralateral control. In the lower graph, incorporation per muscle is expressed as cpm × 10.

This increase in RNA appears to result from *de novo* synthesis, and appears to be an essential aspect of the growth process. Treatment of the animals with actinomycin D blocked work-induced growth (Goldberg and Goodman, 1969c). Furthermore the hypertrophying soleus incorporated H^3-orotic acid, a precursor of uracil, into RNA more actively than the control muscle (Fig. 5). Within six hours after the operation, the muscles of the tenotomized limb showed greater incorporation, but this effect did not occur if the animals were prevented from using their hind limbs. It is of interest that incorporation into RNA reached its maximal extent three days after operation and began to decrease at least 2 days before growth was complete. Although these data on incorporation do not alone prove increased RNA synthesis, they are highly suggestive of such a conclusion. Furthermore, the increase in incorporation (Fig. 5) appears to obey a "precursor-product" relationship to the buildup of RNA during hypertrophy (Fig. 4).

Regulation of Amino Acid Entry into Muscle

In skeletal muscle, as in certain other tissues the rate of protein synthesis appears to correlate with the rate of entry of amino acids into the tissue (Christensen, 1962; Riggs, 1964). For example, muscles from hypophysectomized animals show a reduced ability to concentrate amino acids. Similarly, insulin which promotes protein synthesis in muscle, markedly increases amino acid transport by muscle, while cortisone, which promotes muscle wasting leads to a reduced ability of the muscle to concentrate amino acids. We carried out a series of experiments on the transport of amino acids during compensatory growth (Goldberg and Goodman, 1969c). Our experiments employed the nonmetabolized amino acid analog, α-amino isobutyric acid (AIB) in order to study transport as an isolated process. At various times after tenotomy of the gastrocnemius, AIB was injected intravenously into the rats and 1 hr later, the amount of ^{14}C-AIB in the contralateral hypertrophying and control muscle cells was measured.

As shown in Fig. 6, the hypertrophying soleus and plantaris accumulated AIB more rapidly than the contralateral muscles. In addition, the maximal distribution ratio, i.e., intracellular/extracellular concentration gradient achieved by the hypertrophying muscles was several times greater than that of the controls. Thus, greater AIB uptake could not be accounted for simply by an increased blood flow to the hypertrophying muscle. Even though insulin and growth hormone have marked effects on amino acid transport by muscle, increased accumulation of AIB during hypertrophy was observed in diabetic, hypophysectomized, and normal animals. Following the period of rapid growth, amino acid transport returned slowly to control levels.

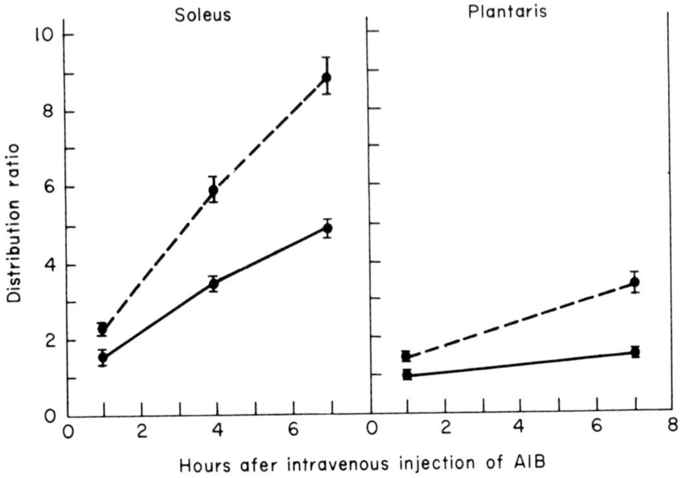

FIG. 6. Rate of accumulation of AIB by hypertrophying and control muscles of hypophysectomized rats 1 day after tenotomy of the gastrocnemius. The rate of uptake by the hypertrophying muscles estimated by the method of least squares is significantly increased ($p < 0.001$). Each point is the mean ±S.E.M. of at least five observations. (—) Control group; (---) hypertrophying.

Increased accumulation of AIB became evident surprisingly quickly after tenotomy of the synergistic gastrocnemius. Within 4 hr of this operation (the earliest time examined *in vivo*), the soleus and plantaris showed increased accumulation of AIB. This rapid increase could not be prevented with antibiotic inhibitors of RNA or protein synthesis. However, if the animals were not allowed to use their hind limbs following tenotomy, no difference between the contralateral muscles was obtained. Thus, altered amino acid transport appears to result from increased work of the soleus and plantaris and is independent of protein synthesis.

Related studies were carried out on muscles atrophying because of denervation or disuse (Goldberg and Goodman, 1969d). Section of the sciatic nerve reduced transport of amino acids into the soleus and plantaris within three hours (the shortest period studied *in vivo*). Decreased uptake also was found in muscles made inactive either by anesthesia of the motor neuron or sectioning of the spinal cord. Such changes were only found in the paralyzed muscles. These experiments and the earlier data on hypertrophied muscles led us to suggest that the level of muscular activity is a major determinant of amino acid transport. Additional evidence supporting this view, was the observation that the basal rate of amino acid uptake by red muscles, which the organism uses continuously, is greater than that of the pale muscles which are used less frequently (Dreyfus, 1967; Goldberg, 1967b).

More direct evidence of the relationship between muscular activity and amino acid transport has been obtained recently by Dr. Jablecki in our laboratory. These studies employed the rat diaphragm, maintained *in situ* in Krebs-Ringer Bicarbonate buffer and stimulated to contract electrically. In these experiments, both hemidiaphragms of the rat were suspended in an experimental chamber. One side was stimulated for varying periods of time, whereas the contralateral hemidiaphragm was inactive, and served as a control. Following this period of exercise both muscles were incubated with AIB-^{14}C, and the rate of transport studied.

When the diaphragm was stimulated at a rate of 2 shocks/sec (approximately the rate of respiration of the rat) or faster, it accumulated AIB significantly more rapidly than the unexercised control (Fig. 7). This difference was evident $\frac{1}{2}$ hr after stimulation and lasted for several hours. As was found in the earlier *in vivo* studies, the ability of the muscle to accumulate amino acids increased with activity even when protein and RNA synthesis were prevented.

The actual increase in AIB transport was found to be a function of the muscular work. (Goldberg, A. L., and Jablecki, C. M., unpublished data). Stimulation at greater frequencies for a specific time increased the magnitude of this effect, while longer periods of stimulation at a given frequency also led to greater uptake. However, any simple relationship between the extent

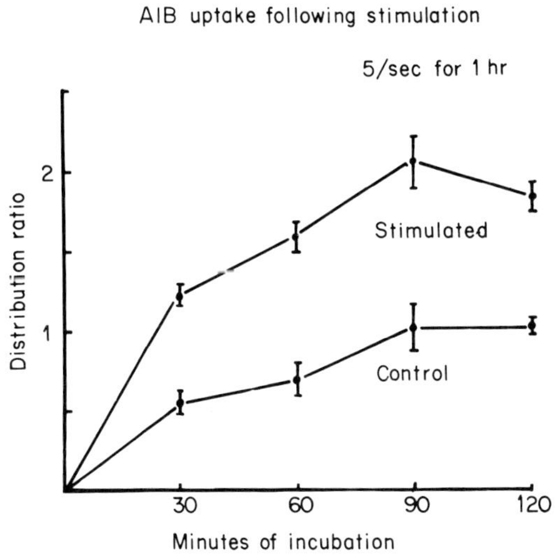

FIG. 7. AIB accumulation by rat diaphragm following electrical stimulation. The two hemidaphragms were removed from the body and maintained in Krebs–Ringer bicarbonate solution. One was stimulated repetitively at the rate of 5 shocks/sec for 1 hr, and both muscles were incubated in buffer containing AIB^{14}C. At subsequent times, the AIB content was compared in the contralateral stimulated and unstimulated muscles. Each point represents the mean ±S.E.M. of six muscles. Distribution ratio equals intracellular concentration/concentration in the medium.

of AIB accumulation and the number of contractions could not be demonstrated. In general, it did appear that if a given number of contractions occurred in rapid succession, they had greater effect on transport than if they occurred more slowly. However, the following experiment did prove that contractile work, rather than the frequency of muscle action potentials or the frequency of release of some neurotransmitter, is the major signal for AIB uptake. Both halves of the diaphragm were stimulated at the same rate; one hemidiaphragm was left free to contract unopposed, while the contralateral muscle was stretched so that it had to contract isometrically. It was found consistently that the muscle, which contracted isometrically, concentrated AIB more rapidly.

Although these findings appear quite exciting and finally demonstrate a direct effect of activity on muscle protein metabolism, it certainly can not be concluded that changes in amino acid transport are the initial event in compensatory hypertrophy. Much further work will be necessary to determine the physiological significance of the work-induced transport system. Further experiments are now in progress with this experimental system in an attempt to determine: (1) the cellular signal relating the contractile activity to rates of AIB transport; (2) the effects of muscle stimulation on entry and metabolism of the natural amino acids; and (3) the relationship of these changes in transport to RNA and protein synthesis in the stimulated muscle.

Protein Catabolism during Hypertrophy

One other area that we have been investigating is the turnover of muscle proteins during growth and atrophy. Although it has long been realized that proteins in mammalian cells are continually being degraded and replaced, surprisingly little is known of the mechanisms of protein degradation in cells. In fact until recently most studies of the control of enzyme levels and of cell growth have concerned only the regulation of protein biosynthesis and have generally ignored the process of protein catabolism (Shimke *et al.*, 1968). In most mammalian tissues, average protein half-lives are far shorter than the half-lives of cells, and as a result, changes in rates of intracellular catabolism theoretically can influence organ size.

At the outset of these investigations, we believed that our only goal in understanding compensatory growth was to learn how increased work causes greater protein synthesis. We were led, however, to investigate protein breakdown during work-induced hypertrophy by the unexpected finding that our data on amino acid incorporation did not appear able to account completely (1) for the net increase in muscle mass, and (2) for the qualitative changes in muscle protein that occur during such growth. Although the absolute growth during hypertrophy is directly proportional to an increase in amino acid incorporation (Fig. 3), the net increase in incorporation (i.e., the slope of Fig. 3) appeared insufficient to account for the growth actually observed (Goldberg, 1968). This argument was based upon previous measures of protein degradation and the assumption that degradative rates were similar in hypertrophying and control muscles. In addition, although amino acid incorporation into soluble and myofibrillar proteins increased in parallel during hypertrophy, the relative amount of soluble protein in the muscle appeared to increase disproportionately (Table I).

One possible explanation for these difficulties was that rates of protein catabolism might be reduced during compensatory growth. Such a decrease in catabolism would permit greater accumulation of proteins during hypertrophy and would thus augment the effects of the increase in protein synthesis. There is experimental precedent for believing that catabolic rates of enzymes can vary under different physiological conditions (Schimke *et al.*, 1968; Mandelstam, 1960), and we had previously discovered that basal rates of protein catabolism must differ in different skeletal muscles (Goldberg, 1967b).

Rates of protein breakdown were therefore compared in hypertrophying and control muscles (Goldberg and Goodman, 1969a). Muscle proteins of hypophysectomized rats were initially labeled with ^{3}H-leucine 2 days prior to tenotomy of the gastrocnemius, and the loss of labeled proteins was compared in the contralateral muscles. The major objection to this approach is the possibility of reincorporation into protein of ^{3}H-leucine released by the catabolism of labelled proteins. To minimize this possibility, the animals received large doses of unlabeled leucine daily beginning 24 hr after injection of radioactivity. In addition, the animals were maintained on a high protein diet (containing at least 64% casein) until the end of the experiment. As a result of these procedures no TCA-soluble radioactivity could be found in the muscle either at the time of operation or at the end of the experiment.

Six days after tenotomy of the gastrocnemius, the hypertrophied soleus was found to contain more labeled protein than the contralateral control (Fig. 8). This result is consistent with decreased breakdown of the prelabeled proteins during the growth process. Although this apparent decrease in the catabolism of the sarcoplasmic proteins was highly significant, the loss of prelabeled myofibrillar proteins did not differ significantly from controls. In fact, the ratio of soluble cpm/myofibrillar cpm significantly increased during hypertrophy.

Several observations suggest that the finding of more counts in the proteins of the hypertrophied muscle actually reflects a decrease in protein turnover rather than increased reutilization of amino acids released from labeled proteins. (1) Although the extent of reutilization of labeled amino acids should vary markedly with the specific amino acid used, results similar to Fig. 8 were obtained when proteins were prelabeled with either glutamic acid or

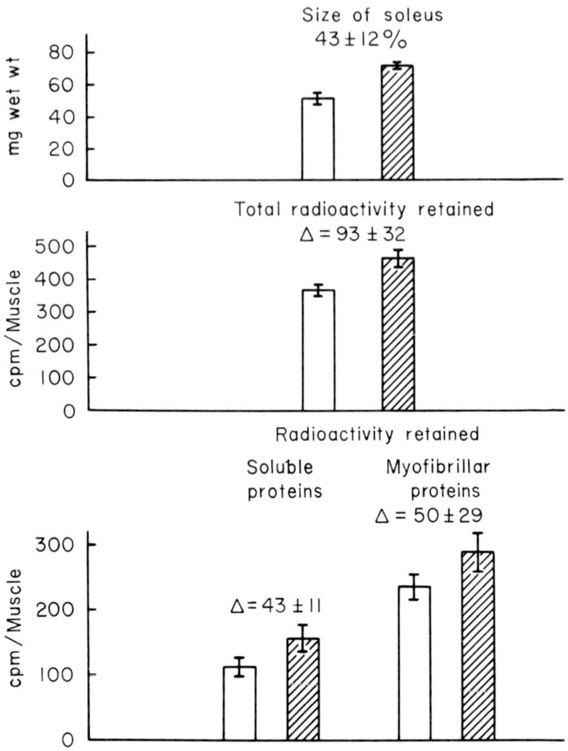

Fig. 8. Rate of protein degradation in hypertrophying and control muscles. Animals were sacrificed 6 days after unilateral tenotomy of the gastrocnemius and 8 days after injection of ^{3}H-leucine. The bars represent the mean values ± S.E.M. found in the control and in hypertrophying muscles of eight animals. Also presented are the average differences ±S.E.M. between the contralateral muscles. The hypertrophied soleus retained significantly more radioactivity per muscle ($p < 0.01$) and more radioactivity in soluble proteins ($p < 0.001$). This result suggests decreased degradation of the labeled protein. The amount of myofibrillar radioactivity retained by the hypertrophied muscle is not significantly greater than that of the control. Open bar represents the control group; striped bar, hypertrophied group.

alanine. (2) If these results were merely artifacts of increased reutilization of label, they should be obtained whenever increased synthesis of protein occurs. Analogous experiments were carried out on muscles induced to grow following treatment with growth hormone. This hormone can induce muscle growth independently of muscular work (Goldberg and Goodman, 1969a). Although the soleus increased in mass upon treatment with growth hormone, these muscles did not retain more of the prelabeled protein than controls. The specific activities of the muscle proteins decreased upon hormone treatment and the ratio of soluble to myofibrillar cpm did not change. These results are in clear contrast with our findings on work-induced growth and indicate that growth hormone, unlike muscular activity leads to increased protein synthesis without affecting protein breakdown. (3) Since soluble and myofibrillar proteins are synthesized in the same proportions in hypertrophying and control muscles, a disproportionate decrease in the catabolism of the soluble components, as suggested by Fig. 8, should result in a disproportionate accumulation of the soluble proteins. These observations on catabolism can thus account for the relative increase in the soluble fraction of the hypertrophied muscle (Table I); by contrast, treatment with growth hormone, which did not appear to alter rates of protein catabolism also did not affect the relative proportions of these two cell fractions.

The finding that regulation of protein turnover might constitute a major determinant of muscle size led us to investigate the mechanism of muscle atrophy following denervation or following treatment with large doses of cortisone. In both these types of atrophy, the average half-lives of muscle proteins were found to decrease, while protein synthesis in muscle was reduced (Goldberg and Goodman, 1969b). As in the case of work-induced hypertrophy, data on turnover was necessary to account for the qualitative changes in muscle composition, and the net changes in muscle weight.

Decreased protein catabolism is probably not unique to work-induced hypertrophy of skeletal muscle and probably also constitutes an important component of other types of cell growth. To test this possibility, we have carried out similar studies of rates of protein breakdown in the kidney, undergoing compensatory growth induced by unilateral nephrectomy. During such growth, average rates of protein catabolism were also found to decrease (Goldberg, A. L., unpublished data). Finally in bacteria and yeast, it has long been known that protein degradation occurs far more slowly in exponentially growing cells than in nongrowing ones (Mandelstam, 1960).

It is of further interest that the decrease in protein catabolism, which occurs during compensatory hypertrophy of muscle and kidney and in exponentially growing bacteria, coincides with increased protein and RNA synthesis. These changes have combined additive effects in promoting cell growth. On the other hand, in atrophying muscle acceleration of catabolism occurs concurrently with a decrease in synthesis. These effects are additive in producing loss of weight. It thus appears possible that the biochemical factors which regulate the synthetic and catabolic aspects of protein metabolism are interrelated. Studies in our laboratory in recent months have been concerned with the mechanisms of protein turnover in bacteria, and have, in fact, demonstrated feedback relationships between the pathways for protein catabolism and biosynthesis mediated by levels of aminoacyl-tRNA (Goldberg, A. L., 1971).

ACKNOWLEDGMENTS

These studies have been supported through grants from the Berkshire County Chapter of the Massachusetts Heart Association, the Air Force of Scientific Research, and from the Milton Fund of Harvard University. Many of the experiments described herein were carried out in the laboratory of Dr. H. M. Goodman. The author is deeply grateful to Dr. Goodman for his expert advice and encouragement.

REFERENCES

Christensen, H. W. (1962). "Biological Transport." Benjamin, New York.
Dreyfus, J. C. (1967). *Revue Fran. Etud. Clin. Biol.* **XII,** 343.
Goldberg, A. L. (1967a). *Amer. J. Physiol.* **213,** 1193.
Goldberg, A. L. (1967b). *Nature* (*London*) **216,** 1219.
Goldberg, A. L. (1968a). *J. Cell Biol.* **36,** 653.
Goldberg, A. L. (1969a). *J. Biol. Chem.* **244,** 3217.
Goldberg, A. L. (1969b). *J. Biol. Chem.* **244,** 3223.
Goldberg, A. L. (1971). *Proc. Nat. Acad. Sci. Wash.* (**68**, in press).
Goldberg, A. L., and Goodman, H. M. (1969a). *J. Physiol.* **200,** 655.
Goldberg, A. L., and Goodman, H. M. (1969b). *J. Physiol.* **200,** 667.
Goldberg, A. L., and Goodman, H. M. (1969c). *Amer. J. Physiol.* **216,** 1111.
Goldberg, A. L., and Goodman, H. M. (1969d). *Amer. J. Physiol.* **216,** 1116.
Hamosh, M., Lesch, M., Baron, J., and Kaufmann, S. (1967). *Science* **159,** 35.
Korner, A. (1967). *Progr. Biophys. Mol.* **17,** 61.
Mandelstam, J. (1960). *Bacteriol. Rev.* **24,** 289.
Riggs, T. (1964). *In* "Action of Hormones on Molecular Processes" (G. Litwack and D. Kritchevsky, eds.). Wiley, New York.
Schimke, R. T., Ganshow, R., Doyle, D., and Arias, I. M. (1968). *Fed. Proc. Fed. Amer. Soc. Exp. Biol.* **27,** 1223.

ALTERATION IN THE CONTRACTILE PROTEIN IN HYPERTROPHIED GUINEA PIG HEARTS

Milton Draper, Natsu Taylor, and Norman R. Alpert

In a previous report from this laboratory, it was shown that myofibrils isolated from failing hearts have a low ATPase activity (Alpert and Gordon, 1962). These results were obtained in patients who succumbed to congestive heart failure following chronic benign essential hypertension. The failing hearts were from an older group of patients and weighed more than the normals. Two important questions were unanswered: (1) Is the diminished ATPase activity associated with the age or the heart weight? (2) Is the dimunition in myofibrillar ATPase activity associated with the contractile protein or the noncontractile structure of the myofibril? Experiments were designed to answer these questions using a model of congestive failure, produced experimentally in guinea pigs, which is similar to the type studied in humans (Gertler, 1959).

Methods

Operative Procedure

Experimental hypertrophy of the heart (congestive heart failure) was produced in guinea pigs by constricting the ascending aorta (Gertler, 1959). Controls were treated in the same manner except that the tie was cut and left in place after the aorta was temporarily constricted. The animals were paired preoperatively according to weight and age. When the animals exhibited obvious signs of weakness, rales and anorexia, they were sacrificed along with the paired control. This occurred 17–33 days after the operative procedure.

Preparation of Myofibrils

Myofibrils were isolated from the left ventricle in a manner similar to the method developed by Perry and Grey (1956) for skeletal muscle. The animals were sacrificed by a sharp blow to the head, the rib cage was rapidly opened and the heart was removed along with the constricted portion of the aorta. The heart was immediately plunged into an ice cold solution of 0.05 *M* KCl–0.01 *M* imidazole at pH 7.1. After washing the heart in this solution, the extraneous tissue was trimmed away from the left ventricle. Eight hundred milligrams of left ventricular tissue were minced and homogenized in 20 ml of 0.05 *M* KCl for one minute in a Waring blender. The homogenate was centrifuged for 15 min at 600 × gravity (G), the supernatent discarded and the myofibrillar paste homogenized in 20 ml of 0.05 *M* KCl–0.01 *M* imidazole for 2 min. Following this centrifugation period, the heavy cell fragments and other extraneous matter were removed from the bottom of the cell, and the remaining myofibrillar paste was washed four more times by means of resuspension in the KCl solution and centrifugation at 600 × G. Finally, the washed myofibrils were suspended in 45 ml of 0.05 *M* KCl–0.01 *M* imidazole for myofibrillar ATPase analyses. The isolation procedure was carried out near 0°C.

Three modifications were made in the method described by Perry and Grey (1956). (1) According to their procedure, a light-colored upper layer of sediment was present following the second centrifugation period when skeletal muscle was used. Upon microscopic examination, they found this layer to be richest in myofibrils. The light-colored layer was therefore retained while the remainder of the sediment was discarded. However, this layer was not observed with the guinea pig hearts. The left ventricular homogenate exhibited a uniform flesh-color throughout the sediment except for a small residue of heavy material at the bottom which appeared to consist of light-colored stringy connective tissue mixed with dark-colored cellular fragments. This heavy residue was discarded. A microscopic examination revealed no difference in myofibrillar concentration in any part of the flesh-colored sediment. The myofibrillar ATPase activities were thus carried out on this portion of the sediment. (2) A considerable amount of connective tissue was present in 200 gm of rabbit skeletal muscle and the Perry and Grey procedure included a step for its removal. This was accomplished by centrifuging the homogenate for three minutes at 400 × G and removing the sediment. However, in the present case the bulk of this material had been trimmed away prior to homogenization, and the amount which remained in the 800 mg of ventricular tissue used was so small that its removal was effected quite easily by means of a suctioning pipette lowered to the cell bottom following the 15-min centrifugation period. The three minute period of centrifugation was therefore omitted. (3) Preliminary studies on the choice of buffers and KCl concentrations were made by substituting imidazole-KCl (0.01 *M* imidazole and 0.05 *M* KCl) for borate-KCl (0.039 *M* borate and 0.025 *M* KCl). When this was done, no significant differences were observed either microscopically or enzymatically. The imidazole–KCl solution was chosen for the current experiments.

Experiments were carried out on four animals in which the modified procedure was compared with the original Perry and Grey method. Because of the absence of a distinct upper light-colored layer of sediment, an arbitrary part of the uppermost portion of the sediment (about $\frac{1}{4}$) was chosen to represent the upper layer of the Perry and Grey method. When the two methods were compared with respect to myofibrillar ATPase activity, no differences were observed either qualitatively or quantitatively (Table I).

TABLE I

MYOFIBRILLAR ATPASE ACTIVITY
A STUDY OF MYOFIBRILLAR ISOLATION TECHNIQUES[a]

		$MgCl_2$				$CaCl_2$			
		1.00 m*M*		2.00 m*M*		1.00 m*M*		2.00 m*M*	
Exp.	Tech.	S	X	S	X	S	X	S	X
1	PG	1.119	0.833	1.197	0.800	0.627	0.417	0.749	0.484
	M	1.125	0.856	1.197	0.811	0.651	0.432	0.722	0.489
2	PG	0.976	0.761	1.021	0.795	0.647	0.380	0.692	0.469
	M	0.965	0.776	0.987	0.787	0.646	0.328	0.692	0.437

[a] Two experiments are represented in which the left ventricular myofibrillar ATPase activities (μmoles) PO_4/mg protein × 2 min) of sham-operated (S) and experimental (X) animals are compared using the myofibrillar isolation techniques of Perry and Grey (PG) and a modification (M) of their method. Each experiment contained one pair of animals. The incubation vessels contained 1.00 m*M* ATP, 0.05*M* KCl, 0.01*M* imidazole, protein concentrations of 0.529 and 0.549 mg/ml and cations as indicated. The assay was run at pH 7.1 and 35°C.

MYOFIBRILLAR ATPASE MEASUREMENTS

The myofibrillar ATPase activity was determined at varying concentrations of ATP, $MgCl_2$ and $CaCl_2$; that is, 0.25, 0.50, 1.00, 1.50, 2.00, and 4.00 m*M*. When the activity was studied at varying ATP concentrations, the $MgCl_2$ concentration was 1.00 m*M*. The initial concentration of ATP in the activating solutions was 1.00 m*M* when the activity was studied at varying divalent cation concentrations. The reaction was run at 35°C, pH 7.1 with a protein concentration of 1 mg/ml and stopped after two minutes by the addition of TCA. The concentration of KCl and imidazole in all of the solutions was 0.05 *M* and 0.01 *M*, respectively.

Reaction vessels containing 1 ml of the washed myofibrillar suspension were equilibrated in a shaking water bath at 35°C for 5 min. Four milliliters of 12% TCA were added to the "zero-time" vessels near the end of the equilibration period. Immediately following the equilibration period, 1.0 ml of the appropriate activating solution was added to the "zero-time" and "two-minute" vessels. To stop the reaction in the "two-minute" vessels at 2.0 min, 4 ml of 12% TCA were used. All containers were quickly cooled on ice before the mixture was centrifuged and the denatured protein removed. The supernatant was used for inorganic phosphate analysis which was carried out by the method of Fiske and Subbarow (1925). The myofibrillar protein concentration was measured according to the procedure of Lowry *et al.* (1951).

This procedure is based on the color reaction of proteins with phospho-18-molybdictungstic acid (Folin and Wu, 1920; Wu, 1922) and is due largely to the protein tyrosine content. In the present experiments, crystalline bovine albumin was used as the standard for measuring myofibrillar protein concentration. Since the nitrogen content of bovine albumin (Neurath and Bailey, 1954) and myofibrillar proteins (Bailey, 1948; Kominz *et al.*, 1954) was shown to be similar, the Lowry method was first standardized to the Kjeldahl method for protein determination. The myofibrillar protein concentration (P) was calculated as follows: $P = KP_L$, where $K = P_{Kj}/P_L$, P_{Kj}, the myofibrillar protein concentration calculated by the Kjeldahl method using bovine albumin as the standard, and P_L is the myofibrillar protein concentration according to the lowry method with bovine albumin as the standard. It was assumed that the tyrosine content was not significantly different in the hypertrophied and control hearts.

Extraction of Actomyosin and ATPase Determination

Actomyosin (myosin B) was prepared by a 5-hr extraction of minced left ventricular muscle with cold Weber-Edsall solution (Szent-Györgi, 1951), after which the mixture was centrifuged and the supernatant diluted with 10 vol of water. The resulting suspension was centrifuged, the actomyosin precipitate washed with water and redissolved in 5 vol of 0.5 *M* buffered KCl. Purification of the actomyosin was carried out by precipitating, washing and redissolving the protein three times.

The purified actomyosin was dissolved in 0.5 *M* or suspended in 0.05 *M* KCl buffered with 0.01 *M* imidazole at pH 7.1. The ATP concentration used in studying Mg^{2+} and Ca^{2+} activated ATPase activity was 1 m*M*. Assays for ATPase activity were run at both 0.5 *M* and 0.05 *M* KCl. The assay was run in the absence of divalent cation and in the presence of 1.00 m*M* Mg^{2+} and Ca^{2+}. 1 ml of enzyme solution (or suspension) was placed in a 10 ml test tube and equilibrated by shaking 5 min in a water bath at 37°C. The reaction was started by adding cation and ATP, and stopped by adding 4 ml of 12% trichloracetic acid at 2 min. Control measurements were made by adding 4 ml of 12% trichloracetic acid at zero time and 1 ml of the appropriate activating solution at 2 min. The final protein concentration was 1.21 (0.96–1.49) mg/cc. Following centrifugation, the denatured protein was discarded and the supernatant analyzed for inorganic phosphate.

Viscosity Measurements

Viscosity measurements were determined in 5 ml samples at 27°C using an Ostwald viscosimeter. Actomyosin was dissolved in buffered KCl to give a protein concentration of approximately 2 mg/ml (Table VI). Specific viscosities were calculated from the relation

$$\text{Specific viscosity} = (t - t_o)/t_o$$

where t_o is the outflow time of the solvent and t is the outflow time of the solvent + actomyosin (Bull, 1964).

ATP sensitivity is defined by the following relationship (Portzehl *et al.*, 1950)

$$\text{ATP sensitivity} = \frac{\log t/t_o - \log {}^t\text{ATP}/t_o}{\log {}^t\text{ATP}/t_o} \times 100$$

where ^{t}ATP is the outflow time measured immediately after the addition of 0.05 ml of 0.1 M $MgCl_2$ and 0.05 ml of 0.1 *M* ATP to 5 ml of the actomyosin solution.

Protein Determination

Protein was determined with the Folin phenol reagent using bovine albumin as the standard (Lowry *et al.*, 1951).

Results

Separate groups of animals were used for the myofibril and actomyosin studies.

Animals Used for Myofibrillar ATPase Analyses

Effects of Aortic Stenosis

Surgery was performed on 60 male guinea pigs; 40 were used as experimentals and 20 as controls. Nineteen experimentals died within 5 days of the operation and two more at 11 and 14 days after surgery. Some animals showed signs of dyspnea and weakness as early as 11 days following aortic stenosis. Others did not develop these symptoms for as long as 24 days after surgery and some never developed signs of ill health. The experimental animals were chosen for sacrifice between 16 and 24 days after surgery when exhibiting signs of weakness, dyspnea, rales, and anorexia. Those surviving more than 24 days (up to 33 days) were sacrificed regardless of their condition of health. An experimental heart was used for analysis if the left ventricular weight was above 125% (calculated as percent body weight on the day of analysis) of its paired control. This criteria was met in 11 of the 40 guinea pigs with aortic stenosis.

The control and experimental animals were operated on and sacrificed together whenever possible. In 9 of the 11 pairs, the experimentals were operated on within 24 hr of the controls. In the other two pairs, the controls which were originally intended to complete the pair could not be used. Therefore, the controls with the next nearest date of operation were used.

There were no significant differences between experimental and control animals, with respect to body weights, when operated on or when sacrificed. The controls weighed 626 ($\pm$ 38) gm at surgery and 730 ($\pm$ 40) gm when sacrificed and the experimentals weighed 622 ($\pm$ 40) gm and 649 ($\pm$ 90) gm, respectively.

The lung, liver, and spleen weights of experimental animals were not significantly different from those of the controls. Calculated as per cent body weight on the day of analysis, the lungs were 1.19 ($\pm$ 0.38)% and 0.88 ($\pm$ 0.27)%, the livers were 3.25 ($\pm$ 0.78)% and 3.27 ($\pm$ 0.42)% and the spleens were 0.19 ($\pm$ 0.11)% and 0.15 ($\pm$ 0.04)% for experimental and control animals, respectively.

There were highly significant differences between the left ventricular weights of experimentals and controls ($p < 0.001$); they were 0.36 ($\pm$ 0.06)% and 0.19 ($\pm$ 0.01)%, respectively, when calculated as percent body weight on the day of analysis (Table II).

Myofibrillar ATPase Analyses

The myofibrillar ATPase activities were evaluated by the standard analysis of variance (Batson, 1956). Eleven pairs were analyzed at each level of ATP, $MgCl_2$ and $CaCl_2$ studied. Representative values for individual animals are shown in Table II. The average ATPase activities obtained at each level of ATP, $MgCl_2$, and $CaCl_2$ studied are recorded in Table III and are plotted in Figs. 1–3. It can be seen that the qualitative pattern of activity in the hypertrophied hearts is similar to that of the control hearts. When analyzed at various concentrations of ATP (in mM/l) there was a rise in activity from 0.25 to 1.50–2.00 and a subsequent fall above this level. As the concentration of $MgCl_2$ (in mM/l) was raised, there was a rise in activity from 0.25 to 1.00

TABLE II

LEFT VENTRICLE WEIGHTS AND REPRESENTATIVE MYOFIBRILLAR ATPASE ACTIVITIES[a]

	Left ventricle			Ratio (%A)	ATPase activity	
Exp. No.	mg	%O	%A	X/S	$MgCl_2$ (1 mM)	$CaCl_2$ (1 mM)
S100	1300	0.19	0.18	1.50	1.173	0.635
X102	1865	0.30	0.27		0.767	0.379
X117	2158	0.34	0.36	1.80	0.640	0.368
S116	1400	0.22	0.20		0.795	0.412
S113	1416	0.22	0.19	1.63	0.864	0.431
X114	1730	0.27	0.31		0.845	0.392
X120	1961	0.36	0.44	2.44	0.733	0.333
S119	1085	0.20	0.18		1.000	0.516
S107	1490	0.25	0.20	1.45	1.537	0.669
X105	2150	0.35	0.29		0.995	0.443
X106	2170	0.35	0.31	1.55	0.693	0.459
S125	1430	0.24	0.20		0.919	0.589
S131	1350	0.20	0.18	1.61	1.089	0.580
X121	1960	0.35	0.29		1.043	0.509
X139	2360	0.37	0.41	2.27	0.911	0.339
S137	1260	0.20	0.18		1.297	0.627
S134	1470	0.24	0.19	1.47	1.173	0.544
X138	2121	0.35	0.28		0.915	0.361
X144	2550	0.39	0.38	1.90	0.901	0.368
S140	1430	0.23	0.20		1.129	0.481
S149	1460	0.22	0.18	1.88	1.029	0.459
X156	2400	0.35	0.34		0.948	0.356
Mean Values						
%O:	S	0.22(± 0.02)			1.091	0.540
	X	0.34(± 0.03)			0.854	0.392
		$p < 0.001$			$p < 0.001$	$p < 0.001$
%A:	S	0.19(± 0.01)				
	X	0.36(± 0.06)				
		$p < 0.001$				

[a] ATPase = μmoles PO_4/mg protein × 2 min, S = control, X = experimental, O and A — body weight at operation and analysis, respectively, p = probability value [from the standard analysis of variance (Batson, 1956) pairs are grouped]. X156. Conditions: as described in the text.

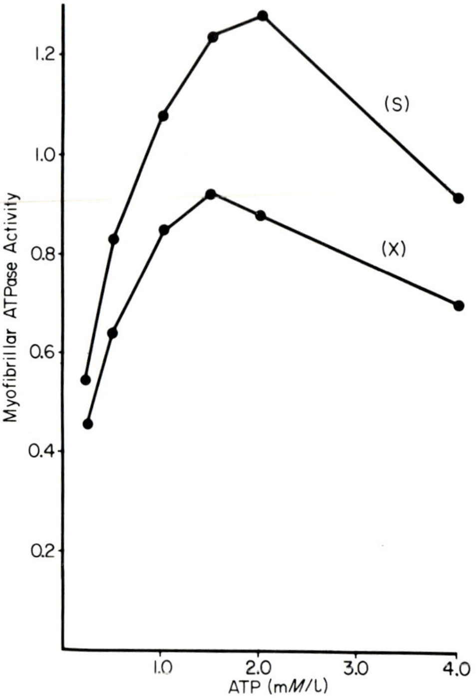
Myofibrillar ATPase Activity
1.2
1.0
0.8
0.6
0.4
0.2
(S)
(X)
1.0
2.0
3.0
4.0
ATP (mM/L)

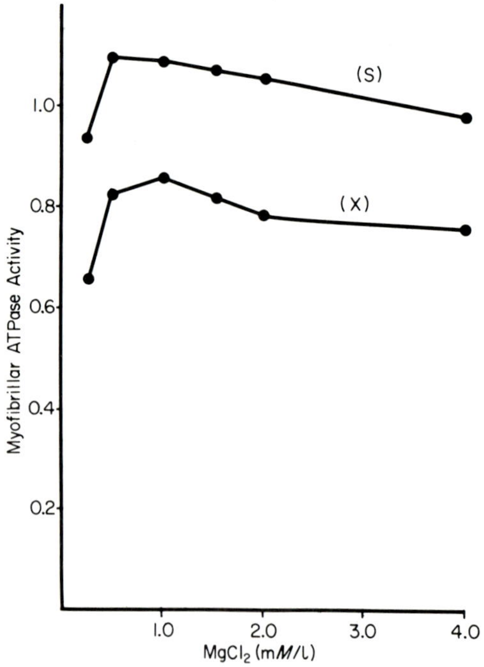
Myofibrillar ATPase Activity
1.0
0.8
0.6
0.4
0.2
(S)
(X)
1.0
2.0
3.0
4.0
$MgCl_2$ (mM/L)

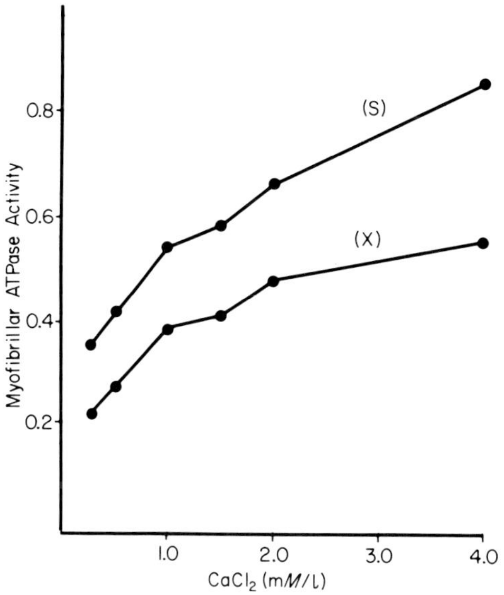

FIG. 3. Myofibrillar ATPase activity as a function of $CaCl_2$ concentration. The average left ventricular myofibrillar ATPase activities (μM PO_4/mg protein × 2 min) are plotted at varying $CaCl_2$ concentrations for 11 sham-operated (S) and 11 experimental (X) animals. Incubation vessels contained 0.05M KCl, 0.01M imidazole, 1.00M ATP and the assays were run at pH 7.1 and 35°C.

and a gradual decline with higher concentrations. When $CaCl_2$ was used as the activator, the activity rose with the $CaCl_2$ concentration.

Quantitatively there was a highly significant difference between the experimental and control hearts with respect to their myofibrillar ATPase activities. The hypertrophied hearts exhibited a reduction in activity at every level of ATP, $MgCl_2$, and $CaCl_2$ studied. This reduction amounted to 24.2 (19.3–25.6)%, 30.6 (27.5–33.7)% and 24.9 (20.3–31.4)%, respectively.

The protein concentrations used for the ATPase analyses were 1.02 (± 0.09) and 1.02 (± 0.06) mg/ml for the experimental and control groups, respectively.

FIG. 1. Myofibrillar ATPase activity as a function of ATP concentration. The average left ventricular myofibrillar ATPase activities (μM PO_4/mg protein × 2 min) are plotted at varying ATP concentrations for 11 sham-operated (S) and 11 experimental (X) animals. Incubation vessels contained 0.05M KCl, 0.01M imidazole, 1.00 mM $MgCl_2$ and the assays were run at pH 7.1 and 35°C.

FIG. 2. Myofibrillar ATPase activity as a function of $MgCl_2$ concentration. The average left ventricular myofibrillar ATPase activities (μM PO_4/mg protein × 2 min) are plotted at varying $MgCl_2$ concentrations for 11 sham-operated (S) and 11 experimental (X) animals. Incubation vessels contained 0.05M KCl, 0.01M imidazole, 1.00M ATP and the assays were run at pH 7.1 and 35°C.

TABLE III

MYOFIBRILLAR ATPASE ACTIVITIES[a]

mM/l	S	X	p
ATP			
0.25	0.549(± 0.072)	0.450(± 0.050)	< 0.001
0.50	0.850(± 0.162)	0.636(± 0.065)	< 0.001
1.00	1.091(± 0.209)	0.854(± 0.129)	< 0.001
1.50	1.241(± 0.289)	0.928(± 0.126)	< 0.01
2.00	1.267(± 0.293)	0.889(± 0.113)	< 0.001
4.00	0.924(± 0.329)	0.688(± 0.134)	< 0.05
$MgCl_2$			
0.25	0.935(± 0.174)	0.634(± 0.120)	< 0.001
0.50	1.096(± 0.171)	0.811(± 0.102)	< 0.001
1.00	1.091(± 0.209)	0.854(± 0.129)	< 0.001
1.50	1.057(± 0.194)	0.817(± 0.086)	< 0.01
2.00	1.041(± 0.194)	0.785(± 0.077)	< 0.001
4.00	0.971(± 0.208)	0.737(± 0.085)	< 0.001
$CaCl_2$			
0.25	0.355(± 0.066)	0.237(± 0.048)	< 0.001
0.50	0.428(± 0.088)	0.298(± 0.060)	< 0.001
1.00	0.540(± 0.087)	0.392(± 0.055)	< 0.001
1.50	0.588(± 0.085)	0.419(± 0.052)	< 0.001
2.00	0.672(± 0.088)	0.479(± 0.059)	< 0.001
4.00	0.850(± 0.134)	0.564(± 0.082)	< 0.001

[a]ATPase = μmoles PO_4/mg protein × 2 min, S = control, X = experimental, p = probability value [from the standard analysis of variance (Batson, 1956) using 11 pairs of animals]. Each figure in columns S and X represents the average activity of 11 animals for the corresponding treatment indicated at the far left. Conditions as described in the text.

ANIMALS USED FOR ACTOMYOSIN ATPASE AND VISCOSITY ANALYSES

Effects of Aortic Stenosis

Surgery was performed on 83 animals; 44 were used as experimentals and 39 as controls. Twenty-five experimentals survived at least 23 days and were chosen for sacrifice between 23 and 27 days after surgery. Experimentals were paired with controls, i.e., an experimental and control were operated on, sacrificed and analyzed together. A heart was used for analysis if the left ventricular weight was above 125% (calculated as per cent body weight on the day of analysis) of its paired control. This criteria was met in nine cases.

TABLE IV

ACTOMYOSIN GROUP: BODY WEIGHTS, LEFT VENTRICULAR WEIGHTS AND ACTOMYOSIN YIELDS

Exp. No.	O/gm	A/gm	t/D	Left ventricle mg	Left ventricle %O	Left ventricle %A	Ratio (%A) X/S	Ratio (%A) %AM
X8	356	380	23	1349	0.37	0.36		2.58
S17	354	440	22	816	0.23	0.18	2.00	
S16	360	500	22	909	0.25	0.18		2.86
S18	338	430	23	876	0.25	0.20		3.16
S24	353	530	23	835	0.23	0.16	1.44	
X15	350	505	24	1314	0.37	0.26		3.11
X14	350	415	25	1091	0.31	0.26		2.59
S20	330	365	24	808	0.24	0.22	1.30	
S22	335	440	24	788	0.23	0.18		2.54
S51	360	520	20	987	0.27	0.19		3.35
S55	355	475	20	806	0.22	0.17	1.38	
X10	316	468	26	1170	0.37	0.25		3.08
X4	355	520	27	1417	0.39	0.27		3.76
S52	340	450	21	772	0.22	0.17	1.58	
S56	320	380	21	642	0.20	0.17		3.55
S59	320	405	22	817	0.26	0.20		3.53
S57	335	470	22	812	0.24	0.17	1.35	
X31	340	430	24	1083	0.32	0.25		2.79
X32	370	430	24	1236	0.33	0.29		2.67
S53	325	470	22	844	0.26	0.18	1.65	
S58	355	580	22	968	0.28	0.17		3.30
S54	350	535	23	962	0.27	0.18		3.12
S63	370	540	22	999	0.27	0.18	1.83	
X42	380	370	24	1227	0.32	0.33		1.93
X41	380	535	24	1495	0.39	0.28		2.75
S61	355	505	22	770	0.22	0.15	1.60	
S62	340	530	22	1053	0.31	0.20		3.02

Mean values

O:	S	344(± 15)	%O:	0.25(± 0.03)	3.16(± 0.33)
	X:	355(± 20)		0.35(± 0.03)	2.81(±0.50)
		$p > 0.05$		$p < 0.001$	$p < 0.05$
A:	S	476(± 59)	%A:	0.18(± 0.02)	
	X	450(± 60)		0.28(± 0.04)	
		$p > 0.05$		$p < 0.001$	

Notation: S = control, X = experimental, O and A = body weight at operation and analysis, respectively, %AM = actomyosin (% of wet weight), p = probability value [from standard analysis of variance (Batson, 1956); pairs are grouped]. Time (t) = days (D) post-op.

The control animals weighed 344 (± 15) gm at surgery and 476 (± 59) gm when sacrificed; experimentals weighed 355 (± 20) gm and 450 (± 60) gm at sacrifice. These differences were not significant.

There were highly significant differences in the left ventricular weights of experimentals and controls ($p < 0.001$); they were 0.28 (± 0.04)% and 0.18 (± 0.02)%, respectively, when calculated as percent body weight on the day of analysis (Table IV). The quantity of contractile proteins obtained by the five hour actomyosin extraction technique, expressed as wet weight, was 2.81 (± 0.50)% and 3.16 (± 0.33)% for the experimental and control hearts, respectively ($p < 0.05$, Table IV).

Actomyosin ATPase Analyses

Previous experiments had shown that the quantity of tissue obtained from one control heart was inadequate for carrying out all of the desired measurements. Therefore, left ventricles of two controls were pooled and used as one part of a pair. Because of its larger mass, only one experimental heart was needed to complete the pair.

The actomyosin ATPase activity was studied in the absence of divalent cations and in the presence of 1 m*M* $MgCl_2$ and $CaCl_2$. When studied at high ionic strength (0.5 *M* KCl–0.01 *M* imidazole), there were no significant differences between the hypertrophied and nonhypertrophied hearts with respect to their actomyosin ATPase activities in the absence of divalent cations or in the presence of 1.00 m*M* $MgCl_2$. However, when the divalent cation was

TABLE V

ACTOMYOSIN ATPASE ACTIVITIES

KCl (*M*/l)	Me (m*M*/*L*)	S	X	*p*
0.5	absent	0.162	0.150	> 0.05
0.5	$MgCl_2$ 1.00	0.068	0.052	> 0.05
0.5	$CaCl_2$ 1.00	0.346	0.264	< 0.01
0.05	absent	0.244	0.198	< 0.01
0.05	$MgCl_2$ 1.00	0.243	0.175	< 0.05
0.05	$CaCl_2$ 1.00	0.372	0.316	< 0.05

Notation: ATPase = μmoles PO_4/mg protein × 2 min; Me = divalent cation; S = control; X = experimental; p = probability value [from the standard analysis of variance (Batson, 1956), using 9 "pairs" of animals]. Each figure in columns S and X represents the average activity of 9 animals for the corresponding KCl and Me concentrations. Conditions as described in the text.

TABLE VI

ACTOMYOSIN VISCOSITY STUDIES

Exp. No.	η_{sp}	P(mg/ml)	ATP Sensitivity
X8	0.95	2.34	90
S 16, 17	0.90	1.91	109
S 18, 24	0.84	1.95	124
X15	0.92	2.16	91
X14	0.65	1.86	73
S 20, 22	0.68	1.74	150
S 51, 55	0.93	1.98	114
X10	0.91	2.03	99
X4	0.84	2.10	103
S 52, 56	0.87	2.41	111
S 57, 59	0.88	1.80	125
X31	0.83	2.10	88
X32	0.88	1.98	96
S 53, 58	0.94	1.89	132
S 54, 63	0.66	1.62	85
X42	0.49	1.96	54
X41	0.88	2.09	105
S 61, 62	0.80	2.34	146
Mean values			
S	0.83($\pm$ 0.10)	1.96($\pm$ 0.26)	122($\pm$ 20)
X	0.82($\pm$ 0.15)	2.07($\pm$ 0.14)	89($\pm$ 16)
	$p > 0.05$	$p > 0.05$	$p < 0.01$

Notation: S = control, X = experimental, η_{sp} = specific viscosity, P = protein concentration, p = probability value [from the standard analysis of variance (Batson, 1956); pairs are grouped]. Conditions as described in the text.

Ca (1.00 mM $CaCl_2$), actomyosin from hypertrophied hearts had an ATPase activity 23.7% lower than ($p < 0.01$) than that of nonhypertrophied hearts (Table V). When studied at low ionic strength (0.05 M KCl–0.01 M imidazole), hypertrophied heart actomyosin exhibited a significantly lower ATPase activity in the absence of divalent cations ($p < 0.01$), in the presence of 1.00 mM $MgCl_2$ ($p < 0.05$) and in the presence of 1.00 mM $CaCl_2$ ($p < 0.05$) than nonhypertrophied heart actomyosin (Table V). These reductions averaged 8.9%, 28.0%, and 15.1%, respectively.

The protein concentrations used for determining the actomyosin ATPase activities were not significantly different for the experimental and control groups. When studied at 0.5 *M* KCl, the concentrations were 1.21 ($\pm$ 0.18) mg/ml for the experimentals and 1.34 ($\pm$ 0.10) mg/ml for the controls; they were 1.22 ($\pm$ 0.20) and 1.32 ($\pm$ 0.11) mg/ml, respectively, when studied at 0.05 *M* KCl.

Actomyosin Viscosity Analyses

There were no significant differences between the specific viscosities of actomyosin from hypertrophied and nonhypertrophied hearts. However, actomyosin from hypertrophied hearts exhibited an average ATP sensitivity 27% beneath that of nonhypertrophied hearts ($p < 0.01$) (Table VI).

Discussion

Guinea pig left ventricles undergo marked hypertrophy following experimental aortic stenosis. Although there is a question that this procedure produces a syndrome comparable to human congestive heart failure, it is interesting that the findings presented in this paper show a remarkable similarity between myofibrils from hypertrophied ventricles isolated from either guinea pigs or man (Alpert and Gordon, 1962). In the study on human congestive failure, the age of the patients was a problem. Under the circumstances of this experiment, decreased ATPase activity of the myofibrils is associated with the hypertrophy despite the fact that the animals are all of the same age.

The decreased activity may result from alterations in the subcellular particles adhering to the cardiac myofibril, the noncontractile protein of the myofibril, or the contractile protein in the myofibrils. Evidence pointing to a change in the contractile proteins of the myofibril lies in the fact that actomyosin isolated from hypertrophied left ventricles of guinea pigs has lower ATPase activity than actomyosin isolated from sham-operated animals (Table V). In addition, the ATP sensitivity of actomyosin from hypertrophied hearts is lower when compared to actomyosin from hearts of sham-operated animals despite the fact that the specific viscosity is unchanged (Table VI).

Davis reported no difference in ATP sensitivity, but suggested there may be a decrease in ATPase activity of actomyosin isolated from dog hearts in failure induced by pulmonary stenosis and tricuspid insufficiency (Davis *et al.*, 1959). In these experiments it was difficult to evaluate the extent and rate of hypertrophy. Furthermore, the variability was large, the number of animals small, and the experiments were not paired. Findings from other laboratories indicate a change in actomyosin isolated from failing hypertrophied hearts. Benson *et al.* (1958) report that actomyosin ATP sensitivity is down while Meerson as well as Miyahara showed a decreased actomyosin ATPase activity whether reported on a nitrogen basis or per unit of DNA (Meerson, 1962; Meerson *et al.*, 1964; Miyahara, 1962; Miyahara *et al.*, 1962). The differences among these results, those of Davis and our results, may relate to the rate of cardiac hypertrophy as well as the extent of failure. In these guinea pigs, enlargement occurs faster than was recorded for the dogs, and accordingly, the rate as well as the pattern of protein synthesis could be different.

Since a substantial portion of myofibrillar protein is actomyosin, the implication is that the actomyosin in the hypertrophied failing ventricle is faulty, or that some other protein which is inhibitory to ATPase activity or inactive, with solubility characteristics similar to actomyosin, is deposited in the myofibril. Ebashi and Ebashi (1964) have isolated a new protein (other than actin, myosin, or tropomyosin) which sensitizes actomyosin to Ca^{2+}. In addition, Maruyama (1965a,b) has discovered another protein which hinders network formation of F-actin in solution. Variations in the relative amounts of these proteins may influence the physical and enzymatic properties of actomyosin. It is conceivable that hypertrophied heart muscle has different ratios of myofibrillar proteins (actin, myosin, tropomyosin, actinin, troponin) which could alter the capacity of actomyosin to hydrolyze ATP. The difference noted between ATPase activities determined at low and high ionic strength may have some bearing. The depression of ATPase activity at high ionic strength occurs in the presence of Ca^{2+}, but not in its absence or in the presence of Mg^{2+} (Table V). Thus, these changes may be caused by a decreased Ca^{2+} sensitivity or an alteration in myosin binding sites. Alternatively, the actin myosin ratio may be changed. This appears unlikely in view of the similarity of the specific viscosity of actomyosin from experimental and control hearts (Table VI). Another possibility is the extraction of inert proteins with the same solubility characteristics as actomyosin but with no ATPase activity. Such was the case in studies on developing tadpoles and frog muscle (Nass, 1962). Despite the uncertainty of the cause, in hypertrophied guinea pig hearts, there is a decreased ability of the contractile machine to utilize ATP.

What are the consequences of a decreased cardiac myofibrillar and actomyosin ATPase activity in these hypertrophied hearts? Actomyosin bands from failing hearts shorten less than those from normal hearts, whereas tension development of glycerinated fibers from failing hearts is depressed (Kako and Bing, 1958; Olson and Piatnek, 1959). Under physiological conditions the velocity at which heart muscle shortens and develops tension is directly related to its ATPase activity (Alpert *et al.*, 1965, 1967). Furthermore, Hasselbach (1956) and Barany (1967) demonstrated that a decrease in the rate of hydrolysis was always associated with a decrease in power output.

Thus the power output may be markedly depressed as a result of the inability of the actomyosin in the myofibril to hydrolyze ATP. This agrees with classical concepts of the failing heart. Patterson and Starling (1914) and Patterson *et al* (1914) pointed out that normal hearts when subjected to venous filling followed one curve whereas the failing heart was on an entirely different curve, developing less tension for any given length, and shortening less rapidly at any given force. This last point is extremely important in terms of the metabolism of the heart. It was demonstrated in skeletal muscle that when the same amount of work is performed on a slower force–velocity curve, the cost of that work is greater (McCrorey and Alpert, 1963). Thus one may speculate that because of the deficient energy utilization, namely the decreased myofibrillar ATPase activity, the failing heart develops force less rapidly at any given length, contracts more slowly for any given force, and must expend more energy for any given amount of work carried out.

Acknowledgment

Supported in part by Grant PHS 5 R01 11611.

References

Alpert, N. R., and Gordon, M. S. (1962). *Amer. J. Physiol.* **202,** 940.

Alpert, N. R., Gale, H. H., and Taylor, N. (1965). *The Physiologist* 8, 100.

Alpert, N. R., Gale, H. H., and Taylor, N. (1967). *In* "Factors Influencing Myocardial Contractility" (R. D. Tanz, F. Kavaler, and J. Roberts, eds.) pp. 127–133. Academic Press, New York.

Bailey, K. (1948). *Biochem. J.* **43,** 271.

Batson, H. C. (1956). "An Introduction to Statistics in the Medical Sciences." Burgess Publishing Co., Minneapolis, Minnesota.

Barany, M. (1967). *J. Gen. Physiol.* **50,** 197.

Benson, E. S. (1955). *Circ. Res.* **3,** 221.

Benson, E. S., Holloway, B. E., and Turbak, C. E. (1958). *Circ. Res.* **6,** 122.

Bull, H. B. (1964). "Physical Biochemistry" T. A. Davis, Philadelphia.

Davis, J. O., Tregasso, M., and Yankopoulos, N. (1959). *Circ. Res.* **7,** 957.

Ebashi, S., and Ebashi, F. (1964). *J. Biochem.* **55,** 604.

Finkel, R. M., and Gergely, J. (1961). *J. Biol. Chem.* **236,** 1458.

Fiske, C. H., and Subbarow, Y. (1925). *J. Biol. Chem.* **66,** 375.

Folin, O., and Wu, H. (1920). *J. Biol. Chem.* **41,** 367.

Gertler, M. M. (1959). *Proc. Soc. Exp. Biol. Med.* **102,** 396.

Hasselbach, W. (1956). *Biochem. Biophys. Acta* **20,** 355.

Kako, K., and Bing, R. J. (1958). *J. Clin. Invest.* **37,** 465.

Kominz, D. R., Hough, A., Symonds, P., and Laki, K. (1954). *Arch. Biochem. Biophys.* **50,** 148.

Lowry, O. M., Rosenbrough, N. J., Farr, A. L., and Randall, R. J. (1951). *J. Biol. Chem.* **193,** 265.

Maruyama, K. (1965a). *Biochim. Biophys. Acta* **94,** 208.
Maruyama, K. (1965b). *Biochim. Biophys. Acta* **102,** 542.
McCrorey, H. L., and Alpert, N. R. (1963). *Fed. Proc. Fed. Amer. Soc. Exp. Biol.* **22,** 403.
Meerson, F. Z. (1962). *Circ. Res.* **10,** 250.
Meerson, F. Z., Beloshapkins, T. D., Lushnikov, E. F., Liekma, E. M., Mavkovskaya, G. N. and Chernyshova, G. V. (1964). *Fed. Proc. Transl. Suppl.* **23,** T667. From Vestn. Akad. Meditsinsikikh Nauk SSSR **18,** 27, 1963.
Miyahara, M. (1962). *Jap. Circ. J.* **26,** 8.
Miyahara, M., Yokoyama, M., Nogasaki, Y., and Kinjo, K. (1962). *Jap. Heart J.* **3,** 46.
Mommaerts, W. F. H. M. (1958). *Methods Med. Res.* **7,** 8.
Nass, M. (1962). *Devlop. Biol.* **4,** 289.
Neurath, H., and Bailey, K. (1954). "The Proteins," Vol. 2, pt. B, p. 68. Academic Press. New York.
Olson, R. E., and Piatnek, D. (1959). Conservation of energy in cardiac muscle. *Ann. N.Y., Acad. Sci.* **72,** 466.
Patterson, S. W., and Starling, E. H. (1914). *J. Physiol.* **48,** 357.
Patterson, S. W., Piper, H., and Starling, E. H. (1914). *J. Physiol.* **48,** 465.
Perry, S. V., and Grey, T. C. (1956). *Biochem. J.* **64,** 184.
Portzehl, H., Schramm, G., and Weber, H. H. (1950). *Z. Naturswschung.* **56,** 61.
Szent-Györgi, A. (1951). "Chemistry of Muscular Contraction," 2nd Ed. Academic Press, New York.
Wu, H. (1922). *J. Biol. Chem.* **51,** 33.

THE ATPase ACTIVITY AND Ca^{2+} *AFFINITY OF MYOSIN B FROM HYPERTROPHIED NONFAILING CAT HEARTS*

Paul F. Hoar, Kathleen T. Shiverick, Burt B. Hamrell, and Norman R. Alpert

Introduction

Muscle hypertrophy is a response to stress which provides the animal with an increased muscle mass capable of developing more total force. However, hypertrophied heart and skeletal muscle exhibit a decrease in active tension and velocity of shortening when these parameters are normalized for cross-sectional area and length (Grimm *et al.*, 1963; Lesch *et al.*, 1968; Meerson and Pshennikova, 1965; Spann *et al.*, 1967). The changes may be explained in terms of theories of muscle contraction where the development of force and power depend on the interaction of myosin, actin, ATP, Mg^{2+}, and Ca^{2+}. The most compelling view of this relationship, the sliding filament hypothesis, describes the interaction of actin and myosin by means of cross-bridges which extend from myosin to actin. This interaction produces force or displacement by the cyclic binding of the myosin cross bridges to actin. A prerequisite for activity in this model is the hydrolysis of ATP in the presence of Mg^{2+} and Ca^{2+} by the contractile protein complex actomyosin. In this context, the ATPase activity of myosin has been correlated with velocity of shortening and tension development in a number of different muscles from several animals (Barany, 1967; Barany *et al.*, 1967; Brahms and Kay, 1962). A decrease in the normalized mechanical response of compensated-hypertrophied and failing muscle has been consistently demonstrated (Grimm *et al.*, 1963; Lesch *et al.*, 1968; Meerson and Pshennikova, 1965; Spann *et al.*, 1967); however, the ATPase activity of myofibrils, actomyosin, and myosin from these preparations has variously been reported as unchanged, increased, or decreased (Table I). This mechanical–biochemical discrepancy may result from differences in the cationic milieu in which the protein ATPase

TABLE I

ATPase Activity of Myofibrillar, Actomyosin, and Myosin Preparations from Failing and Hypertrophied Hearts

Species	Preparation	Conditions and results	Author
		Cardiac failure	
Human	Myofibrils	Mg^{2+}-activated ATPase activity decreased at low ionic strength	Alpert and Gordon (1962)
Human	Myofibrils	Mg^{2+}-activated ATPase activity decreased; Ca^{2+} activated ATPase activity unchanged at low ionic strength	Aras and Haas (1962)
Human	Myofibrils	Ca^{2+}-activated ATPase activity decreased at low ionic strength	Gordon and Brown (1966)
Guinea pig	Myofibrils	Mg^{2+}- and Ca^{2+}-activated ATPase activity decreased at low ionic strength	Alpert and Draper (1965); Draper *et al.*, this volume
Cat	Myofibrils	Mg^{2+}-activated ATPase activity decreased in presence and absence of azide at low ionic strength	Chandler *et al.* (1967)
Dog	Myofibrils	No change in ATPase activity (histochemical evaluation)	Sommers and Spach (1964)
Dog	Actomyosin	$0.01M$ Ca^{2+}-activated ATPase decreased; $0.1M$ Ca^{2+}-activated ATPase in no change at low ionic strengths	Davis *et al.* (1959)
Dog	Actomyosin	Ca^{2+}-activated ATPase activity increased	Benson (1955)
Dog	Actomyosin	ATPase activity decreased at low ionic strength	Miyahara (1962)
Guinea pig	Actomyosin	Ca^{2+}-activated ATPase activity decreased at high ionic strength; Mg^{2+}- and Ca^{2+}-activated ATPase activity decreased at low ionic strength	Draper *et al.*, this volume
Human	Myosin	ATPase activity increased	Nebel and Bing (1963)
Dog	Myosin	ATPase activity unchanged	Olson (1961)
Dog	Myosin	Ca^{2+}-activated ATPase activity depressed	Luchi *et al.* (1969)
		Cardiac hypertrophy	
Human	Myofibrils	No change in Mg^{2+}-activated ATPase activity	Brown *et al.* (1959)
Human	Myofibrils	No change in Mg^{2+}-activated ATPase activity	Gordon and Brown (1966)
Cat	Myofibrils	No change in Mg^{2+}-activated ATPase activity	Chandler *et al.* (1967)
Dog	Actomyosin	Depressed ATPase activity	Meerson *et al.* (1969)

activity is assayed. To evaluate this problem the ATPase activity of myosin B from normal and hypertrophied hearts was studied in the presence of an inert cation, TMA^+ (tetramethylammonium ion), which permits the evaluation of the separate effects of K^+ and Ca^{2+} activation. Our results demonstrate depression of Ca^{2+}-activated ATPase activity and Ca^{2+} affinity of myosin B from hypertrophied-compensated hearts studied in a high ionic strength medium.

Methods

Experimental left ventricular hypertrophy was produced in seven cats by constriction of the ascending aorta to 50% of its original diameter. Surgical intervention was carried out under pentobarbital anesthesia with positive pressure ventilation via tracheostomy. Seven cats were sham operated and served as control animals. Each cat was terminally studied under barbiturate anesthesia, 6–8 months postoperatively. The chest was opened and intraventricular pressures were measured with a Statham P23Dd pressure transducer connected to an 18-gauge trocar by a short length of polyethylene tubing. Pressure was recorded on a Beckman Dynograph polygraph.

Immediately following the hemodynamic measurements the heart was removed. The myocardium was weighed and the left ventricle (including the septum) was excised. Myosin B was isolated by the method of Maruyama with some modifications (Maruyama and Watanabe, 1962). After initial extraction in Weber–Edsall EDTA solution, the crude myosin B was divided into two fractions and solubilized in either 0.6 *M* KCl or 0.6 *M* TMAC (tetramethylammonium chloride). Further purification of the two fractions was carried out concurrently in their respective salts. The protein was stored at 0°–4°C and measurements of ATPase activity were made within 12 days of isolation.

ATPase activity was assayed titrimetrically with an automatic pH-stat (Eisenberg and Moos, 1967). The reaction mixture at 25°C contained 10 m*M* imidazole, 5 m*M* ATP, either 0.6 *M* KCl or TMAC and $CaCl_2$ as indicated. The reaction was stopped by addition of per chloric acid. Inorganic phosphate was determined by the standard Fiske and Subbarow method (Morales and Hotta, 1967). Protein concentration was determined by the method of Lowry, *et al.* (1951).

Data were statistically evaluated by means of Student's *t*-test and analysis of variance. Measurements on the effects of varying activator concentrations involve factorial analysis in which the same experimental unit is observed under more than one treatment condition. For these studies a repeated-measure design was used to evaluate the correlation between experimental errors inherent in this type of analysis (Winer, 1962). Maximum ATPase and apparent dissociation constants for the activator–myosin B complex were estimated from Lineweaver–Burk plots modified to relate the double reciprocals of enzyme activity and activator concentration. Unfortunately there is no way to treat extrapolated intercepts statistically, but this form of analysis provides a qualitative evaluation of enzyme parameters.

Results

Expermental Model

A comparison of left and right ventricular weights normalized for body weight is presented in Table II. The experimental animals showed significantly higher left and right ventricular weight/body weight ratios when compared

TABLE II

Ventricular Weight/Body Weight Ratios[a]

LV wt/body wt × 10^3		RV wt/body wt × 10^3	
Control	Experimental	Control	Experimental
2.08	3.33	1.38	1.28
1.74	4.56	0.87	1.33
2.33	3.72	1.38	1.57
1.83	2.93	0.96	1.66
2.40	3.48	1.33	1.43
2.55	3.22	1.45	2.06
2.52	2.78	1.17	1.44
2.21 ± 0.12	3.43 ± 0.22	1.22 ± 0.09	1.54 ± 0.10

[a] Mean ± S.E. shown at foot of each column. LV wt/body wt: $p < 0.001$; RV wt/body wt: $p < 0.05$.

with sham-operated controls ($p < 0.001$ and $p < 0.05$). Using these ratios as an index of stress-induced growth, the data indicate that there was substantial hypertrophy in both left and right ventricles of the myocardium in cats with constriction of the ascending aorta.

The experimental animals exhibited no clinical manifestations of heart failure, i.e., ascites, pleural effusion, peripheral edema, or dyspnea and in clinical appearance could not be differentiated from the control population. Data on hemodynamic measurements from four sham-operated and five experimental animals are presented in Table III. Although the left ventricular systolic pressure in hypertrophied animals was significantly elevated ($p < 0.05$)

TABLE III

LEFT VENTRICULAR PRESSURE (mm Hg)[a,b]

Control[a]			Experimental[a]		
Animal No.	Systolic	Diastolic	Animal No.	Systolic	Diastolic
1338	100	8	1334	110	12
1339	90	0	1336	129	3
1343	74	5	1340	136	11
1344	113	4	1341	132	3
			1342	123	6
	94.2 ± 8.2	4.25 ± 1.65		126.0 ± 4.5	7.0 ± 2.0

[a] Mean ± S.E. shown at foot of each column.
[b] Control vs. experimental, evaluated by means of unpaired t-test. Systolic: $p < 0.05$; diastolic $p > 0.10$.

over the sham-operated control animals, the end-diastolic pressures were not statistically different. The lack of elevation of end-diastolic pressure coupled with the excellent clinical state of the cats and the absence of pleural effusion and ascites at autopsy indicate that congestive heart failure was not present. Our weight and hemodynamic data establish that following experimental overload of the left ventricle, substantial stress-induced growth occurs and the ventricle is functionally characterized by development of elevated systolic pressure. This picture is consistent with that defined by Meerson as a model for compensatory hypertrophy (Meerson, 1969).

ATPASE MEASUREMENTS

Initially, we defined several parameters of normal cardiac myosin B ATPase activity in the presence of the inert cation TMA^+ (Morales and Hotta, 1967); in the pH range of 6.0–8.5 there was no splitting of ATP. The effects of K^+ on enzyme activity in the presence of a constant salt concentration are shown in Fig. 1. The ATPase activity of the enzyme bears a linear relationship to K^+ concentration. V_{max} values calculated from double reciprocal plots for Ca^{2+} and K^+ activation are similar (Fig. 2); however, K^+ binding to the enzyme is approximately 1/700 that of Ca^{2+}. Since high concentrations of K^+ activate the myosin B ATPase activity to the same extent as Ca^{2+}, studies were carried out in the presence of TMA^+ to prevent the K^+ from masking the Ca^{2+} effects.

The ATPase activity of cardiac myosin B from control and hypertrophied left ventricles was evaluated as a function of Ca^{2+} concentration in the presence of KCl and TMAC.

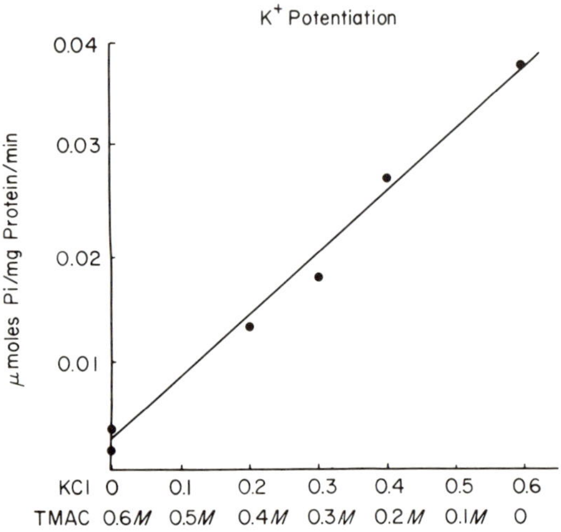

FIG. 1. Effect of increasing K^+ concentration on the ATPase activity of cardiac myosin B at constant total molarity. Conditions for enzyme assay were 5 m*M* ATP, 10 m*M* imidazole, 0.6 *M* salt (KCl and/or TMAC), pH 7.0, 25°C.

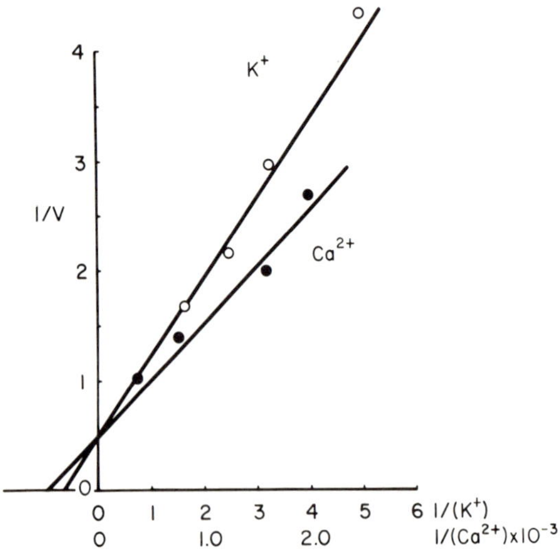

FIG. 2. The double reciprocal plot of cardiac myosin B ATPase activity. The cation concentration is in moles per liter and the velocity in μmoles Pi/mg protein/5 min. Conditions for enzyme assay are 0.6 *M* TMAC, 5 m*M* ATP, 10 m*M* imidazole, and activating cation as indicated pH 7.0, 25°C.

TABLE IV

CALCIUM-ACTIVATED ATPase ACTIVITY IN THE PRESENCE OF 0.6 *M* KCl[a]

	Calcium conc. (m*M*)					
Myosin B	0.00	0.25	0.50	0.63	1.25	2.50
Control LV	0.50	0.57	0.47	0.30	0.63	0.72
	0.22	0.18	0.18	0.18	0.27	0.46
	0.36	0.42	0.27	0.36	0.39	0.41
	0.20	0.24	0.44	0.42	0.39	0.40
Hypertrophied LV	0.12	0.17	0.23	0.12	0.43	0.39
	0.28	0.32	0 36	0 31	0.33	0.33
	0.39	0.35	0.41	0.29	0.46	0.47
	0.21	0.43	0.32	0.28	0.39	0.62

[a] Control vs. experimental, evaluated by analysis of variance (multifactor experiment with repeated measures on the same element). $F < 1$; not significantly different. Values are in μmoles Pi/mg protein/5 min. Each value was randomly selected from multiple series of experiments from various animals.

Data in Table IV show that enzyme activity in 0.6 *M* KCl was not significantly different between groups. However, in 0.6 *M* TMAC myosin B ATPase activity from hypertrophied left ventricles as compared with controls was significantly decreased in all Ca^{2+} concentrations studied (Table V). The regression line for these data (Fig. 3) shows a linear activation

TABLE V

CALCIUM-ACTIVATED ATPase ACTIVITY IN THE PRESENCE OF 0.6 *M* TMAC[a]

	Calcium conc. (m*M*)					
Myosin B	0.00	0.25	0.50	0.63	1.25	2.50
Control LV	0.04	0.05	0.08	0.14	0.15	0.36
	0.04	0.07	0.09	0.17	0.29	0.38
	0.05	0.05	0.05	0.10	0.18	0.31
	0.03	0.08	0.26	0.04	0.16	0.29
Hypertrophied LV	0.01	0.07	0.04	0.06	0.14	0.30
	0.01	0.05	0.10	0.09	0.18	0.27
	0.03	0.03	0.06	0.07	0.08	0.33
	0.07	0.06	0.03	0.05	0.14	0.27

[a] Control vs. experimental, evaluated by analysis of variance (multifactor experiment with repeated measures on the same element). $F = 10.62$; $p < 0.05$. Values are in μmoles Pi/mg protein/5 min. Each value was randomly selected as in Table IV.

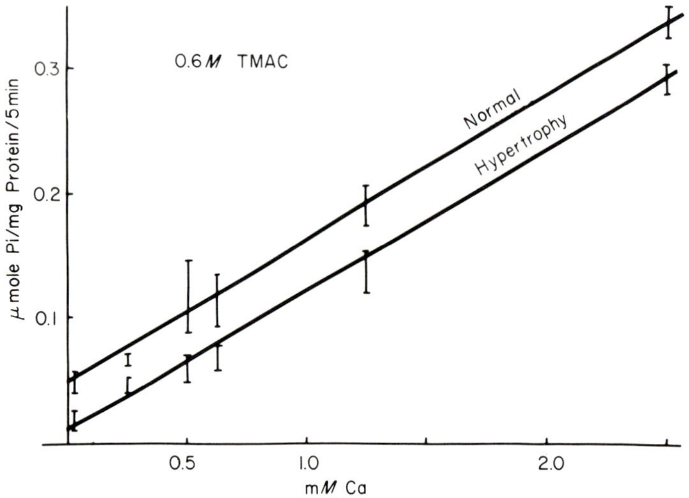

FIG. 3. ATPase activity of myosin B from sham-operated control and hypertrophied left ventricies as a function of Ca^{2+} concentrations. Conditions for enzyme assay were 0.6*M* TMAC, 10 m*M* imidazole, 5 m*M* ATP, pH 7.0, 25°C. I ± SEM.

of enzyme activity for myosin B from sham-operated control and hypertrophied hearts.

Maximum ATPase rates and apparent dissociation constants for the Ca^{2+}–myosin B complex were calculated from double reciprocal plots of enzyme activity as a function of activator concentration. V_{max} values in the control group ranged from 0.30 to 0.62 μmoles Pi/mg protein/5 min (mean 0.47 ± 0.05 S.E.)* and hypertrophied left ventricles ranged from 0.29 to 0.90 μmoles Pi/mg protein/5 min (mean 0.68 ± 0.08 S.E.). The K_s values ranged from 1.42 to 2.20 × 10^{-3} *M* (mean 2.03 ± 0.25 S.E. × 10^{-3} *M*) in the controls as compared to 2.70 to 9.17 × 10^{-3} *M* (mean 5.36 ± 0.74 S.E. × 10^{-3} *M*) in the hypertrophy group.†

Thus, in the presence of an inert salt environment, there is a significantly decreased ability of myosin B protein from hypertrophied as compared with control left ventricles to split ATP when Ca^{2+} is the activating agent (see Table V). This depressed activity is not found when large concentrations of K^+ are present (see Table IV). The depressed enzyme activity found over all Ca^{2+} concentrations studied suggests two possible alterations in contractile

* (±1 S.E.M.)

† Although V_{max} and K_s values are extrapolated theoretical numbers and are not subject to simple statistical evaluation, the ranges of the binding constants from control and experimental animals is strongly suggestive of two separate populations.

protein from hypertrophied myocardium: (1) lower intrinsic velocity of the enzyme, or (2) altered Ca^{2+} binding. The apparent dissociation constants for calcium-myosin B complex support the latter case.

Discussion

Alterations in protein metabolism occur rapidly after a sustained increase in ventricular intraluminal pressure (Schreiber *et al.*, this volume). Then, following an initial alteration in water metabolism resulting in fluid accumulation, the dry weight mass of the heart increases (Meerson, 1969; Spann *et al.*, 1967). The increase in tissue mass allows the heart to meet the long-term demands for increased work in spite of a tissue unit decrement in functional capacity (Spann *et al.*, 1967). However, it is clear that in an animal model in which stress is chronic, cardiac decompensation will eventually appear. Thus, it would seem that pressure overload is an initial stimulus for a metabolic chain of events that culminates in increased but functionally faulty tissue. The purpose of these experiments was to examine the chemical integrity of the contractile protein complex in hypertrophied myocardium to test the validity of the above scheme.

The course of the changes in myocardial tissue during the onset and development of hypertrophy has not been examined in detail. It may be that the unit myocardial decompensation that underlies congestive heart failure differs only quantitatively from unit changes that accompany chronic hypertrophy. If this is true, the elucidation of the fundamental mechanisms of muscle tissue response to chronic stress is best sought in the course of development of hypertrophy prior to the onset of decompensation. With this in mind, we can state that the experimental animals in this study were free of overt symptoms or signs of congestive cardiac failure. There was no pathological or hemodynamic evidence of decompensation although we are aware of the problems in using end-diastolic pressure as a functional criterion (Braunwald and Ross, 1963).

The significantly larger left ventricular weight/body weight ratios in the experimental as compared to the sham-operated control animals indicates the degree of chronic hypertrophy obtained. Since Meerson's (1969) data demonstrate that edema following overload occurs early and is transient, the heart-weight data observed in this study clearly relate to myocardial constituents other than water. The significantly greater right ventricular weight/body weight ratios in the experimental group as compared to the sham-operated animals is puzzling, in light of the normal right ventricular systolic pressures (< 30 mm Hg).

In view of the divergent reports of changes in ATPase activity following the development of cardiac hypertrophy (Table I), it was essential to use a study design in the evaluation of contractile protein ATPase activity, in which the activating effects of each cation could be examined separately. For this reason, we used TMA^+ to replace K^+. This cation proved to be as inert in its interaction with cardiac muscle as with skeletal muscle proteins (Morales and Hotta, 1967). Under comparable conditions of Ca^{2+} activation, cardiac myosin B has a V_{max} of 0.5 (0.6 *M* TMAC) and 0.7 (0.6 *M* KCl) μmoles Pi/mg protein/5 min, whereas calculations from the data of Morales and Hotta (1967) indicate a V_{max} of 1.8 in TMAC and 1.2 μmoles Pi/mg protein/5 min in KCl for white skeletal muscle myosin B. Myosin B at high ionic strength exhibits enzyme activity resembling that of myosin alone; hence the above data are in agreement with kinetic analyses of cardiac and white skeletal myosin which report the V_{max} of the cardiac enzyme to be 1/3–1/2 that of the skeletal enzyme (Brahms and Kay, 1962, 1963). Apparent binding constants for Ca^{2+} were found to be 2×10^{-3} *M* (in TMAC) and 1×10^{-3} *M* (in KCl) for cardiac myosin B, as compared with values of 2×10^{-4} *M* (in TMAC) and 1×10^{-4} (in KCl) calculated from data of Morales and Hotta (1967) for skeletal muscle. A lower affinity for Ca^{2+} in cardiac muscle compared with skeletal muscle protein is consistent with findings which indicate that higher Ca^{2+} concentrations are needed to achieve maximal cardiac myosin ATPase activity (Mueller *et al.*, 1964), while the extent of activation of cardiac myosin by Ca^{2+} is less than that of white skeletal myosin (Katz *et al.*, 1966). These reports of kinetic parameters which establish a lower V_{max} and Ca^{2+} binding for cardiac myosin than for white skeletal myosin probably reflect structural differences between the two proteins (Locker and Hagyard, 1968).

The data presented here on myosin B from hypertrophied, nonfailing myocardium show an unequivocal decrease in Ca^{2+}-activated ATPase activity at high ionic strengths when measured in the presence of TMA^+. Comparable V_{max} values between experimental and control preparations indicate that decreased Ca^{2+} activation cannot be attributed to a lower myosin content of the experimental myosin B protein complex. At the same time, the apparent affinity constant for Ca^{2+} of myosin B from experimental myocardium is less than that of controls. A possible explanation may be found in a tighter binding of free Ca^{2+} by the actin–troponin receptors in the experimental preparations. As actin and myosin are functionally dissociated at high ionic strength, this activity would effectively reduce the free Ca^{2+} available for direct activation of the myosin enzyme. Fuchs and Briggs (1968) found two classes of Ca^{2+} binding sites for myosin B with apparent affinity constants of 2.1×10^6 M^{-1} (Class I) and approximately 3×10^4 M^{-1} (Class II), respectively. These workers present strong evidence for the location of Class I sites on the actin–troponin complex which would identify them as the physiologic Ca^{2+} receptors. Since the experiments presented in this chapter employed Ca^{2+} concentrations in the range of 0.25–2.5 × 10^{-3} *M*, the Class I receptors would be saturated and therefore ineffective in altering the free Ca^{2+} concentration. The lower-affinity Class II sites were not identified by Fuchs and Briggs, but may be associated with the lower affinity of myosin for Ca^{2+} recorded by Nanninga (1957).

Thus, an alternative explanation for our findings would be an alteration in the myosin molecule which interferes with Ca^{2+} binding and/or hinders enzyme activation by bound Ca^{2+}. This implies that at any given Ca^{2+} concentration, the contractile protein complex exhibits a lower ATPase activity, or to achieve the same activity more Ca^{2+} must be moved to and from the myofibrils. Either phenomenon could serve as a model for the functionally deficient contractile protein that is synthesized during the progressive hypertrophic pathophysiological state leading to decompensation.

In this regard, it is interesting to note that the affinity constants of myosin B for Ca^{2+} in the presence of 0.6 *M* KCl is the same for the experimental and control groups. This might well account for those reports indicating no difference or an increase in ATPase activity following hypertrophy and failure.

Our experiments support previously noted findings that hypertrophied hearts have an enzymological deficiency. There are many similarities in the changes noted above and those enzymological deficiencies found in failing hearts (Table I). In view of this, it would appear that a hypertrophied heart is part of a continuum that leads to failure.

Acknowledgment

This work was supported in part by grant R0 111611.

References

Alpert, N. R., and Draper, M. (1965). *23rd Int. Congr. Physiol. Sci.*

Alpert, N. R., and Gordon, M. S. (1962). *Amer. J. Physiol.* **202,** 940.

Aras, A., and Haas, G. (1962). *Fed. Proc. Fed. Amer. Soc. Exp. Biol.* **21,** 132.

Barany, M. (1967). *J. Gen. Physiol.* **50,** 197.

Barany, M., Conover, T. E., Schliselfeld, L. H., Gaetjens, E., and Goffard, M. (1967). *Eur. J. Biochem.* **2,** 156.

Benson, E. S. (1955). *Circ. Res.* **3,** 221.

Brahms, J., and Kay, C. M. (1962). *J. Mol. Biol.* **5,** 132.

Brahms, J., and Kay, C. M. (1963). *J. Biol. Chem.* **238,** 198.

Brown, A., Aras, A., and Haas, G. (1959). *Fed. Proc. Fed. Amer. Soc. Exp. Biol.* **18** 471.

Braunwald, E., and Ross, J. (1963). *Amer. J. Med.* **34,** 147.

Chandler, B. M., Sonnenblick, E. H., Spann, J. F., and Pool, P. E. (1967). *Circ. Res.* **21,** 717.

Davis, J. O., Trapasso, M., and Yankopoulos, N. (1959). *Circ. Res.* **7,** 957.

Eisenberg, E., and Moos, C. (1967). *J. Biol. Chem.* **242,** 2945.

Fuchs, F , and Briggs, F N. (1968). *J. Gen. Physiol.* **51,** 655.

Gordon, M., and Brown, A. L. (1966). *Circ. Res.* **18,** 534–542.
Grimm, A., Kubota, R., and Whitehorn, W. V. (1963). *Circ. Res.* **12,** 118.
Katz, A. M., Repke, D. I., and Rubin, B. B. (1966). *Circ. Res.* **19,** 611.
Lesch, M., Parmley, W., Hamosh, S., Kaufman, B., and Sonnenblick E. (1968). *Amer. J. Physiol.* **214,** 685.
Locker, R. H., and Hagyard, C. J. (1968) *Arch. Biochem. Biophys.* **127,** 370.
Lowry, O. H., Rosebrough, N. J., Farr, A. L., and Randall, R. J. (1951). *J. Biol. Chem.* **193,** 265.
Luchi, R. J., Kritcher, A. B., and Thyrum, P. T. (1969). *Circ. Res.* **24,** 513.
Maruyama, K., and Watanabe S. (1962). *J. Biol. Chem* **237,** 3437.
Meerson, F. Z. (1969). *Circ. Res.* **24,** Suppl. 2, 82.
Meerson, F. Z., and Pshennikova, M. G. (1965). *Fed. Proc. Fed. Amer. Soc. Exp. Biol.* **24,** T957.
Meerson, F. Z., Beloshapkina, T. D., Lushnikov, E. F., Markovskaya, G. N., and Chernyshova, G. V. (1964). *Fed. Proc. Fed. Amer. Soc. Exp. Biol.* **T,** 667.
Miyahara, M. (1962). *Jap. Circ. J.* **26,** 8.
Morales, M., and Hotta, K. (1967). *J. Biol. Chem.* **235,** 1979.
Mueller, H., Franzen, J., Rice, R. V., and Olson, R. E. (1964). *J. Biol. Chem.* **239,** 1447.
Nanninga, L. B. (1957). *Arch. Biochem. Biophys.* **70,** 346.
Nebel, M. L., and Bing, R. J. (1963). *Arch. Intern. Med.* **111,** 190.
Olson, R. E., Ellenbogen, E., and Iyengar, R. (1961). *Circulation* **24,** 471.
Sommers, J. R., and Spach, M. S. (1964). *Amer. J. Pathol.* **44,** 491.
Spann, J. F., Buccino, R. A., Sonnenblick, E. H., and Braunwald, E. (1967). *Circ. Res.* **21,** 341.
Winer, B. J. (1962). "Statistical Principles in Experimental Designs" (B. J. Winer, ed.), Chapt. 7. McGraw-Hill, New York.

EFFECTS OF ANOXIA ON PROTEIN SYNTHESIS IN HEART MUSCLE

L. S. Jefferson, E. B. Wolpert, K. E. Giger, L. W. Forney, and H. E. Morgan

The regulation of protein synthesis in heart muscle is not well defined. The three steps which are considered to constitute possible control sites in the synthetic pathway are (1) amino acid transport, (2) activation of the amino acid, and (3) translation of the mRNA to form protein. The overall rate of protein synthesis can be assessed by measuring the incorporation of a radioactive amino acid into protein if the specific activity of the precursor pool and the form of the label in the protein are known. The importance of membrane transport in protein synthesis can be evaluated through the measurement of the intracellular levels of free amino acid. Since it is possible that any one of the 20 amino acids could be rate-limiting for the overall synthetic rate, the assessment of the role of membrane transport is difficult. In the present study we have attempted to define the site of the anaerobic inhibition of synthesis of whole heart protein and, in some experiments, of myosin. Myosin was selected because it is present in large amounts in the heart and is characteristic of the muscle cell.

Experimental Procedures

For the investigation of protein synthesis isolated rat hearts were perfused, as previously described (Neely *et al.*, 1967), by a modified Langendorff technique using Krebs-Henseleit bicarbonate buffer containing glucose and various amino acid concentrations. At the end of the perfusion, hearts were cut from the cannula into a beaker of cold saline, rinsed, blotted, and frozen with Wollenberger tongs cooled in liquid nitrogen. When nucleotide levels were to be measured, hearts were frozen while still being perfused.

Frozen heart samples were powdered in a percussion mortar at the temperature of liquid nitrogen, a portion of this powder being used to quantitate the incorporation of radioactive amino acid into protein after the sample was freed of amino acids, RNA and lipid (Munro *et al.*, 1964). Powdered tissue samples from pooled hearts were treated with picric acid to extract the free amino acids from the tissue as described by Tallan *et al.* (1954). Amino acids were quantitated using a Beckman amino acid analyzer. A portion of the effluent from the column of the analyzer was collected and used in determining the specific activity of the radioactive amino acid that was used as label in the perfusion experiments. Under all of the conditions tested, more than 95% of the radioactivity in the picric acid extract could be recovered in the phenylalanine peak. Myosin was prepared from powdered heart samples by the procedure of Perry (1955) as modified by Weeds and Hartley (1968).

Results

Selection of the amino acid to be used for estimating the rate of synthesis was based on the following considerations: (1) lack of production or degradation of the amino acid by the heart, (2) rapid equilibration of the free amino acid pool in the tissue with the amino acid in the perfusate, and (3) stable distribution of the amino acid under various perfusion conditions. Phenylalanine was found to meet these requirements. A stable distribution of phenylalanine was found over perfusion periods from 15 min to 3 hr. In addition, phenylalanine rapidly equilibrated across the cell membrane, so that the ratio of the specific activities of heart and perfusate phenylalanine was ~ 1 over perfusion periods from 30 min to 3 hr. The volume of distribution of phenylalanine was reduced when other amino acids were added, presumably a result of competition for entry into the cell.

Earlier studies of Manchester and Young (1959) demonstrated that incorporation of amino acid into protein was inhibited when diaphragms were incubated under anaerobic conditions. As shown in Table I, incorporation of ^{14}C-phenylalanine into heart protein was inhibited $\sim 60\%$ when the buffer was gassed with $N_2:CO_2$, rather than $O_2:CO_2$. This inhibition was observed when only phenylalanine, all amino acids at normal plasma levels* or $5\times$ normal plasma amino acid levels were added to the perfusate. This effect was not produced by a lower specific activity of heart phenylalanine in the anaerobic muscle, since no significant difference in the specific activity of

* The mixture of amino acids that was used was based on our analyses of the amino acid composition of serum from normal rats that were fasted overnight. The normal plasma levels were as follows for each amino acid (concentration, 10^2 mM): Alanine, 40; arginine, 8; aspartic acid, 5; asparagine, 7; cysteine, 10; glutamic acid, 12; glutamine, 35; glycine, 30; histidine, 10; isoleucine, 10; leucine, 15; lysine, 35; methionine, 5; phenylalanine, 8; proline, 20; serine, 20; threonine, 25; trypotophan, 10; tyrosine, 8; valine, 20.

TABLE I

EFFECT OF ANOXIA ON INCORPORATION OF PHENYLALANINE INTO HEART PROTEIN[a]

Amino acid mixture	Gas phase	^{14}C-Phenylalanine incorporation: μmoles/gm protein	^{14}C-Phenylalanine incorporation: μmoles/gm myosin
Only ^{14}C-Phe, 0.08 mM	O_2: CO_2	0.44 ± 0.05	—
	N_2: CO_2	0.19 ± 0.02[b]	—
All amino acids at normal plasma levels including ^{14}C-Phe, 0.08 mM	O_2: CO_2	0.55 ± 0.05	—
	N_2: CO_2	0.24 ± 0.03[b]	—
All amino acids at 5× normal plasma levels including ^{14}C-Phe, 0.4 mM	O_2: CO_2	0.62 ± 0.03	0.27 ± 0.01
	N_2: CO_2	0.28 ± 0.02[b]	0.12 ± 0.01[b]
+ Cycloheximide $2 \times 10^{-5} M$	O_2: CO_2	0.07 ± 0.01	—
	N_2: CO_2	0.05 ± 0.01	—
+ Tetrodotoxin 9 μg/ml	O_2: CO_2	0.63 ± 0.04	—
	N_2: CO_2	0.35 ± 0.02[b]	—

[a] Hearts were removed from rats that were fasted overnight, heparinized, and anesthetized with Nembutal. A preliminary perfusion by the Langendorff technique was begun using Krebs-Henseleit bicarbonate buffer gassed with O_2: CO_2 and containing glucose (15 mM), ^{12}C-phenylalanine, and the other amino acids at the concentrations employed during the subsequent period of recirculation. The buffer passed through the heart a single time and was discarded. Before recirculation of buffer containing ^{14}C-phenylalanine (^{14}C-Phe) was begun, 10 ml of the buffer was perfused through the heart and discarded. When only phenylalanine and normal concentrations of all amino acids were employed, 125 ml of buffer were recirculated; 25 ml of buffer were recirculated in experiments involving 5× normal plasma levels of amino acid. Recirculation of buffer was continued for 30 min in each case. The buffer was equilibrated with the gas mixture listed in the table. The number of μmoles of phenylalanine incorporated into whole heart protein or myosin was calculated by the following formula.

$$\text{Incorporation, } \mu\text{moles/gm protein} = \frac{\text{Incorporation, cpm/gm}}{\text{Average specific activity of heart phenylalanine, cpm}/\mu\text{mole}}$$

The means ± S.E.M. are presented. At least six hearts were perfused under each condition.

[b] $p < 0.01$ vs. aerobic control.

heart phenylalanine was observed under any of the conditions studied. The anaerobic effect was associated with a reduced rate of myosin synthesis. The extent of inhibition was similar to that observed with whole heart protein indicating that the anaerobic inhibition was a property of the muscle cells. Addition of cycloheximide to either aerobic or anaerobic hearts resulted in ~90% inhibition of protein synthesis suggesting that protein synthesis was predominantly cytoplasmic rather than mitochondrial under both conditions. Cycloheximide had no effect on the mechanical performance of the heart.

When hearts are perfused under anaerobic conditions, beating ceases after ~5 min. However, it was possible to demonstrate that cessation of beating did not account for the inhibition of protein synthesis. When tetrodotoxin was added to the perfusate to completely stop contractions in aerobic hearts, no reduction in phenylalanine incorporation was observed, nor did tetrodotoxin modify the incorporation rate in anaerobic muscle.

The anaerobic inhibition of phenylalanine incorporation could be reversed by returning the heart to an aerobic environment. In a time course study, the incorporation of phenylalanine was observed to be constant over 1 hr of perfusion in aerobic hearts. Under anaerobic conditions, the degree of inhibition increased from 40% during the first 30 min to 76% during the second 30 min of perfusion. When the gas bubbled through, the perfusate was changed from $N_2:CO_2$ to $O_2:CO_2$ during the second 30 min of perfusion, beating was restored after ~10 min, and the rate of phenylalanine incorporation increased nearly threefold. This rate of protein synthesis was ~70% of that observed in hearts that had been perfused under aerobic conditions from the outset.

The anaerobic inhibition of protein synthesis could be demonstrated with amino acids other than phenylalanine. The incorporation of ^{14}C-lysine, ^{14}C-glycine or ^{14}C-aspartic acid into whole heart protein was inhibited by 55%, 63%, and 70%, respectively, within 15 min of perfusion under anaerobic conditions.

The anaerobic inhibition of protein synthesis could be attributed to either an inhibition of the entry of amino acid into the cell, resulting in low intracellular free amino acid levels, or to an inhibition of activation or translation. As shown in Table II, the intracellular levels of five amino acids rose in anaerobic hearts, two fell, and the remainder were unchanged. The increase in intracellular levels of valine, leucine, and isoleucine probably resulted from an inhibition of the oxidation of these compounds since a net uptake of these three amino acids could be observed in aerobic heart. The rise in alanine levels was coupled with the faster production of pyruvate. Although aspartic acid and glutamic acid levels fell, they were still among the highest in intracellular concentration and this fall appeared unlikely to explain the anaerobic inhibition of protein synthesis.

The role of amino acid transport in the anaerobic inhibition of protein synthesis was explored further by measuring the rate of entry of ^{14}C-amino acids into the cell. As can be seen in Table III, transport of phenylalanine and isoleucine, substrates for the L-transport system, was unaffected by perfusion under anaerobic conditions. These results would indicate that the increase in heart isoleucine concentration that was noted in anaerobic muscle resulted

TABLE II

EFFECT OF ANOXIA ON INTRACELLULAR CONCENTRATIONS OF AMINO ACIDS IN THE PERFUSED RAT HEART[a]

Amino acid	Initial perfusate concentration (10^2 mM)	Final intracellular concentration, 10^2 mM	
		Aerobic	Anaerobic
Asparagine	35	47 ± 4	117 ± 7[b]
Alanine	200	354 ± 50	812 ± 73[b]
Valine	100	28 ± 4	71 ± 4[b]
Isoleucine	50	20 ± 1	47 ± 4[b]
Leucine	75	31 ± 4	74 ± 5[b]
Aspartic acid	25	475 ± 127	253 ± 38
Glutamic acid	60	981 ± 54	610 ± 42[b]
Serine	100	68 ± 12	93 ± 6
Threonine	125	99 ± 14	109 ± 12
Glutamine	175	1885 ± 93	1652 ± 132
Glycine	150	166 ± 19	171 ± 7
Methionine	25	24 ± 1	31 ± 3
Tyrosine	40	35 ± 4	34 ± 3
Phenylalanine	40	32 ± 7	32 ± 3
Lysine	175	186 ± 40	202 ± 32
Histidine	50	40 ± 1	34 ± 5
Arginine	40	56 ± 15	37 ± 9
Proline	100	—	—
Cysteine	50	—	—
Tryptophan	50	—	—

[a] Hearts were perfused with buffer containing 5× normal plasma levels of amino acid for 30 min under aerobic and anaerobic conditions as described in the footnote to Table I. The means ± S.E.M. are presented. Three pools of six hearts were analyzed.

[b] $p < 0.01$ vs. aerobic control.

from a change in the utilization of isoleucine rather than its entry into the cell. Entry of glycine and α-aminoisobutyric acid, substrates for the A-transport system, was stimulated in anaerobic hearts. As noted earlier, the intracellular level of glycine was not higher in anaerobic muscle. The entry of lysine was stimulated and the entry of aspartic acid unaffected by anoxia, although the intracellular level of aspartic acid was reduced almost 50% under anaerobic conditions. Taken together, these results suggested that amino acid transport was not the site of the anaerobic inhibition of protein synthesis, and that some intracellular step such as amino acid activation or translation was responsible for the reduced rate of synthesis.

If the anaerobic effect on protein synthesis were on the translation step,

TABLE III

EFFECT OF ANOXIA ON THE TRANSPORT OF SEVERAL AMINO ACIDS[a]

^{14}C-Amino acid	Period of perfusion (min)	Gas phase	Distribution ratio
Phenylalanine (0.08 m*M*)	2	$O_2: CO_2$	0.98 ± 0.06
		$N_2: CO_2$	1.11 ± 0.13
Isoleucine (0.1 m*M*)	3	$O_2: CO_2$	0.85 ± 0.04
		$N_2: CO_2$	0.86 ± 0.06
Glycine (0.3 m*M*)	60	$O_2: CO_2$	1.66 ± 0.11
		$N_2: CO_2$	2.48 ± 0.08[b]
α-Aminoisobutyric acid	60	$O_2: CO_2$	0.83 ± 0.06
(0.05 m*M*)		$N_2: CO_2$	1.57 ± 0.25[b]
Lysine (0.35 m*M*)	15	$O_2: CO_2$	2.52 ± 0.19
		$N_2: CO_2$	3.21 ± 0.16[b]
Aspartic acid (0.05 m*M*)	60	$O_2: CO_2$	1.54 ± 0.20
		$N_2: CO_2$	1.64 ± 0.20

[a] Hearts were removed from rats that had been fasted overnight, heparinized, and anaesthetized with Nembutal. A preliminary perfusion by the Langendorff technique was begun using Krebs-Henseleit bicarbonate buffer containing glucose (15 m*M*). In the phenylalanine experiments, preliminary perfusion took 10 min with buffer equilibrated with $O_2: CO_2$ and an additional 15 min with buffer equilibrated with either $O_2: CO_2$ or $N_2: CO_2$ preceding the period of amino acid accumulation. In experiments with all of the other amino acids that were studied, the buffer used for preliminary perfusion (10 min) was gassed with the same mixture utilized during the period of amino acid accumulation. The buffer used for preliminary perfusion passed through the heart a single time and was discarded. In all experiments in which the period of amino acid accumulation was 10 min or less, the buffer containing the ^{14}C-amino acid passed through the heart a single time and was discarded. In experiments in which the period of amino acid accumulation was more than 10 min, 10 ml of radioactive buffer was perfused through the heart, followed by recirculation of 40 ml of buffer containing ^{14}C-amino acid and glucose.

At the end of perfusion, hearts were frozen and powdered as described in the text and the powder homogenized with 2 ml of 1 *N* perchloric acid to extract the ^{14}C-amino acid. After centrifugation, the radioactivity in an aliquot of the supernatant was determined. An aliquot of the perfusate was also analyzed for radioactivity. The distribution ratio of ^{14}C-amino acid between the intracellular and extracellular fluid was calculated by the following formula.

$$\text{Distribution ratio} = \frac{^{14}\text{C-amino acid space, ml/gm—sorbitol space, ml/gm}}{\text{total water, ml/gm—sorbitol space, ml/gm}}$$

The means ± S.E.M. are presented. At least six hearts were perfused in each group.

[b] $p < 0.01$ vs. aerobic control.

this might be reflected in a decrease in the number of large ribosomal aggregates and a concomitant increase in the number of small ribosomal aggregates, particularly monomeric ribosomes. Sucrose density-gradient analysis of the postmitochondrial supernatant from nonperfused, perfused aerobic, and perfused anaerobic hearts produced ribosomal profiles similar to those shown in Fig. 1. It can be seen that when hearts were perfused under aerobic or

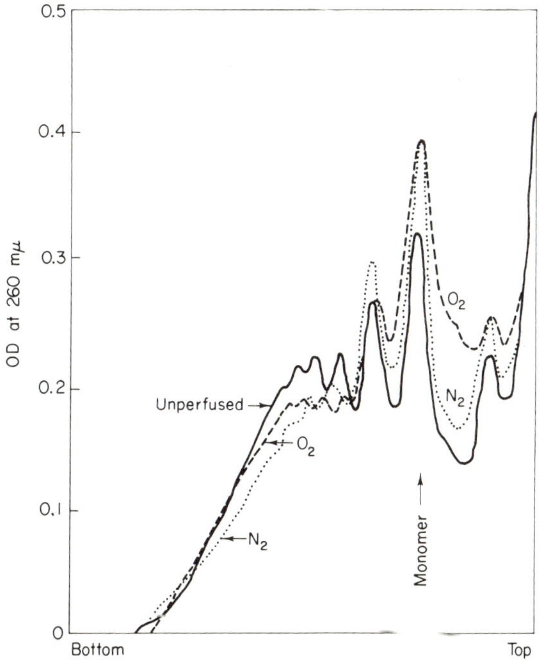

FIG. 1. Effect of anoxia on aggregation of heart ribosomes. Hearts were perfused with buffer containing glucose (15 mM) and 5 × normal plasma levels of amino acids for 1 hr under aerobic and anaerobic conditions as described in the footnote to Table I. At the end of perfusion, hearts were homogenized in 3 volumes of a solution containing 0.25 M KCl, 0.01 M tris, pH 7.4, and 10 mM $MgCl_2$. A Dounce homogenizer fitted with a lucite ball was used. Homogenates were spun for 10 min at 10,000 × G in a refrigerated centrifuge. Triton-X-100 was added to the supernatant to give a concentration of 0.3%. The supernatant was layered on to exponential gradients of 15% to 2 M sucrose prepared by the method of Noll (1967, 1969). The gradients were centrifuged at 40,000 rpm for 3¼ hr in a SW 40 rotor of a Spinco ultracentrifuge. Unperfused hearts were treated in the same manner. Sedimentation of ribosomes was monitored by pumping the gradients through the flow-cell of a Gilford Spectrophotometer. Patterns of aggregation seen in unperfused hearts are indicated by the solid line. Patterns of aerobic hearts are indicated by a broken line and anaerobic hearts by a dotted line. At least six experiments were carried out for each condition and the distribution of ribosomes on the gradients in all experiments was similar to that shown above.

anaerobic conditions, the percentage of small aggregates increased somewhat, but the pattern was similar in homogenates from aerobic or anaerobic muscle with the exception of a peak appearing near the top of the gradient. This peak sedimented at approximately the rate of a 60 S particle and may represent the larger ribosomal subunit. It appeared to be increased significantly in aerobic heart. These results indicated that ribosomal aggregation was similar in homogenates prepared from aerobic or anaerobic muscle.

Oxidative metabolism is necessary to maintain tissue levels of high-energy phosphate compounds. Tissue levels of ATP, GTP, and creatine phosphate are shown in Table IV. The levels of ATP, GTP, and creatine phosphate were

TABLE IV

EFFECT OF ANOXIA ON TISSUE LEVELS OF NUCLEOTIDES IN THE PERFUSED RAT HEART[a]

	Heart content (μmoles/gm)		
Nucleotide	Initial	Aerobic	Anaerobic
ATP	20.6 ± 0.8	20.3 ± 1	11.6 ± 3[b]
GTP	1.53 ± 0.14	1.46 ± 0.04	0.78 ± 0.06[b]
Creatine-P	29.5 ± 2.2	23.5 ± 1.8	6.7 ± 0.6[b]

[a] Perchloric acid extracts of hearts perfused with buffer containing 5× normal plasma levels of amino acid and glucose (15 m*M*) were prepared from 10 gm of heart powder and the nucleotides estimated as described earlier (Wood and Morgan, 1969). Initial heart contents were determined after 10 min of perfusion with buffer gassed with O_2: CO_2; this buffer was not recirculated. Aerobic and anaerobic contents were estimated after 30 min of additional perfusion with buffer gassed with either O_2: CO_2 or N_2: CO_2. The means ± S.E.M. are presented. Three pools of six hearts were analyzed in each group.

[b] $p < 0.01$ vs. aerobic control.

substantially reduced in the anaerobic muscle. These reductions were accompanied by increased levels of AMP and GMP. Reduced levels of these high-energy phosphates may inhibit protein synthesis either by interfering with amino acid activation or by slowing the rate of translation.

Discussion

Protein synthesis in heart muscle is regulated by a number of factors, both hormonal and nonhormonal. Availability of amino acids as substrates for protein synthesis limits the aerobic rate when normal plasma levels of amino acids are present. As shown in Table I, this restriction is small during the first 30 min of perfusion. Where perfusion was continued for 3 hr, the rate of synthesis was increased ~30% when 5× normal plasma levels of amino acid were employed. In preliminary experiments, amino acid levels have been found to affect aggregation of heart ribosomes. When only phenylalanine or normal plasma levels of amino acids were present, large aggregates were lost during 1 hr of perfusion and increased numbers of monomeric and dimeric ribosomes appeared. Perfusion with 5× normal plasma levels of all amino acids prevented polysome disaggregation. Similar effects of amino acid levels on ribosomal aggregation have been found in the perfused rat liver (Jefferson and Korner, 1969).

Decreased intracellular levels of free amino acids did not appear to account for the anaerobic inhibition of protein synthesis. As shown in Table I, inhibition was seen when high levels of amino acid were added to the perfusate; as demonstrated in Table II, inhibition of protein synthesis was accompanied by either an increase or no change in the intracellular level of most amino acids. The entry of amino acid into the cell was either stimulated or unaffected in anerobic muscle.

The anaerobic inhibition of protein synthesis was associated with reduced levels of high energy phosphates, ATP, GTP, and creatine-P. A fall in these levels could result in an inhibition of either amino acid activation or of ribosomal activity. Levels of activated amino acids have not been measured, but the levels of ATP, AMP, and pyrophosphate that occur in heart would suggest that more than 90% of sRNA would be in the aminoacyl form. As shown in Table IV, the ATP concentration in aerobic muscle was about 8 m*M* and fell to 5 m*M* under anaerobic conditions. AMP levels increased from 0.2 m*M* to 0.8 m*M* with this transition. In other experiments, levels of inorganic pyrophosphate have been measured in aerobic and anaerobic hearts. In both experimental situations, the intracellular concentration was estimated to be 0.05 m*M*. The high levels of ATP and low levels of AMP and pyrophosphate would favor aminoacyl sRNA formation under both aerobic and anaerobic conditions.

Ribosomal aggregation was similar under aerobic and anaerobic conditions. Since the extent of aggregation is a balance of the rates of chain initiation and mRNA reading, initiation of chains on the ribosomes must have occurred at a rate sufficient to maintain the number of larger aggregates. Recently, Friedman *et al.* (1969) have reported a preferential inhibition of chain initiation in *E. coli* during incubation at 4°C. Under these circumstances, large numbers of ribosomal subunits were found indicating an inhibition of chain initiation that was proportionally greater than translation of mRNA. These considerations would suggest that translation of mRNA may be the site of the anaerobic inhibition of protein synthesis in heart muscle.

Summary

The synthesis of either whole heart protein or myosin was inhibited in anaerobic muscle. The degree of inhibition, ~60%, was similar in each case. In association with this inhibition, intracellular levels of five amino acids rose, two fell, and the remainder were unchanged. These changes appeared to result principally from changes in the metabolism of these compounds since the rate of amino acid transport was either unchanged or increased. Polyribosome aggregation was unaffected in anaerobic muscle and the anaerobic effect appeared to be caused by decreased levels of either ATP or GTP, or both, which are required for either amino activation or for translation.

Acknowledgments

Supported by Grants from the National Institutes of Health (HE-11534-03), American Heart Association, and Life Insurance Medical Research Fund.

References

Friedman, H., Lu, P., and Rich, A. (1969). *Nature (London)*, **233,** 909.
Jefferson, L. S., and Korner, A. (1969). *Biochem. J.* **111,** 703.
Manchester, K. L., and Young, F. G. (1959). *J. Endocrinol.* **18,** 381.
Munro, A. J., Jackson, R. J., and Korner, A. (1964). *Biochem. J.* **92,** 289.
Neely, J. R., Liebermeister, H., Battersby, E. J., and Morgan, H. E. (1967). *Amer. J. Physiol.* **212,** 804.
Noll, H. (1967). *Nature (London)*, **215,** 360.
Noll, H. (1969). *Anal. Biochem.* **27,** 130.
Perry S. V. (1955). *Methods Enzymol.* **2,** 583.
Tallan, H. H., Moore, S., and Stein, W. H. (1954). *J. Biol. Chem.* **211,** 927.
Weeds, A. G., and Hartley, B. S. (1968). *Biochem. J.* **107,** 531.
Wood, R. E., and Morgan, H. E. (1969). *J. Biol. Chem.* **244,** 1951.

ALTERATIONS AMONG MYOSINS FROM DIFFERENT TYPES OF MUSCLE

John Gergely

That myosin from hypertrophied or failing heart may differ in its chemical structure from the normal protein, has been suggested elsewhere in this volume and by Chandler *et al.*, 1967; I should like to discuss briefly some observations made in our laboratory (Nakamura *et al.*, 1969) that may have a bearing on detecting differences among myosins from different types of muscles.

Proteolytic enzymes split myosin into two fragments, a highly α-helical rod—light meromyosin (LMM), and a globular portion—heavy meromyosin (HMM)—that retains the enzymatic activity of myosin and its ability to combine with actin (for a recent summary, see Lowey *et al.*, 1969). LMM is insoluble at low ionic strength and forms aggregates that usually revealed a 430-A periodicity (Philpott and Szent-Györgyi, 1954; Huxley, 1963) when examined with the electron microscope.

In our studies we compared the LMM aggregates, or paracrystals, prepared from white and red skeletal muscle myosin and from cardiac muscle myosin. Aggregates of white muscle LMM stained with uranyl acetate show the typical 430-A period with a subperiod consisting of a 100-A lightly stained band, and a 330-A period with a subperiod consisting of a 100-A lightly stained band and a 330-A heavily stained band. In contrast, LMM paracrystals from cardiac or red skeletal muscle myosin, although revealing the same 430-A main period, show a completely different band pattern; there is a wider, 250–280 A, lightly stained band and a narrower, 150–180 A, dark band. Within the lightly stained band, two pairs of 25–30 A wide dark lines are seen. It should be added that white muscle LMM paracrystals often show a repeat of ~145-A, which has been described by Lowey *et al.* (1967) for the helical portion (subfragment 2) of heavy meromyosin; we never found this pattern in cardiac and red muscle LMM aggregates (Fig. 1).

These results indicate that differences between cardiac and red muscle myosin and its white muscle counterpart are not restricted to the heavy

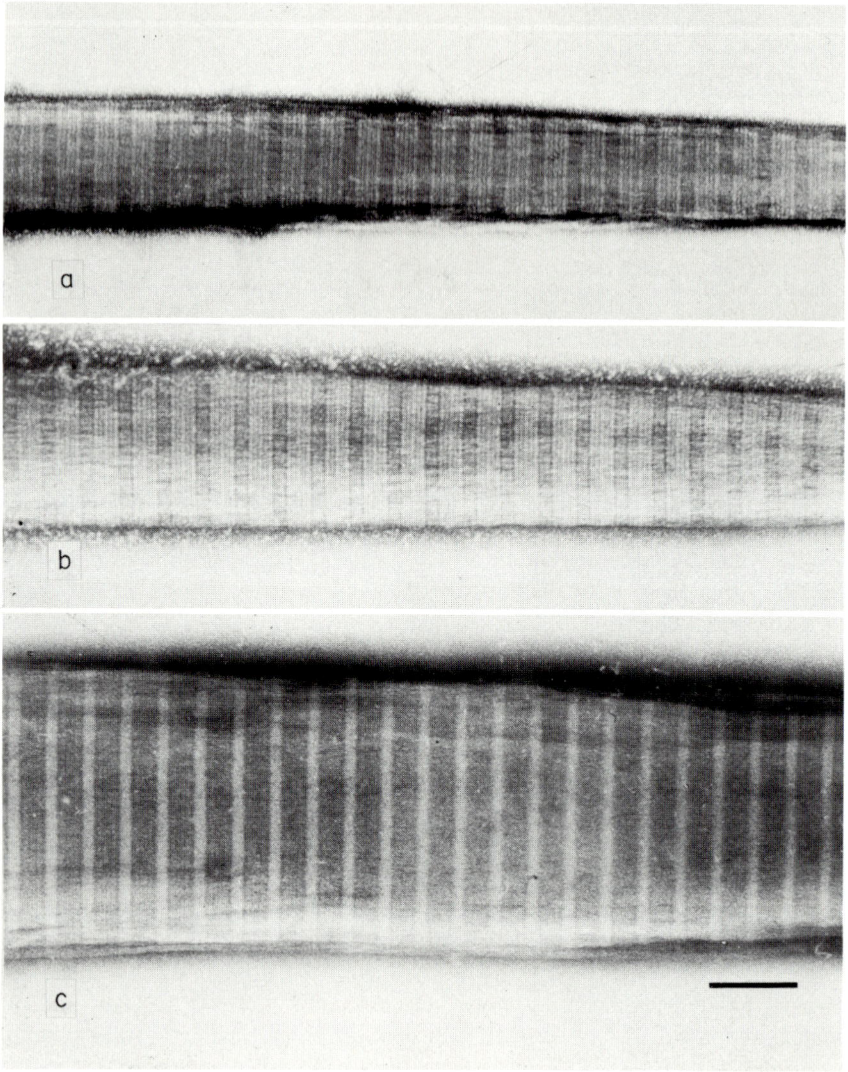

FIG. 1. Comparison of band patterns of tryptic light meromyosin paracrystals: (a) Cardiac muscle; (b) red muscle; (c) white muscle. Negative staining with 1% uranyl acetate. The bar indicates 1000 A.

meromyosin portion, reflected in differences in ATPase activity and stability at pH 9 (Sreter *et al.*, 1966; Seidel, 1967), but extend into the helical portion of the molecule.

This approach to examining the molecular, "fingerprinting" of cardiac myosin revealed by electron microscopy of negatively stained LMM aggregates may be useful in the study of changes in myosin.

References

Chandler, B. M., Sonnenblick, E. H., Spann, J. J. and Pool, P. (1967). *Circ. Res.* **21,** 717.
Huxley, H. E. (1963). *J. Mol. Biol.* **7,** 281.
Lowey, S., Goldstein, L., Cohen, C., and Luck, S. (1967). *J. Mol. Biol.* **23,** 287.
Lowey, S., Slayter, H. S., Weeds, A. G., and Baker, H. (1969). *J. Mol. Biol.*, **42,** 1.
Nakamura, A., Sreter ,F. A., and Gergely, J. (1969). *Abstract, Biophys. Soc.*, A-11 and *J. Cell. Biol.* (in press).
Philpott, D. E., and Szent-Györgyi, A. G. (1954). *Biochim. Biophys. Acta* **15,** 165.
Seidel, J. C. (*J. Biol. Chem.* **242,** 5623.
Sreter, F. A., Seidel, J. C., and Gergely, J. (1966). *J. Biol. Chem.* **241,** 5772.

Part V
The Mechanical Characteristics of Hypertrophied Heart Muscle

The studies presented here extend from analyses of the mechanical performance of isolated hypertrophied ventricular muscle strips to evaluation of left ventricle performance in conscious humans with hypertrophied hearts. The intent of these investigations was to provide a better understanding of myocardial mechanics as affected by ventricular hypertrophy.

Although it has been repeatedly suggested in the past that at some stage hypertrophy of the heart may actually be beneficial and enhance cardiac performance, a survey of the studies presented here do not lend support to this view. A thorough and conclusive evaluation of the mechanical characteristics and the performance of hypertrophied hearts as contrasted to normal hearts can not be made at this time. More studies are needed. Furthermore, the role of changes in wall tensile stress as the stimulus for the development of hypertrophy, though attractive, has not been proven.

Edward W. Hawthorne

MECHANICAL PROPERTIES OF RAT CARDIAC MUSCLE DURING EXPERIMENTAL HYPERTROPHY

Oscar H. L. Bing, Satoru Matsushita, Barry L. Fanburg, and Herbert J. Levine

Introduction

Although the overall performance of the hypertrophied heart may be improved, studies comparing the mechanical properties of hypertrophied cardiac muscle per unit mass have yielded conflicting results. Kerr *et al.* (1961) found the maximum tension developed per unit weight of hypertrophied rat left ventricle to be increased. On the other hand, Grimm and associates (1963) found no change in peak isometric force of hypertrophied rat papillary muscle when hypertrophy was induced by either exercise or aortic constriction. More recently, having analyzed force–velocity curves from the papillary muscle of the hypertrophied cat right ventricle, Spann and co-workers (1967) have reported a reduction in contractility with no significant change in peak isometric force. In an effort to resolve some of these apparent discrepancies, we have performed a detailed analysis of the mechanical properties of the trabecular muscle of the hypertrophied rat left ventricle.

Materials and Methods

In these studies, 77 inbred Charles River CD® rats were subjected to constriction of the aortic arch as described previously (Fanburg and Posner, 1968) with 77 animals serving as unoperated or sham-operated controls. Animals were sacrificed at 1, 3, 7, 14, and 28 days after operation. The chest was opened, and the heart removed rapidly and placed in an oxygenated Krebs-Henseleit solution (Krebs and Henseleit, 1932). The columnar carneal muscle of the left ventricle was dissected free and mounted in an isolated muscle chamber equipped with tension and displacement transducers for force and velocity measurements. The remainder of the heart was blotted, weighed, and frozen for later analyses of dry weight, hydroxyproline content, and lactic dehydrogenase (LDH) isoenzymes. Muscles placed in the chambers were stimulated 12×/min at 28°C by parallel platinum electrodes delivering 7-msec square-wave pulses at voltages just above threshold. After a 1-hr period of equilibration, an isotonic force–velocity curve was obtained for each muscle that had been carefully stretched to the apex of its length-active tension curve. All values were normalized for muscle length and cross-sectional area. When muscles were stretched to the peak of their active tension curves, resting tension represented about twenty percent of total tension. At this load, contractile element velocity is relatively distant from true V_{max} or the extrapolated y axis intercept of a curve connecting measured force–velocity points. To obtain an additional point nearer the velocity axis, a velocity measurement was made using the lightest possible preload, which represented a load of less than 5% of total tension for a muscle of average cross-sectional area. Whereas the muscle length is somewhat shorter at this lighter preload than at peak-active tension, contractile element velocity approaches V_{max}, which is itself independent of muscle length. Since an error in determining the true V_{max} might have been introduced by using this point to extrapolate to the y axis, extrapolation was not performed, and the measured velocity will be referred to herein as V_{max}.

Each experiment was carried out with four muscles contracting simultaneously in four separate chambers, with common temperature regulation and oxygenation. The experiment was designed so that each set of four muscles included those from an unoperated animal, a sham-operated animal, and two animals with aortic constriction. Cases in which there was no significant difference between sham-operated and unoperated animals are either referred to interchangeably as controls, or are combined to increase the sample size.

Results and Discussion

Heart weights and left ventricle-to-body weight ratios of animals with aortic constriction increased significantly above controls by seven days following operation and remained relatively constant thereafter to 28 days (Fig. 1). The cross-sectional area of the trabecular muscles showed similar changes during the experimental period.

Although left ventricular end diastolic pressures were not measured in these experiments, the lungs and livers did not appear to be congested. The water content of hearts and lungs from animals with aortic constriction was not significantly different from that of controls. Trabecular muscles were too small for the determination of water content, but the constancy of the protein

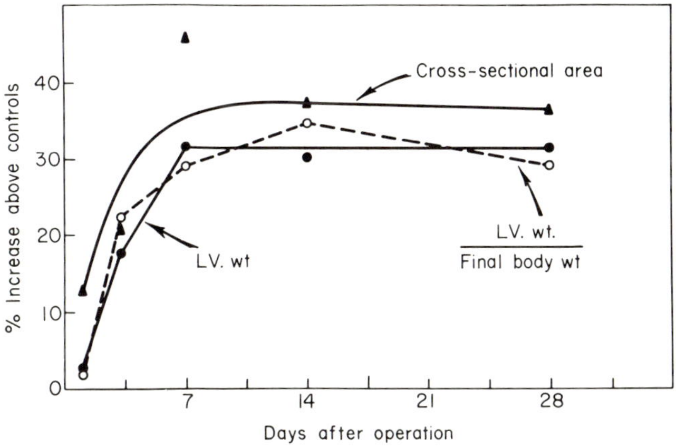

FIG. 1. The effects of aortic constriction on left ventricular weight, left ventricular–body weight ratio, and trabecular muscle cross-sectional area.

content indicated that no water retention had taken place in these muscles. These findings indicated that the group of animals with aortic constriction was primarily one with hypertrophy in the absence of congestive heart failure.

The average force–velocity curve of animals with aortic constriction did not differ from that of controls at 1 and 3 days after operation. However, at 7 days after operation, downward displacement of the entire curve was evident (Fig. 2). No further changes were seen in the force–velocity curves at 2 and 4 weeks after operation. Since some of the mechanical changes subsequent to aortic constriction might be the result of an increased cross-sectional area of the hypertrophied trabecular muscle, the mechanical parameters were plotted against cross-sectional area. A highly significant correlation was found for muscles from both hypertrophied and control hearts when developed tension was plotted against cross-sectional area (Fig. 3, bottom). On the other hand, no significant correlation was found between V_{max} and cross-sectional area, except when the two groups of animals were combined (Fig. 3, top).

To definitively separate the effects of muscle thickness from the mechanical alterations of the hypertrophied muscle, a group of 19 muscles from hypertrophied hearts was compared with 14 muscles with the same cross-sectional area from control hearts. The force–velocity curves for these muscles are shown in Fig. 4. Although the V_{max} of muscles from hypertrophied hearts was depressed when compared with controls, there was no significant difference between the two groups in peak isometric tension. The V_{max} for these muscles

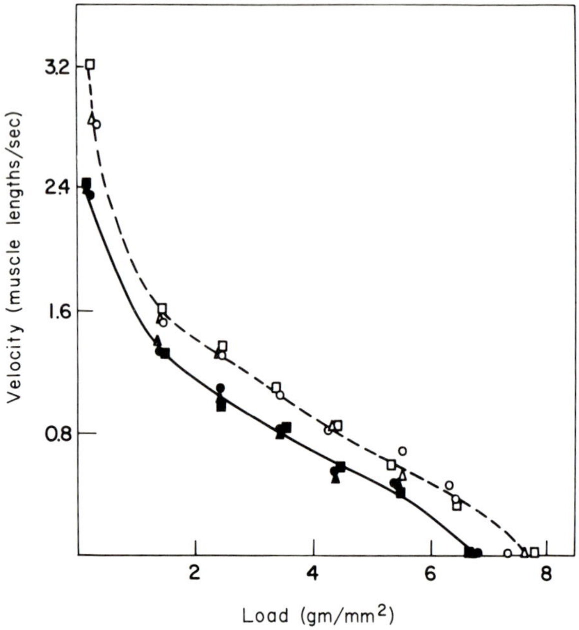

FIG. 2. The effect of hypertrophy on the force–velocity relationship of trabecular muscles obtained from all animals studied. Each point is an average of 7–28 trabecular muscles. The curves were obtained from a total of 54 muscles of animals with cardiac hypertrophy (●, ▲, ■—1, 2, 4 weeks, respectively), and 53 muscles of unoperated and sham-operated animals (○, △, □—1, 2, 4 weeks, respectively).

with the same cross-sectional area showed a high inverse correlation with the extent of hypertrophy as reflected by the left ventricular-to-body weight ratio (Fig. 5). Thus, changes in developed tension noted in the total group of hypertrophied muscles could be explained by changes in muscle cross-sectional area, whereas the decrease in V_{max} appeared to be related to some other property of the hypertrophied muscle.

The comparison of muscles with similar cross-sectional areas from hypertrophied and control hearts is summarized in Fig. 6. Whereas V_{max} fell 24%, developed tension remained unchanged. The maintenance of an unchanged developed tension may be explained, at least in part, by a prolonged contraction time. It is of interest that these findings are very similar to those described by Alpert *et al.* (1967) for rat heart muscle during aging.

Since a chronic increase in work load or an increase in muscle mass might produce a relative hypoxia of the muscle cell, which might, in turn, contribute

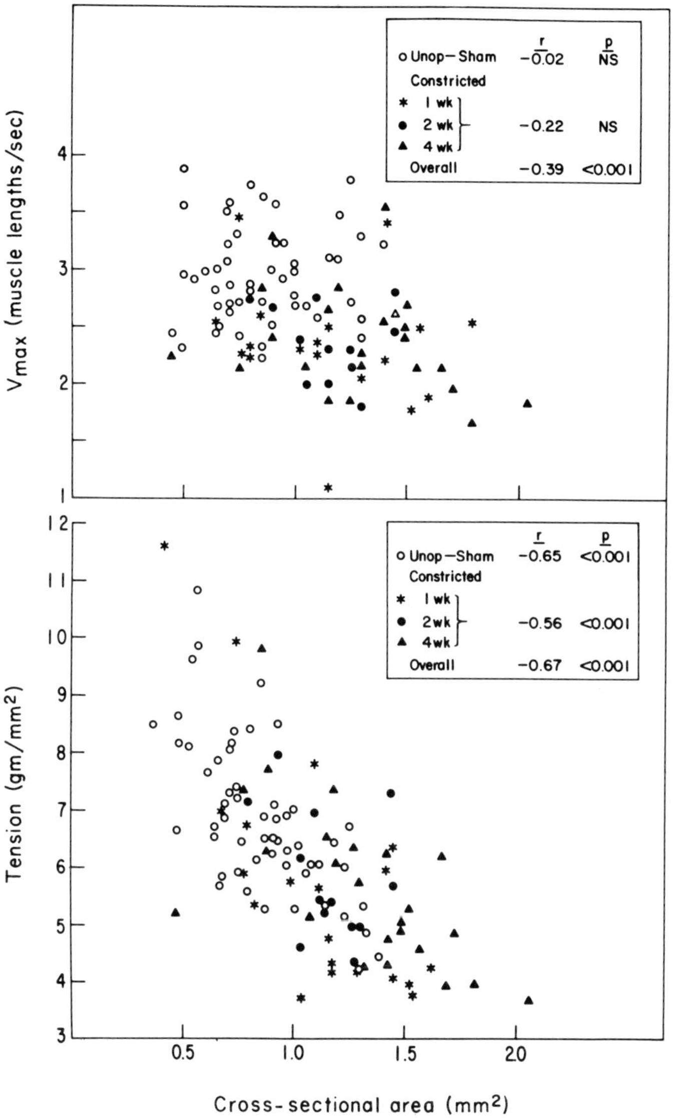

FIG. 3. Correlation of muscle cross-sectional area with V_{max} (upper) and tension development (lower). Each point represents a determination from a single muscle.

to a decrease in contractility, we were interested to learn if there was any evidence for hypoxia as reflected by increased anaerobic activity of the hyper-

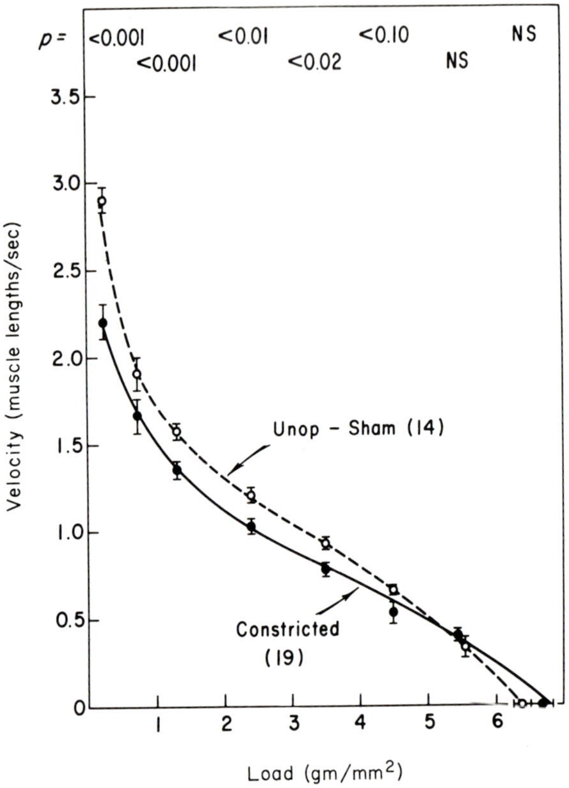

FIG. 4. Force–velocity curves from trabecular muscles of similar cross-sectional areas. Each point represents an average value and the standard error is indicated with brackets.

trophied hearts in our studies. Hearts from rats subjected to chronic hypoxia have been shown to exhibit an increased mechanical tolerance to hypoxia (McGrath and Bullard, 1968). As noted by Mager and co-workers (1968), they also have a shift in the LDH subunit distribution toward the "M" type of LDH.

Muscles in our study were examined for the possible occurrence of the above changes. Trabecular muscles from hearts of animals at 4 weeks after operation were subjected to a Krebs solution gassed with 95% N and 5% CO_2, and the time course of changes in developed tension was measured. In hypertrophied hearts, we found no enhanced ability of muscles to develop tension in a hypoxic environment when compared with controls. In addition, there was no increase in LDH concentration as determined by the method of Kornberg (1955) or shift in the electrophoretically determined isoenzyme pattern. Thus, if the degree of hypertrophy observed in these experiments is

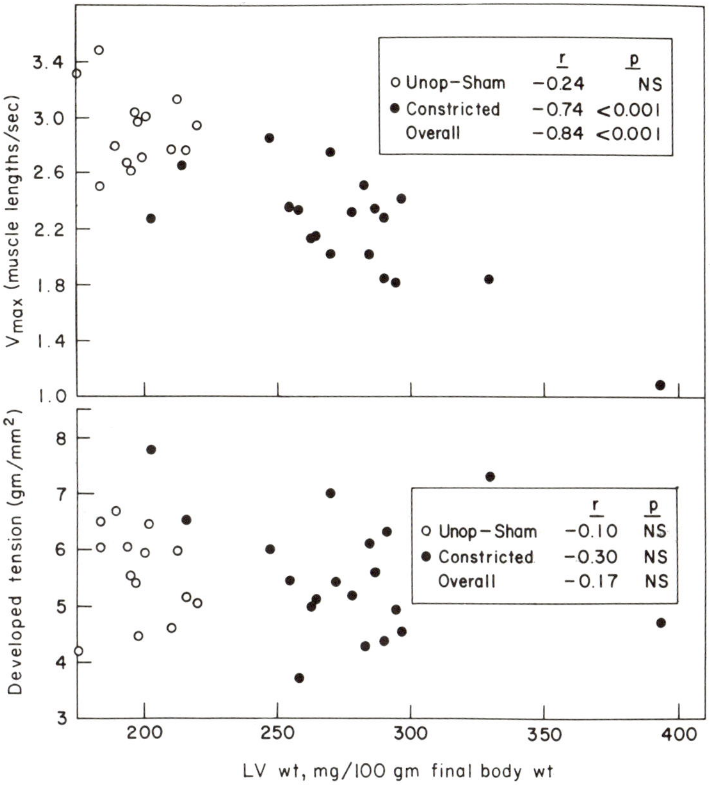

FIG. 5. Correlation of left ventricular–body weight ratio with V_{max} (upper) and developed tension (lower) in trabecular muscles of similar cross-sectional area. Each point represents a determination from a single muscle.

associated with hypoxia of the muscle, no evidence for this was found in the form of adaptive changes of the LDH isoenzymes or increased mechanical tolerance to hyoxia.

We have found, as have others (Bertosŏvá *et al.*, 1969; Buccino *et al.*, 1969), that hypertrophied muscle contains an increased collagen content and concentration as reflected by an elevation of hydroxyproline. In our studies, the hydroxyproline concentration of the free wall of the left ventricle, measured by the method of Prockop and Udenfriend (1960), showed a significant inverse correlation with V_{max}. However, a depression in V_{max} often occurred in muscles from hearts that had a collagen concentration within the normal range. We concluded from this that our findings failed to delineate a clear-cut relationship between a depression in contractility and an increase in collagen concentration. Others have tried to correlate myofibrillar ATPase activity with

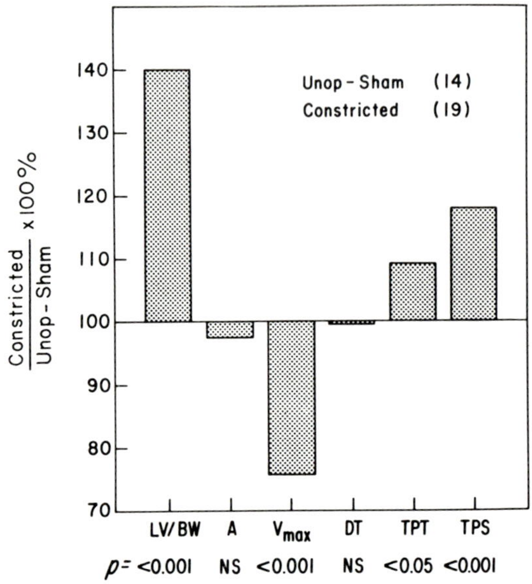

FIG. 6. Summary of the effects of hypertrophy on cardiac muscle mechanics in trabecular muscles of similar cross-sectional area (A). (DT), developed tension; (TPT), time-to-peak isometric tension; and (TPS), time-to-peak "unloaded" isotonic shortening. The number of animals used in each group is indicated in parentheses.

alterations in contractility (Alpert and Gordon, 1962; Chandler, 1967; Gordon and Brown, 1966). Further investigation is necessary to clearly define the cause for the depressed contractility in myocardial hypertrophy.

Summary

In summary, the results of this study indicate that there is a fall in contractility in cardiac hypertrophy that appears to be related more to the degree than the duration of hypertrophy. Developed tension appears to be maintained, at least partially, by a prolonged contraction time. It might be anticipated that with more extensive hypertrophy, aging, and other factors, contractility would fall further, and the compensatory prolongation of contraction time would be inadequate to sustain tension development leading ultimately to a decreased cardiac performance. With hypertrophy of the degree produced in these experiments, no evidence for myocardial hypoxia was found. An increase in tissue hydroxyproline concentration was present in hypertrophied heart muscle.

Acknowledgments

This investigation was supported by grants nos. HE-6924 and HE-7139 from the National Heart Institute, National Institutes of Health, United States Public Health Service. Dr. O. H. L. Bing is a former trainee of graduate training program No. HE-5391, National Heart Institute. Dr. B. L. Fanburg is a recipient of a Research Career Development Award from the National Institutes of Health, United States Public Health Service. We would like to acknowledge the work of Dr. Arvind Inamdar, who performed the lactic dehydrogenase assays.

References

Alpert, N. R., and Gordon, M. S. (1962). *Amer. J. Physiol.* **202,** 940.

Alpert, N. R., Gale, H. H., and Taylor, N. (1967). *In* "Factors Influencing Myocardial Contractility" (R. D. Tanz, F. Kavaler, and J. Robert, eds.), pp. 127–133. Academic Press, New York.

Bertosŏvá, D., Chvepil, M., Korecký, B., Poupa, O., Rakŭson, K., Taurek, A., and Vizek, M. (1969). *J. Physiol.* **200,** 285.

Buccino, R. A., Harris, E., Spann, J. F., Jr., and Sonnenblick, E. H. (1969). *Amer. J. Physiol.* **216,** 425.

Chandler, B. M., Sonnenblick, E. H., Spann, J. F., and Pool, P. E. (1967). *Circ. Res.* **21,** 717.

Fanburg, B. L., and Posner, B. I. (1968). *Circ. Res.* **23,** 123.

Gordon, M. S., and Brown, A. L., Jr. (1966). *Circ. Res.* **18,** 534.

Grimm, A. F., Kubota, R., and Whitehorn, W. V. (1963). *Circ. Res.* **12,** 118.

Kerr, A., Jr., Winterberger, A. R., and Giambattista, M. (1961). *Circ. Res.* **9,** 103.

Kornberg, A. (1955). *In* "Methods in Enzymology" (S. B. Colowick and N. O. Kaplan, eds.), Vol. I, p. 441. Academic Press, New York.

Krebs, H. A., and Henseleit, K. (1932). *Physiol. Chem.* **210,** 33.

McGrath, J. J., and Bullard, R. W. (1968). *J. Appl. Physiol.* **25,** 761.

Mager, M., Blatt, W. F., Natale, P. J., and Blatteis, C. M. (1968). *Amer. J. Physiol.* **215,** 8.

Prockop, O. J., and Udenfriend, S. (1960). *Anal. Biochem.* **1,** 228.

Spann, J. F., Jr., Buccino, R. A., Sonnenblick, E. H., and Braunwald, E. (1967). *Circ. Res.* **21,** 341.

MAXIMAL FORCE DEVELOPMENT BY HYPERTROPHIED RIGHT VENTRICULAR PAPILLARY MUSCLES REMAINING IN SITU

Vincent J. Fisher and Frederic Kavaler

Myocardial hypertrophy is a compensatory adjustment of the cardiac muscle cell to chronic increase in load. The increase in muscle mass of the stressed cardiac ventricle is often sufficient to permit it to handle the increased load, sometimes for prolonged periods of time. However, most hearts that fail after moderate to prolonged imposition of an increased load show evidence of hypertrophy (Friedberg, 1966). It is of importance to determine whether there may be some intrinsic functional defect in the hypertrophied cell that makes it less effective than the normal cell and that may eventually lead to cellular failure. Prior studies have differed in experimental animal used, manner of causing hypertrophy, duration of hypertrophy, and method of measuring and expressing contractile function (Badeer, 1967). As a result, no clear statement can be made as to whether hypertrophied cardiac muscle functions normally, subnormally or supernormally.

We have reexamined the question of contractile force development by hypertrophied cardiac muscle using a technique that permits the measurement of isometric force from individual right ventricular papillary muscles remaining attached to the septum and perfused by the coronary circulation. Force can thus be related to the size of the contracting muscle mass. The distance for diffusion of oxygen and metabolites during the study is no greater than that existing prior to it. Our study leads us to the conclusion that canine right ventricular papillary muscles with moderately severe degrees of cellular hypertrophy of short duration (less than 4 months) are capable of normal force development. Nevertheless, we feel that this statement cannot be applied to other species with the same degree and duration of hypertrophy, nor to the same species with either greater hypertrophy or with the same degree of hypertrophy of longer duration.

Methods

A total of 46 normal dogs and 26 dogs with right ventricular hypertrophy are included in this study. Ventricular hypertrophy was induced by partial banding of the pulmonary artery to the extent that the systolic pressure developed by the right ventricle increased to between 40 and 60 mm Hg. Dogs with right ventricular hypertrophy were studied between 6 and 16 weeks after pulmonary artery banding. None of the dogs had hepatomegaly, ascites, or pleural effusion at the time of study. The average right ventricular pressure at the time of study was 50/2 mm Hg with a range in systolic pressure of 26–78 mm Hg.

Procedures for studying papillary muscle mechanics have been described previously (Fisher *et al.*, 1969), and were the same for both groups of dogs. Animals were anesthetized with 25 mg/kg of sodium pentobarbital given intravenously. Anesthesia was maintained with supplementary pentobarbital as needed. They were ventilated by a Bird positive-pressure respirator through an endotracheal tube using a 40% oxygen–room air mixture. A lead II electrocardiogram was monitored continuously by an Electronics for Medicine DR-8 photographic recorder. Aortic pressure was measured by a Statham AA pressure transducer. In the dogs with ventricular hypertrophy, right ventricular pressure was measured prior to commencing the study. The chest was opened by a bilateral thoracotomy and the dogs were placed upon complete cardiopulmonary bypass. The venous blood was oxygenated in a Rygg-Kyvsgaard disposable bag oxygenator by a 97% O_2–3% CO_2 mixture. Arterialized blood was pumped into the right common carotid artery by an American Optical Company roller pump at a flow rate of 100 ml/kg/min. Complete atrioventricular block was induced by severing the bundle of His (Pruett and Woods, 1967). Ventricles were stimulated through an electrode sewed to the epicardial surface of the right ventricle. All studies were performed at 27°C.

The free wall of the right ventricle was incised and retracted backward. One of the papillary muscles arising from the septum was selected and a 3–0 silk thread was tied to the apex of the muscle at the attachment of the chorda. The chorda was cut and the circular base of the gauge slipped over the muscle (Fig. 1). With the removable circular bases, it was possible to select for each muscle a gauge base that was just slightly larger than the base of the muscle. The apical end of the muscle was tied to the platform of the gauge. To the upper and lower surfaces of this platform were bonded Baldwin-Lima-Hamilton C-7 gauges which formed adjacent resistance arms of a Wheatstone bridge. During continuous single-pulse stimulation at a ventricular rate ranging from 56 to 95 beats/min, the papillary muscle was progres-

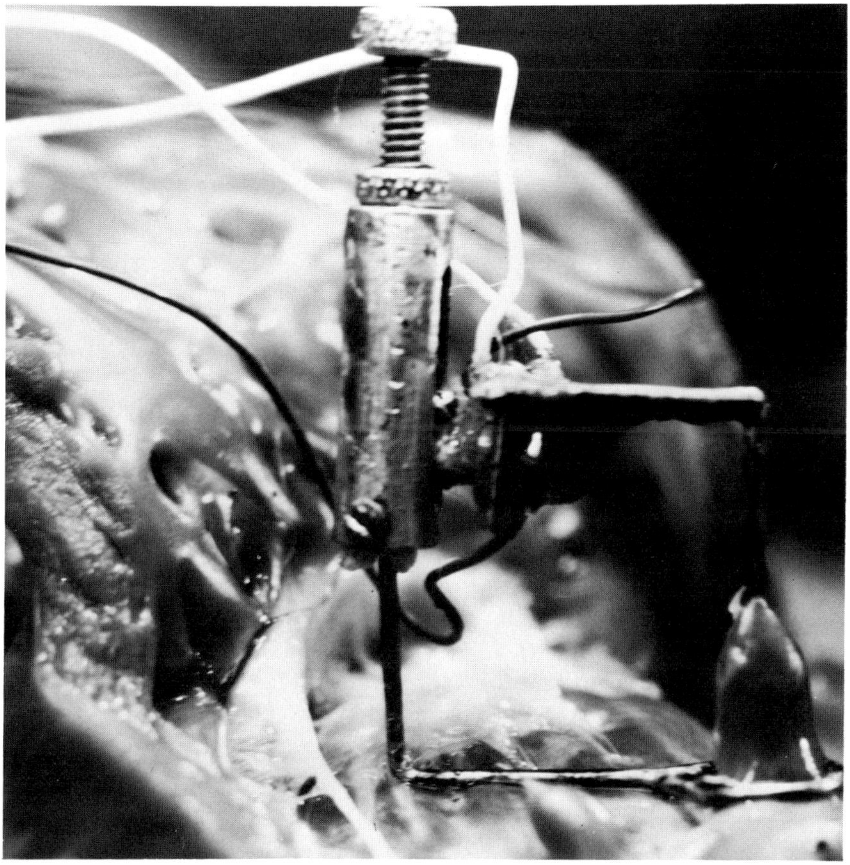

FIG. 1. A photograph of a right ventricular papillary muscle in the *in situ* papillary muscle gauge. The gauge takes origin from the septum and its base is encircled by a ring. The purpose of the ring is to exclude the septal muscle mass from altering the force exerted by the papillary muscle on the gauge platform. The ventricle is more widely incised than is usually the case.

sively stretched in increments of 0.32–0.64 mm by turning the central screw of the gauge. In several studies, continuous paired pulse stimulation was used because of difficulty in pacing the ventricles by single-pulse stimulation. Force was recorded at each length and active systolic force (peak systolic force minus diastolic force) was observed to increase, peak and fall as the length–tension curve was defined (Fig. 2). When the optimal length of the muscle was determined, it was left at this length for the remainder of the study.

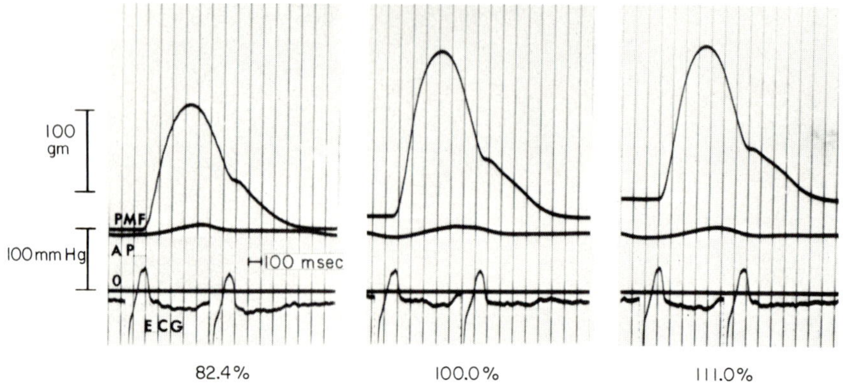

FIG. 2. Three records from a study of a hypertrophied right ventricular papillary muscle showing forces developed during the recording of the length–tension curve. This is one of the few studies where the length–tension curve was recorded during paired stimulation of the ventricles. The center record was made with the muscle at its optimal length (100%). The left record was made with the muscle at 82.4% of optimal length and the right record with the muscle at 110.0% of optimal length. (PMF) Papillary muscle force; (AP) aortic pressure; (0) zero pressure line; (ECG) lead II electrocardiogram.

A maximal contraction was induced by paired pulse stimulation of the ventricles at a ventricular rate between 18 and 45 paired beats/min (Fisher *et al.*, 1967; Kavaler *et al.*, 1968). Various rates and pairing intervals were tested until a peak contraction was obtained. The stiffness of the gauge platform was such that the average normal muscle shortened by only 3.2% during maximal contraction and the average hypertrophied muscle shortened by 3.3%. No muscle shortened more than 5% of its optimal length.

At the conclusion of the study the heart was depolarized by injection of 5–20 ml of a 25% solution of potassium chloride into the coronary arteries through a large catheter, the tip of which lay just above the aortic valve. This was followed by infusion of 700 ml of a 10% solution of formaldehyde under an average pressure head of 70–100 mm Hg. Perfusion was limited to the heart by ligating the brachiocephalic and left subclavian arteries at their origins, and by ligating the aorta just below the left subclavian artery. Papillary muscle force was measured during KCl and formaldehyde infusion; no significant increase over the level of diastolic force occurred. At the conclusion of the formaldehyde infusion, the rigid muscle was cut free at its base, weighed, and its length measured. Average cross-sectional area was calculated assuming the muscle to be a cylinder with a specific gravity of 1.000.

After 1–2 weeks of additional fixation in 10% formaldehyde solution muscles were cut into two longitudinal halves. Longitudinal sections 5 μ thick were cut from one of the halves and cross sections 8 μ thick were cut from the other. All sections were stained with Gomori trichrome stain. Microscopy was performed using a Leitz Ortholux microscope or a Nikon LB research microscope. Photomicrographs were made of the cross sections of the muscle cells at a magnification of 1000×. Cross-sectional area of the muscle cells was determined by planimetry of cells on 8 × 10 inch prints (average total magnification, 3450×). In order to insure measurement at a uniform site in the cells, only cells with a centrally located nucleus were measured. Diameter was calculated from area assuming the cell to be circular in cross section. Cell length was measured from longitudinal sections at a magnification of 400× using an eyepiece filar micrometer. The length of the cell was considered to be the distance between two consecutive intercalated discs provided a nucleus was visible between the two discs. Lengths of sarcomeres of 11 normal and 15 hypertrophied muscles were also measured. An eyepiece filar micrometer was used at a magnification of 1250×. The total length of five sarcomeres in series was measured to the nearest 0.04 μ and the average was taken. Forty such measurements were made in each of five areas for each muscle. The details of the measurement technique and its interpretation have been described previously.

Results

Cellular cross-sectional areas of six normal muscles and 13 muscles with right ventricular hypertrophy (RVH) were measured (Table I). The cross-

TABLE I

CELLULAR DIMENSIONS

Measurements	Normal	RVH	% Increase	p Value
Area, μ^2	212 ± 75	438 ± 93	106.6	< 0.001
Diameter, μ	16.2 ± 2.8	23.4 ± 2.4	44.4	< 0.001
Length, μ	71.4 ± 4.1	93.5 ± 8.8	31.0	< 0.001
Volume, $\mu^3 \times 10^3$	15.1	41.0	173	–

sectional area of hypertrophied cells was twice as great as that of normal cells. The cellular lengths of 15 normal muscles and 12 hypertrophied muscles were compared. The length increased by an average of 31% in the process of hypertrophy. When the average cell volume of each group of cells is calculated from the average length and average cross-sectional area, the volume of hypertrophied cells is seen to be increased by 173% over normal. Since the mass is proportional to the volume, the weight of the hypertrophied ventricles almost tripled.

When maximal force developed by the 46 normal muscles is plotted against cross-sectional area a linear relationship is found (Fig. 3). The line is described by the equation $y = 46.0 + 2.4 \times$. The standard error of the estimate is $\pm$ 20.2 gm and the coefficient of correlation is 0.665 ($p < 0.01$). The scatter of points is greatest for muscles of greater than 25.0 mm^2 cross-sectional area. Five of these six points fall below the regression line for the 40 muscles of less than 25.0 mm^2 cross-sectional area (described by the equation $y = 30.6 + 3.8 \times$). Since 10 of the 26 hypertrophied muscles were of greater than 25.0 mm^2 cross-sectional area, comparisons will be made with the entire group of normal muscles rather than with the 40 smallest muscles.

A plot of force against the wet weight of the muscles closely resembled plots of force against cross sectional area. This suggests that little error was introduced by the assumptions involved in calculating the average cross-sectional area of the muscles. No relationship was found between force and muscle length. The subsequent discussion will deal only with the relationship of force to cross-sectional area.

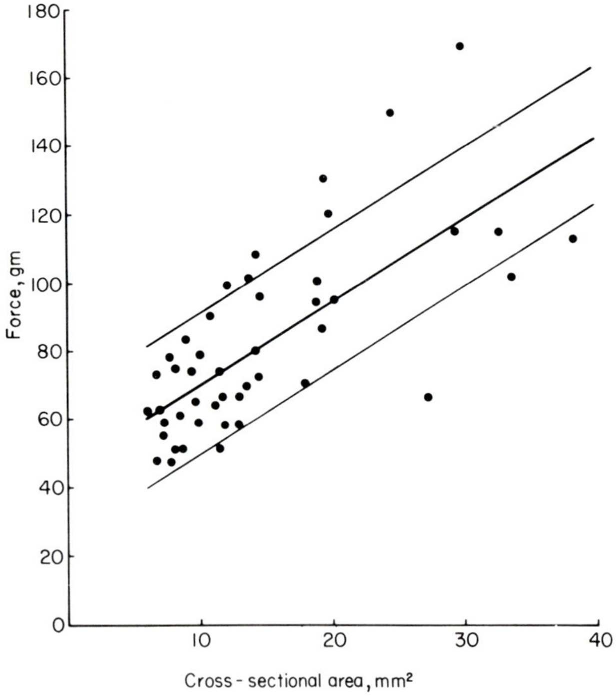

FIG. 3. A plot of maximal force against cross-sectional area for 46 normal right ventricular papillary muscles. The thick line is the regression line and the thin lines represent 1 S.E. of the estimate above and below the regression line.

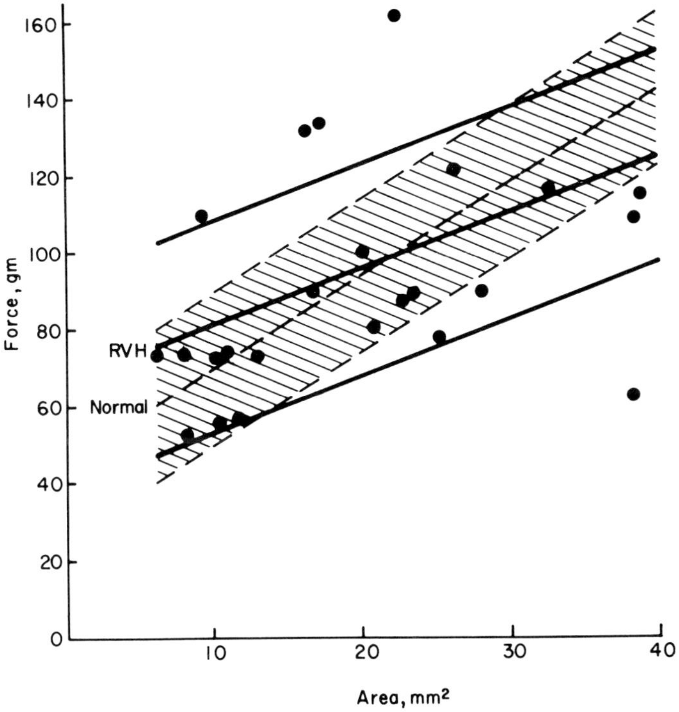

FIG. 4. A plot of maximal force against cross-sectional area for 26 hypertrophied right ventricular papillary muscles. Each muscle is represented by a closed circle. The thick line is the regression line and the thin lines represent 1 S.E. of the estimate above and below the regression line. The shaded area represents the regression line $\pm$ 1 S.E. of the estimate for 46 normal muscles.

When the maximal force developed by the 26 hypertrophied muscles is plotted against their cross-sectional areas, the relationship is again found to be linear (Fig. 4). The line is described by the equation $y = 67.1 + 1.36\times$. The standard error of the estimate is ± 27.4 gm, and the coefficient of correlation is 0.482 ($p < 0.01$). There is no significant difference in the relationship of maximal force to cross-sectional area between the normal and hypertrophied muscles ($p > 0.10$).

A surprising finding for both groups of muscles was that thick muscles developed less force per milligram of wet weight than did thin muscles (Table II). Muscles were arbitrarily divided into three groups according to their cross-sectional areas: < 10.1 mm^2, between 10.1 and 15.0 mm^2, and > 15.0 mm^2. The differences in force development per mm^2 of cross-sectional area between the three size groups of muscles was statistically significant for

TABLE II

RELATIONSHIP OF FORCE TO MUSCLE SIZE
(gm/mm^2 $\pm$ 1 sd)

Group	Size (mm^2)	Normal[a]	RVH[a]
1	$<$ 10.1	7.96 $\pm$ 1.69 ($n = 16$)	8.94 $\pm$ 3.25 ($n = 5$)
2	10.1–15.0	6.00 $\pm$ 1.25 ($n = 16$)	6.24 $\pm$ 0.77 ($n = 4$)
3	$>$ 15.0	4.54 $\pm$ 1.32 ($n = 14$)	4.32 $\pm$ 1.81 ($n = 17$)
	p 1 vs 2	$<$ 0.005	$>$ 0.10
	p 1 vs 3	$<$ 0.001	$<$ 0.001
	p 2 vs 3	$<$ 0.01	$>$ 0.05

[a] n = number of muscles in each group.

normal muscles. The difference between the smallest and largest groups of muscles was significant for the hypertrophied muscles. However, no significant difference in maximal force development was found between normal and hypertrophied muscles for any size group (Fig. 5).

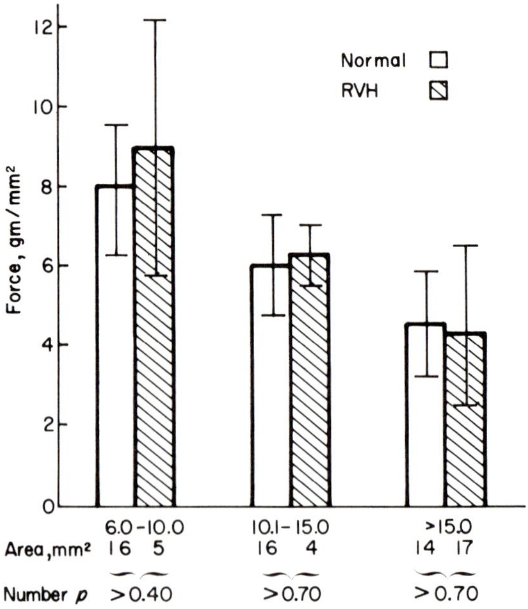

FIG. 5. Maximal force per mm^2 of cross-sectional area developed by three different size groups of normal (open area) and hypertrophied right ventricular (shaded area) papillary muscles. Each column represents the average force for the group. The bar at the top represents $\pm$ 1 sd.

The reason for the relative weakness of thick muscles is not clear. A reasonable partial explanation could be offered, based on the uneven distribution of sarcomere lengths in muscles stretched to optimal length by the present technique (Table III). There was a highly significant difference between the lengths of sarcomeres in the basal and apical segments of normal muscles ($p < 0.005$), with the basal sarcomeres being shorter than the apical ones. The same pattern was found in hypertrophied muscles, although basal and apical sarcomeres were less divergent in size than in normal muscles, and the difference was not statistically significant ($p > 0.20$). It is felt, however, that the apparent uniformity of sarcomeres in hypertrophied muscles may be an artifact of the measuring technique. In order to avoid overestimation of sarcomere length due to nonparallel cutting of myofibrils, the experimental protocol required that the five sacromeres whose length was measured have at least five to eight additional sarcomeres in series on each end. This limited the overestimation of sarcomere length resulting from nonparallel sectioning to less than 2%. Hypertrophied muscles had many more fibrous tissue bundles than normal muscles. Fibrils adjacent to these bundles tended to be buckled and the sarcomeres appeared to be shorter than those located in taut fibrils. Since our criteria excluded the former group of sarcomeres from measurement, an impression is created of more uniformity than actually exists. It is thus uncertain, as to whether the explanation of the relative weakness of the thick hypertrophied muscles included in this study is the same as that for the thick normal muscles.

TABLE III

SARCOMERE LENGTHS[a]

Area	Normal (μ)[a]	RVH (μ)
1 (base)	1.95 ± 0.07	2.03 ± 0.14
II	1.98 ± 0.07	2.05 ± 0.11
III (mid)	1.99 ± 0.07	2.05 ± 0.12
IV	2.05 ± 0.07	2.06 ± 0.10
V (apex)	2.07 ± 0.09	2.09 ± 0.09

[a] Mean distribution for muscles from 11 normal hearts was 2.01 ± 0.07 μ; for 12 with RVH, 2.05 ± 0.10 μ.
[b] Mean ± 1 sd.

The maximal rate of rise of force (dF/dt_{max}) of both groups of muscles was measured at the optimal heart rate and pairing interval. This rate varied from 18 to 45 beats/min. The maximal rate of rise of force increased with both heart rate and muscle size, but the increase was not statistically significant. Comparisons of the maximal rate of rise of force in normal and hypertrophied muscles should be made between muscles of comparable size stimulated at the same rate. Because there were five different optimal rates and because muscles were divided into three groups according to size, individual groups of normal and hypertrophied muscles contained too few muscles to permit statistical comparison. The optimal heart rate for the largest number of normal and hypertrophied hearts was 35 paired beats/min. All muscles stimulated at this rate were therefore grouped together to permit comparison of the maximal rate of rise of force of normal and hypertrophied muscles. The dF/dt_{max} of 21 normal muscles was 35.8 ± 14.4 gm/sec/mm^2 and that of 14 hypertrophied muscles was $36.2 + 26.9$ gm/sec/mm^2. The difference was not statistically significant ($p > 0.90$). Within this group of hearts stimulated at 35 paired beats/min, the six normal muscles of over 15 mm^2 cross-sectional area had a dF/dt_{max} of 25.4 ± 9.4 gm/sec/mm^2, whereas the eight hypertrophied muscles of similar size had a dF/dt_{max} of 24.4 ± 9.7 gm/sec/mm^2 ($p > 0.80$). Thus, even when muscles of comparable size are compared, maximal rate of rise of force is not found to be depressed.

Discussion

The common association of hypertrophy of ventricular muscle and failure of the ventricle (Friedberg, 1966) raises the question of the interrelationship of myocardial hypertrophy and myocardial failure. The mechanical function of hypertrophied, nonfailing cardiac muscle has been the subject of a number of investigations. Major differences in the experimental subjects and the experimental approach have yielded results that often appear divergent and sometimes contradictory. Perhaps the principal difficulty that investigators face is how to characterize myocardial function.

One approach is to study the cardiac output of normal and hypertrophied ventricles an index of the pumping ability of the chamber. Such an approach was used by Beznak (1958) who found that cardiac output was normal 3 weeks after constriction of the upper abdominal aorta of rats. The maximum cardiac output was determined in this study by loading the circulation with a polyvinylpyrrolidone solution. Whereas the normal ventricle could increase its output from 48 ml/min to 131 ml/min, the hypertrophied ventricle could increase its output to 178 ml/min. Since the mass of these ventricles was increased by 45%, this study indicates that the larger than normal mass of ventricular muscle is capable, at least for a limited time, of an increase in total cardiac function. The important question of whether there is any gain or loss in the contractile capability of the individual unit of cardiac muscle in the process of hypertrophy can only be answered, however, by relating the measured index of function to muscle mass.

Geha and coworkers (1966) caused a 40% increase in the right ventricular mass of dogs by partially banding the pulmonary artery for 6–12 weeks. They acutely stressed the right ventricles of control dogs by partial occlusion of the pulmonary artery and simultaneous catecholamine infusion. Ventricles of experimental animals were stressed by catecholamine infusion only. The maximal stroke work of the latter group was increased by 275% over that of the normal group. Thus they felt that hypertrophied cardiac muscle is capable of performing more work per unit of muscle mass than normal muscle) Contradictory results were found by Meerson and Pshennikova (1965) studying left ventricular hypertrophy in rabbits and Krames *et al.* (1967) studying left ventricular hypertrophy in rats. Both groups measured the maximal pressure developed by the left ventricle of normal and experimental animals during transient complete occlusion of the aorta. When pressure was related to ventricular weight the peak pressure developed by hypertrophied ventricles was less than that developed by normal ventricles. The left ventricle had increased its mass by 75–80% in the study of Meerson and Pshennikova and by 13–36% in the study of Krames *et al.* The duration of hypertrophy was between $4\frac{1}{2}$ and 5 months in the former study, and 24 days in the latter.

Another approach to the assessment of function of hypertrophied cardiac muscle is to excise a sample after a period of development of hypertrophy *in vivo*, and to study some aspect of contractile function *in vitro*. This permits much greater control of the experimental conditions than studies *in vivo*, but it introduces the problem of oxygenation and removal of metabolic wastes by a nonphysiological system. In studying murine left ventricular papillary muscles contracting 6 times/min under isometric conditions at 27°C, Kerr *et al.* (1961) reported an increase in force from a normal value of 1.28 gm/mg dry weight to 1.95 gm/mg dry weight with hypertrophy. The duration of aortic occlusion was 21–90 days and the weight of the ventricles was increased by 30%. Grimm and coworkers (1963), however, studying isolated papillary muscles of rats under comparable conditions found no significant difference in force development/mg weight between normal muscles and muscles from ventricles with a 20–40% increase in mass due to exercise. The duration of the exercise was 8 weeks.

Spann *et al.* (1967) produced right ventricular hypertrophy by banding the pulmonary artery of cats. At the time of study 20–85 days after banding the right ventricles had about doubled their weight. Excised papillary muscles were stimulated 12 times/min at 30°C. At optimal length, there was a small but statistically insignificant reduction in isometric force developed by hypertrophied muscles. The maximal rate of rise of tension was reduced below normal particularly at the faster rates. More significantly, the maximal force developed by hypertrophied muscles during continuous paired stimulation was significantly reduced below that developed by normal muscles (10.6 ± 0.4 gm/mm^2 for normals; 8.5 ± 1.0 gm/mm^2 for hypertrophy; $p < 0.05$).

Thus, prior studies have indicated that hypertrophied muscles develop more force than normal muscles, less force, and the same amount of force per unit of muscle mass. One limitation of all the studies referred to, with the exception of that of Spann *et al.* (1967), is that the maximal contractile capability was not studied. The isolated tissue studies compared normal and hypertrophied muscles contracting at a slow, regular rate. Previous studies in our laboratory (Fisher *et al.*, 1967; Kavaler *et al.*, 1968) have shown that isolated papillary muscles driven by single pulse stimulation in normal Tyrode's solution develop a force below that developed in a high calcium, low sodium medium (contractile maximum) and randomly related to it. A variety of factors which influence adrenergic and inotropic activity of heart muscle *in vivo* may vary the contractile response of the subsequently excised muscle to single pulse stimulation without altering the maximal contraction. This is even more true of the heart which is studied *in situ*. The ventricle which contracts isovolumically at the peak of its pressure–volume curve does not ordinarily contract with maximal force. Paired pulse stimulation can usually cause such a ventricle to contract even more forcefully (Fisher *et al.*, 1967). We feel that all comparisons of normal and hypertrophied cardiac muscle should include a comparison with the muscles in a maximal inotropic state.

Our study utilized a relatively new preparation which combines many of the advantages of isolated tissue techniques with the retention of the capillary circulation for oxygen supply and waste disposal. Among the advantages are maintenance of the isometric state at an optimal muscle length, fairly precise definition of the mass of muscle giving rise to the force, and a relatively parallel arrangement of the muscle fibers. Foremost among the disadvantages is the potential of the large number of latent pacemakers of the ventricles for causing arrhythmia during pacing of the heart. Using this technique we find that *in situ* cardiac muscle develops an amount of force when maximally stimulated that is comparable to that reported of isolated cardiac muscle in a maximal inotropic state (Fisher *et al.*, 1967; Spann *et al.*, 1967; Kavaler *et al.*, 1968; Sonnenblick *et al.*, 1968). In addition, right ventricular papillary muscles that have been subjected to an increased pressure load for 6–16 weeks and have increased their mass almost threefold are capable of the same magnitude of maximal contraction as normal muscles. The maximal rate of rise of force appears to be normal in the group of hypertrophied muscles included in this study, but a larger number of muscles of comparable size should be studied at the principal optimal heart rates to confirm this observation.

This observation appears to be contrary to that of Spann and coworkers (1967) and, since they were first in print, it is incumbent upon us to offer some explanation. One possibility that immediately presents itself is that their hypertrophied muscles, being thicker than thin normal muscles, had their maximal contractile capacity limited by the greater distance for diffusion between the surface and the center of the muscles. The work of Pool *et al.* (1968) indicated that oxidative phosphorylation is normal for isolated muscles of moderately large diameter (mean equals 1.3 mm). The hypertrophied muscles studied by Spann *et al.* (1967) were of smaller diameter than this and presumably had normal oxidative phosphorylation. Muscle contraction, however, produces a number of products that have a negative inotropic action (Buckley *et al.*, 1968). Since these molecules are larger than those in oxygen, it is possible that they may accumulate in thick, nonperfused muscles and depress contraction without affecting oxidative phosphorylation.

We found in our optimally stretched normal muscles a significant variation of sarcomere lengths between the apical and the basal segments. We postulated that this, in addition to the conical shape of the muscle, which gave the segment with the shortest sarcomeres the largest surface area, was mainly responsible for the considerable relative weakness of our thick muscles. However, we had previously found (Fisher *et al.*, 1967; Kavaler *et al.*, 1968) that isolated, isometrically contracting normal muscles of over a critical thickness developed less force than thin muscles. Similar observations had been made by Kelly and Hoffman (1960) and it was assumed to be a result of inadequate diffusion of oxygen (Cranefield and Greenspan, 1960). The possibility also exists that sarcomere heterogeneity may play a role in reducing the force developed by isolated, optimally stretched thick muscles. Although our observations apply only to our specific preparation, the findings of Huxley and Peachey (1961) with highly stretched single skeletal muscle fibers suggests that significant sarcomere heterogeneity may exist in thin strips of isolated cardiac muscle. For the present, it is best to compare contractile performance of normal and hypertrophied muscles of comparable size.

One interesting finding in this study was the increased length of hypertrophied muscle cells without a singificant increase in sarcomere length. This observation has been reported previously by Laks and coworkers (1969), and had been predicted by the angiocardiographic studies of Grant *et al.* (1965), indicating that in the process of hypertrophy, additional sarcomeres are laid down not only in parallel, but also in series. The implication for the cardiac chamber surrounded by hypertrophied muscle cells is that the chamber is chronically dilated without any increase in sarcomere length. In the example of a thin-walled sphere, a 31% increase in circumference (the average increase in cell length in this study) results in more than a doubling of chamber volume. A further implication of chronic dilatation of a chamber is that, when compared with a normal chamber, a given change in diastolic volume causes a smaller change in circumference and therefore in sarcomere lengths. This is a correlate of the observations by Burch *et al.* (1952) that in order to eject a given stroke volume, a dilated chamber needs to alter its volume (and therefore its sarcomere lengths) less than a normal chamber. The type of hypertrophy seen in this study will be accompanied by dilatation. This makes the heart less dependent upon, but also less able to make use of, the Frank-Starling mechanism.

A final consideration relates to the comparative sizes of the cells of the normal and hypertrophied muscles included in this study. The average cell diameters in our hypertrophied muscles ranged from 20.6 to 27.4 μ. In the absence of failure, the cells of the hypertrophied human ventricle seldom enlarge to over 27 μ diameter (Harrison *et al.*, 1932; Lowe and Bate, 1948) and even in the presence of failure they may be within this limit (Roberts and Wearn, 1941). Harrison and co-workers (1932) found the diameters of normal and canine heart-muscle cells to be of the same order of magnitude. Differences in histological technique, differences in species tolerance of hypertrophy, and the difficulty in defining heart failure in autopsy studies dictate caution in making comparisons of our findings with these prior studies. We have nevertheless observed an average increase in cellular diameter of 44% without any decline in cardiac function. An average increase of diameter of 51% in the smaller muscle cells of feline ventricles studied by Spann *et al.* (1967) was associated with a decline in maximal force development. The duration of hypertrophy in their study and in ours was comparable. It is possible that the reaction of various species of animals to hypertrophy is different. It is also possible that with additional cellular enlargement or with the same degree of enlargement for a larger duration, our canine papillary muscles would have shown a decline in function prior to the development of clinical heart failure.

ACKNOWLEDGMENTS

This work was supported by a grant-in-aid from the American Heart Association. Dr. Kavaler is a Career Scientist of the Health Research Council of the City of New York, Contract No. 1-376. We thank Pedro Dedos, Emiladis Torres, and David Rosa for technical assistance during the experiments. We also thank Miss Gloria R. Ferris for the histologic preparations and microscopic measurements and Miss Barbara A. Fisher for microscopic measurements.

REFERENCES

Badeer, H. S. (1967). *Amer. Heart J.* **73,** 693.
Beznak, M. (1958). *Circ. Res.* **6,** 207.
Buckley, N. M., Sussman, I., Frasier, I., and Singleton, A. (1968). *Proc. Int. Un. Physiol. Sci.* **7,** 65.
Burch, G. E., Ray, C. T., and Cronvich, J. A. (1952). *Circulation* **5,** 504.
Cranefield, P. F., and Greenspan, K. (1960). *J. Gen. Physiol.* **42,** 235.
Fisher, V. J., Lee, R. J., Marlon, A. M., and Kavaler, F. (1967). *Circ. Res.* **20,** 520.

Fisher, V. J., Martino, R. A., Harris, R. S., and Kavaler, F. (1969). *Amer. J. Physiol.*
Friedberg, C. J. (1966). "Diseases of the Heart," 3rd ed., pp. 195–202. Saunders, Philadelphia, Pennsylvania.
Geha, A. S., Duffy, J. P., and Swan, H. J. C. (1966). *Circ. Res.* **19,** 255.
Grant, C., Greene, D. G., and Bunnell, I. L. (1965). *Amer. J. Med.* **39,** 895.
Grimm, A. F., Ryo, K., and Whitehorn, W. V. (1963). *Circ. Res.* **12,** 118.
Harrison, T. R., Ashman, R., and Larson, R. M. (1932). *Arch. Int. Med.* **49,** 151.
Huxley, A. F., and Peachey, L. D. (1961). *J. Physiol.* (*London*) **156,** 150.
Kavaler, F., Marlon, A., Harris, R. S., and Fisher, V. J. (1968). *In* "Paired Pulse Stimulation of the Heart" (P. F. Cranefield and B. F. Hoffman, eds.), pp. 72–81. Rockefeller Univ. Press, New York.
Kelly, J. J., and Hoffman, B. F. (1960). *Amer. J. Physiol.* **199,** 157.
Kerr, A. Jr., Winterberger, A. R., and Giambattista, M. (1961). *Circ. Res.* **9,** 103.
Krames, B. B., Northup, D. W., and Van Liere, E. J. (1967). *Proc. Soc. Exp. Biol. Med.* **124,** 150.
Laks, M. M., Morady, F., and Swan, H. J. C. (1969). *Circ. Res.* **24,** 705.
Lowe, T. E., and Bate, E. W. (1948). *Med. J. Austral.* **1,** 467.
Meerson, F. Z., and Pshennikova, M. G. (1965). *Fed. Proc. Fed. Amer. Soc. Exp. Biol.* **24,** T957.
Pool, P. E., Chandler, B. M., Sonnenblick, E. H., and Braunwald, E. (1968). *Circ. Res.* **22,** 213.
Pruett, J. K., and Woods, E. F. (1967). *J. Appl. Physiol.* **22,** 830.
Roberts, J. T., and Wearn, J. T. (1941). *Amer. Heart J.* **21,** 617.
Sonnenblick, E. H., Parmley, W. W., Buccino, R. A., and Spann, J. F., Jr. (1968). *Nature* (*London*) **219,** 1056.
Spann, J. F. Jr., Buccino, R. A., Sonnenblick, E. H., and Braunwald, E. (1967). *Circ. Res.* **21,** 341.

METHODS FOR ASSESSING PERFORMANCE FOR THE INTACT HYPERTROPHIED HEART

M. Lucius Walker, Jr., Edward W. Hawthorne, and Harold Sandler

SYMBOLS

P	ventricular pressure, gm/cm^2
σ_m	meridional stress, gm/cm^2
σ_h	hoop stress, gm/cm^2
H	wall thickness, cm
r_m	radius of curvature in meridional direction, cm
r_h	radius of curvature in circumferential direction, cm
R_i	inside radius at equator, cm
R_o	external radius at equator, cm
$2B$	aorta to apex length, cm
L_{CF}	mean circumference, cm
l_{SE}, l_{CE}	mean series elastic element length and mean contractile element length at equator, cm
L_0	mean circumference (constant) corresponding to zero diastolic ventricular pressure, cm
n	number of sarcomeres contained in circumferentially oriented muscle fibers at the equator
V_{CF}, V_{SE}, V_{CE}	contractile fiber, series elastic, and contractile element velocities, respectively, cm/sec
t	time of measurement, sec
Δt	time interval between recorded measurements, sec
A	area, cm^2
w	work per unit volume of muscle fiber, gm·cm/cm^3
E_{SE}	stored energy in series elastic per unit volume of muscle fiber, gm·cm/cm^3
η	efficiency

It has long been recognized that heart volume and ventricular shape are important variables in determining cardiac function in animals and man. These principles are part of the Frank-Starling mechanism for cardiac function (Sarnoff and Berglund, 1954) and LaPlace's Law of the heart (Burch *et al.*,

1952; Burton, 1957). The exact mechanisms that cause cardiac enlargement and hypertrophy in man still remain unclear. The purpose of this chapter is to review those mechanisms that are postulated to be associated with hypertrophy, and to present the latest methods available for assessing the effects of hypertrophy in the intact heart. It is clear that hypertrophy may be associated with gross changes in chamber size, shape, or wall thickness. Such changes may produce marked alterations in cardiac performance and its regulation when the heart is considered as a hydraulic pump or a shell of contracting muscle. In either case, it is important to realize that the heart is a part of the overall circulation and that hydraulic or muscle performance is altered by a variety of regulating mechanisms that affect peripheral resistance, venous return, and myocardial contractility (Gorlin and Sonnenblick, 1968).

Prolonged and persistant elevation of intracavitary pressure (hypertension, aortic stenosis) or flow (valvular insufficiency, severe anemia arteriovenous fistula) are regularly associated with hypertrophy. Pronounced hypertrophy is also known to occur in patients with coronary artery disease. Many cases have been reported in which hypertrophy has been present in the absence of clinical and postmortem evidence of increased cardiac work (Van Pennen and Geistl, 1962), as may be associated with mitral regurgitation resulting from cardiac dilatation or papillary muscle dysfunction. There is also ample evidence that patients with moderate aortic stenosis often have hearts with normal X-ray silhouettes, but have angiocardiographic and electrocardiographic indication of left ventricular hypertrophy.

Various causes have been postulated to explain the hypertrophy noted in these conditions. The LaPlace equation has been used by most investigators to relate chamber dimensions, pressure, and wall thickness to the force per unit cross-sectional area of muscle wall (Sandler and Dodge, 1963). An increase in ventricular pressure has been postulated as an important stimulus to hypertrophy by increasing the load that must be supported by the ventricular wall. Several groups of investigators have now calculated the average force per unit cross-sectional area of ventricular wall (stress) for subjects with heart disease of varied etiologies and have found similar values for various groups (Sandler and Dodge, 1963; Sandler and Ghista, 1969; Hood *et al.*, 1968). These findings suggest that hypertrophy is an adaptive mechanism, as suggested by Bohnenkamp (1929) and Linzbach (1960). It is postulated that an increase in mural force of contraction leads to an increase in wall thickness to maintain stress at some relatively fixed value.

Recent studies have demonstrated that a distinction must be made between an increased wall stress caused by change in size or shape and that caused by an elevated intracavitary pressure. For a given end-diastolic pressure, the principles of LaPlace's Law will explain an increase in wall stress by increasing chamber volume, changing shape (increase in wall curvature), or thinning of the ventricular wall. Such hearts are usually said to be "preloaded" or dilated and are regularly seen in situations associated with heart failure (increased end-systolic volume) or with an increase in end-diastolic volume such as may occur with valvular insufficiency or other conditions necessitating an increased stroke volume (without decrease in end-systolic volume). This situation will not explain hypertrophy in the undilated heart of a subject with aortic stenosis with a normal end-diastolic pressure. The heart in this latter condition must contain elevated wall forces resulting from the associated elevated systolic pressure that is generated.

More recently, investigators have determined force–velocity relationships for the pumping heart (Levine and Britman, 1964; Fry *et al.*, 1964; Ross *et al.*, 1966; Taylor *et al.*, 1967; Glick, 1965; Covell *et al.*, 1966). It has been found that at any instantaneous muscle length, there is a reciprocal relationship between stress or tension and the velocity of shortening, similar to that of isolated muscle. Many investigators have found difficulty in applying these approaches to the intact heart due to difficulties in extrapolating the force–velocity relationships to determine isometric force (P_o) and/or maximal velocity of contraction (V_{max}).

The technique of studying maximal peak ventricular pressure (P_{max}) as determined by complete aortic occlusion, has been used by several investigators as a means of assessing muscle performance before and after hypertrophy (Kramer and Northrup, 1964; Meerson and Pshennekova, 1965). Hawthorne has presented results of such studies elsewhere in this volume. The tension–time index (TTI) has also been used for these purposes. A higher TTI and P_{max} have been found regularly in the hypertrophied ventricle However, neither ventricular size and shape and not wall thickness have been documented in most studies, making it impossible to calculate wall forces or stress, or to assess the significance of these pressure rises with respect to chamber geometry. Furthermore, P_{max} has not been found to increase linearly with respect to muscle mass in hypertrophy, as commented upon by Badeer (1967). The role of rate of rise of intraventricular pressure (*dp/dt*) is discussed in the chapter by Mason *et al.*, pages 433–444. It will suffice here to state that Mason (1969) has been able to demonstrate *dp/dt* to be a measure of contractile state in animals and man. Change in preload or afterload (aortic root impedance) may cause significant alterations in a given subject, as may change in chamber size. In practice, *dp/dt* is used in a given patient for the assessment of directional changes in contractility associated with a known intervention (exercise or drug). Most investigators have not used *dp/dt* to compare responses for large groups of individuals or from patient to patient (Mason, 1969).

We shall now present a review of those techniques currently available for studying cardiac mechanics in the intact heart, with an emphasis directed toward newer methods that show promise for application to the intact hypertrophied heart. From the material presented above, it is clear that further work is necessary to document the dynamic geometry of the hypertrophied hearts, determine the material properties of hypertrophied muscle and obtain the force–velocity–length relationships for the intact hypertrophied ventricle.

Determination of Ventricular Size and Wall Thickness

Gauer and Wieckert (1944) and later Rushmer and Thal (1951) were the first to report qualitative studies of ventricular dimensions in experimental animals. The first reports of ventricular volume in man were presented by Dodge and Tannenbaum (1956), Arvidsson (1958), and Chapman *et al.* (1958). The methods presently used for determining ventricular dimensions in animals range from the use of mercury-in-silastic strain gauges to implanted beads or screws (Mitchell *et al.*, 1969; Hinds *et al.*, 1969). Radiographic methods are by far the most frequently used techniques for measuring volume and dimensions in man (Dodge *et al.*, 1966).

The complex configuration of the internal cardiac chambers of the heart precludes accurate computation of chamber dimensions or volume without simplifying assumptions. It has been assumed for these purposes that the heart chambers can be represented as a sphere, cylinder, or ellipse. In human subjects such analog models have been applied to measurements obtained from single or biplane angiographic or cineangiographic films. Figure 1 is an illustration of ventricular dimensions and pressure obtained from a cineangiocardiographic study in a subject with valvular insufficiency and an increased left ventricular mass. Measurements such as these can now be used to determine ventricular mass and to quantify the degree of left ventricular hypertrophy in patients with heart disease as demonstrated by Rackley *et al.* (1964) and Kennedy *et al.* (1967). The detailed use of these methods is presented elsewhere in this volume. Wall thickness has now been measured by several techniques in intact animals (Hawthorne, 1966; Mitchell *et al.*, 1969; Feigl and Fry, 1964). Change in wall thickness during the cardiac cycle has ranged from 30% to 75% in these studies. Similar changes have been determined from angiocardiographic measurements when calculated ventricular mass has remained constant from diastole to systole (Sandler and Ghista, 1969; Bunnell *et al.*, 1968; Hugenholtz, 1969). To date, there is no evidence that chamber dimensions other than wall thickness are inappropriate for the hypertrophied heart. Studies of chest-wall motion and chamber motion during the heart cycle show characteristic abnormalities for the hypertrophied heart as reported by Deliyannis *et al.* (1964) and Sandler and Dodge (1968).

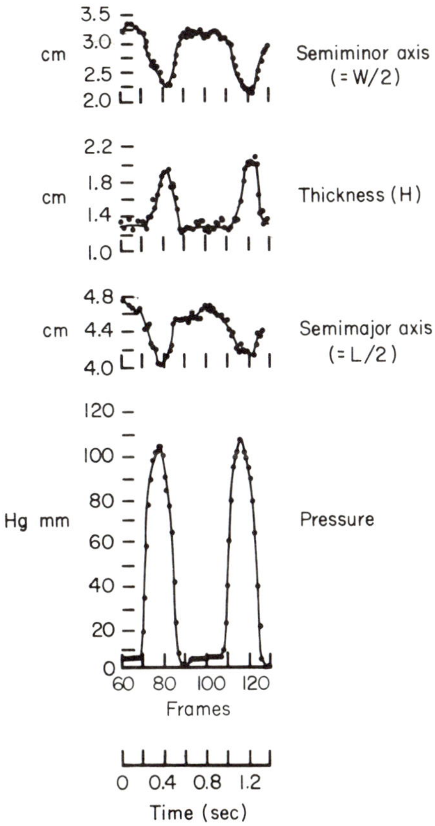

FIG. 1. Variations of the dimensions of the left ventricle during the cardiac cycle of a patient.

Determination of Ventricular Wall Stresses

The wall of the intact ventricle differs from isolated strips of cardiac muscle in that it possesses a finite curvature, thickness, and fibers of varying orientations. The application of LaPlace's principle to the heart recognizes the importance of size and shape in determining the force operating within the ventricular wall, as discussed above.

The myocardium is subject to stresses owing to the transmural pressure acting upon it during systole and diastole. The stresses during systole originate from active contraction of the muscles against the load presented by the impedance of the peripheral circulation starting with that of the aorta and the inertia of the blood in the ventricular chamber. The stress during diastole originates from the distention of the elastic components of the heart wall as a result of the blood filling the ventricular chamber and that forced into the ventricle by the contraction of the atria.

Two wall stresses which may be readily derived from ventricular pressure and chamber dimensions are the average meridional stress and the average hoop stress at the equator of the heart.

The average meridional stress, which is the force per unit area acting at midplane of the heart in the direction of the apex to base length, may be derived simply by equating the meridional wall forces to the pressure loading, assuming that the ventricle is a surface of revolution (Fig. 2).

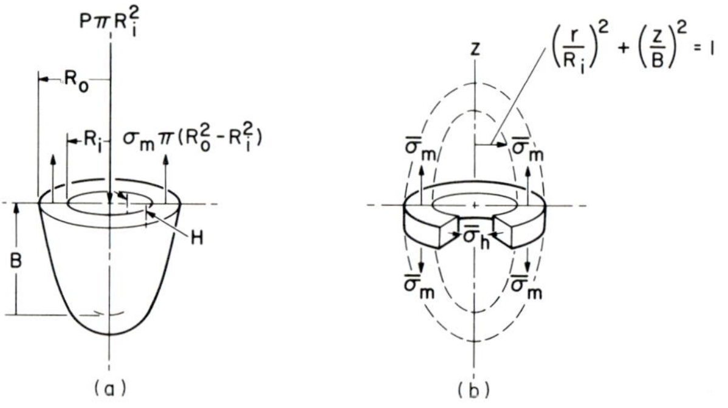

FIG. 2. Forces, stresses, and dimensions, left ventricle model.

Mathematically, this equilibrium condition may be written as

$$\sum F_m = \bar{\sigma}_m \pi (R_o^2 - R_i^2) - P\pi R_i^2 = 0 \tag{1}$$

Rearranging Eq. (1) gives

$$\bar{\sigma}_m = PR_i^2/(R_o^2 - R_i^2) \tag{2}$$

or in terms of wall thickness,

$$\bar{\sigma}_m = PR_i/2H(1 + H/2R_i) \tag{3}$$

The average hoop stress, which is the force per unit area in the circumferential direction, is not so easily derived, because it varies from station to station from the apex to the base of the heart [Fig. 2(b)]. In order to estimate this stress, a particular geometric shape must be assumed for the ventricle. Spherical and ellipsoidal shapes have been assumed by investigators for these purposes. Although these shapes have been demonstrated to be inexact representations of the left ventricle in experimental animals (Hawthorne 1966; Gribbe *et al.* (1959), this is not the case for man (Sandler and Dodge, 1968).

The major axis of the ellipsoid is taken to equal the inner radius measured at the midplane of the heart. Based on these assumptions, the average hoop stress, neglecting radial shear stresses, may be derived from a modified form of LaPlace's Law. The pressure loading on any elemental area of a shell must be equilibrated by the normal components of the hoop and meridional stresses acting upon the element.

From Fig. 3 it can be seen that this equilibrium condition may be expressed

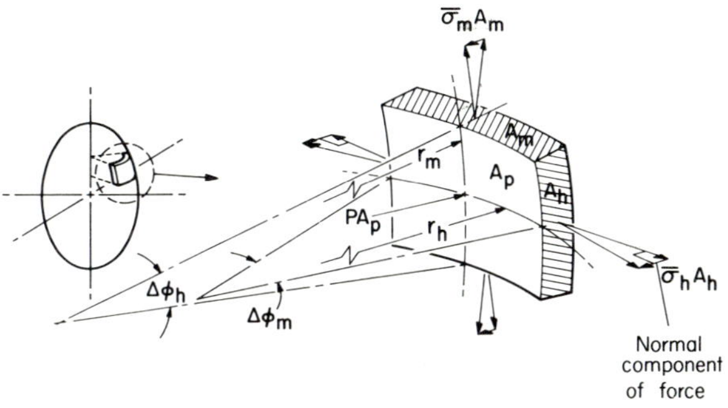

FIG. 3. Force equilibrium on elemental volume of myocardium.

mathematically as

$$PA_P = 2\,(\bar{\sigma}_m A_m\,\Delta\phi_m/2) + 2\,(\bar{\sigma}_h A_h\,\Delta\phi_h/2) \tag{4}$$

where

$$\begin{aligned} A_P &= (r_m \Delta\phi_m)(r_h \Delta\phi_h) \\ A_m &= (r_m + H/2)\Delta\phi_m H \\ A_p &= (r_h + H/2)\Delta\phi_h H \end{aligned} \tag{5}$$

by substuting Eq. (5) into Eq. (4) and then rearranging, a modified form of LaPlace's Law for thin-walled shells is obtained:

$$\frac{\bar{\sigma}_m}{r_m}\left(\frac{r_h + H/2}{r_h}\right) + \frac{\bar{\sigma}_h}{r_h}\left(\frac{r_m + H/2}{r_m}\right) = \frac{P}{H} \tag{6}$$

This modified form of LaPlace's Law has been developed to replace the traditional thin-walled equations employed by many investigators (Sandler and Ghista, 1969; Levine and Britman, 1964; Covell *et al.*, 1966). Mirsky (1969) and Sandler and Ghista (1969) pointed out previously that thin-walled equations can lead to errors in calculating stress on the order of 40% to 100% for thick shells. By comparing Eq. (6) with LaPlace's original equation,

$$\sigma_m/r_m + \sigma_h/r_h = P/H \tag{7}$$

The effective radii of curvatures for a thick-walled shell are given by

$$(r_m)_{\text{eff}} = r_m\,[(r_h/(r_h + H/2)] = a_m r_m$$

$$(r_h)_{\text{eff}} = r_h[(r_m/(r_m + H/2)] = a_h r_h \tag{8}$$

where

$$a_m = [r_h/(r_h + H/2)] \quad \text{and} \quad a_h = [r_m/(r_m + H/2)]$$

are actually less than either the midwall or inner radii of curvature, since

$$a_m, a_h < 1$$

These equations explain the error that results if midwall or inner radii are used to calculate average wall stress for a thick-walled shell.

Equation (9) represents the expressions for the radii of curvature at the equator of the ellipsoid (Sandler and Dodge, 1969). If these equations

$$r_h\Big|_{z=0} = R_i\sqrt{1 + \left[\left(\frac{R_i}{B}\right)^2 - 1\right]\left(\frac{Z}{B}\right)^2}\Bigg|_{z=0} = R_i$$

$$r_m\Big|_{z=0} = \left(\frac{B}{R_i}\right)^2 \frac{r_h^{\,3}}{R_i^{\,2}}\Bigg|_{z=0} = \left(\frac{B}{R_i}\right)^2 R_i \tag{9}$$

and Eq. (3) for average meridional stress are substituted into Eq. (6), the following equation is obtained for the average hoop stress at the equator:

$$\bar{\sigma}_h = \frac{PR_i}{H}\left[\frac{1}{1 + (H/2R_i)\left(\dfrac{R_i}{B}\right)^2}\right]\left[1 - \frac{1}{2}\left(\frac{R_i}{B}\right)^2\right] \tag{10}$$

or

$$\bar{\sigma}_h = (PR_i/H)a_h[1 - \tfrac{1}{2}(R_i/B)^2] \tag{11}$$

Equations (3)–(10) are exact equations for the average meridional and hoop stresses at the equator, assuming that bending moments and shear stresses may be neglected. Equation (3) has previously been given in the literature by Sandler and Dodge (1963) and Mirsky (1969); however, Eq. (10), derived from an exact-force balance on an element of volume, has not been previously presented. Both of these equations necessarily are in exact agreement with thick-wall theories which are based on the same assumptions of negligible shear stresses and bending moments such as those developed by Wong and Rautaharju (1968) and Ghista and Sandler (1969).

Although the present theory has its limitations, its simplicity and kinship with the well-understood and documented basic law of LaPlace should render it a valuable tool in studies concerned with the assessment of myocardial performance. When sarcomere structures and fiber orientation are to be correlated with stress patterns, the considerably more complex equations for estimating local stresses may be obtained from the articles of Mirsky (1969), Ghista and Sandler (1969), and Wong and Rautaharju (1968). It should be appreciated that, in general, a complete stress–strain distribution of the myocardium may be analytically obtained only when (1) the geometry of the ventricle may be exactly described, (2) constitutive equations accounting for the nonhomogeneity, anisotropy, and large deformations during the passive and active states can be determined, and (3) the exact boundary conditions or stresses and displacement can be established. The constitution of the ventricle, involving complex patterns and interstitial arrangements of arteries, veins, capillaries, muscle fibers, Purkinje fibers, nerves, trabeculae carnae, and connective tissues renders these determinations formidable if not impossible at the present time.

Contraction Velocities

In relating the gross dynamic characteristics of the intact heart to the characteristics of isolated muscle fibers, it is important to determine the series elastic and contractile element velocities. Changes in the velocity of these elements will be used to assess the state of contractility of the active fibers of the heart during systole (Levine and Britman, 1964; Fry *et al.*, 1964; Ross *et al.*, 1966; Taylor *et al.*, 1967; Glick, 1965; Covell *et al.*, 1966). Equations for estimating these velocities from ventricular dimensional and pressure measurements derive from the following assumptions.

(1) The heart is an ellipsoid of revolution.

(2) The net effect of the distribution of orientations of muscle fibers across the heart wall of the equator is equivalent to a series of circumferentially oriented muscle fibers at the same location where the wall thickness and circumference are measured.

(3) The parallel elastic element in the Hill model of muscle fiber makes a negligible contribution to the instantaneous stress during systole (Hill, 1949).

From Fig. 4, the length of the midwall circumference at the equator is the

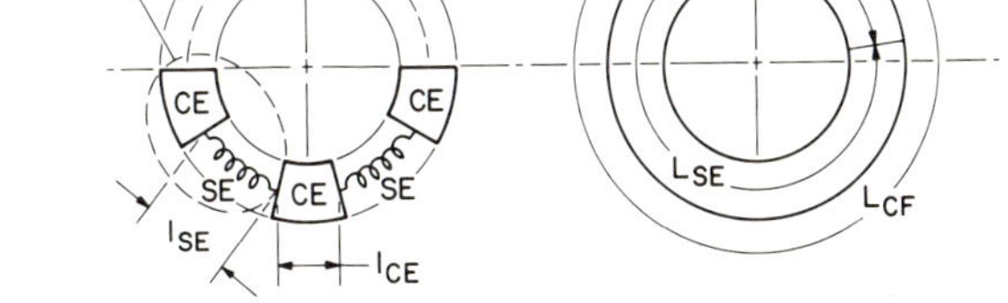

FIG. 4. Model of circumferential muscle fibers at equator of heart.

sum of the lengths of the individual contractile elements and the series elastic springs:

$$L_{CF} = nl_{CE} + nl_{SE} \tag{12}$$

where L_{CF} is the circumferential fiber length, n is the number of sarcomeres and l_{SE}, l_{CE} are the respective lengths of the series elastic spring and the contractile element. The circumferential fiber length is taken to be the mean of the epi- and endocardial circumference as calculated from measurements of the outer circumference and the wall thickness at the equator of the heart.

Differentiating Eq. (12) with respect to time yields a kinematical expression relating circumferential fiber velocity of shortening (V_{CF}), contractile element velocity (V_{CE}), and sereis elastic velocity (V_{SE}):

$$V_{CF} = nV_{CE} + nV_{SE} \tag{13}$$

in which V_{CF}, V_{CE}, $V_{SE} < 0$ imply shortening of the circumference, the series elastic elements, and the contractile elements, respectively.

By determining the circumferential velocity from measurements of circumferential radius and wall thickness and determining the series elastic velocity from a Hill model using the instantaneous measured stress, Eq. (13) may be used to calculate the contractile element velocity (V_{CE}).

First, the circumferential velocity is calculated by using a finite difference representation of the time derivative of the midwall circumference:

$$V_{CF}(t) = [L_{CF}(t + \Delta t) - L_{CF}(t - \Delta t)]/2\Delta t \tag{14}$$

The series elastic velocity may then be calculated from the time rate of change of the average hoop stress in the heart wall and the stiffness of the series elastic component in Hill's model. By the chain rule of the basic calculus, V_{SE} is given by

$$V_{SE} = (d\bar{\sigma}h/dt)/(d\bar{\sigma}h/dl_{SE}) \tag{15}$$

where $\bar{\sigma}_h$ is given by Eq. (11). The time derivative of $\bar{\sigma}_h$ appearing in Eq. (11) is calculated either by using the same finite difference representation as for V_{CF} or by first mathematically differentiating Eq. (10) with respect to time, and then evaluating the terms involving pressure with the electronically measured value of dP/dt and the term involving dimensions by finite differences. The two alternatives may be written, respectively, as

$$d\bar{\sigma}_h/dt = [\bar{\sigma}_h(t + \Delta t) - \bar{\sigma}_h(t - \Delta t)]/2\Delta t \tag{16a}$$

or

$$d\bar{\sigma}_h/dt = (dP/dt)F(t) + P[F(t + \Delta t) - F(t - \Delta t)]/2\Delta t \tag{16b}$$

where

$$F(t) = (R_i/H)a_h[1 - \tfrac{1}{2}(R_i/B)^2]$$

The relationship between stress and deformation of the series elastic component is assumed to be the same as that obtained from systolic quick release experiments on isolated cat papillary muscle for which recent experiments by Hefner and Bowen (1967) give

$$\bar{\sigma}_h = 19[e^{34(L_{CF}/L_o - 1.02)} - 1] \tag{17}$$

where L_o is the resting length at barely detectable stresses or equivalently, in the intact heart, diastolic pressure.

Substituting Eq. (12) for the circumferential fiber length expressed in terms of contractile and series elastic lengths, Eq. (17) becomes

$$\bar{\sigma}_h = 19[e^{34((nl_{SE} + nl_{CE})/L_o - 1.02)} - 1] \tag{18}$$

Differentiating Eq. (18) with respect to the series elastic element length yields the stiffness of the element

$$d\bar{\sigma}_h/dl_{SE} = (34n/L_o)19\ e^{34((nl_{SE} + nl_{CE})/L_o - 1.02)} \tag{19}$$

A more convenient form for evaluating the stiffness at a particular stress is obtained by eliminating the common exponential term appearing in Eqs. (18) and (19) which gives

$$d\bar{\sigma}_h/dl_{SE} = (34n/L_o)(\bar{\sigma}_h + 19) \tag{20}$$

One very important consideration to the validity of this stiffness formula is whether or not area changes were accounted for in its emperical development, a point which is not clear in the paper of Hefner and Bowen (1967). Assuming that it has not been taken into account, its influence on stiffness can easily be evaluated by considering that the muscle is incompressible, i.e.,

$$\text{Volume} = L_o A_o = L_{CF} A = \text{Constant} \tag{21}$$

then the actual stress, $\bar{\sigma}_h'$ existing at a given length would be given by

$$\sigma_h' = (A_o/A)\bar{\sigma}_h \tag{22}$$

or by substituting Eq. (21):

$$\bar{\sigma}_h' = (L_{CF}/L_o)\bar{\sigma}_h = [((nl_{SE} + nl_{CE})/L_o)]\bar{\sigma}_h \tag{23}$$

Differentiating Eq. (23) with respect to l_{SE} yields:

$$d\bar{\sigma}_h'/dl_{SE} = n\bar{\sigma}_h/L_o + (L_{CF}/L_o)/d\bar{\sigma}_h/dl_{SE} \tag{24}$$

Substituting Eqs. (20)–(22) for $(d\bar{\sigma}_h/dl_S l)$ and $\bar{\sigma}_h$, respectively, in terms of the actual stress gives

$$d\bar{\sigma}_h'/dl_{SE} = (34n/L_o)[(L_o/34L_{CF} + 1)\bar{\sigma}_h' + 19(L_{CF}/L_o)] \tag{25}$$

Using this as a model of fibers at the equator, Eq. (25) demonstrates that the maximum change of stiffness for a normal heart beat including area change, will be on the order of 5%. During isovolumic systole $L_{CF} \simeq L_o$ $(L_o/34L_{CF} + 1) \simeq 1.03$, this could result at best in a 3% correction, and virtually no correction would result from the term, 19.0 L_{CF}/L_o. During systole, the midwall circumference in the above formlas experiences a much similar change (usually 5–10%) compared to changes in the inner wall circumference (as much as 20%). Since the terms in the stiffness formula tend to negate each other, corrections for area in this model will make a negligible difference in the calculations. However, it would be appropriate for investigators studying isolated muscle mechanics to clarify their definitions of stress since large deformations and area changes are involved in normal muscle contractions.

Since the influence of area changes on stiffness are small in this model, the velocity of the contractile element is expressed in terms of the somewhat simple formula for stiffness which does not account for area changes. The substitution of Eqs. (15) and (20) into Eq. (13) yields the following expression for contractile element velocity:

$$nV_{CE} = V_{CF} - L_o(d\bar{\sigma}_h/dt)/34(\bar{\sigma}_h + 19) \tag{26}$$

Of course, the average number of individual sarcomeres contained in the circumference of a length of isolated muscle fiber is not actually known and therefore results generally given in the units of cm/sec or mm/sec are apparently not consistent (Levine and Britman, 1964; Fry *et al.*, 1964; Ross *et al.*, 1966; Taylor *et al.*, 1967; Glick, 1965; and Covell *et al.*, 1966). By making the reasonable assumption that the number of elements is proportional to some reference length of the muscle fiber, preferably L_o, Eq. (26) is normalized with respect to this length, which should tend to make the results in intact dogs as well as isolated muscle preparations consistent in magnitude:

$$\overline{\overline{V}}_{CE} = nV_{CE}/L_o = V_{CF}/L_o - (d\bar{\sigma}_h/dt)/34(\bar{\sigma}_h + 19) \tag{27}$$

where $\overline{\overline{V}}_{CE}$ is the contractile element velocity in muscle circumferences or lengths per unit time.

The effects of the parallel elastic component on the calculated values of the velocities of the contractile and series elastic elements can be easily determined from experimental measurements of ventricular pressure and dimensions as demonstrated for isolated muscle by Hefner and Bowen (1967). By considering the diagram of the model of the circumferential fibers including the parallel elastic components (Fig. 5), it is recognized that the difference between it and the first model (Fig. 1) is that some of the load is now carried by the parallel elastic element.

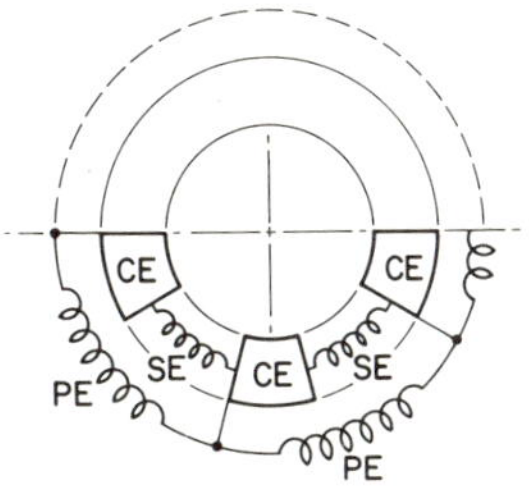

FIG. 5. Hill's model with parallel elastic component.

Mathematically,

$$\bar{\sigma}_h = \bar{\sigma}_h(\mathrm{PE}) + \bar{\sigma}_h(\mathrm{SE}) \tag{28}$$

Differentiating with respect to time and rearranging Eq. (28) gives

$$(d\bar{\sigma}_h/dt)(\mathrm{SE}) = d\bar{\sigma}_h/dt - (d\bar{\sigma}_h/dt)(\mathrm{PE}) \tag{29}$$

Now the previous Eq. (15) for the series elastic velocity becomes

$$nV_{\mathrm{SE}} = [(d\bar{\sigma}_h/dt) - (d\bar{\sigma}_h/dt)(\mathrm{PE})]/(d\bar{\sigma}_h/dl)(\mathrm{SE}) \tag{30}$$

In addition to the kinematic equation relating V_{CF}, V_{CE}, and V_{SE}, which applies to both models, another kinematical equation can be written relating V_{PE} and V_{CF}, which enables one to conveniently account for $(d\sigma_h/dt)(\mathrm{PE})$ appearing in Eq. (30). The total length of the parallel elastic components equals the length of the muscle fiber; thus,

$$V_{\mathrm{CF}} = nV_{\mathrm{PE}} \tag{31}$$

By the chain rule of elementary calculus $(d\bar{\sigma}_h/dt)(\mathrm{PE})$ may now be written as

$$(d\bar{\sigma}_h/dt)(\mathrm{PE}) = (V_{\mathrm{CF}}/n)/(d\bar{\sigma}_h/dl)(\mathrm{PE}) \tag{32}$$

The velocity of the series elastic may now be written in terms of known physical quantities. Substituting Eq. (32) into Eq. (30) gives

$$nV_{\mathrm{SE}} = n(d\bar{\sigma}_h/dt)/d\bar{\sigma}_h/dl(\mathrm{SE}) - V_{\mathrm{CF}}(d\bar{\sigma}_h/dl)(\mathrm{PE})/(d\bar{\sigma}_h/dl)(\mathrm{SE}) \tag{33}$$

From this equation, it can be seen that as one might expect, the parallel elastic does not affect nV_{SE} during an isometric contraction ($V_{\mathrm{CF}} = 0$) but during auxotonic or isotonic contractions, the inclusion of this component serves to augment nV_{SE}, which would normally be assumed to be zero in this latter case.

Substituting Eq. (33) into the kinematical Eq. (13) relating V_{CF}, V_{CE}, and V_{SE} gives the following expression for contractile element velocity:

$$nV_{CE} = V_{CF}[1 + (d\bar{\sigma}_h/dt)(\mathrm{PE})/(d\bar{\sigma}_h/dt)(\mathrm{SE})] - n(d\bar{\sigma}_h/dt)/(d\bar{\sigma}/dt)(\mathrm{SE}) \quad (34)$$

The only difference between the Eq. (34) for V_{CE} and Eq. (26), neglecting the parallel elastic elements, is the first term including a ratio of stiffnesses. As in the case of the series elastic velocity, there is no correction during isometric contraction, whereas during isotonic of auxtonic contraction the effect is to give higher values for contractile element velocities then obtained from Eq. (26). Correction for this overestimation would depend on the magnitude of the preload when studying isolated muscle preparation or end-diastolic pressure in the intact heart. The ratio of stiffness may be expressed as

$$(d\bar{\sigma}_h/dl)(\mathrm{PE})/(d\bar{\sigma}_h/dl)(\mathrm{SE}) = (K_{PE}/K_{SE})[\bar{\sigma}_h(\mathrm{PE}) + C(\mathrm{PE})]/\bar{\sigma}_h(\mathrm{SE}) + C(\mathrm{SE})] \quad (35)$$

where K and C, are constants of the stress-deformation relationships. When end-diastolic pressure is normal, or the preload is light, σ_h(PE) is much smaller than σ_h(SE) and the need for correction may be neglected. In a typical case, $K_{PE} \simeq K_{SE}$; $C(\mathrm{PE}) = 10$ gm/cm^2; $C(\mathrm{SE}) = 20$ gm/cm^2; $\bar{\sigma}_h(\mathrm{PE}) = 5$ gm/cm^2; and $\bar{\sigma}_h(\mathrm{SE}) = 200$ gm/cm^2. If the contractile element velocity at the beginning of systolic ejection is calculated from these values, the use of a ratio of stiffness results in a 10% correction in V_{CE}. For the intact heart, such corrections can be included in the calculations provided a resting length tension curve is established. Once this is accomplished, the hoop stress associated with the series elastic component can be obtained by subtracting the parallel elastic component of the total hoop stress from the total hoop stress. This latter adjusted hoop stress is then used to calculate the velocities of the contractile and series elastic elements. The outstanding unknown which cannot be easily determined for the intact heart is the stress–strain relationship of the series elastic component.

Power, Work, Mechanical Efficiency

The totality of the contractile elements in the myocardial wall serve as the prime mover or energy source for the purpose of pumping blood from the left ventricle against the load presented by the circulatory system.

The series elastic elements connecting the contractile elements serve a very important function as the transmission of energy which enables the prime mover to be matched with the load from moment during the systolic phase of the heart cycle. When the load is too great for the heart wall to follow the contraction of the sarcomere, the series elastic elements store energy and elongate, thereby developing force and correspondingly ventricular pressure to match the load resisting the displacement.

When the blood is moving more rapidly than the sarcomeres tend to contract, the series elastic elements proceed to shorten and release energy and thereby assist in the maintenance of pressure in the ventricle.

From the contraction velocities and stresses derived from ventricular dimensional and pressure measurements, several energy quantities can be derived which serve as useful indices of the heart's performance. These quantities indicate answers to questions which logically follow from considering the heart as a prime mover-transmission-pumping system.

(1) How much work is available per cardiac cycle to pump blood from the heart?

(2) Of the work available, how much actually delivered to the blood in a cycle?

(3) Of the energy stored in the series elastic element, how much it is recovered during its period of recoil?

Energy quantities serving to answer these questions are respectively, the work of contractile element shortening, the work of circumferential fiber shortening, and the energy stored in the series elastic element, all on a per unit volume of muscle fiber basis (Britman and Levine, 1964). However, it must be emphasized that these quantities can only serve as indices of the answers to the questions posed. In addition to work and energy storage associated with the hoop stress, there is work and energy storage associated with the meridional stress which cannot be readily accounted for by the simplified model of circumferential fibers at the equator. An estimate of this work and energy is obtained from the pressure and radial displacement at the equator.

A relationship between the power or the time rate at which work is being done is obtained simply by multiplying the equation relating to contractile velocities by the hoop stress:

$$\bar{\sigma}_h V_{\mathrm{CF}}/L_{\mathrm{CF}} = \bar{\sigma}_h n V_{\mathrm{CE}}/L_{\mathrm{CF}} + \bar{\sigma}_h n V_{\mathrm{SE}}/L_{\mathrm{CF}} \tag{36}$$

where dividing by L_{CF} places all quantities on a per unit volume of muscle fiber basis, $\bar{\sigma}_h V_{\mathrm{CF}}/L_{\mathrm{CF}}$ is the power per unit volume of circumferential fibers which is being delivered to the blood in the ventricle (or to distort the myocardial wall during the isovolumic phase), $\bar{\sigma}_h V_{\mathrm{CE}}/L_{\mathrm{CF}}$ is the power per unit volume of circumferential fibers being delivered by the contractile elements, and $\bar{\sigma}_h n V_{\mathrm{SE}}/L_{\mathrm{CF}}$ is the rate of energy storage per unit volume of circumferential fibers in the series of elastic elements.

Now, the work per unit volume from the beginning of isovolumic contraction ($t = 0$) to any instant of time during systole may be obtained by integrating the Eq. (36) for power with respect to time:

$$\int_0^t \frac{\bar{\sigma}_h V_{\text{CF}}}{L_{\text{CF}}}\,dt = \int_0^t \frac{\bar{\sigma}_h n V_{\text{CE}}}{L_{\text{CF}}}\,dt + \int_0^t \frac{\bar{\sigma}_h n V_{\text{SE}}}{L_{\text{CF}}}\,dt$$

circumferential fiber work per unit volume of muscle fiber (w_{CF})	contractile element work per unit volume of muscle fiber (w_{CE})	energy stored in the series elastic elements per unit volume of muscle fibers (ΔE_{SE})

The evaluation of W_{CF} and W_{CE} requires numerical integration of the integrals and may be accomplished using the following algorithm based on the trapezoid rule:

$$w(t) = w(t - \Delta t) + (\Delta t/2)/[\sigma_h(t)V(t)/L_{\text{CF}}(t) + \sigma_h(t - \Delta t)V(t - \Delta t)/L_{\text{CF}}(t - \Delta t)] \qquad (38)$$

As pointed out in the section dealing with wall stresses, the midwall circumference experiences a very small change over the period of systole (5% or less) and therefore in evaluating Eq. (36) it is reasonable to assume $L_{\text{CF}} \cong L_o$. This assumption allows the energy stored in the series elastic (ΔE_{SE}) to be evaluated analytically. Substituting the term for V_{SE} given in Eq. (26) into the expression for ΔE_{SE} gives:

$$\Delta E_{\text{SE}} = \int_0^t \frac{\bar{\sigma}_h \cancel{L_o}\, d\bar{\sigma}_h / \cancel{dt}\, \cancel{dt}}{\cancel{L_o} 34(\bar{\sigma}_h + 19)} \qquad (39)$$

and then carrying out the indicated integration gives

$$\Delta E_{\text{SE}} = \frac{\bar{\sigma}_h(t) - \bar{\sigma}_h(o)}{34} - (19/34)LN\left(\frac{\bar{\sigma}_h(t) + 19}{\bar{\sigma}_h(o) + 19}\right) \qquad (40)$$

Now the overall mechanical efficiency of the prime mover-transmission-pump system would be the ratio of the mechanical work done by circumferential fiber shortening to the work made available by contractile element shortening:

$$\eta_{\text{mech.}} = W_{\text{CF}}/W_{\text{CE}} \qquad (41)$$

And of course, $1 - \eta_{\text{mech.}}$ would be the fraction of the available energy dissipatedafter end ejection as the series elastic and contractile element return to their initial states.

Another ratio of interest is the percentage of energy stores in the series elastic up to peak systolic stress which is recovered as useful work during the recoil period of ejection. The following analytical expression may be written for the efficiency of recoil:

$$\eta_{\text{recoil}} = [\Delta E(\bar{\sigma}_{h_{\max}}) - \Delta E(\bar{\sigma}_h \text{ES})]/\Delta E(\bar{\sigma}_{h_{\max}}) \tag{42}$$

or by substituting Eq. (40):

$$\eta_{\text{recoil}} = 1 - \frac{(\bar{\sigma}_h(\text{ES}) - \bar{\sigma}_h(o) - 19LN\,[(\bar{\sigma}_h(\text{ES}) + 19)/(\bar{\sigma}_h(o) + 19)]}{\bar{\sigma}_{h_{\max}} - \bar{\sigma}_h(o) - 19LN\,[(\bar{\sigma}_{h_{\max}} + 19)/(\bar{\sigma}_h(o) + 19)]} \tag{43}$$

An estimate of the total work per unit volume of circumferential fiber at the equator can be made based on the ventricular pressure. Considering a circumferential ring at the circumference of unit height, the differential work done would be

$$dW_T = P\,dv = P\,2\pi R_i\,dR_i \tag{44}$$

dividing by the corresponding volume of the circumferential fibers

$$dw_T = P2\pi R_i\,dR_i/L_{\text{CF}}H = PL_i\,dL_i/2\pi L_{\text{CF}}H \tag{45}$$

or integrating with respect to L_i

$$w_T \cong \int \frac{PL_i\,dL_i}{L_{\text{CF}}H2\pi} \tag{46}$$

This equation must be numerically integrated by the algorithm given in Eq. (38).

Whole-Heart Geometry and Energy Quantities

Although the response of the myocardium to various inotropic interventions can best be understood in terms of the stress–velocity–length relationship of its muscle fibers, the extent to which the heart is satisfying its overall function as a positive displacement pump forcing blood through the circulatory system is best measured by physical quantities related to the whole left ventricle—internal volume, stroke volume, ejection fraction, flow rate, power, stroke work, flow work, filling work and cardiac work (Franklin *et al.*, 1962). When applied to the human left ventricle these estimates are based on the assumption that the endocardial surface can be represented by an ellipsoid of revolution.

Formulas have been presented and derived in this article which permit the calculation of variables involved in the various methods used to assess left ventricular contractility and performance. The derivation of these formulas have been based on three major assumptions.

(1) The internal volume of the heart can be approximated as an ellipsoid of revolution.

(2) The wall thickness of the heart is uniform around the midplane.

(3) The circumferentially oriented muscle fibers prevail in the determination of dimensional changes at the midplane of the heart.

Undoubtedly, these assumptions place some limitation on the degree of accuracy of the physical quantities calculated. However, very often in assessing the performance of the heart, the most important concerns are the consistency with which a given calculation or measurement can be made and the degree to which they correlate with the actual values.

With regard to the use of the various variables, measured and derived, it should be appreciated that there are basically only two sets of independent variables for characterizing the heart's performance. For the basic macroscopic unit of the heart, the muscle fibers, the primary variables are stress (or tension), length and velocity and for the whole left ventricle, the primary variables are pressure, volume and rate of change of volume. At a particular level of observation, all other variables may be derived from these more basic quantities—power, work, etc. Further, there exists a geometric transformation which relates corresponding variables in each of these sets. This idea is simply illustrated by the relationships herein derived between pressure and the average wall stresses [Eqs. (3)–(10)] and between internal volume and internal dimensional changes.

Ventricular hypertrophy is a common feature of heart disease. It is possible to assess the appropriateness of such changes by using the methods outlined in this study. As pointed out by Dodge (1968), an increased mass is correlated with an increased stroke work, increased end-diastolic volume and increased left ventricular oxygen consumption in patients with chronic heart disease. Pugh *et al.* (1964) have also uniformly demonstrated for such subjects an increased ventricular mass in relationship to a low work efficiency and increased total oxygen consumption. It appears at present, as stated by Dodge (1968), that one of the best gauges for the appropriateness for hypertrophy is the relationship of the increase in muscle weight to the work that the ventricle must perform. Myocardial failure in these terms would be a state of relative or absolute excess of muscle for the required work load.

References

Arvidsson, H. (1958). *Circulation* **18,** 1958.

Badeer, H. S. (1967). *Amer. Heart J.* **73,** 693.

Bohnenkamp, H. (1929). *Klin. Wochschr.* **8,** 433.

Britman, N. A., and Levine, H. J. (1964). *J. Clin. Invest.* **43,** 1397.

Bunnell, I. L., Shapiro, S. H., Falsetti, H. L., Grant, C., and Green, D. G. (1968). *Circulation* **38,** VI-3.

Burch, G. E., Ray, C. T., and Cronvich, B. S. (1952). *Circulation* **5,** 504.

Burton, A. C. (1957). *Amer. Heart J.* **54,** 801.

Chapman, C. B., Baker, O., Reynolds, J., and Bonte, F. J. (1958). *Circulation* **18,** 1105.
Covell, J. W., Ross, J., Jr., Sonnenblick, E. H., and Braunwald, E. (1966). *Circ. Res.* **19,** 364.
Deliyannis, A. A., Gillam, P. M., and Mousey, J. P. (1964). *Brit. Heart J.* **26,** 396.
Dodge, H. T., and Tannenbaum, H. L. (1956). *Circulation* **14,** 927.
Doge, H. T., Sandler, H., Baxley, W. A., and Hawley, R. R. (1966). *Amer. J. Cardiol.* **18,** 10.
Dodge, H. T. (1968). *Ann. Int. Med.* **69,** 941.
Feigl, E. O., and Fry, D. L. (1964). *Circ. Res.* **14,** 541.
Franlin, O. L., Van Citters, R. L., and Rushmer, R. F. (1962). *Circ. Res.* **71,** 702.
Fry, D. L., Griggs, D. M., Jr., and Greenfield, J. G., Jr. (1964). *Circulation Res.* **14,** 73.
Gauer, O., and Wieckert, H. (1944). *Luftfahrtmed.*, IX, 121, as cited by O. Gauer, German Aviation Medicine, World War II, V. 1, p. 565 (1950).
Ghista, D. N., and Sandler, H. (1969). *J. Biomech.* **2,** 35.
Glick, G. E. (1965). *J. Clin. Invest.* **44,** 978.
Gorlin, R., and Sonnenblick, E. H. (1968). *Amer. J. Cardiol.* **22,** 16.
Gribbe, P., Hirvonen, L., Lind, J., and Wegelius, C. (1959). *Cardiologia* **34,** 348.
Hawthorne, E. W. (1966). *Amer. J. Cardiol.* **18,** 566.
Hefner, L. L., and Bowen, T. E., Jr. (1967). *Amer. J. Physiol.* **212,** 1331.
Hill, A. V. (1949). *Proc. Roy. Soc. (London), Ser. B.* **136,** 399.
Hinds, J. E., Hawthorne, E. W., Mullins, C. B., and Mitchell, J. H. (1969). *Fed. Proc. Fed. Amer. Soc. Exp. Biol.* **28,** 1351.
Hood, W. J., Jr., Rackley, C. E., and Rolett, E. L. (1968). *Amer. J. Cardiol.* **22,** 550.
Hugenholtz, P. G. (1969). *Amer. Heart J.* **7,** 513.
Kennedy, J. W., Reichenbach, D. D., Baxley, W. A., and Dodge, H. T. (1967). *Amer. J. Cardiol.* **19,** 221.
Kramer, B., and Northrup, D. W. (1964). *Fed. Proc. Fed. Amer. Soc. Exp. Biol.* **23,** 358.
Levine, H. R., and Britman, N. A. (1964). *J. Clin. Invest.* **43,** 1383.
Linzbach, A. J. (1960). *Amer. J. Cardiol.* **5,** 370.
Mason, D. T. (1969). *Amer. J. Cardiol.* **23,** 516.
Meerson, F. Z., and Pshennekova, M. G. (1965). *Fed. Proc. Trans. Suppl.* **24,** T957.
Mirsky, I. (1969). *Biophys. J.* **9,** 139.
Mitchell, H., Wildenthal, K., and Mullins, C. B. (1969). *Fed. Proc. Fed. Amer. Soc. Exp. Biol.* **28** (4), 1334.
Pugh, D. M., Dodge, H. T., Rackley, C. E., and Sandler, H. (1964). *Clin. Res.* **12,** 191.
Rackley, C. E., Dodge, H. T., Coble, Y. O., and Hay, R. E. (1964). *Circulation* **29,** 666.
Ross, J., Jr., Covell, J. W., Sonnenblick, E. H., and Braunwald, E. (1966). *Circ. Res.* **18,** 149.
Rushmer, R. F., and Thal, N. (1951). *Circulation* **4,** 219.
Sandler, H., and Dodge, H. T. (1963). *Circ. Res.* **13,** 91.
Sandler, H., Pugh, O. M., Dodge, H. T. (1964). *Circulation* 30. *Suppl.* **111,** 151.
Sandler, H., and Dodge, H. T. (1968). *Amer. Heart J.* **75,** 325.
Sandler, H., and Ghista, D. N. (1969). *Fed. Proc. Fed. Amer. Soc. Exp. Biol.* **28,** 1344.
Sarnoff, S. J., and Berglund, E. (1954). *Circulation* **9,** 706.
Taylor, R. R., Ross, J., Jr., Covell, J. W., and Sonnenblick, E. H. (1967). *Circ. Res.* **21,** 99
Van Peenen, H. J., and Geistl, B. (1962). *J. Amer. Ger. Soc.* **10,** 505.
Wong, Y. K., and Rautaharju. (1968). *Amer. Heart J.* **75,** 649.

EARLY VENTRICULAR ADJUSTMENTS TO A CHRONICALLY INCREASED AFTERLOAD

Frances Kraft-Hunter, LaVal N. Cothran, and Edward W. Hawthorne

Introduction

The afterload against which a ventricle contracts is determined by the resistance to outflow it encounters upon contracting from any given end-diastolic volume.

It is well known that stenosis of the ascending aorta will increase left ventricular afterload. In experimental animals, left ventricular hypertrophy will develop in time after 50–60% constriction of the ascending arota (Alexander *et al.*, 1962; Clatworthy *et al.*, 1950; Grant *et al.*, 1968; Meerson, 1965; Pearse, 1928, 1940). In dogs with this type of severe left ventricular outflow obstruction peak systolic left ventricular pressure is chronically increased. They can be expected to have developed a significant ventricular hypertrophy in from 12 to 20 weeks after the stenosis has been produced (Alexander *et al.*, 1962; Spann *et al.*, 1967). However, it is not known just how soon after the aortic stenosis has been produced that hypertrophy can be detected. The acute effects on ventricular function of increasing left ventricular afterload have been studied (Blumenthal *et al.*, 1962; Clancy *et al.*, 1968; Dow, 1940; Katz, 1928; Levine *et al.*, 1966; Meerson and Pshennikova, 1965; Meerson, 1965, 1969). Some investigators suggest that myocardial contractile capability can be enhanced by ventricular hypertrophy (Alexander *et al.*, 1962; Beznak, 1958; Geha *et al.*, 1966). Others who customarily have studied animals with a greater degree of hypertrophy suggest that myocardial function and contractility is depressed (Meerson and Pshennikova, 1965; Spann *et al.*, 1967). Thus there is some support for the view that myocardial contractility is enhanced in the early phases of ventricular adjustment to a chronically increased afterload; that is, the affected ventricle can develop a higher peak tension from a given end-diastolic volume.

Ventricular hypertrophy is first detectable at this time. Later on as hypertrophy progresses myocardial contractility becomes depressed and myocardial failure subsequently develops.

The stimulus for the development of left ventricular hypertrophy in dogs with aortic stenosis is not known. Since these animals invariably have elevated peak-systolic ventricular pressures the wall stresses would be expected to be increased. However, Sandler and Dodge (1963) found that in patients with left ventricular hypertension and hypertrophy resulting from aortic stenosis, ventricular wall stress values during systole were either similar to or less than those for subjects without ventricular hypertension, This caused them to suggest that in spite of elevated ventricular tension, force per unit area of ventricular wall, or wall stress, may be relatively normal as a result of increased ventricular wall thickness from ventricular hypertrophy. One might hypothesize that in some way the increased peak wall tensile stresses (radial, longitudinal, latitudinal) trigger the development of left ventricular hypertrophy so as to restore wall tension to within normal limits through thickening of the ventricular wall. In fact, it has been suggested by Wong and Rautaharju (1968) that ventricular hypertrophy is an adaptive mechanism which, through contributing to an increase in wall thickness, is the means by which the ventricle can reduce to near normal values, wall tensile stresses in hearts that are subjected to a chronic ventricular systolic and/or diastolic pressure overload. It is recognized that this mechanism is only effective within certain limits and that these limits have not been defined.

We know very little about the changes in ventricular performance that occur in the interim between the experimental production of the aortic stenosis in animals and the development of hypertrophy of the left ventricle. Most often animals were studied for a control period, prior to receiving aortic stenosis and then several weeks or a month later, when ventricular hypertrophy is assumed to be present. These animals were studied in ways designed to evaluate the functional capacity of the hypertrophied ventricle. As a result of this approach serious study of the early phases of ventricular response to the increased afterload has been bypassed. Early levels of hypertrophy go unnoticed and the experimental animals are frequently allowed to increase their left ventricular muscle mass, well beyond minimal values which may be of physiologic significance before they are studied. Perhaps the major reason for this has been the lack of techniques for semicontinuous monitoring over long periods (weeks or months) in conscious, instrumented animals whose primary variables required to make any serious evaluation of ventricular function possible at any given time.

It is difficult to obtain a severe ascending aortic stenosis in dogs that is compatible with survival of the animal for long periods of time (Pearse, 1928; 1940). Such animals usually die suddenly as a result of rupture of the aorta. We have recently solved this technical problem by first wrapping the ascending aorta with dacron* and then placing about this wrapping an inflatable cuff of special design. The latter is inflated, after the animal recovers from the surgery, to produce the desired degree of aortic stenosis. Dogs survive with 50–60 % reduction in cross-sectional area of the ascending aorta produced in this manner for long periods and are not subject to rupture of the aorta.

The detection of the early hemodynamic consequences of chronically and, significantly increasing left ventricle afterload needs further study. Perhaps this can only be accomplished by studying the progressive changes in ventricular dimensions and function starting at an early period after introduction of an intervention such as aortic stenosis in animals.

In the past, there has been a lack of (1) techniques for the chronic semicontinuous monitoring of the primary variables necessary for analysis of ventricular function in experimental animals, and (2) adequate mathematical methods for making reliable estimates of wall tensile stresses in the thick-walled ellipsoidal left ventricle.

However, techniques are now available for following chronically in conscious animals changes in flows (Noble *et al.*, 1967), pressures (Fryer, *et al.*, 1969), and various ventricular dimensions (Cothran *et al.*, 1967; Hawthorne, 1961, 1966; Hawthorne and Ison, 1965; Hinds *et al.*, 1969; Perry and Hawthorne, 1958a,b). In our laboratory we have developed the transducing devices and have used the appropriate analog techniques for monitoring the left ventricular dimensions of length (aorta-apex), equatorial external circumference or cross-sectional area, and wall thickness, in experimental animals. These variables are recorded simultaneously with left ventricular pressure, aortic pressure, and ECG. The techniques used permit semicontinuous monitoring of these primary variables for long periods of time (days, weeks, or month) during cardiac cycles, from instrumented conscious animals. At present dogs are used. With the aid of an analog to digital converter, a high-speed digital computer, and the use of a specially developed program (written in either FORTRAN or BASIC language), both the primary and a selected set of derived variables are digitized, and an on-line printout of the quantities is made available to the investigator. This information is then used to evaluate ventricular performance at any desired time.

Derivations of significant physical quantities in each of the following categories have been made for (1) wall stresses, (2) contraction velocities at the equator of the left ventricle, (3) mechanical energy quantities at the equator, and (4) whole heart geometry.

Formulas have been derived which permit the calculation of variables

* DeBakey TM Seamless Arterial Graft. C. R. Bard, Inc., Murray Hill, New Jersey.

involved in assessing left ventricular contractility and performance (Walker *et al.*, pages 387–405. Primarily the derivation of the formulas has been based on three major assumptions: (1) The internal volume of the left ventricle can be approximated as an ellipsoid of revolution; (2) The wall thickness of the heart is uniform around the midplane; (3) The circumferentially oriented muscle fibers prevail in the determination of dimensional changes at the midplane of the left ventricle. Undoubtedly these assumptions place some limitation on the degree of accuracy of the physical quantities calculated. However, very often in assessing the performance of the heart, the most important concerns are the consistency with which a given calculation or measurement can be made and the degree to which they correlate with the actual values.

As a result of these developments, in our laboratory, we have begun a study of the progressive alterations that occur in ventricular performance in dogs in response to a chronically sustained increase in left ventricular afterload. This report describes the experimental approach we have taken and our observation that dogs during the first 14 days after induction in them of a chronically maintained 55% reduction of ascending aortic cross-sectional area adjust to this intervention primarily as a result of an increase in end-diastolic left ventricular volume. The adjustment seems to be primarily through the well known Frank-Starling mechanism (Starling, 1918). These animals develop a greater peak left ventricular tensile stress during isovolumic contractions after 14 days of stenosis than during the control period. Myocardial contractility was depressed by the intervention. Left ventricular stroke work and stroke power increased with the increases in end-diastolic volume that occurred over this period of study.

Methods

Studies were performed on more than 12 mongrel dogs weighing from 20.0 to 30.0 kg. Each of the dogs was instrumented with catheters for making pressure measurements, a strain gauge for measuring left ventricular circumference, induction coils to measure left ventricular wall thickness, and an inflatable cuff for constricting the aorta. Every animal has the aorta constricted to 55% for prolonged periods.

The surgery for implantation of these devices was performed through a standard left thoracotomy under sterile operating conditions. The diagram of the instrumentation is shown in Fig. 1(a). Left ventricular pressure and aortic pressure were obtained through polyvinyl catheters inserted into the apical dimple and the descending aorta (Hinds *et al.*, 1969) and were attached to P23Db or P23Gb Statham pressure transducers.

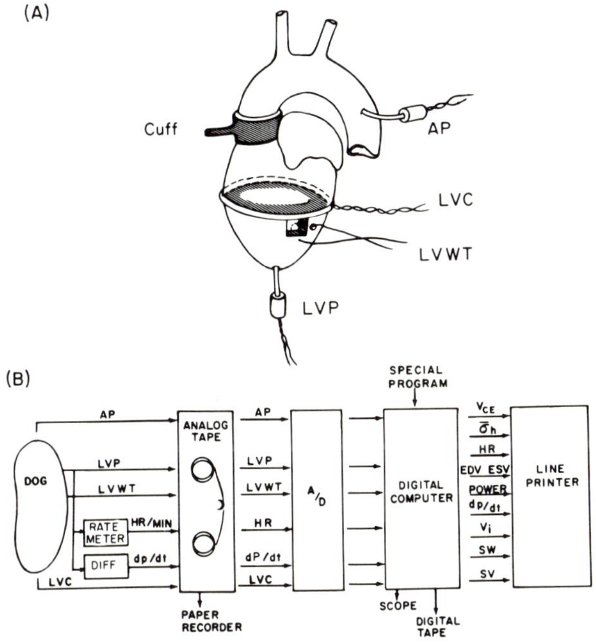

FIG. 1. (a) Schematic diagram of instrumentation for primary variables. The silastic cuff is placed on the ascending aorta just above the aortic valve and is used to produce various levels of aortic constriction. AP, aortic pressure; LVWT, left ventricular wall thickness; LVC, left ventricular circumference; LVP, left ventricular pressure. (b) Schema of the total system for continuous monitoring of primary and derived variables in the intact animal V_{CE} represents velocity of contractile element shortening $\bar{\delta}_h$ = hoop stress; HR = heart rate; EDV, end diastolic volume; ESV, end systolic volume; V_i, left ventricular internal volume; SW, stroke work; SV, stroke volume.

A specially designed inflatable silastic cuff* was placed on the ascending aorta just above the aortic valve and coronary vessels. Left ventricular wall thickness was measured by the use of coaxially placed coils, attached one to each side of an appropriate section of the wall of the left ventricle near its equator. One coil was used as the exciting coil and it was energized by an oscillating current of a chosen constant frequency, voltage, and amperage. The oscillating magnetic field thus produced induced an EMF in the other coil, the magnitude of which was solely a function of the separation of the two coils, and therefore provided the measure of the wall thickness at any instant (Perry and Hawthorne, 1958a,b).

External left ventricular circumference was measured by means of a mercury-

* Hazen Everett Company, Inc., 192 Kinderkamack Rd., Park Ridge, New Jersey.

in-silastic strain gauge (Hinds *et al.*, 1969) positioned about the equator of the left ventricle.

After surgery, a postoperative recovery period of 5 to 7 days was allowed. To fix settings of the cuff to desired degrees of constriction, the cuff was first completely occluded with saline solution and the amount of fluid required for total occlusion measured. Henceforth, the amount of fluid necessary to produce a desired degree of constriction was taken as that per cent of the total volume required for complete occlusion. Initially, 55% constriction of the aortic cuff was set, left on for 24 hr, checked, and reset. In a 24-hr period, less than 0.1 cc of fluid was lost. After several 24-hr tests of cuff stability at 55% constriction, the animals were studied every 48 hr, while monitoring heart rate (HR), dP/dt, aortic pressure (AP), left ventricular pressure (LVP), left ventricular wall thickness (LVWT) and left ventricular circumference (LVC) during various levels of occlusion—25%, 55%, 75%—and complete occlusion. After each recording session aortic constriction was reset at 55%.

All beats studied after complete occlusion (isovolumic beats) (Blumenthal *et al.*, 1962), produced during diastole, were required to meet the following criteria: (1) The first isovolumic beat after occlusion had the same end diastolic pressure base as the control beat; (2) Concomitant and progressive fall in the aortic pressure; (3) Smooth contour of left ventricular pressure tracings; and (4) Steady uninterrupted fall in left ventricular dP/dt following its peak. An acceptable isovolumic beat is shown in Fig. 7.

All primary variables, and their calibrations, were recorded on a multichannel, direct writing Sanborn recorder and on analog tape. The data were sampled at 10-msec intervals, digitized, then analyzed (Fig. 1(b). The computer used was Hewlett-Packard model 2116B, with A-D converter. Primary variables recorded were aortic pressure (AP), left ventricular pressure (LVP), left ventricular wall thickness (LVWT), and left ventricular circumference (LVC).

By appropriate programming of digital and analog computers derived variables obtained in this study included hoop stress ($\bar{\sigma}_h$), velocity of the contractile element shortening (V_{CE}), instantaneous and total stroke volume, ejection fraction (EF), heart rate (HR), midwall circumference, end diastolic volume (EDV), end systolic volume (ESV), and stroke power. Typical, randomly sampled cardiac cycles during steady state conditions were chosen for analysis.

Average hoop stress in gm/cm^2 was calculated by the equation

$$\bar{\sigma}_h = \left(\frac{PR_i}{H}\right)\alpha_h\left[1 - \frac{1}{2}\left(\frac{R_i}{B}\right)^2\right] \tag{1}$$

where P equals left ventricular pressure in gm/cm^2; R_i, left ventricular internal radius (cm); B, $\frac{1}{2}$ aorta to apex length (cm); H, left ventricular wall thickness (cm).

$$\alpha_h = \left\{\frac{1}{(1 + H/2R_i)(R_i/B)^2}\right\}$$

a parameter which accounts for thickness of heart wall, dimensionless.

Velocity of the contractile element in muscle lengths per second was calculated using the formula

$$V_{\mathrm{CE}} = (V_{\mathrm{CF}}/L_o - d\bar{\sigma}_h/dt)/34(\bar{\sigma}_h + 19) \tag{2}$$

where L_o equals mean left ventricular circumference; V_{CF}, velocity of contractile fiber (muscle lengths/sec). Stroke work is equal to the time integral of the power over the period of ejection in gm · cm.

$$\text{S.W.} = \int_{teivc}^{tes} PQ\,dt \tag{3}$$

where S.W. represents stroke work; P, ventricular pressure; Q, rate of blood flow leaving left ventricle (cm^3/sec); PQ, myocardial power (gm·cm/sec); *tes*, time at end systole; *teivc*, time at end isovolumic contraction.

The internal volume of the left ventricle is approximated by the ellipsoid of revolution using the formula

$$V_o = \tfrac{4}{3}\Pi R_i^3(B/R_i) \tag{4}$$

Stroke volume was determined by integrating rate of flow (where flow rate is considered the time rate of change of left ventricular volume) between end diastole and end systole.

$$\text{S.V.} = \int_{eivv}^{esv} Q\,dt \tag{5}$$

The ejection fraction (E.F.) was determined by the relationship

$$\text{E.F.} = 1 - ESV/EDV \tag{6}$$

Results and Discussion

Chronic Aortic Constriction

After a suitable postoperative recovery period each animal was recorded every other day for 3 weeks. Figure 2 shows the typical type of recording obtained for a dog in the early postoperative period. In addition, the effect of 55% aortic constriction is seen. The 55% constriction was maintained in the animal over 48-hr periods between recording sessions. This degree of

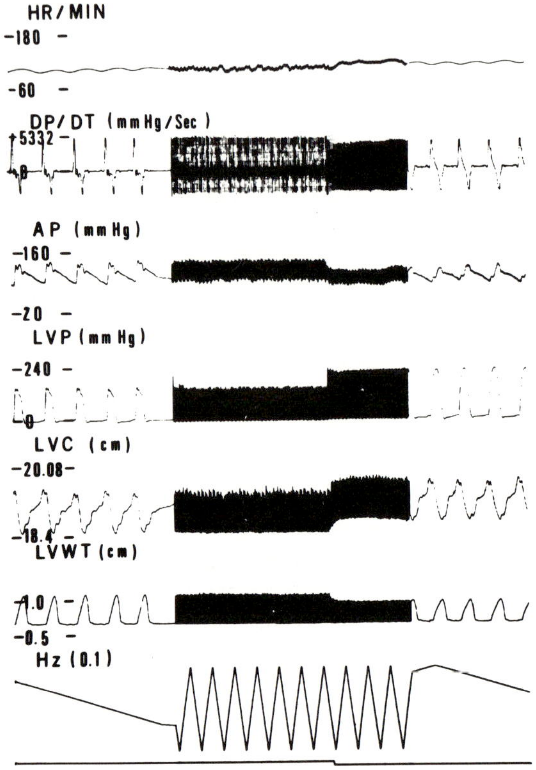

FIG. 2. Response obtained on the second day to 55% aortic constriction.

constriction regularly resulted in little or no increase in heart rate, a decrease in peak *dP/dt*, a decrease in aortic pressure of approximately 40 mm Hg, a rise of an average of 60 mm Hg in peak systolic ventricular pressure (with no obvious change in end-diastolic ventricular pressure), a decrease in end-diastolic wall thickness, and an increase in both end-diastolic and end-systolic circumference. A systolic ventricular–aortic pressure gradient of 100 m Hg was observed. By the 7th day, this had reduced to 20–25 mm Hg and held stable in this range.

These changes in dimensions and pressure were usually maintained over the 48-hr period. At each recording session the alteration in the primary and derived variables [Fig. 1(b)] were monitored on-line and the digital printouts of these data were produced by the computer for several typical cardiac cycles during control periods, and during periods of aortic constriction at various degrees.

The effect of temporary 75% aortic constriction is shown in Fig. 3, for 3 days of 14 days of continuous 55% aortic constriction. On the 2nd day

[Fig. 3(a)] there is a marked increase in heart size as evidenced by decreased peak systolic wall thickness and increased end-diastolic and end-systolic external circumference. In addition, left ventricular end-diastolic pressure increased in excess of 20 mm Hg, while aortic pressure was reduced by approximately 80 mm Hg during the time of constriction. In spite of the considerable lowering of central aortic pressure associated with the aforementioned volume and pressure changes, it is of interest to observe that peak *dP*/*dt* and heart rate were both decreased. This observation suggests that myocardial contractility was decreased by this intervention, a finding that was unexpected since such a decrease in aortic pressure should classically have resulted in a reflex increase in cardiac sympathetic nerve activity. On succeeding days, increased ventricular systolic pressure was associated with little or no increase in end-diastolic ventricular pressure and heart rate. The dimensional changes were directionally the same but smaller in magnitude. Although peak *dP*/*dt* declined with the intervention on the 7th day [Fig. 3(b)]

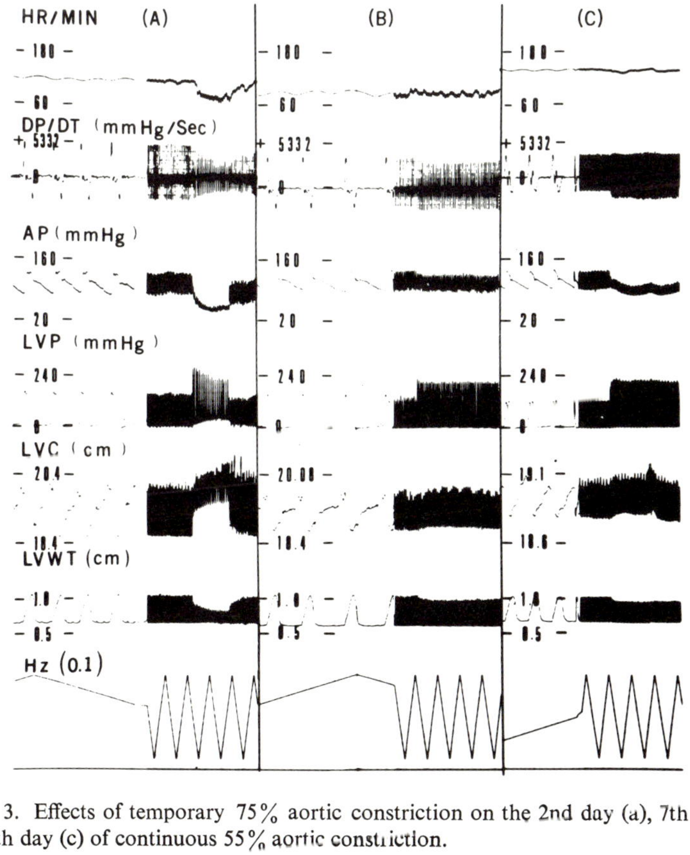

FIG. 3. Effects of temporary 75% aortic constriction on the 2nd day (a), 7th day (b), and 14th day (c) of continuous 55% aortic constriction.

no change occurred on the 14th day. Heart rate did not change significantly with temporary 75% aortic constriction on either the 7th [Fig. 3(b)] or 14th day [Fig. 3(c)].

It might be argued that the degree of aortic constriction accomplished was not the same on each of these 3 days in view of the difference in aortic pressure response [Figs. 3(b) and (c) vs (a)]. It must be pointed out, in this regard, that 75% aortic constriction in this study is defined as that degree of constriction of the aorta which occurred when the fluid-filled aortic cuff was inflated to 75% of the total volume required for complete occlusion. This is not the same criterion as constricting to a constant ventricular–aortic pressure gradient, for it is clear that if the maintenance of a constant ventricular–aortic pressure gradient had been the criterion for constriction, on each successive day this could have required a larger amount of inflation of the aortic cuff and consequently a progressively greater reduction in aortic cross-sectional area. The experimental design adopted was to attempt to maintain aortic cross-sectional area constant, rather than to hold to a near constant pressure gradient.

Both representative control cardiac cycles and cycles during 75% aortic constriction selected from the recordings shown in Fig. 3 were analyzed and the derived data are presented in Fig. 4. In Fig. 4(a), the most impressive changes seen are the progressive increase in peak stroke work and power that occurred over the 14-day period during the intervals while the left ventricle was exposed to the forcing function, namely, temporary 75% aortic constriction.

It can further be observed [Fig. 4(b)] that end-diastolic pressure and volume also were increased to greater degrees by this intervention as time progressed.

Changes in Muscle Volume

An index of muscle volume was determined by subtraction of the calculated internal volume from the calculated external volume of the left ventricle. When the study of each animal was completed, whether the experiment was acute or chronic, carefully the left ventricle was weighed, and its volume displacement determined. Thus for each animal the calculated muscle volume from dimensional measurement can be compared to left ventricular muscle volume and muscle weight. For 22 dogs, a plot of left ventricular muscle volume calculated from dimensional measurements versus actual displaced volume of the same left ventricular muscle mass revealed a significant linear relationship (correlation coefficient, 0.94). On the basis of this correlation, changes in calculated muscle volume obtained by the use of dimensional measurements were considered to provide a reliable estimate of true muscle mass. Furthermore, muscle volume changes are probably a more accurate index of hypertrophy than wall thickness since wall thickness can change according to the shape and size of the ventricle with the same muscle mass.

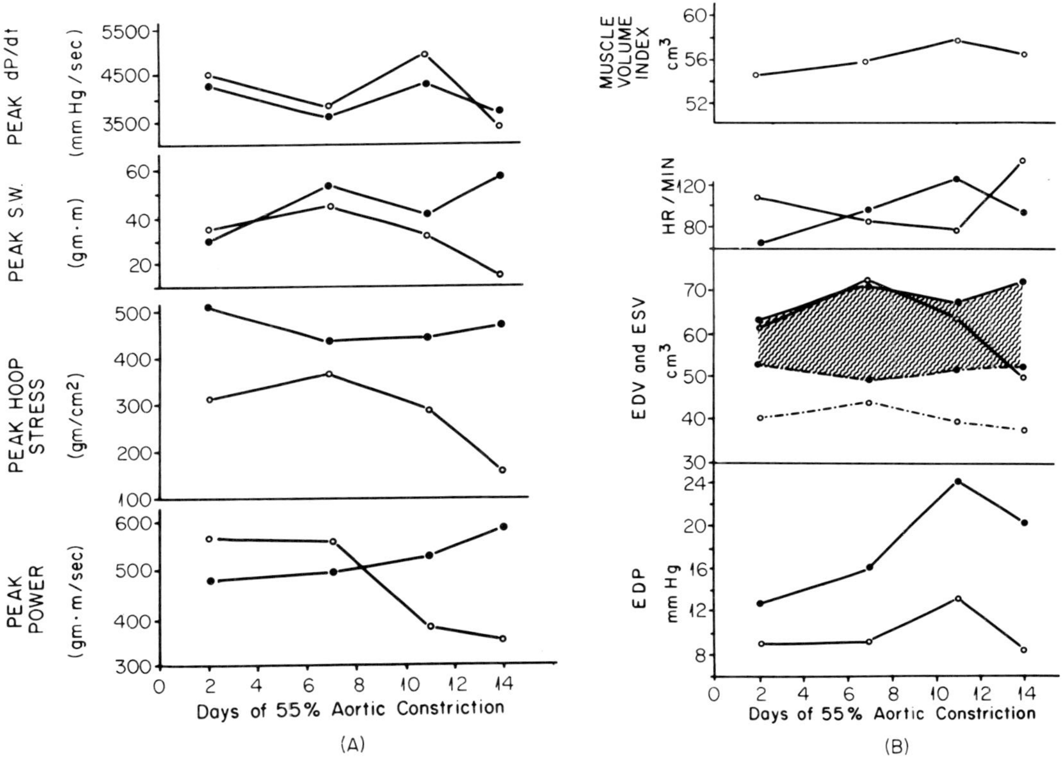

FIG. 4. The pattern of the changes of a selected set of primary and derived variables designed to portray ventricular function over 14 days of continued 55% aortic constriction. The values presented for the 2nd, 7th, and 14th days were taken from the analysis of typical cycles of the control period and the period of 75% aortic constriction as shown in Fig. 3.

Changes in Stroke Work and Volume

Figure 5 and the tabulation below show the pattern of change in left ventricular internal volume and stroke work during the ejection phase of typical cardiac cycles selected from the recordings indicated in Fig. 3. For this purpose a representative cycle was chosen from each control period and during the periods of 75% aortic constriction.

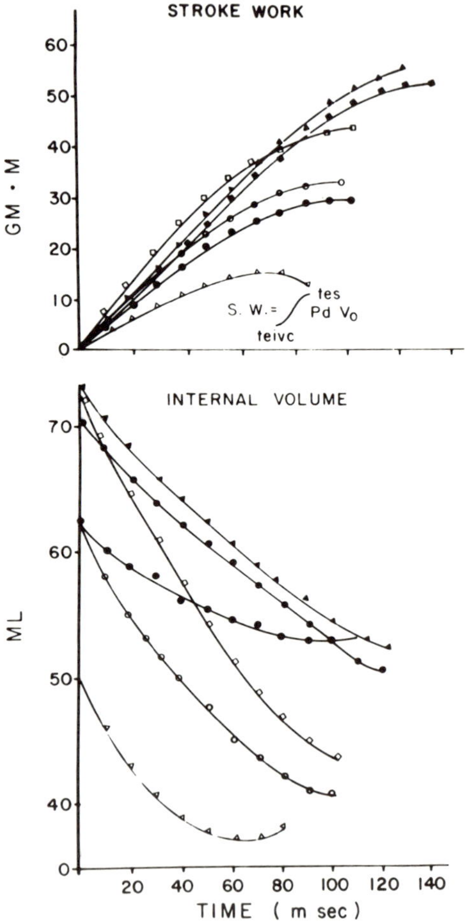

FIG. 5. Changes in stroke work and internal volume of left ventricle during the ejection phase of selected cardiac cycles taken from (a), (b), and (c) in Fig. 3, where (*teivc*) represents time at end of isovolumic contraction; (*tes*) time at end systole; (V_o) volume of the ventricle (cm^3); (%EF) percent ejection fraction. (○, □, and △) represent control groups on 2nd, 7th, and 14th days, respectively; (●, ■, and ▲) 75% aortic constriction.

Day	HR	EDP	EDV	SV	%EF
○	105	9	61	21	34
●	96	13	62	10	16
□	84	9	72	28	39
■	94	16	71	21	30
△	138	8	49	12	24
▲	91	20	72	21	30

Of interest is the observation that on the 7th and 14th days temporarily increasing the ventricular afterload, by 75% aortic stenosis, resulted in prolongation of ejection time and an increase in peak stroke work. As shown in Fig. 6, there was a good relationship between the peak stroke work accomplished and end-diastolic volume from which a particular ejection occurred.

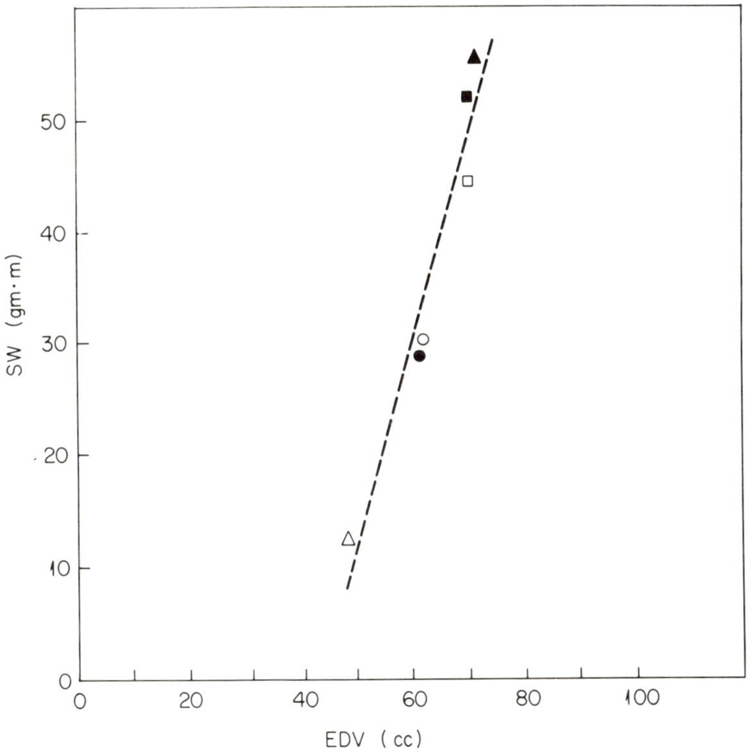

FIG. 6. Relation between end-diastolic volume and stroke work. (○, □, and △) represent control groups on 2nd, 7th, and 14th days, respectively; (●, ■, and ▲) 75% aortic constriction

Thus, all stroke work values, even though they were obtained on different days and with the ventricle contracting against different afterloads, fell on the same curve.

These observations suggest that the observed changes in stroke work were not due to increased myocardial contractility but rather are the simple expression of heterometric autoregulation (Sarnoff *et al.*, 1960).

The mere observation, however, of the relationship between stroke work and end-diastolic volume as presented in Fig. 6 does not permit a conclusion that changes in contractility did not occur. Each stroke work value could have been a point on a different stroke work–end-diastolic volume curve of a family of such curves according to the concepts set forth by Sarnoff and Mitchell (1962).

Changes in Myocardial Contractility

The observation that raising left ventricular afterload by the 75% aortic stenosis (Fig. 3) decreased peak dP/dt, whereas end-diastolic volume increased and heart rate fell (or held stable), indicates that this intervention caused a decrease in myocardial contractility.

Another way of evaluating the contractile state of the heart is that expressed by the force–velocity relation (Covell *et al.*, 1966; Levine and Britman, 1964; Sonnenblick, 1962; Sonnenblick *et al.*, 1960). This approach presumes that the estimation of V_{max} produces a measure of the contractile state of the ventricle which is independent of the end-diastolic myocardial fiber length (Sonnenblick *et al.*, 1960). Perhaps the simplest and most direct way for analysis of the force–velocity relation is in its use in studying isovolumic beats.

Figure 7 shows a typical isovolumic beat. All isovolumic beats studied were always the first beat after complete aortic occlusion. In association with each isovolumic beat the aortic pressure shows a progressive fall and the dP/dt following its peak has a steady uninterrupted fall. The dimensional changes observed here are due, largely, to changes in the shape of the ventricle.

Figure 8 presents the hoop stress–velocity relation as derived from selected control cycles and the following isovolumic beat for the 2nd and 7th days. Attempts at extrapolation for obtaining values for V_{max} on these curves was difficult. Inspection of these curves, however, reveals that the simple extension of each of the force–velocity curves onto the ordinate would provide estimates of V_{max} which are different on the 2nd and the 7th day. Furthermore, the V_{max} obtained in this way was found to be lower on the 7th day than on the 2nd day. Curves of this type comparing the 2nd day to the 14th day also showed a depression of V_{max}. Thus, these observations offer further evidence that increases in afterload, as studied in these experiments, depress myocardial contractility.

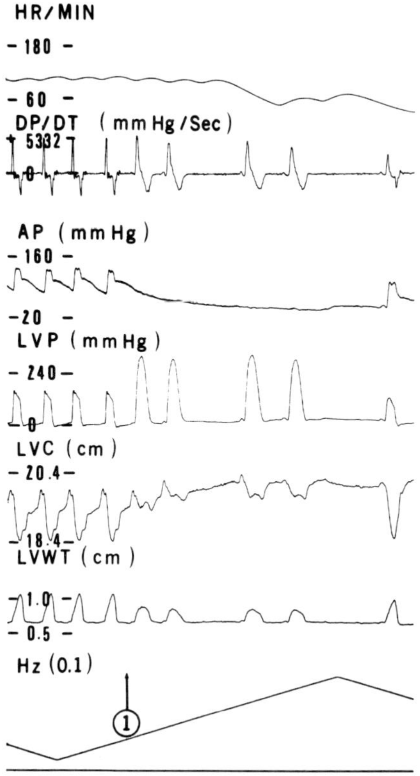

FIG. 7. Typical isovolumic beat is shown, beginning at the arrow. The isovolumic beat studied is always the first after complete aortic occlusion. During the contraction the aortic pressure shows a progressive fall and *dP/dt* a steady uninterrupted fall following its peak.

Summary

These studies illustrate the use of techniques for chronic and semicontinuous monitoring from conscious dogs of primary and derived variables that are indicative of ventricular performance and an approach to evaluating the long term effects of a particular intervention on left ventricular dynamics. The estimated normal values for all the derived variables were well within the limits of values reported by other investigators (Mitchell and Mullins, 1967; Noble *et al.*, 1966, 1967; Sanmarco, 1966).

A study was made of the changes in left ventricular function occurring in dogs during the first two weeks of exposure to a moderately severe aortic stenosis. The results obtained in one of these animals has been analyzed. These responses were typical of the animals we have studied to this point.

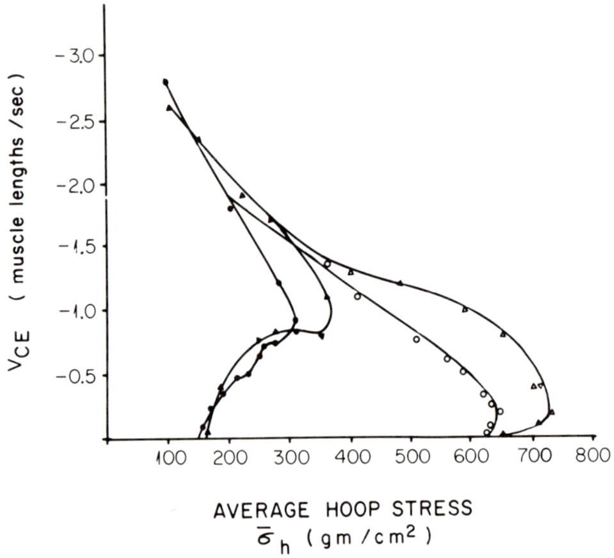

FIG. 8. Changes in stress–velocity relations during control periods and during complete aortic occlusion on the 2nd and 7th days of 55% aortic constriction. Control group: (●) 2nd day; (▲) 7th day. Isovolumic group: (○) 2nd day; (△) 7th day.

An attempt was made to evaluate the performance of the ventricle at regular intervals through observing its pattern of adjustment in response to a sudden and temporary 75% aortic constriction, where the latter was used as a forcing function. The primary responses to this forcing function were (1) regular depression of myocardial contractility and (2) increased peak stroke work. In addition, the peak hoop stress developed during isovolumic contractions was greater on successive days. The latter could be explained to be entirely a function of the increased end-diastolic volume at the time of producing the isovolumic contraction. In like manner, the findings that stroke work and power were increased by 75% aortic constriction the 7th day of aortic stenosis and thereafter can be explained to be a result of the increased end-diastolic volume, that is, a result of heterometric autoregulation (Sarnoff *et al.*, 1960).

Other investigators (Alexander *et al.*, 1962; Beznak, 1958; Geha *et al.*, 1966) have suggested that the basic contractile state of the ventricular myocardium might either be increased or unchanged in animals exposed to a chronically increased left ventricular afterload. Our studies do not support this view. Rather, they suggest that, even in the absence of a demonstrable ventricular hypertrophy, a left ventricle which is chronically exposed to an increased afterload against which it must contract has a reduced myocardial contractility and responds when challenged with a sudden and severe increase in afterload primarily through use of the Frank-Starling mechanism.

ACKNOWLEDGMENTS

Supported in part by National Aeronautics and Space Administration Grant NGR 09-011-018 and National Institutes of Health Grant HE 01015-19.

REFERENCES

Alexander, N., Toldfarg, T., and Dury, D. R. (1962). *Circ. Res.* **10,** 11.

Beznak, M. (1958). *Circ. Res.* **6,** 207.

Blumenthal, M. R., Hsush-Hwa Wang, M. D., and Wang, S. C. (1962). *Circ. Res.* **11,** 727.

Clancy, R. L., Graham, T. P., Jr., Ross, J., Sonnenblick, E. H., and Braunwald, E. (1968) *Amer. J. Physiol.* **214,** 1186.

Clatworthy, H. W., Jr., Sako, Y., Chisholm, T. C., Culmer, C., and Varco, R. L. (1950). *Surgery* **28,** 245.

Cothran, L. N., Bowie, W. C., Hinds, J. E., and Hawthorne, E. W. (1967). *In* "Factors Influencing Myocardial Contractility" (R. D. Tanz, F. Kavaler, and J. Roberts), p. 163. Academic Press, New York.

Covell, J. W., Ross, J., Sonnenblick, E. H., and Braunwald, E. (1966). *Circ. Res.* **29,** 364.

Dow, P. (1940). *Amer. J. Physiol.* **131,** 432.

Fryer, T. B., Sandler, H., and Datnow, B. (1969). *Med. Res. Eng.* **8,** 9.

Geha, A. S., Duxxy, J. P., and Swan, H. J. C. (1966). *Circ. Res.* **19,** 255.

Grant, C., Raphael, M. J., Steiner, R. E., and Goodwin, J. F. (1968). *Cardiovasc. Res.* **4,** 346.

Hawthorne, E. W. (1961). *Circ. Res.* **9,** 110.

Hawthorne, E. W. (1966). *Amer. J. Cardiol.* **18,** 566.

Hawthorne, E. W., and Ison, E. L. (1965). *In* "Shock and Hypotension," p. 45. Grune and Stratton, New York.

Hinds, J. E., Hawthorne, E. W., Mullins, C. B., and Mitchell, J. H. (1969). *Fed. Proc. Fed. Amer. Soc., Exp. Biol.* **28,** 1351.

Katz, L. N., Ralll, E. P., and Cheer, S. (1928). *J. Clin. Invest.* **5,** 205.

Levine, H. J., and Britman, N. A. (1964). *J. Clin. Invest.* **43,** 1383.

Levine, H. J., Forwand, S. A., McIntyre, K. M., and Schecter, E. (1966). *Circ. Res.* **18,** 729.

Meerson, F. Z. (1965). *Amer. J. Cardiol.* **15,** 755.

Meerson, F. Z. (1969). *Circ. Res.* **25,** (Suppl. II), II, 115.

Meerson, F. Z., and Pshennikova, M. G. (1965). *Bull. Exp. Biol. Med. USSR.* **5,** 32.

Mitchell, J. H., and Mullins, C. B. (1967). *In* "Factors Influencing Myocardial Contractility" (R. D. Tanz, F. Kavaler, and J. Roberts, eds.), pp. 177–188. Academic Press, New York.

Noble, M. I. M., Trenchard, D., and Guz, A. (1966). *Circ. Res.* **19,** 139.

Noble, M. I. M., Gabe, I. T., Trenchard, D., and Guz, A. (1967). *Cardiovasc. Res.* **1,** 9.

Perry, S. L. C., and Hawthorne, E. W. (1958a). *J. Nat. Med. Ass.* **50,** 117.

Perry, S. L. C., and Hawthorne, E. W. (1958b). *Fed. Proc. Fed. Amer. Soc. Exp. Biol.* **17,** 123.

Pearse, H. E. (1928). *Surg. Gynecol. and Obstet.* **46,** 411.

Pearse, H. E. (1940). *Ann. Surg.* **112,** 923.

Sandler, H., and Dodge, H. T. (1963). *Circ. Res.* **13,** 91.
Sanmarco, M. E., Fronek, K., Philips, C. M., and Davila, J. C. (1966). *Amer. J. Cardiol.* **18,** 584.
Sarnoff, S. J., and Mitchell, J. H. (1962). *In* "Handbook of Physiology," Section 1, *Circulation,* p. 489. Amer. Physiol. Soc., Wash. D.C.
Sarnoff, S. J., Mitchell, J. H., Gilmore, J. P., and Remensynder, J. P. (1960). *Circ. Res.* **8,** 1077.
Sonnenblick, E. H. (1962). *Fed. Proc. Fed. Amer. Soc. Exp. Biol.* **21,** 1975.
Sonnenblick, E. H., Parmley, W. W., and Urschell, C. W. (1960). *Amer. J. Cardiol.* **23,** 488.
Spann, J. F., Buccino, R. A., Sonnenblick, E. H., and Braunwald, E. (1967). *Circ. Res.* **21,** 341.
Starling, E. H. (1918). "The Law of the Heart" (Linacre Lecture, 1915). Longmans, London.
Walker, M. L., Hawthorne, E. W., and Sandler, H., this volume.
Wong, A. Y. K. and Rautaharju, P. M. (1968). *Amer. Heart J.* **75** 649.

RELATIONSHIP OF LEFT VENTRICULAR PERFORMANCE AND HYPERTROPHY IN HUMANS

William A. Baxley and Harold T. Dodge

In 1964 Rackley *et al.*, reported a method for directly determining the mass or weight of the human left ventricle *in vivo* from biplane angiocardiograms. The method involves measurements of the left ventricular wall thickness from the antero-posterior film, correction for nonparallel X-ray beams, and calculation of the left ventricular cavity volumes utilizing an ellipsoid reference figure as described earlier by Dodge and co-workers (1960). The calculated weight and actual weight of the left ventricle compared favorably in 23 postmortem hearts (standard error of estimate 23 gm) (Rackley *et al.*, 1964). A later report compared the left ventricular mass as determined from the angiocardiograms with postmortem left ventricular weights in 28 patients who had subsequently died; the correlation coefficient was 0.97 with a standard error of estimate 33 gm, and ranges of values to nearly 600 gm (Kennedy *et al.*, 1967). Kennedy *et al.* (1966) established the average normal value for left ventricular mass determined by these methods in adults as 167 ± 42 gm or 92 ± 16 gm/m^2 body surface area; such values agree within 10% of the normal values of left ventricular weight predicted from other postmortem studies. These methods, which permit the measurement of left ventricular mass along with chamber volumes in living patients with heart disease, have permitted a wide range of investigation pertinent to the subject of myocardial hypertrophy; the results of some of these studies form the basis of the work described in this chapter.

Left Ventricular Mass and Volume

A significant relationship exists between left ventricular mass and end-diastolic volume in chronic heart disease. Figure 1 shows this relationship in 226 patients with various forms of disease, studied in the resting state.

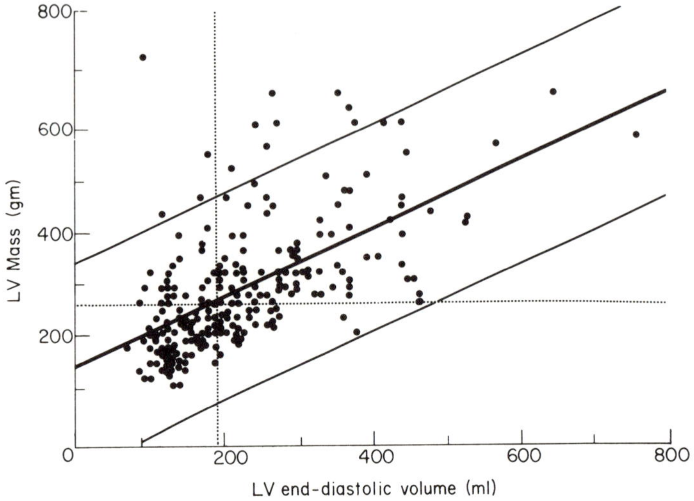

FIG. 1. The relationship between left ventricular (LV) end-diastolic volume and mass in 226 patients. The dashed lines indicate the upper limits of normal for the variables; the solid diagonal lines are the line of best fit and standard error of estimate. $n = 226$; $r = 0.59$; $p < 0.01$.

The correlation is not close ($r = 0.59$), primarily in patients who have excessive mass values relative to end-diastolic volume. Such patients usually have pressure overloads of the left ventricle in the form of aortic or subaortic stenosis, or systemic arterial hypertension with thick left ventricular walls but little or no chamber enlargement. However, it is noteworthy that generally those patients with increased end-diastolic volumes also have increased mass values, indicating that dilatation of the ventricle in the absence of hypertrophy does not occur in chronic heart disease. Some of the patients with enlarged end-diastolic volumes have the dilatation on the basis of increased volume work load from mitral or aortic valve incompetence with consequent large stroke volumes, but also some of these patients have dilatation as a result of myocardial disease which is either primary or in association with long-standing ventricular work overload. Those with poor ventricular function have dilatation out of proportion to the volume work overload. Ventricular dilatation, whether a result of volume overload or decreased myocardial performance, appears to be associated with hypertrophy. Figure 1 includes patients with various types of abnormalities; patients may have left ventricular pressure-work overload, volume-work overload, and decreased myocardial function either primarily or associated with pressure or volume overloads.

Left ventricular mass, in addition to being related to end-diastolic volume is also significantly related to left ventricular stroke work, as shown in Fig. 2. The correlation coefficient is 0.60 ($p < 0.01$) in 170 adults with various chronic heart diseases, which is consistent with the theory that one stimulus to left ventricular hypertrophy is work overload. However, the degree of scatter evident on the graph suggests that some patients have inappropriate or excessive hypertrophy relative to the imposed work load. As suggested previously, such inappropriate hypertrophy in some patients may be a result of chronic myocardial functional abnormality. In this regard, one index of left ventricular function is the ejection fraction, or ratio of stroke volume to end-diastolic volume. The mean normal value of ejection fraction is 0.67 ± 0.08, and low values even in the presence of a ventricular work overload are generally regarded as an indication of decreased myocardial function (Dodge *et al.*, 1966). Accordingly, the patients represented in Fig. 2 were arbitrarily divided into three groups by drawing radial lines through the origin as shown, with the mean ejection fractions for these resulting three groups found to be significantly diffierent. The lowest value, 0.41, was present in the group with the largest ventricular mass for any given work load, and the highest mean ejection fraction, 0.63, in the group with the lowest left ventricular mass value for any given work load. This relationship appears to be perhaps analogous to the Frank-Starling relationship; thus patients with depressed left ventricular function have high mass values relative to

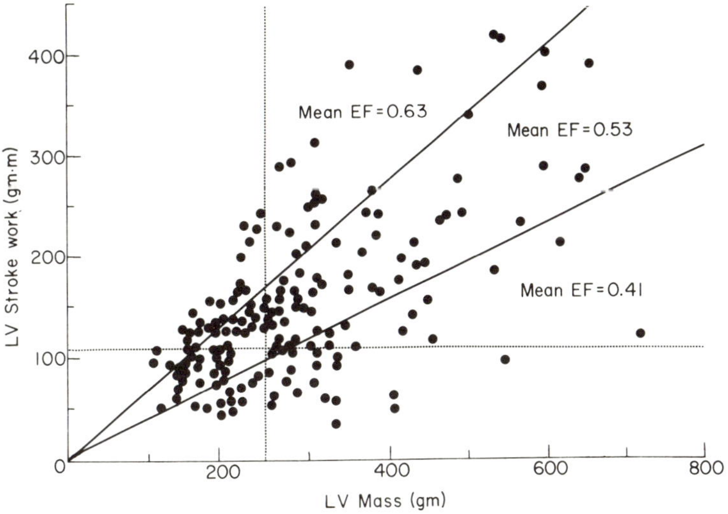

FIG. 2. Left ventricular (LV) stroke work and mass in 170 patients. The dashed lines indicate upper normal values for the variables. The diagonal lines were drawn arbitrarily as described in the text. EF = ejection fraction; $n = 170$; $r = 0.60$; $p < 0.01$.

work. Studies of the Frank-Starling relationship have demonstrated large diastolic volume and high diastolic pressure relative to levels of work in the presence of depressed myocardial function. In fact, the ejection fraction is a numerical expression of the Frank-Starling mechanism with stroke volume considered with respect to diastolic volume. These relationships demonstrate that left ventricular hypertrophy may be in part a compensation for decreased left ventricular function. These associations between left ventricular work, mass, and function are further demonstrated in Fig. 3, which shows ejection fraction related to stroke work/mass, or work per gram of ventricular myocardium. It can be seen that all patients with low ejection fractions also have low work values per gram of muscle. However, many patients with low work values per gram have normal ejection fractions; this particular association has been observed in patients with idiopathic hypertrophic subaortic stenosis in whom there is characteristically excessive hypertrophy in relation to the work load in the presence of normal or even high ejection fraction. Yet the meaning of this combination of left ventricular dynamic features in other types of heart disease is unclear.

In another study to more precisely define the dynamic properties of *in vivo* human myocardium and their relationship to hypertrophy, the cyclic characteristics of a 1 cm cube of muscle, or segment, located in the midwall equator of the left ventricle were calculated from volume and pressure data obtained during quantitative biplane angiography. Stress (σ) or force per unit area in the longitudinal and equatorial directions is a continuous function and is calculated for the 1 cm cube utilizing the law of La Place with

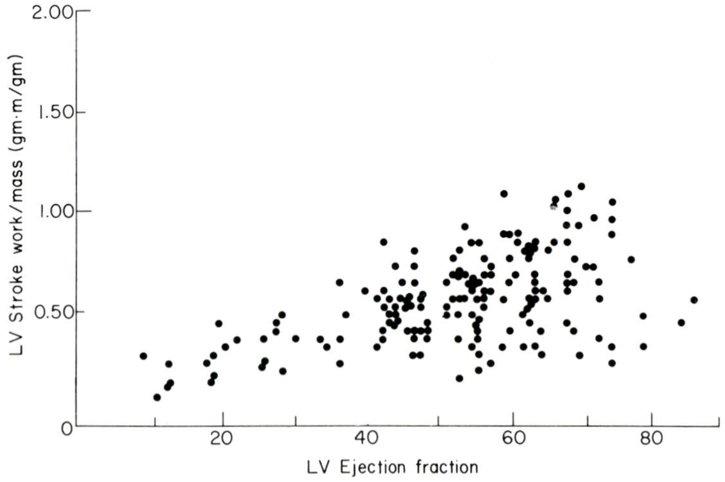

FIG. 3. Left ventricular (LV) stroke work/mass compared to ejection fraction in 170 patients: $n = 170$; $r = 0.54$; $p < 0.01$.

mathematical input data including ventricular chamber pressure and dimensions and wall thickness as determined from the angiocardiograms. Methods for calculation of left ventricular wall stress have been published previously (Sandler and Dodge, 1963).

Strain (E), or time–rate of deformation of the 1 cm cube in either the longitudinal or equatorial directions, is calculated as the time–rate of change of the midwall circumference of the left ventricle which is considered as an ellipsoid,

$$E = (1/C)\, dC/dt$$

where C equals the midwall circumference in either the longitudinal or equatorial directions.

The work (W) of the 1 cm cube during the systolic portion of the cardiac cycle is then the sum of these instantaneous stress–strain products,

$$W = \int_{ED}^{ES} \sigma_1 E_1 + \int_{ED}^{ES} \sigma_2 E_2$$

where ED equals end-diastole and ES equals end-systole; σ_1 and E_1 are longitudinal stress and strain and σ_2 and E_2 are circumferential stress and strain.

Power (P_o) is the time–rate of work production and is thus represented as the first derivative of work with respect to time:

$$P_o = dW/dt$$

Figure 4 illustrates the systolic work of the 1 cm cube or segment compared

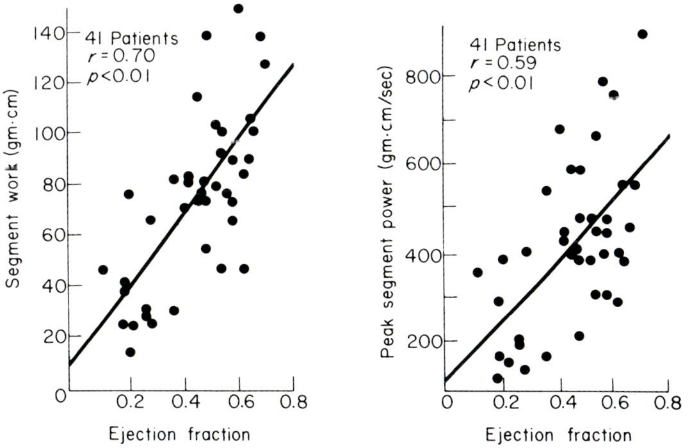

FIG. 4. Segment work and peak segment power compared to left ventricular ejection fraction in 41 patients.

to ejection fraction in 41 patients with chronic heart disease. This significant relationship is also consistent with the supposition that ventricular dilatation associated with decreased left ventricular function may be a stimulus to hypertrophy, since those patients with low ejection fraction tend to have low work values for the segment.

Also in Fig. 4 is seen the relationship between peak systolic segment power and ejection fraction. The relationship is close, suggesting that in decreasing left ventricular function the time–rate of work production is diminished.

In addition to determination of the causes of left ventricular hypertrophy in humans with heart disease, it is of interest to consider the degree of regression of hypertrophy after removal of a stimulus to hypertrophy. Accordingly we have determined the left ventricular mass by quantitative biplane angiocardiography preoperatively in ten adults with chronic valvular disease, and then have repeated the studies some months postoperatively. These patients represented excellent surgical results with correction of the mechanical defect associated with the valve disease and with marked clinical improvement after surgical replacement of mitral or aortic valves, and in one case combined mitral, aortic, and tricuspid valves. The results of these preoperative and postoperative left ventricular mass studies are shown in Fig 5. It can be seen that no significant regression of left ventricular hypertrophy occurred in this group 4–14 months after successful removal of the left ventricular work overloads. In addition, there was little decrease in left ventricular end-diastolic volume postoperatively. However, in a similar type of study, Kennedy and

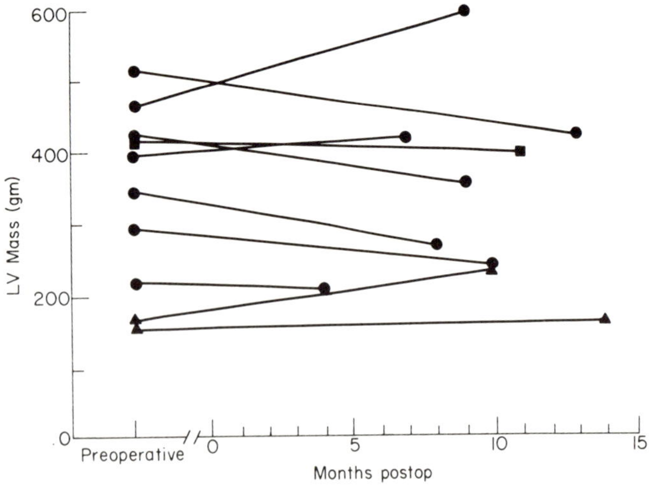

Fig. 5. Left ventricular (LV) mass preoperatively and postoperatively in ten patients with valve replacement: ●, aortic; ▲, mitral; ■, triple.

coworkers (1968) did find regression of elevated left ventricular mass values significant at $p < 0.05$ in a group of patients a year following aortic valve homograft replacement. Whether a more consistent decrease in left ventricular mass will be observed over a longer period of time after acute removal of a chronic left ventricular work overload is unknown at present.

In summary, quantitative biplane angiocardiography has been utilized to determine left ventricular mass in patients with chronic heart disease. Such studies indicate that hypertrophy results from both pressure and volume overload but it is also associated with ventricular dilatation, which is a consequence of volume overload or diminished myocardial function. Accordingly analysis of ventricular performance in chronic heart disease should consider not only ventricular volume or Starling effect as in acute studies, but also the ventricular hypertrophy associated with heart disease.

Acknowledgments

This study was supported in part by grants HE 11310, HE 05080, and 2 M01 FR 3209 from the U.S. Public Health Service; RD 2219-M from the Vocational Rehabilitation Administration of the Department of Health, Education, and Welfare; and from the U.S. Veterans Administration.

References

Dodge, H. T., Sandler, H., Ballew, D. W., and Lord, J. D. (1960). *Amer. Heart J.* **60,** 762.

Dodge, H. T., Sandler, H., Baxley, W. A., and Hawley, R. R. (1966). *Amer. J. Cardiol.* **18**, 10.

Kennedy, J. W., Baxley, W. A., Figley, M. M., Dodge, H. T., and Blackmon, J. R. (1966). *Circulation* **34,** 272.

Kennedy, J. W., Reichenback, D. D., Baxley, W. A., and Dodge, H. T. (1967). *Amer. J. Cardiol.* **19,** 221.

Kennedy, J. W., Twiss, R. D., Blackmon, J. R., and Merendino, K. A. (1968). *Circulation Suppl.* **2,** 110.

Rackley, C. E., Dodge, H. T., Coble, Y. D., and Hay, R. E. (1964). *Circulation* **29,** 666.

Sandler, H., and Dodge, H. T. (1963). *Circ. Res.* **13,** 91.

COMPARISON OF THE CONTRACTILE STATE OF THE NORMAL, HYPERTROPHIED, AND FAILING HEART IN MAN

Dean T. Mason, James F. Spann, Jr., Robert Zelis, and Ezra A. Amsterdam

The development of myocardial hypertrophy provides one of the fundamental mechanisms that permits the heart to maintain cardiac output in the face of abnormal volume or pressure load (Braunwald *et al.*, 1966; Spann 1969; Spann *et al.*, 1969a). Despite considerable interest in experimentally produced cardiac hypertrophy and failure (Spann *et al.*, 1967a,b; Bing *et al.*, 1969; Hawthorne, this volume), there has been little quantitative information available concerning the contractile state of the myocardium in ventricular hypertrophy in man. Accordingly, the present study was carried out in patients in order to define the contractile state of cardiac muscle in the hypertrophied left ventricle of patients with circulatory compensation and in the hypertrophied left ventricle of patients with overt congestive heart failure. Recent developments in the assessment of cardiac function in man utilizing the relationship between isovolumic intraventricular systolic pressure and the rate at which intraventricular pressure rises or *dP/dt* now have made it possible to examine directly the inotropic state of the left ventricle in conscious patients (Braunwald *et al.*, 1969; Mason, 1969; Mason *et al.*, 1970a).

Clinical and Hemodynamic Data: Definition of Patient Groups

High-fidelity left ventricular pressure and corresponding *dP/dt* were recorded in 44 conscious patients at the time of diagnostic cardiac catheterization. Whereas it is realized that the definition between normal, hypertrophied, and failing ventricles is not rigid and that these groups represent a continuum, it is possible to establish clinical and hemodynamic criteria in order to facilitate comparison. Thus, these patients included 18 without left ventricular disease, 17 with left ventricular hypertrophy without circulatory decompensation who had symptoms of shortness of breath only with more than ordinary activity, and nine patients with congestive heart failure who had symptoms of dyspnea and fatigue at rest or with ordinary activity. Their ages were 20 to 65 years and there was no significant difference ($p > 0.4$) between the three groups. The patients without left ventricular disease included five with functional heart murmurs, five with idiopathic chest pain, three with mild isolated fixed infundibular pulmonic stenosis, three with uncomplicated atrial septal defects, and two with pure mitral stenosis in normal sinus rhythm. Patients with ventricular hypertrophy without failure included eight with idiopathic left ventricular hypertrophy, seven with valvular aortic stenosis, one with idiopathic hypertrophic subaortic stenosis, and one with coarctation of the aorta. The group of patients with left ventricular hypertrophy and congestive heart failure comprised seven with idiopathic cardiomyopathy, one with valvular aortic stenosis, and one with patent ductus arteriosus. In each patient, selective left ventricular cineangiography was carried out following the recording of the routine hemodynamic data and the special measurements of contractility described herein; left ventricular hypertrophy was identified by wall thickness in end-diastole of greater than 1 cm, corrected for distortion and magnification, at the minor axis of the chamber in the right anterior oblique position (Rackley *et al.*, 1964, Kennedy *et al.*, 1967, Baxley *et al.*, 1968). None of the patients had valvular regurgitation, ventricular septal defect, or segmental disease in the left ventricle.

In Fig. 1 are shown the average values of the left ventricular end-diastolic pressure and the cardiac index in the groups of patients studied. Patients with ventricular hypertrophy without failure had moderate elevations of left ventricular end-diastolic pressure of 17.4 ± 1.7 mm Hg (SEM); four of these

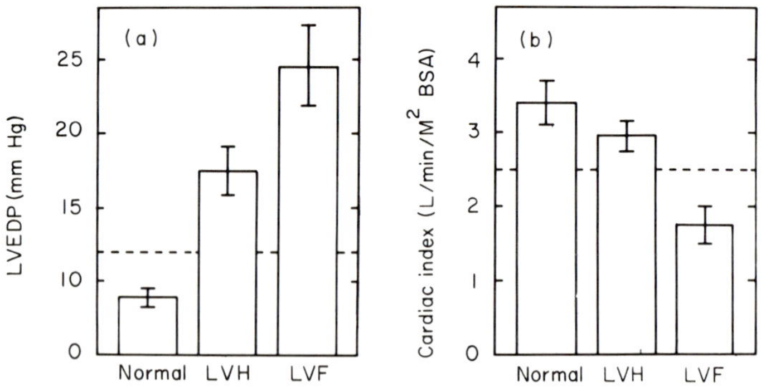

FIG. 1. Average values (± SEM) of left ventricular end-diastolic pressure (LVEDP) in (a), and of the cardiac index in (liter/min/m²) (b) in the three groups of patients studied. LVH represents left ventricular hypertrophy; LVF, left ventricular failure. (a) $p < 0.01$; $p < 0.05$; (b) $p > 0.02$; $p < 0.01$.

patients had normal left ventricular end-diastolic pressures of 12 mm Hg or less [Fig. 1(a)]. The cardiac index in each patient of this group was normal and averaged 2.95 ± 0.20 l/min/m^2 body surface area (lower limit of normal 2.50 l/min/m^2); there was no significant difference between normal patients and those with hypertrophy ($p > 0.2$) [Fig. 1(b)]. In contrast to patients with hypertrophy, each patient with left ventricular failure had a diminished cardiac index which averaged 1.75 ± 0.25 l/min/m^2 ($p < 0.01$) [Fig. 1(b)], despite marked elevations of left ventricular end-diastolic pressure in each instance which averaged 24.6 ± 2.9 mm Hg and was significantly greater than in hypertrophy alone ($p < 0.05$) [Fig. 1(a)]. Left ventricular end-diastolic volume index was 70 ± 4 ml/m^2 in the normal left ventricles, 87 ± 8 ml/m^2 in the hypertrophied ventricles, and 155 ± 21 ml/m^2 in the hypertrophied and failing ventricles measured by selective left ventricular cineangiography in the right anterior oblique position (Sandler and Dodge, 1968) at the conclusion of the study.*

Peak *dP/dt*

Peak *dP/dt* itself reflects the contractile state of the intact ventricle (Mason, 1969). However, *dP/dt* is a complex function dependent upon the loading conditions in which cardiac muscle performs in addition to the contractile state (Mason, 1969). Thus, an increase of end-diastolic pressure or preload

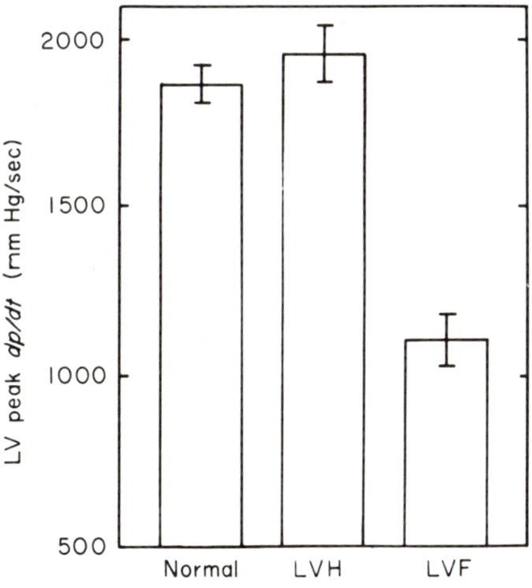

FIG. 2. Average values of left ventricular (LV) peak *dP/dt* in the three groups of patients, where $p > 0.4$ and $p < 0.01$.

* *Note*: ml represents milliliter; ML is muscle length.

of the ventricle, or of arterial diastolic pressure, a principal determinant of ventricular afterload, results in a rise of peak *dP/dt*. Figure 2 indicates the peak *dP/dt* developed by the left ventricle in the three groups of patients studied. Peak *dP/dt* was reduced in ventricular failure, 1219 $\pm$ 155 mm Hg/sec, compared to hypertrophy without failure, 1915 $\pm$ 175 mm Hg/sec, and normal ventricles, 1738 $\pm$ 111 mm Hg/sec ($p < 0.01$, $p < 0.02$). These observations are consistent with those of other workers (Gleason and Braunwald, 1962). Thus it appears that in the presence of heart disease with ventricular hypertrophy without decompensation, the increased preload or Frank-Starling mechanism and ventricular hypertrophy maintain peak *dP/dt* at normal levels despite the presence of any reduction of contractility.

Contractile State

dP/dt at Common Isovolumic Ventricular Pressure Related to Ventricular End-Diastolic Volume

It has recently been shown in our laboratories that when ventricular end-diastolic pressure is relatively constant with a change of arterial diastolic pressure, the relation of *dP/dt* to peak common developed isovolumic intraventricular pressure is an accurate measurement of the contractile state of the intact ventricle, independent of variations in afterload of the ventricle (Mason *et al.*, 1967b, Mason, 1969). In the present study among different patients, *dP/dt* was determined at the total isovolumic ventricular pressure of 50 mm Hg, which was common to each of the different ventricles. Since the preload of these different ventricles varied widely, *dP/dt* at common isovolumic pressure was modified by relating this ratio to left ventricular end-diastolic volume (Mason *et al.*, 1969a). This ratio of *dP/dt* at a given isovolumic pressure between patients is analogous to a common point at isopressure on the pressure–velocity curve, described in the next section of this chapter, which is normalized to a certain extent for the influence of preload on the vertical position of the curve by relating the ratio to the end-diastolic volume of the ventricle. The values of the measure of contractility obtained in this manner are shown in Fig. 3. The ratio of *dP/dt* at 50 mm Hg to end-diastolic volume in patients with hypertrophy without failure was 9.8 $\pm$ 1.4 (mm Hg/sec)/ml, and in those with ventricular failure was 4.1 $\pm$ 0.9 (mm Hg/sec)/ml and, thus were observed to be considerably reduced compared to the values of the normal ventricles of 14.8 $\pm$ 1.8 (mm Hg/sec)/ml ($p < 0.05$ with hypertrophy, $p < 0.01$ with failure). Similar conclusions were able to be derived when these determinations were carried out utilizing common developed isovolumic pressure. Thus, it appears that contractility was significantly

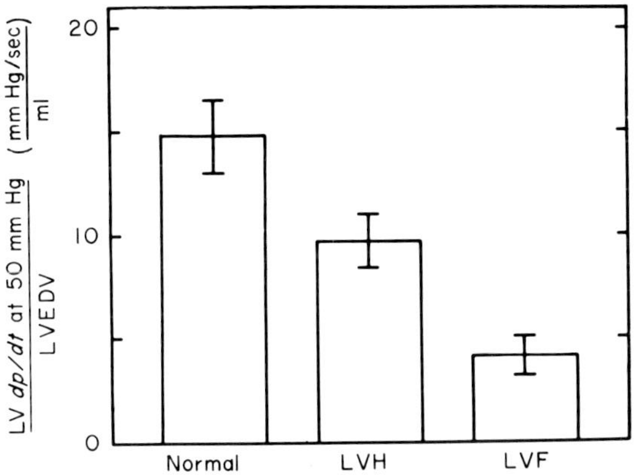

FIG. 3. Average value of the ratio of left ventricular dP/dt at the common isovolumic pressure of 50 mm Hg related to left ventricular end-diastolic volume (LVEDV) in the three groups of patients, where $p < 0.05$ and $p < 0.01$.

diminished both in patients with ventricular hypertrophy without failure and those with failure, the most severe depression occurring in patients with congestive heart failure ($p < 0.01$ between failure and hypertrophy).

MAXIMUM VELOCITY OF CONTRACTILE ELEMENT SHORTENING

In order to extend the observation that contractility is reduced in hypertrophy before the onset of failure, this fundamental property of the myocardium was examined directly in terms of the force–velocity concept. It has been shown in our laboratories that the instantaneous velocity of shortening of the contractile elements (V_{CE}) of the intact left ventricle during the isovolumic portion of ejecting beats can be determined as the relation of ventricular dP/dt to the product of the corresponding isovolumic ventricular pressure and the series elastic constant (Mason *et al.*, 1968; Mason, 1969; Mason *et al.*, 1970a, b). In brief, since alterations in ventricular geometry are small in the intact heart during isovolumic contraction with V_{CE} equaling series eleastic elongation, it follows that V_{CE} during the isovolumic portion of ejecting beats can be determined entirely from isovolumic ventricular pressure (IP) and its dP/dt without requiring knowledge of tension. Further, assuming minor alterations in geometry during isovolumic systole as in methods utilizing tension, it can be shown mathematically that IP and its dP/dt are the only independent variables and thus knowledge of ventricular radius and wall thickness are not necessary in the determination of instantaneous V_{CE} and the extrapolated value of V_{max} (Mirsky *et al.*, 1969; Mason *et al.*, 1970a). From these observations, the rational basis for the accurate calculation of instantaneous isovolumic V_{CE} in the spherical or ellipsoidal ventricle was established by the equation $(dP/dt)/(k \cdot \mathrm{IP})$, where k is the series elastic constant of 32 per muscle length at body temperature (Yeatman *et al.*, 1969). Further, it was recognized that V_{CE} at the ordinate is identical when derived from pressure–velocity or tension–velocity curves, and since the left ventricular pressure–velocity relation can be determined precisely, construction of the inverse IP to V_{CE} relation and extrapolation to zero load permitted determination of maximum V_{CE} (V_{max}), the measure of contractility which has been shown to be independent of loading changes (Sonnenblick, 1962; Sonnenblick and Downing, 1963; Braunwald *et al.*, 1967; Braunwald *et al.*, 1969; Sonnenblick *et al.*, 1969).

In order to examine the usefulness and validity of instantaneous V_{CE} and V_{max} determined in this manner from recordings of ventricular pressure and dP/dt alone, the effects of inotropic agents and loading conditions were determined in conscious patients (Mason *et al.*, 1967b; Mason, 1969). Increasing contractility by leg exercise or by the administration of isoproterenol resulted in an upward shift of the pressure–velocity curve and the elevation of the estimated value of V_{max}. In contrast, increases of left ventricular end-diastolic pressure produced by leg raising or elevation of aortic diastolic pressure induced by methoxamine did not alter the pressure–velocity curve or value of V_{max}. In addition, it is important to point out that the studies of other investigators now have attested to the validity of the determination of V_{CE} and V_{max} entirely from intraventricular pressure and dP/dt during isovolumic systole as a means of quantifying contractility (Mirsky *et al.*, 1969; Wolk *et al.*, 1969; Finkelstein *et al.*, 1969).

In addition, since V_{max} is expressed in terms of muscle units and is independent of variables of left ventricular loading and wall thickness, this method of determining the pressure–velocity relation and derivation of V_{max} solely from IP and dP/dt can be extended to the specific comparison of the basal inotropic state of the intact ventricle between different patients (Mason, 1969; Mason *et al.*, 1969b; Mirsky *et al.*, 1969; Mason *et al.*, 1970a). Indeed, comparison of basal contractility among different ventricles has shown the value of V_{max} to be essentially the same whether it is determined from pressure or tension–velocity curves (Mirsky *et al.*, 1969). Furthermore, since (1) instantaneous V_{CE} can be calculated from IP and dP/dt alone, if constant ventricular geometry is assumed during isovolumic systole, and (2) there is a common point of origin on the ordinate (V_{max}) of the pressure–velocity and tension–velocity curves, it appears more rational to determine the extrapolation to zero load from the more precisely defined pressure–velocity curve, rather than from the tension–velocity curve; the latter is obtained with difficulty and is perhaps somewhat inaccurate owing to inherent problems in the measurement of ventricular volume and wall thickness and the assumptions upon which the models and equations for the calculation of tension are based. In addition,

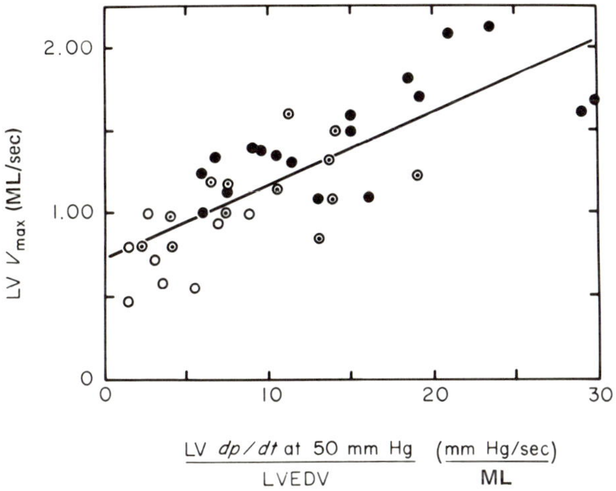

FIG. 4. Relation of left ventricular V_{max} to the ratio of left ventricular dP/dt at the common isovolumic pressure of 50 mm Hg divided by left ventricular end-diastolic volume. ●, Normal; ⊙, LVH; ○, LVF; $r = 0.76$; $p < 0.01$; $n = 39$; x/y slope = 22.2 and the y intercept = 0.73.

there was a positive correlation observed between V_{max} determined from the pressure–velocity data and the ratio of dP/dt at 50 mm Hg divided by left ventricular end-diastolic volume in the 39 patients in whom both of these measurements were obtained ($r = 0.76$ and $p < 0.01$) (Fig. 4). From all of these observations in the present study, instantaneous V_{CE} was determined by the equation given above of the relation of dP/dt to the product of corresponding isovolumic pressure and the series elastic constant, and V_{max} was obtained by extrapolation of the pressure–velocity descending limb to its origin at zero load.

It is recognized that some investigators consider V_{max} determined in the standard manner from force–velocity curves to be somewhat less than true maximum potential V_{CE} (Noble *et al.*, 1969), and thus perhaps traditional V_{max} is best termed V'_{max}. Nevertheless, maximum V_{CE} is the same when derived from tension–velocity or pressure–velocity curves and is influenced only by the contractile state. It is stressed that this method of determining instantaneous V_{CE} and V_{max} entirely from IP and dP/dt requires a truely isovolumic portion of systole, and thus is not applicable in patients with mitral insufficiency, severe aortic insufficiency, ventricular septal defects, and ventricular aneurysms. In addition, this technique should not be utilized in patients with coronary arterial disease with localized fibrosis of the myocardium or in those with infiltrative segmental disease in whom the value of the series elastic modulus might vary throughout the left ventricle. Furthermore, it is essential that IP and *dP/dt* be accurately recorded; thus high-fidelity catheter-manometer systems are necessary such as the intracardiac micromanometer catheter (Gleason and Braunwald, 1962; Mason and Braunwald, 1963; Mason, 1969), direct needle puncture of the left ventricle (Brockenbrough *et al.*, 1961; Mason *et al.*, 1967a), or the newly devised external microdisplacement gauge attached to a cardiac catheter of standard length with a wide lumen and multiple side holes (Spann *et al.*, 1969b). It can be difficult to extrapolate with great accuracy relatively short isovolumic pressure–velocity segments of ejecting beats to zero load. However, this problem is largely obviated by the determination of the average pressure–velocity relation from several beats. Although the pressure–velocity curve is an hyperbola, it was considered most precise in the present study to carry out this extrapolation by the visual fit of a straight line connecting the descending limb to the ordinate axis.

The applicability of the present technique of obtaining instantaneous V_{CE} and V_{max} is also dependent, to some extent, both on the level of ventricular end-diastolic pressure and arterial diastolic pressure (Mason *et al.*, 1970a). If ventricular end-diastolic pressure is considerably elevated and thereby approaches aortic diastolic pressure, the isovolumic portion of systole is abbreviated and thereby might be too brief to allow the relation between instantaneous V_{CE} and isovolumic pressure to describe a pressure–velocity descending segment of sufficient length for analysis. Similar considerations apply when the aortic valve opens at a relatively low pressure. On the other hand, it is important to point out that the present method possesses a number of advantages when compared to force–velocity properties determined during the ejection phase of systole (Mirsky, 1969; Mason *et al.*, 1970a). Thus, the determination of the velocity of shortening of the circumferential ventricular fibers at peak tension (Gault *et al.*, 1968; Braunwald *et al.*, 1969) requires cineangiography and complex analysis, providing only a single point on the force–velocity curve which is considerably distant from zero load, and is thereby markedly influenced by variations in preload, and V_{CE} is not compared at isotension. Further, accurate knowledge of ventricular tension is difficult to obtain owing to assumptions in the measurement of ventricular volume and wall thickness and the model used for the estimation of tension itself. In addition, the number of points on the tension–velocity curve are limited by the film speed, only a few beats can be utilized in averaging the tension–velocity curve, since contractility is altered when the contrast dye reaches the coronary capillary bed (Zelis *et al.*, 1970), and serial studies in an individual patient are not appropriate as a result of alteration of contractility and ventricular loading with the contrast dye (Spann *et al.*, 1968, Zelis *et al.*, 1969).

In Fig. 5 are illustrated the relation between instantaneous V_{CE} and IP

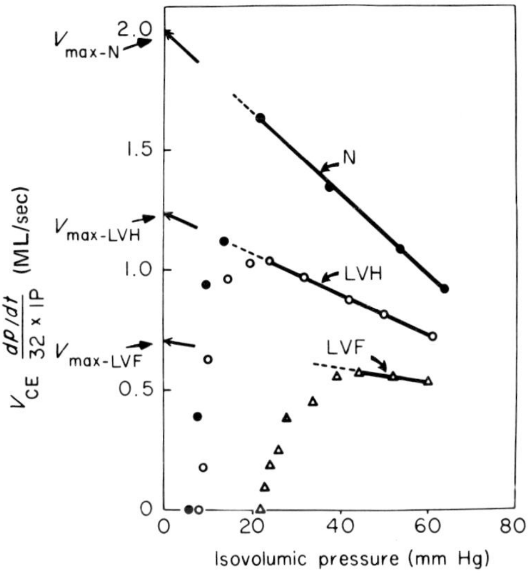

FIG. 5. Representative comparison of the pressure–velocity relation during isovolumic contraction of the left ventricle in a normal patient, a patient with left ventricular hypertrophy in the absence of failure, and a patient with left ventricular failure. The diagonal broken lines indicate extrapolation of the isovolumic segment to V_{max} at zero load, shown by the arrows. Instantaneous V_{CE} and V_{max} are expressed in muscle length/second (ML/sec) as the relation $(dP/dt)/(32 \cdot IP)$, where IP = instantaneous isovolumic left ventricular pressure. ●, Normal; ○, LVH; △, LVF.

determined from a representative patient in each of the three groups studied. The relation is plotted at 5-msec intervals from the closure of the mitral valve to the opening of the aortic valve. The descending limb of the relation between pressure and velocity, shown by the solid diagonal lines, is related to the upper portion of the conventional force–velocity curve relating V_{CE} to tension. Extrapolation of these portions of the pressure–velocity relations to zero load, shown by the broken diagonal lines and arrows, provides determination of V_{max}. In the patient without left ventricular disease, the pressure–velocity curve and extrapolated value of V_{max} were considerably elevated above those of the patient with hypertrophy and those of the patient with failure. Thus, these observations indicate that contractility of ventricular muscle is reduced in ventricular hypertrophy without failure and is severely depressed in overt congestive heart failure.

The average values of V_{max} obtained in each of the three groups of patients are shown in Fig. 6. V_{max} was 1.50 ± 0.09 muscle lengths/sec in normal ventricles, 1.10 ± 0.06 muscle lengths/sec in hypertrophy, and 0.76 ± 0.07 muscle lengths/sec in failing ventricles. The differences between the groups were statistically significant, indicating that contractility is moderately

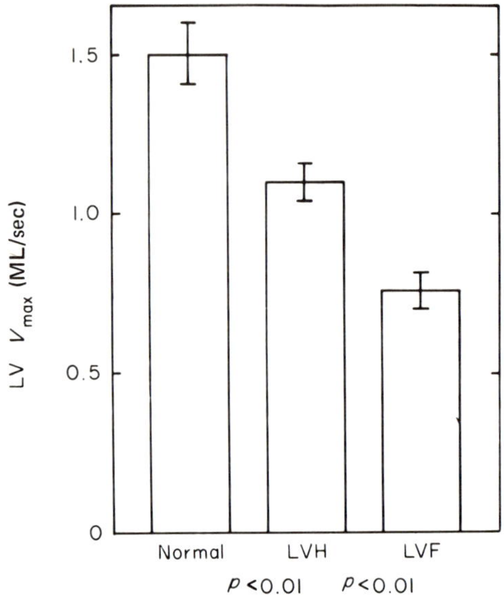

FIG. 6. Average value of left ventricular V_{max} in the three groups of patients.

depressed in hypertrophy and markedly reduced in hypertrophy with failure. These conclusions were found to apply both to patients with primary myocardial hypertrophy and to those with hypertrophy secondary to chronic pressure overloading. In addition to the determination of V_{max}, V_{CE} was examined by certain methods that other workers have considered to provide assessment of contractility. Thus, the value of peak developed contractile element velocity (Mirsky, 1969; Nejad *et al.*, 1969), were found to be reduced in both hypertrophy and in failure, moreso in failure. Furthermore, similar conclusions could be drawn whether instantaneous V_{CE} and V_{max} were calculated utilizing total or developed isovolumic pressure.

Conclusions

In this study, a number of methods in conscious patients have demonstrated that cardiac contractility during basal conditions is depressed both in the hypertrophied nonfailing heart and in the failing ventricle. Thus, the findings in isolated papillary muscle (Spann *et al.*, 1967a; Bing *et al.*, 1969) and the intact ventricle (Spann *et al.*, 1967b; Spann *et al.*, 1969a) of laboratory animals with experimentally induced heart failure can be extended to the understanding of hypertrophy and congestive heart failure in man. In man, left ventricular hypertrophy alone may be associated with depression of ventricular contractility in the absence of alterations in the less sensitive indicators of cardiac performance such as the cardiac output. It is recognized that these velocity data are quantified for a representative muscle unit and not necessarily per identical number of contractile sites. However, the relative increase in noncontractile tissue in experimental hypertrophy is quite small compared to the marked depression in contractile state (Buccino *et al.*, 1969; Spann, this volume). Also in regard to the possibility of a slight decrease of available contractile sites in a segment of representative size of hypertrophied myocardium, quantitative alterations in the components of the contractile apparatus might be of importance in the reduction of contractility and thus true fall in V_{max}, although recent studies suggest qualitative changes in the calcium pump activity of sarcoplasmic reticulum (Suko *et al.*, 1969; Swartz, this volume). It is of interest that studies in experimental animals have suggested that a certain amount of time may be required during the development of ventricular hypertrophy secondary to a chronic pressure or volume overload before the contractile state per unit of muscle is reduced (Taylor *et al.*, 1968; Bing *et al.*, 1969; Hawthorne, page 359). The probability that contractility may be more severely depressed in patients with primary myocardial disease and hypertrophy than in those with secondary hypertrophy is pointed out, and the data obtained in the present study show that V_{max} tended to be more reduced in idiopathic myocardiopathy than in systolic ventricular overload support this view.

From the present clinical observations, it appears that overt congestive heart failure is a late manifestation of the severely depressed heart, and that more subtle losses of ventricular function may precede detectable abnormalities of hemodynamic performance (Spann *et al.*, 1969a; Spann *et al.*, 1970). Thus there appears to be a spectrum of decreasing ventricular function from left ventricular hypertrophy without failure to left ventricular hypertrophy with failure. In hypertrophy without failure, the absolute increase in total muscle mass and elevated ventricular end-diastolic pressure maintain cardiac output at rest, although pulmonary congestion may occur with excessive elevations of end-diastolic pressure and the cardiac output may not increase to a normal extent with exercise. In hypertrophy with failure, despite the striking increase in ventricular end-diastolic pressure and muscle mass, cardiac output falls in the basal state as a result of the markedly reduced level of contractile state.

References

Baxley, W. A., Dodge, H. T., and Sandler, H. A. (1968). *Circulation* **37,** 509.

Bing, O. H. L., Matsushita, S., Fanburg, B. L., and Levine, H. J. (1969). *Cicrulation* **40,** Suppl. 3, 46.

Braunwald, E., Chidsey, C. A., Pool, P. E., Sonnenblick, E. H., Ross, J., Jr., Mason, D. T. Spann, J. F., Jr., and Covell, J. W. (1966). *Ann. Int. Med.* **64,** 904.

Braunwald, E., Ross, J., Jr., and Sonnenblick, E. H. (1967). *N. Engl. J. Med.* **277,** 794.

Braunwald, E., Ross, J. Jr., Gault, J. H., Mason, D. T., Mills, C., and Gabe, I. (1969). *Ann. Int. Med.* **70,** 369.

Brockenbrough, E. C., Morrow, A. G., Talbert, J., and Braunwald, E. (1961). *Brit. Heart J.* **23,** 643.

Buccino, R. A., Harris, E., Spann, J. F., Jr., and Sonnenblick, E. H. (1969). *Amer. J. Physiol.* **216,** 425.

Finkelstein, L. J., Keefe, J. F., Wolk, M. J., Bing, O. H. L., and Levine, J. H. (1969). *Circulation* **40,** Suppl. 3, 80.

Gault, J. H., Ross, J., Jr., and Braunwald, E. (1968). *Circ. Res.* **22,** 451.

Gleason, W. L., and Braunwald, E. (1962). *J. Clin. Invest.* **41,** 80.

Kennedy, J. W., Reichenbach, D. D., Baxley, W. A., and Dodge, H. T. (1967). *Amer. J. Cardiol.* **19,** 221.

Mason, D. T. (1969). *Amer. J. Cardiol.* **23,** 516.

Mason, D. T., and Braunwald, E. (1963). *J. Clin. Invest.* **42,** 1105.

Mason, D. T., Ross, J., Jr., Gault, J. H., Braunwald, E., and Morrow, A. G. (1967a). *Circulation* **35,** Suppl. 1, 15.

Mason, D. T., Sonnenblick, E. H., Covell, J. W., Ross, J., Jr., and Braunwald, E. (1967b). *Circulation* **36,** Suppl. 2, 183.

Mason, D. T., Spann, J. F., Jr., and Zelis, R. (1968). *Circulation* **38,** Suppl. 4, 134.

Mason, D. T., Spann, J. F., Jr., and Zelis, R. (1969a). *J. Clin. Invest.* **48,** 56a.

Mason, D. T., Spann, J. F., Jr., and Zelis, R. (1969b). *Dis. Chest,* **56,** 258.

Mason, D. T., Spann, J. F., Jr., and Zelis, R. (1969c). *Circulation* **40,** Suppl. 3, 141.

Mason, D. T., Spann, J. F., Jr., and Zelis, R. (1970a). *Amer. J. Cardiol.* **26**, 248.

Mason, D. T., Spann, J. F., Jr., Zelis, R., and Amsterdam, E. A. (1970b). *Progr. Cardiov. Dis.* **12**, 507.

Mirsky, I. (1969). *Circulation* **40,** Suppl. 3, 147.

Mirsky, I., Ellison, R. C., and Hugenholtz, P. G. (1969). *Clin. Res.* **17,** 255.

Nejad, N. S., Klein, M. D., Mirsky, I., and Lown, B. (1969). *Physiologist* **12,** 313.

Noble, M. I. M., Bowen, T. E., and Hefner, L. L. (1969). *Circ. Res.* **24,** 821.

Rackley, C. E., Dodge, H. T., Coble, Y. D., Jr., and Hay, R. E. (1964). *Circulation* **29,** 666.

Sandler, H., and Dodge, H. T. (1968). *Amer. Heart J.* **75,** 325.

Sonnenblick, E. H. (1962). *Fed. Proc. Fed. Amer. Soc. Exp. Biol.* **21,** 975.

Sonnenblick, E. H., and Downing, S. E. (1963). *Amer. J. Physiol.* **204,** 604.

Sonnenblick, E. H., Parmley, W. W., and Urschel, C. W. (1969). *Amer. J. Cardiol.* **23,** 488.

Spann, J. F., Jr. (1969). *Amer. J. Cardiol.* **23,** 504.

Spann, J. F., Jr., Buccino, R. A., Sonnenblick, E. H., and Braunwald, E. (1967a). *Circ. Res.* **21,** 341.

Spann, J. F., Jr., Covell, J. W., Eckberg, D. L., Sonnenblick, E. H., Ross, J., Jr., and Braunwald, E. (1967b). *Circulation* **36,** Suppl. 2, 241.

Spann, J. F., Jr., Mason, D. T., Beiser, G. D., and Gold, H. K. (1968). *Circulation* **38,** Suppl. 4, 185.

Spann, J. F., Jr., Mason, D. T., and Zelis, R. (1969a). *Amer. J. Med. Sci.* **258**, 291.

Spann, J. F., Jr., McCusker, D. R., Zelis, R., and Mason, D. T. (1969b). *Circulation* **40,** Suppl. 3, 190.

Spann, J. F., Jr., Mason, D. T., and Zelis, R. (1970). *Mod. Conc. Cardiovasc. Dis.* **39,** 79.

Suko, J., Ito, Y., Vogel, J., and Chidsey, C. (1969). *Circulation* **40,** Suppl. 3, 197.

Taylor, R. R., Covell, J. W., and Ross, J., Jr. (1968). *J. Clin. Invest.* **47,** 1333.

Wolk, M. H., Keefe, J. F., Bing, O. H. L., Finkelstein, L. J., and Levine, H. J. (1969). *J. Clin. Invest.* **48,** 90a.

Yeatman, L. A., Jr., Parmley, W. W., and Sonnenblick, E. H. (1969). *Amer. J. Physiol.* **217,** 1030.

Zelis, R., Mason, D. T., and Spann, J. F., Jr. (1969). *Circulation* **40,** Suppl. 3, 221.

Zelis, R., Mason, D. T., Spann, J. F., Jr., and Amsterdam, E. A. (1970). *Clin. Res.* **18,** 118.

DYNAMICS OF HYPERTROPHY IN THE LEFT VENTRICULAR WALL OF MAN

William P. Hood, Jr.

The development in recent years of angiographic techniques to quantitate left ventricular volume and mass has permitted us to study the magnitude of hypertrophy in the intact human ventricle. In our laboratory, biplane angiocardiography has been used to determine dimensions and volume of the left ventricle by the area–length method of Dodge *et al.* (1960). Details of our techniques have been reported previously (Rackley *et al.*, 1968; Hood *et al.*, 1968). Wall thickness is measured from each AP film as the average thickness of a 4-cm segment of free left ventricular wall immediately below the equator. After correction for X-ray magnification, end-diastolic chamber dimensions and wall thickness are used to estimate left ventricular weight in grams by the method of Rackley *et al.* (1964).

Volume and mass data collected from 99 patients are summarized in Table I. In the 10 subjects with normal left ventricles, end-diastolic volume was 77 ml/m^2, end-diastolic wall thickness 8.2 mm, and left ventricular mass 25×10^{-4} gm/gm body weight (BW). Among 19 patients with mitral stenosis, average volume, wall thickness, and mass values were essentially the same as in normals. In all other groups, end-diastolic wall thickness and left ventricular mass were increased. These other groups included 35 patients with compensated volume overload, 9 with compensated pressure overload, 17 with decompensated volume or pressure overload, 6 with primary myocardial disease of the nonobstructive type, and 3 with idiopathic myocardial hypertrophy of which 2 had dynamic obstruction. In all patients with enlarged chambers, even those with primary myocardial disease, end-diastolic wall thickness and left ventricular mass were significantly increased, indicating that chronic chamber enlargement is not just a consequence of fiber stretching or of fiber slippage, as has been observed in acute dilatation (Linzbach, 1960; Sonnenblick and Ross, 1967), but involves eccentric hypertrophy to some degree.

TABLE I

PARAMETERS OF VENTRICULAR HYPERTROPHY[a]

Physiological group	End-diastolic volume (ml/m²)	End-diastolic wall thickness (mm)	Left ventricular mass (gm/gm BW × 10⁻⁴)	Circumferential stress (dyn/cm² × 10³): Peak	Circumferential stress (dyn/cm² × 10³): End-diastolic
Normal left ventricle (10)	77 ± 4	8.2 ± 0.5	25 ± 2	312 ± 16	32 ± 4
Mitral stenosis (19)	83 ± 6	7.7 ± 0.3	25 ± 2	349 ± 17 ($N = 18$)	36 ± 4 ($N = 17$)
Compensated volume overload (35)	133[d] ± 9	9.3[b] ± 0.3	39[d] ± 3	335 ± 16 ($N = 27$)	47[c] ± 4 ($N = 32$)
Compensated pressure overload (9)	78 ± 7	10.5[b] ± 0.8	31[b] ± 2	385[b] ± 25	40 ± 4
Decompensated volume or pressure overload (17)	211[d] ± 21	12.1[d] ± 0.6	66[d] ± 5	392[c] ± 17 ($N = 16$)	66[c] ± 10 ($N = 15$)
Primary myocardial disease (6)	170[d] ± 14	11.3[b] ± 1.1	55[c] ± 9	364 ± 38	86[c] ± 13 ($N = 5$)
Idiopathic myocardial hypertrophy (3)	78 ± 18	22.2[b] ± 3.7	81[b] ± 16	144[d] ± 21	42 ± 10

[a] Group means ± 1 SE are shown. Values for stress are mean values across the ventricular wall derived using a thick-walled ellipsoidal model. Number in parentheses represent number of patients involved. (See text for further explanation.)

[b] In comparison with normals, $p < 0.05$

Thus, quantitation of left ventricular mass allows us to document the degree of hypertrophy in chronic heart disease. However it does not permit us to say anything about how appropriate this hypertrophy is in terms of anatomy or function. On the assumption that hypertrophy should be appropriate to the existing pressure and volume demands, various indexes of hypertrophy have been studied. For example, in pressure overload, left ventricular wall thickness has been correlated with peak left ventricular pressure (Levine *et al.*, 1963; Wallgren *et al.*, 1965). In volume overload left ventricular wall thickness has been related to chamber radius (Grant *et al.*, 1965). Each of these indexes reflects the factor of pressure or volume but not both. In our laboratory we have attempted to take into account both pressure and volume by quantitating wall stress. Stress (σ), in accordance with the modified law of Laplace, is directly proportional to pressure (P) and radius of curvature (r), and inversely proportional to wall thickness (h).

$$\sigma \sim (P \cdot r)/h$$

If wall hypertrophy is appropriate to the pressure and volume load in chronic heart disease, then stress remains normal. If hypertrophy is inadequate for the pressure–volume demands, stress increases. If the wall thickens out of proportion to pressure and volume, then stress is reduced.

Stress represents force per unit cross-sectional area of wall and in the metric system is expressed as dyn/cm^2. Figure 1 is a diagrammatic representation of a segment of ventricular wall and illustrates that the wall is actually subjected to more than one stress. Radial stress, not shown in the figure, acts

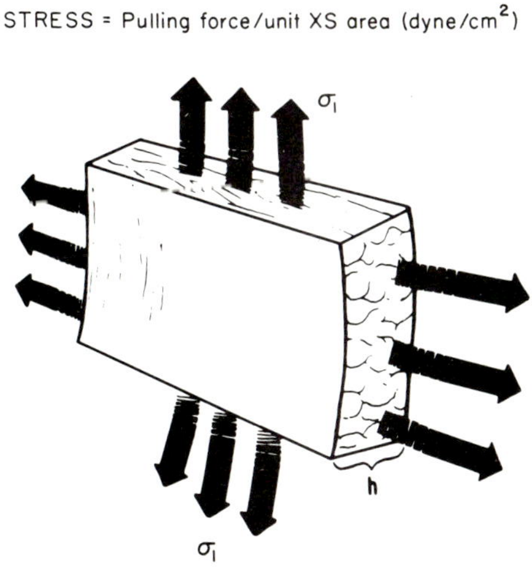

FIG. 1. Stresses acting on a segment of left ventricular wall. σ_1 represents longitudinal stress; σ_2, circumferential stress.

perpendicular to the endocardial surface; longitudinal stress, labeled σ_1, acts within the wall parallel to the long axis of the heart; circumferential stress, labeled σ_2, also acts within the wall but parallel to the short axis. We did not attempt to quantitate radial stress, but we initially calculated both longitudinal and circumferential stress at the ventricular equator. When longitudinal stress proved in most cases to be approximately one-half circumferential stress, we stopped looking at the smaller force and focused our attention entirely on circumferential stress.

Circumferential stress has been derived from simultaneous chamber dimensions, wall thickness measurements, and ventricular pressure in two ways: one based on the thin-walled ellipsoidal model of Sandler and Dodge (1963), the other based on the thick-walled ellipsoidal model of Wong and Rautaharju (1968). The thick-walled model is more sophisticated and theoretically more correct, but both models make the same basic assumptions and regard stress, in its passive sense, as the force opposing ventricular contraction or the force tending to rupture the ventricular wall.

Figure 2 shows the time course of mean circumferential stress as calculated from both thin-walled and thick-walled models in a subject with a normal

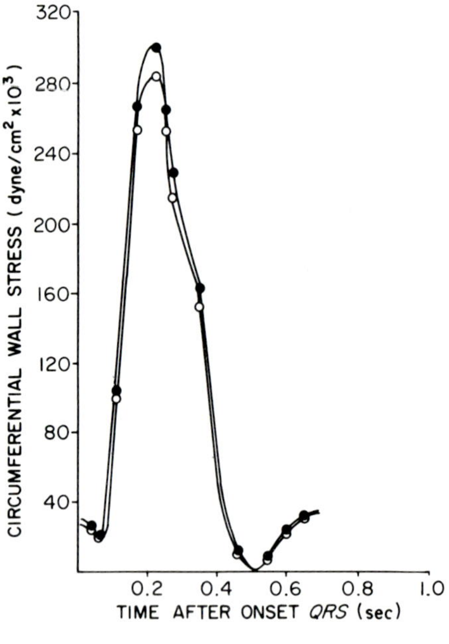

FIG. 2. Time course of mean circumferential stress in a subject with a normal left ventricle (EDV = 109 ml) as calculated using the thin-walled model of Sandler and Dodge (S & D), represented by filled circles, and the thick-walled model of Wong and Rautaharju (W & R) represented by open circles.

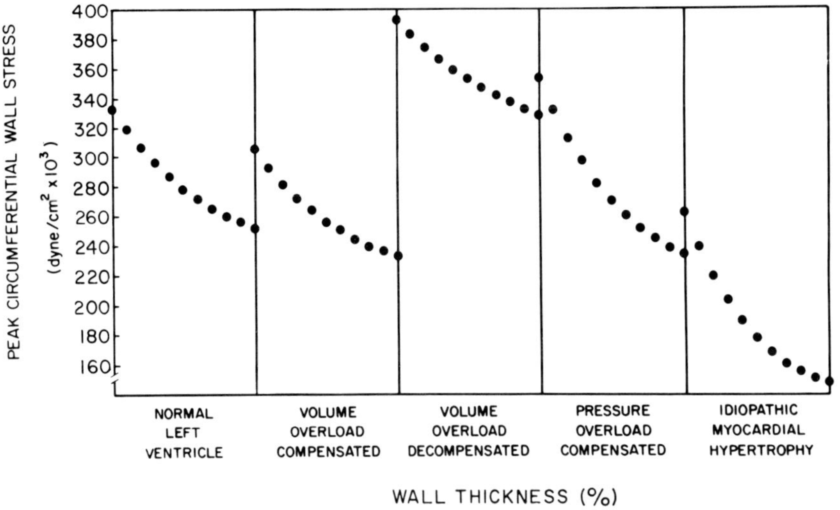

FIG. 3. Thick-wall distribution curves for peak circumferential stress in different physiologic states. Stress is plotted from 0% wall thickness (endocardium, left) to 100% wall thickness (epicardium, right).

left ventricle. In all cases studied, the time course of stress as determined from the two models was virtually identical, but Sandler and Dodge values were, on the average, 10% higher than those of Wong and Rautaharju (Hood *et al.*, 1969). Among 10 normal subjects, end-diastolic stress (thick wall) averaged 32 dyn/cm^2 $\times$ 10^3, and peak systolic stress (thick wall) averaged 312 dyn/cm^2 $\times$ 10^3 (Table I). It should be emphasized that these values represent mean values across the ventricular wall. Utilizing the Wong and Rautaharju model, it is possible to determine actual stress distribution across the wall. Figure 3 shows such distribution curves for peak systolic stress in five representative subjects with varying physiology. In each case illustrated, the endocardium is toward the left and the epicardium is toward the right. It can be appreciated that mean stress underestimates maximal stress, which occurs at the endocardium, and overestimates minimal stress, which occurs at the epicardium, but this fact does not invalidate use of the mean value as an index of the appropriateness of hypertrophy (*vide infra*).

Figure 4 is a bar graph comparing mean thick-wall end-diastolic and peak systolic stress values among the various physiologic categories. It can be seen that values for both end-diastolic and peak systolic stress formed tight groups in the normals. In the patients with mitral stenosis, similar values were obtained. In the group with compensated volume overload, peak stress was normalized but statistically end-diastolic stress was not (Table I). Similar findings were seen in the patients with primary myocardial disease. Within

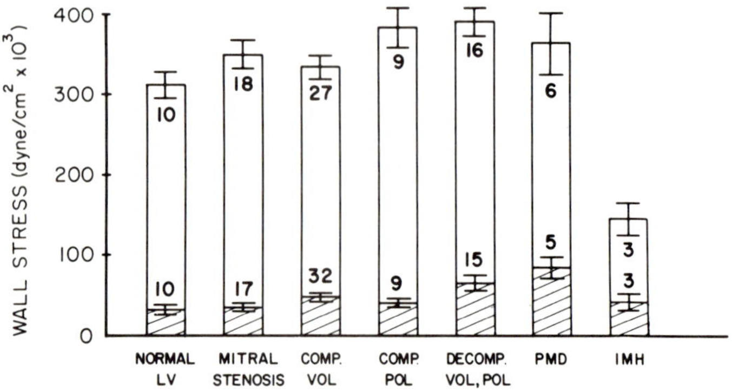

FIG. 4. Comparison of mean thick-wall stress values in different physiologic states. Open bars (top) demonstrate peak systolic stress; cross-hatched bars (bottom), end-diastolic stress. Brackets indicate ± 1 SE. Numbers represent number of observations in each category.

the decompensated group, although left ventricular mass was more than twice normal, the degree of hypertrophy was insufficient to normalize either end-diastolic or peak systolic stress. Among patients with compensated pressure overload, end-diastolic stress was not significantly increased but peak stress was. In the group with idiopathic myocardial hypertrophy, peak stress was greatly reduced.

We may conclude from these observations that the normal left ventricle functions within a narrow range of both end-diastolic and peak systolic stress values. In chronic valvular disease there is a tendency for stress to be normalized by hypertrophy of the ventricular wall appropriate to the pressure and volume demands. The tendency for normalization of peak stress appears to be somewhat greater than that for end-diastolic stress, suggesting that systolic events are more important determinants of myocardial hypertrophy than are diastolic events. In the presence of myocardial disease, the degree of hypertrophy may be inadequate or excessive in terms of peak stress.

Although peak systolic stress is a useful index of the anatomic adaptation in chronic heart disease, this parameter is not a sensitive index of function, as is shown in Fig. 5. This figure plots ejection fraction and peak stress (thick-wall) in all subjects. Correlation was poor, with an r value of -0.272. Whereas a severe degree of decompensation is frequently accompanied by elevated peak stress, because of the tendency for peak stress to be normalized, a lesser degree of dysfunction may be associated with normal peak stress.

In summary, quantitative angiocardiography has demonstrated that left ventricular chamber enlargement in chronic heart disease is characteristically accompanied by hypertrophy of the myocardium. Except in hypertrophic myocardial disease, the magnitude of this hypertrophy appears to be deter-

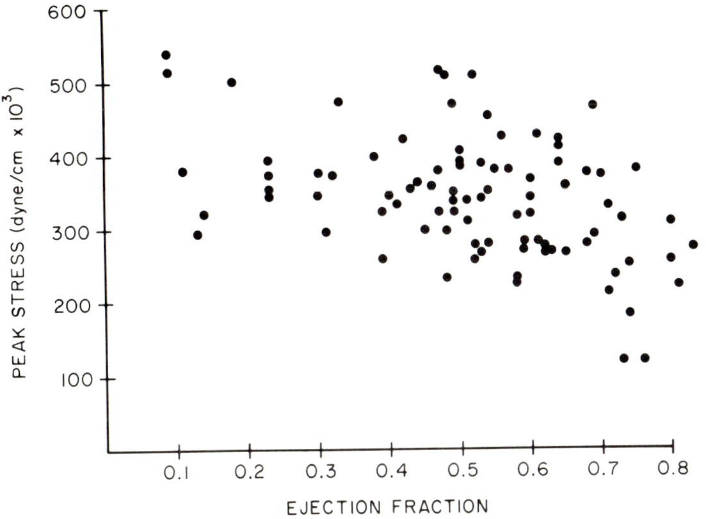

FIG. 5. Relationship of ejection fraction (abscissa) and peak systolic (thick-wall) stress (ordinate) in all subjects. r value is -0.272.

mined by wall stress, especially peak systolic stress, hypertrophy tending to increase appropriate to the pressure–volume load until stress is normalized. In hypertrophic myocardial disease, hypertrophy occurs out of proportion to that which can be explained by the stimulus of stress. "Ideal" anatomical adaptation in terms of stress does not preclude abnormal myocardial function.

ACKNOWLEDGMENTS

These studies were supported in part by USPHS grants HE5186 and FR46, and in part by a grant from the North Carolina Heart Association. Dr. Charles E. Rackley, Dr. Ellis L. Rolett, and Dr. Daniel T. Young collaborated in the performance of these studies. Mrs. Linda Cleveland was responsible for computer programming and operation.

REFERENCES

Dodge, H. T., Sandler, H., Ballew, D. W., and Lord, J. D. (1960). *Amer. Heart J.* **60,** 762.
Grant, C., Greene, D. G., and Bunnell, I. L. (1965). *Amer. J. Med.* **39,** 895.
Hood, W. P., Jr., Rackley, C. E., and Rolett, E. L. (1968). *Amer. J. Cardiol.* **22,** 550.
Hood, W. P., Jr., Thomson, W. J., Rackley, C. E., and Rolett, E. L. (1969). *Circ. Res.* **24,** 575.
Levine, N. D., Rockoff, S. D., and Braunwald, E. (1963). *Circulation* **28,** 339.
Linzbach, A. J. (1960). *Amer. J. Cardiol.* **5,** 370.
Rackley, C. E., Dodge, H. T., and Coble, Y. D., Jr. (1964). *Circulation* **29,** 666.

Rackley, C. E., Hood, W. P., Jr., Cleveland, L., and Stacy, R. W. (1968). *J. Appl. Physiol.* **24,** 254.

Sandler, H., and Dodge, H. T. (1963). *Circ. Res.* **13,** 91.

Sonnenblick, E. H., and Ross, J., Jr. (1967). *In* "Factors Influencing Myocardial Contractility" (R. D. Tanz, F. Kavaler, and J. Roberts, eds.), p. 43. Academic Press, New York.

Wallgren, G., Hatam, K., and Rudhe, U. (1965). *Amer. J. Cardiol.* **15,** 827.

Wong, A. Y. K., and Rautaharju, P. M. (1968). *Amer. Heart J.* **75,** 649.

LEFT VENTRICULAR DILATATION AND HYPERTROPHY IN CORONARY ARTERY DISEASE

Charles E. Rackley, H. Davis Dear, William A. Baxley, William B. Jones, and Harold T. Dodge

Cardiac enlargement is frequently encountered in patients with coronary artery disease and has been attributed to myocardial ischemia (Davis and Blumgart, 1937), hypertension (Zaino and Tabor, 1963), or congestive heart failure (Ellis *et al.*, 1962; Friedberg, 1966). In addition, mitral regurgitation resulting from papillary muscle dysfunction (Burch, De Pasquale, and Phillips, 1963; Bashour, 1965), rupture, or enlargement of the left ventricle (Levy and Edwards, 1962) may provide a volume overload. Accurate clinical and pathological measurements of left ventricular chamber size, mass, and mitral regurgitation have been difficult in these patients. The present investigation was undertaken in patients with coronary artery disease to quantitate left ventricular volume, mass, and mitral regurgitation, to relate these measurements to coronary arteriograms and to examine the mechanisms for ventricular hypertrophy.

Methods

Twenty-three patients with clinical evidence of coronary artery disease underwent selective coronary cineangiography and left ventricular biplane angiocardiography. The clinical indications for catheterization were (1) to select candidates for revascularization operations, and (2) to identify mechanisms for persistent heart failure. Coronary arteriography was performed by the Sones technique (Sones and Shirey, 1962). Cardiac output was measured by the Fick principle at right heart catheterization. Biplane angiocardiography was performed at filming rates of 6 to 12 films per second, and left ventricular volumes were determined by the area length method as previously described (Dodge and Baxley, 1969). Left ventricular wall thickness was added to chamber dimensions to estimate left ventricular mass (Rackley *et al.*, 1964). The difference between the angiographic left ventricular stroke volume and forward stroke volume determined by the Fick output is the regurgitant flow per beat (Sandler *et al.*, 1963). Ejection fraction is the ratio of angiographic left ventricular stroke volume to end-diastolic volume. Patients with aortic valve disease and left ventricular aneurysms were excluded from the present study.

Results

The clinical findings, including the chest roentgenogram and electrocardiogram are recorded in Table I. Neither a history nor clinical evidence for diastolic hypertension was obtained in any of the 23 patients. Seventeen patients described orthopnea and paroxysmal nocturnal dyspnea. Apical systolic murmurs were heard in 14 patients. Radiographic evidence for left ventricular enlargement on conventional anteroposterior and left lateral chest X-rays was observed in 17 patients and left atrial enlargement in 10 patients. Abnormal Q waves consistent with previous myocardial infarction were present in the electrocardiogram in 15 of the 23 patients.

The data from biplane angiocardiography and coronary arteriography are recorded in Table II. End-diastolic volume ranged from 111 to 580 ml and left ventricular mass from 152 to 533 gm. The upper limit for normal end-diastolic volume is 172 ml and for normal ventricular mass 247 gm (Kennedy *et al.*, 1966). A significant correlation (Fig. 1) was found between end-diastolic volume and left ventricular mass ($r = 0.765$, $p < 0.01$). Of 18 patients with complete occlusion of one or more coronary arteries, 10 had mass values larger than normal and 8 were within the normal range. In the 5 patients representing diffuse coronary disease without obstruction, three possessed significantly increased mass values and two were normal. Four electrocardiograms were interpreted by voltage as left ventricular hypertrophy, yet 13 patients possessed left ventricular masses larger than 247 gm.

Fifteen of the 23 patients demonstrated mitral regurgitation by angiocardiography. Apical systolic murmurs were heard in 14 of the 15 patients; but in four patients, the apical murmur was not considered typical of mitral regurgitation. One patient without a murmur exhibited mitral regurgitation by angiography. Apical systolic murmurs were not detected in the 8 patients without angiographic mitral regurgitation. End-diastolic volumes ranging from 200 to 253 ml were found in the presence, as well as the absence of mitral regurgitation. Although a significant relationship between end-diastolic volume and mitral regurgitation was not demonstrated, end-diastolic volumes greater than 255 ml were invariably associated with mitral valve incompetence (Fig. 2).

TABLE I

CLINICAL FINDINGS[a]

Patient	Age	Sex	Symptoms	Physical examination	X-Ray	ECG
1. J. M.	41	M	Dyspnea	III/VI Apical holosystolic murmur	LAE, LVE	LAH, LVH, PMI
2. W. S.	53	M	PND, orthopnea	II/VI Apical holosystolic murmur	LAE, LVE	LAD, LAH, LBBB
3. D. S.	58	F	Angina, dyspnea, orthopnea	I/VI Apical holosystolic murmur	LVE	LVH, PMI
4. R. B.	43	M	PND	No murmur	LAE, LVE	LAD, AMI
5. D. C.	62	F	Fatigue	IV/VI Apical systolic murmur	LAE, LVE	ST depressed $V_4 - V_6$
6. L. M.	56	M	Angina, PND, orthopnea	III/VI Apical systolic murmur	LVE	ST depressed $V_3 - V_6$
7. F. M.	62	M	PND, orthopnea	III/VI Apical systolic murmur	LAE, LVE	LAH, PMI
8. F. N.	62	M	Angina, PND, orthopnea	III/VI Apical systolic murmur	LVE	LAH, LVH, PMI
9. E. S.	49	M	Angina, PND, orthopnea	II/VI Apical systolic murmur	LAE, LVE	LAH, RAH, AMI
10. N. M.	51	M	Angina, PND, orthopnea	II/VI Apical systolic murmur	LAE, LVE	LAH, RAH, PMI
11. L. K.	40	M	Dyspnea, orthopnea	II/VI Apical systolic murmur	Normal	LVH, PMI
12. B. A.	53	M	Angina, PND, orthopnea	III/VI Apical systolic murmur	LAE, LVE	LAH, LVH, LBBB
13. J. S.	46	M	Angina, PND, orthopnea	III/VI Apical systolic murmur	LAE, LVE	LAH, PMI
14. C. H.	53	M	Angina, PND, orthopnea	III/VI Apical systolic murmur	LAE, LVE	LBBB
15. C. M.	51	M	Angina, PND, orthopnea	II/VI Apical systolic murmur	LAE, LVE	AMI
16. O. L.	54	M	Angina, dyspnea, orthopnea	No murmur	LVE	LAH, ST depressed $V_5 - V_6$
17. M. L.	47	F	Angina, PND, orthopnea	No murmur	LVE	RAD, LAH, AMI
18. J. M.	43	M	Angina	No murmur	Normal	Normal
19. A. T.	46	M	Angina	I/VI Systolic murmur left of sternum	LVE	Normal
20. C. D.	56	M	Angina	II/VI Systolic murmur left of sternum	Normal	PMI
21. B. O.	46	M	Angina, dyspnea, orthopnea	No murmur	—	AMI
22. B. D.	38	M	Angina	No murmur	Normal	PMI
23. T. B.	51	M	Angina	I/VI Systolic murmur left of sternum	Normal	PMI

[a] PND, Paroxysmal nocturnal dyspnea; LAE, left atrial enlargement; LVE, left ventricular enlargement; PMI, posterior myocardial infarction; AMI, anterior myocardial infarction; RAH, right atrial hypertrophy; LAH, left atrial hypertrophy; LVH, left ventricular hypertrophy; LBBB, left bundle branch block; LAD, left axis deviation; RAD, right axis deviation.

TABLE II

HEMODYNAMIC AND ANGIOGRAPHIC FINDINGS[a]

Patient	Heart rate Fick/Angio	LV Pressure mm HG	FICK C.O. 1/min	EDV ml (cc)	ESV ml (cc)	LVSV ml (cc)	RV ml (cc)	EF	LV Mass (gm)	Coronary angiograms
1. J. M.	92/93	100/20	4.40	314	215	99	51	0.32	278	RC occluded, LC and LAD narrowed
2. W. S.	79/80	90/22	2.90	573	447	126	89	0.22	533	RC and LAD severely narrowed
3. D. S.	72/52	160/10	5.26	250	158	92	19	0.37	244	RC occluded, main left coronary narrowed at ostium
4. R. B.	82/79	84/36	2.04	179	139	40	15	0.22	152	RC, LC and LAD narrowed
5. D. C.	102/96	115/10	4.90	190	60	130	82	0.68	193	LC and LAD narrowed
6. L. M.	86/86	90/25	2.59	280	168	112	82	0.43	304	RC and LC narrowed
7. F. M.	100/100	80/15	3.10	352	272	80	49	0.23	260	RC and LC occluded
8. F. N.	89/89	100/21	5.0	388	247	91	35	0.27	298	RC occluded, LC and LAD narrowed
9. E. S.	90/75	91/34	2.36	580	505	75	49	0.13	446	RC, LC and LAD narrowed
10. N. M.	107/102	95/40	1.92	250	205	45	37	0.22	180	RC and LAD occluded
11. L. K.	75/76	105/17	5.43	270	168	102	29	0.38	454	RC occluded, LC and LAD narrowed
12. B. A.	76/93	100/22	3.20	524	398	126	84	0.24	406	RC and LAD occluded
13. J. S.	90/83	95/35	3.31	300	188	112	75	0.37	256	RC and LC occluded, LAD narrowed
14. C. H.	94/83	100/25	5.12	434	342	92	37	0.27	408	RC, LC and LAD occluded
15. C. M.	107/94	100/25	2.99	483	416	67	39	0.14	389	LAD occluded, LC narrowed
16. O. L.	88/100	125/10	4.37	202	152	50	0	0.25	412	RC and LC occluded
17. M. L.	88/83	123/38	3.45	233	184	39	0	0.17	191	RC and LAD occluded, LC narrowed
18. J. M.				112	27	85	0	0.75	175	RC occluded, main left coronary narrowed
19. A. T.	/81	116/10		253	158	95	0	0.38	246	LC and LAD occluded
20. C. L.	67/57	110/5	3.85	111	55	56	0	0.50	221	RC occluded, LC narrowed
21. B. O.	75/73	130/10	8.82	215	134	81	0	0.38	305	LAD occluded
22. B. D.	65/73	115/8	4.31	160	100	60	0	0.38	205	RC occluded
23. T. B.	72	120/8	6.65	208	125	83	0	0.40	156	RC occluded, LC narrowed

[a] [illegible] EDV, end-diastolic volume; ESV, end-systolic volume; LVSV, left ventricular stroke volume; RV, regurgitant volume

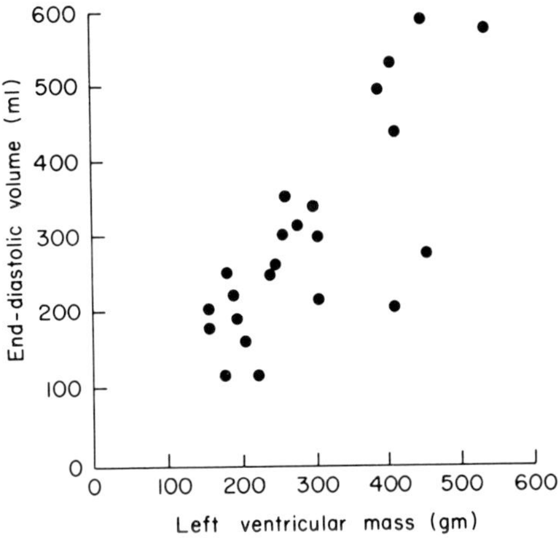

FIG. 1. A significant correlation was found between end-diastolic volume and left ventricular mass in the 23 patients with coronary artery disease. $n = 23$; $r = 0.765$; $p < 0.01$.

Comparison of left ventricular mass in the absence and presence of mitral regurgitation revealed 6 subjects in the former group and 4 in the latter with normal mass values (Fig. 3). Two of the 8 patients without mitral regurgitation and 11 of the 15 patients with mitral regurgitation had left ventricular masses greater than 247 gm.

One patient in the group without mitral regurgitation and one patient possessing mitral regurgitation had normal ejection fractions of 0.75 and 0.68, respectively. The mean ejection fractions were 0.40 in the patients not having regurgitation and 0.30 in those demonstrating mitral regurgitation (Fig. 4). Although the ejection fractions were below the normal range (0.56–0.78) (Kennedy *et al.*, 1966) in 21 of the 23 patients, the values tended to be more reduced in the group with mitral regurgitation. However, the latter group also had more marked ventricular dilatation as shown in Fig. 2.

In the eight patients with coronary artery disease and no angiographic evidence of mitral regurgitation, the coronary arteriograms demonstrated occlusion of the right coronary artery in four, occlusion of the right and left circumflex in one, and occlusion of the right and left anterior descending in one. One patient revealed narrowing of the left circumflex and anterior descending, and one patient exhibited diffuse narrowing of all major coronaries.

In the 15 patients with mitral regurgitation, the right coronary was occluded in three, the right and circumflex left in two, the right and left anterior descending in four and the right with both branches of the left in one. The coronary vessels were significantly narrowed without occlusion in four patients (Fig. 5). The mitral regurgitant volume in these 15 patients ranged

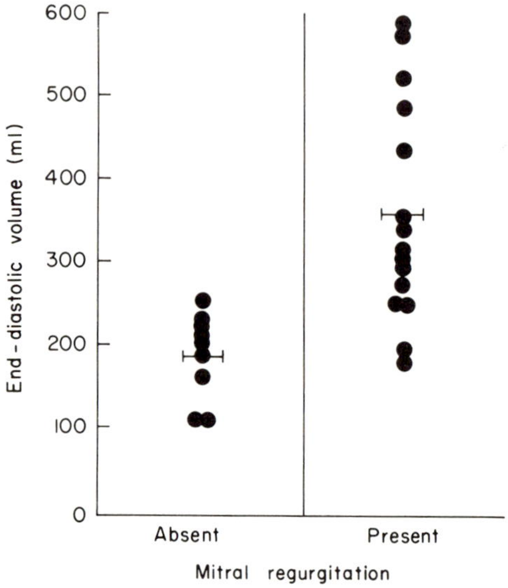

FIG. 2. Fifteen of the 23 patients demonstrated mitral regurgitation and an end-diastolic volume larger than 255 ml was consistently associated with mitral regurgitation.

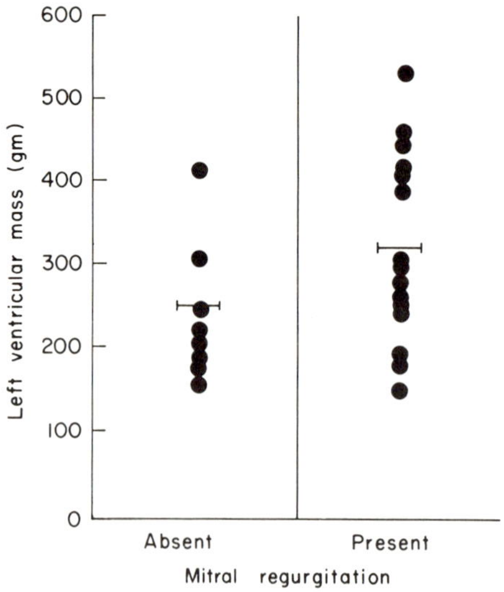

FIG. 3. Patients with mitral regurgitation tended to possess left ventricular masses larger than the upper limit of normal 247 gm.

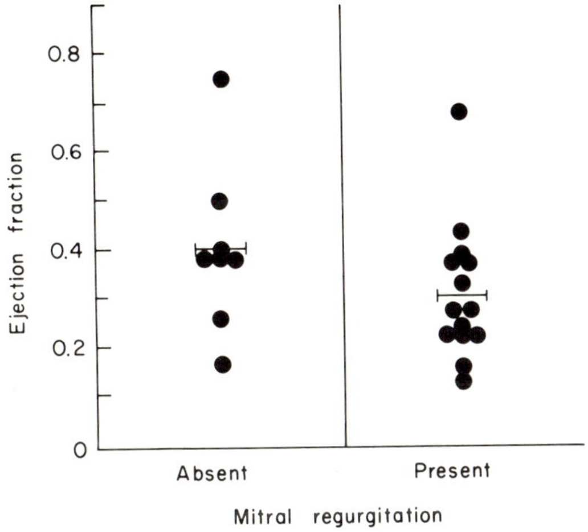

FIG. 4. Ejection fractions were reduced significantly below the normal range of 0.56 to 0.78 in the absence as well as the presence of mitral regurgitation.

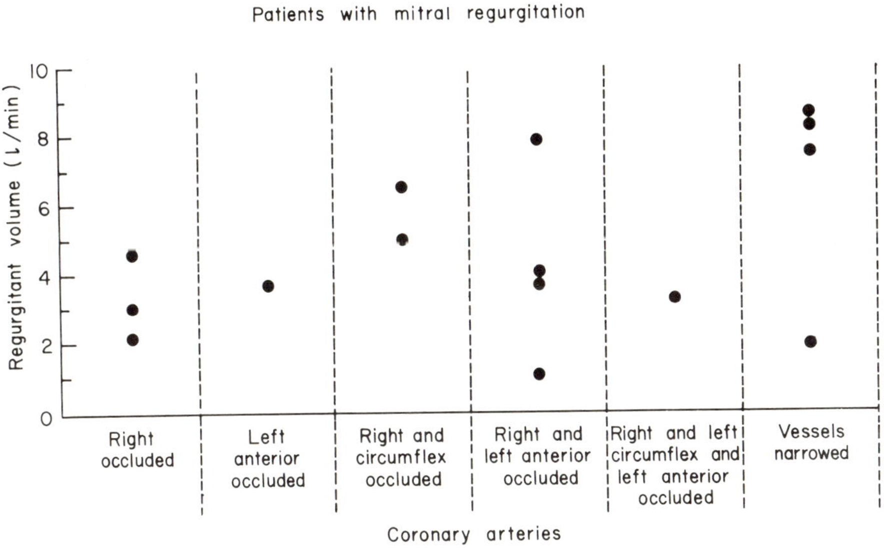

FIG. 5. The mitral regurgitant volume per minute ranged from 1 to 8.5 liter/min. The right coronary artery was occluded alone or in combination with branches of the left coronary in 10 of the 15 patients.

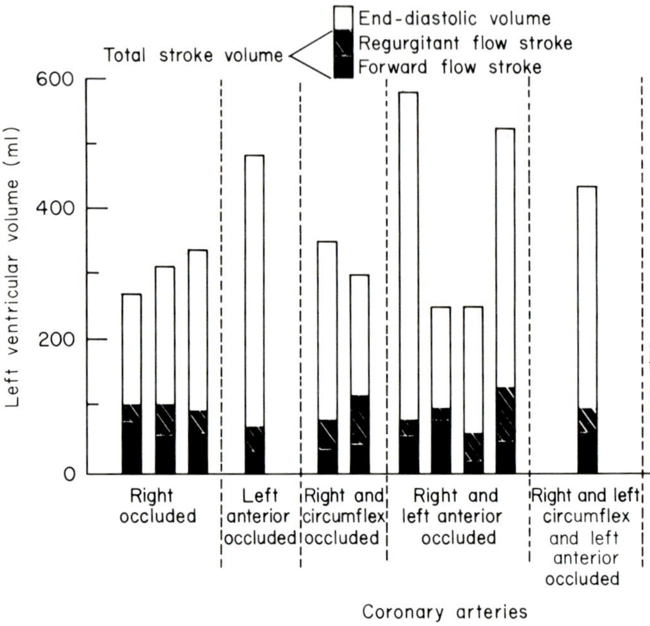

FIG. 6. The end-diastolic volume, regurgitant and forward stroke volumes are illustrated in the 15 patients with mitral regurgitation.

from 1.0 to 8.5 liter/min. For each patient with mitral regurgitation, the end-diastolic volume, the regurgitant and forward flow per beat are illustrated in Fig. 6.

Three patients (1, 2, and 6) underwent surgical repair of the mitral valve, and two others (4 and 13) had postmortem examinations. A dilated mitral annulus with normal papillary muscles was observed in patient No. 1, and the papillary muscles were unremarkable in patient No. 4. Infarcted papillary muscles were observed in 3 patients (Nos. 2, 6, and 13). Coronary occlusions were demonstrated on the arteriograms in patient No. 1 with the dilated mitral annulus and in patient No. 13 with papillary muscle infarctions. In 2 patients (Nos. 2 and 6) with papillary muscle infarctions and in patient No. 4 with unremarkable papillary muscles the coronary arteriograms revealed diffuse coronary disease without occlusions.

Discussion

The incidence of cardiac enlargement in coronary artery disease has been well studied clinically and pathologically. Weiss and Weiss (1957) found radiographic evidence for cardiac hypertrophy in only 8 of 489 patients who survived an acute myocardial infarction. Master (1954) noted clinical cardiac enlargement in 29 hypertensive and 45 normotensive patients out of 500 men followed after coronary occlusions. In a study of cardiac pathology, Davis and Blumgart (1937) found little or no cardiac hypertrophy with lesser degrees of coronary atherosclerosis and a slight degree of hypertrophy with more severe involvement of the coronary arteries. After excluding hypertension and cardiovascular disease, Friedberg (1966) and Sohvol found no evidence of cardiac hypertrophy in 100 pathological cases of coronary occlusion unless congestive heart failure had been present. In the absence of heart failure in subjects with coronary artery disease, Ellis and co-workers (1962) noted cardiac hypertrophy infrequently in those without coronary occlusions or myocardial infarctions, but hypertrophy occurred in about half of the patients with occlusions and infarctions. With a history of heart failure, hypertrophy was found in 50–60% of patients without occlusions and infarctions, and in nearly all those with these lesions. At autopsy, heart weight can be accurately measured. However, accurate estimation of *in vivo* end-diastolic chamber size from post-mortem studies is difficult, if not impossible, because rigor mortis reduces the chamber volume.

In the present investigation 13 of 23 patients with coronary artery disease demonstrated abnormally increased left ventricular mass values. It would be of interest to know to what extent hypertrophy compensated for infarcted muscle, but the techniques employed in the present study do not permit one to differentiate scar and fibrous tissue from muscle. The values for left ventricular weight include scar and fibrous tissue plus myocardium. Although the larger mass values were found in patients with one or more coronary arteries occluded, three patients with nonocclusive coronary disease possessed increased left ventricular masses. The patient exhibiting the largest left ventricular weight of 533 gm demonstrated diffuse coronary narrowing without obstruction. Although hypertension was not present in any patients in the present study, 17 had symptoms compatible with left ventricular failure. A history of heart failure was associated with an increased mass value, yet 5 patients with heart failure revealed normal left ventricular weights. All 5 patients with angina alone demonstrated normal left ventricular masses. In these 23 patients a significant relationship was found between left ventricular dilatation and left ventricular mass. Only one patient revealed an abnormally increased left ventricular mass with a normal end-diastolic volume. In fact, significant dilatation was not observed in the absence of hypertrophy (Fig. 1).

Even though the patients comprising the present study manifested refractory chest pain or congestive heart failure, the incidence of significant mitral regurgitation in 15 of the 23 patients was surprising. The amount of mitral regurgitation ranged from 1 to 8.5 liter/min. Abnormal function of the papillary muscle is commonly invoked to explain apical systolic murmurs in coronary artery disease. However, only 3 of the 5 patients examined at surgery or autopsy demonstrated papillary muscle infarction. In addition to papillary muscle dysfunction or infarction, the enlarged ventricular chamber must contribute to the development of mitral incompetence. An end-diastolic volume greater than 255 ml was invariably associated with mitral regurgitation in the present investigation. The ejection fraction tended to be lower in patients demonstrating mitral regurgitation than those with competent valves. Thus, in patients with coronary artery disease the progressive increase in end-diastolic volume may reflect further impairment of myocardial contractility. Furthermore, left ventricular dilatation in excess of 255 ml is usually associated with mitral insufficiency which imposes an additional burden on a left ventricle with compromised coronary circulation, and leads to further increases in end-diastolic volume and hypertrophy.

In relating end-diastolic volume, ventricular mass, and mitral regurgitation to the coronary arteriograms, no specific vascular lesion consistently resulted in mitral valvular incompetence. Experimentally, acute ligation of the canine circumflex coronary artery produces an increase in end-diastolic and end-systolic volumes, a reduction in ejection fraction and mitral regurgitation (Harley *et al.*, 1968). However, Symbas and co-workers (1969) could not produce mitral valve incompetence in the dog with papillary muscle injury or infarction limited to the base of the anterior papillary muscle. In the present series significant mitral regurgitation was found in patients exhibiting diffuse vessel narrowing by coronary arteriography as well as occlusion of the major coronary vessels. Two patients with infarcted papillary muscles and one with unremarkable papillary muscles demonstrated diffuse coronary narrowing without occlusions. Obstructed coronary arteries were shown on the arteriograms in one patient with a dilated mitral annulus and in another patient with papillary muscle infarction. Interestingly, the right coronary artery was occluded alone or in combination with branches of the left in 11 of the 15 patients with mitral regurgitation. Shelburne *et al.* (1969) have reported an increased incidence of severe right coronary lesions in mitral regurgitation due to papillary muscle dysfunction. A higher incidence of mitral incompetence after myocardial infarction has been reported with posterior infarctions than with anterior location (Heikkila, 1967).

Previously proposed mechanisms for ventricular hypertrophy in coronary artery disease include myocardial injury, hypertension and congestive heart failure. Hypertension was not a contributing factor in the present group of patients. Left ventricular failure was manifested in 17 of the 23 patients by history and each of these patients had an elevated volume with a reduced ejection fraction. Ventricular hypertrophy was present in all, except four patients with a history of heart failure. However, there was a wide variation of end-diastolic pressure volume relationships in comparing individual subjects as is evident in Table II. The association of an increased end-diastolic volume and left ventricular mass with a reduced ejection fraction supports the previous theories that muscle injury (Eyster, 1928) and heart failure (Linzback, 1960) with reduced contractility are responsible for cardiac hypertrophy. Whether the impaired contractility that results from coronary disease is local or generalized, left ventricular end-diastolic volume increases as a result. Although left ventricular stroke volume may be maintained through dilatation and the Frank-Starling mechanism, the stimulus for ventricular hypertrophy may arise from muscle injury as well as increased systolic wall forces in a dilated ventricle (Linzback, 1960; Hood *et al.*, 1968). In addition to the increase in end-diastolic volume to maintain an adequate stroke volume, the development of mitral regurgitation provides a volume overload stimulus for physiologic hypertrophy.

Despite the ventricular hypertrophy in coronary artery disease, the ejection fraction remains significantly reduced and systolic wall forces are correspondingly elevated. Furthermore, the severely reduced ejection fraction indicates intrinsic myocardial disease with diminished contractility. The mitral regurgitation in patients with coronary artery disease is related at least in part to cardiac dilatation and, accordingly, more closely resembles that observed in idiopathic cardiomyopathy than rheumatic heart disease. Coronary cardiomyopathy might be an appropriate classification for such patients. Even though left ventricular dilation and hypertrophy are major compensatory mechanisms for volume overload and diminished contractility, left ventricular mass is an important determinant of coronary blood flow. The increased ventricular mass presents an additional burden to patients with coronary artery disease who have the problem of supplying adequate myocardial blood flow.

In conclusion, observations on 23 patients with coronary artery disease reveal that (1) a dilated left ventricle is hypertrophied and the extent of hypertrophy is proportional to the dilatation; (2) an enlarged left ventricle is frequently associated with mitral regurgitation; and (3) dilatation, hypertrophy and mitral regurgitation are manifestations of reduced left ventricular contractility.

Summary

In 23 patients coronary artery disease was demonstrated by selective coronary arteriograms, and left ventricular volume and mass were determined from biplane angiocardiograms. End-diastolic volume ranged from 111 to 580 ml, left ventricular mass from 152 to 533 gm and ejection fraction from 0.13 to 0.75. An increased end-diastolic volume was associated with an increased left ventricular mass ($r = 0.765$, $p < 0.01$). In 15 of the 23 patients mitral regurgitant volume ranged from 1.0 to 8.5 liter/min and an end-diastolic volume greater than 255 ml was invariably associated with mitral regurgitation. The ejection fraction was significantly reduced in the absence as well as the presence of mitral regurgitation. These observations on 23 patients with coronary artery disease reveal that (1) a dilated left ventricle is hypertrophied and the extent of hypertrophy is proportional to the dilatation; (2) an enlarged left ventricle is frequently associated with mitral regurgitation; and (3) dilatation, hypertrophy and mitral regurgitation are manifestations of reduced left ventricular contractility.

Acknowledgments

Supported in part by Grants HE 11310, and 2 MO1 FR 3209 from the U.S. Public Health Service and Grant RD 2219 M from the Vocational Rehabilitation Administration, Department of Health, Education and Welfare, and Cardiovascular Research, Veterans Administration Hospital, Birmingham, Alabama.

References

Bashour, F. A. (1965). *Dis. Chest* **48,** 113.

Burch, G. E., DePasquale, N. P., and Phillips, J. H. (1963). *Arch. Int. Med.* **112,** 158.

Davis, D., and Blumgart, H. L. (1937). *Ann. Int. Med.* **11,** 1024.

Dodge, H. T., and Baxley, W. A. (1969). *Amer. J. Cardiol.* **23,** 528.

Ellis, L. B., Allison, R. B., Rodrignez, F. L., and Robbins, S. L. (1962). *N. Engl. J. Med.* **266,** 525.

Eyster, J. A. E. (1928). *J. Amer. Med. Ass.* **91,** 1881.

Friedberg, C. K. (1966). "Diseases of the Heart," p. 790. Saunders, Philadelphia.

Harley, A., Behar, V. S., and McIntosh, H. D. (1968). *Amer. J. Cardiol.* **22,** 559.

Heikkila, J. (1967). *Acta Med. Scand. Suppl.* **475,** 1.

Hood, W. P., Jr., Rackley, C. E., and Rolett, E. L. (1968). *Amer. J. Cardiol.* **22,** 550.

Kennedy, J. W., Baxley, W. A., Figley, M. M., Dodge, H. T., and Blackmon, J. R. (1966). *Circulation* **34,** 272.

Levy, M. J., and Edwards, J. E. (1962). *Progr. Cardiov. Dis.* **5,** 119.

Linzback, A. J. (1960), *Amer. J. Cardiol.* **5,** 370.

Master, A. M. (1954). *Amer. Heart J.* **47,** 321.

Rackley, C. E., Dodge, H. T., Coble, Y. D., Jr., and Hay, R. E. (1964). *Circulation* **29,** 666.

Sandler, H., Dodge, H. T., Hay, R. E., and Rackley, C. E. (1963). *Amer. Heart J.* **65,** 501.

Shelburne, J. C., Rubinstein, D., and Gorlin, R. (1969). *Amer. J. Med.* **46,** 862.

Sones, F. M., Jr., and Shirey, E. K. (1962). *Mod. Conc. Cardiov. Dis.* **31,** 735.

Symbas, P. N., Ferrier, F. L., Litman, G. J., and Sybers, R. G. (1969). *Clin. Res.* **17,** 20.

Weiss, M. W., and Weiss, M. W., Jr. (1957). *Amer. J. Med. Sci.* **234,** 129.

Zaino, E. C., and Tabor, S. H. (1963). *Circulation* **28,** 1081.

CARDIAC MUSCLE PERFORMANCE IN VENTRICULAR HYPERTROPHY AND CONGESTIVE HEART FAILURE

James F. Spann, Jr.

Introduction

The clinical manifestations of cardiac hypertrophy and congestive heart failure are well known; the deleterious effects of heart failure on other organ systems such as the kidney have been described in detail and the hemodynamic alterations have been emphasized. The skeletal muscle studies of A. V. Hill (1938) have recently been extended to the understanding of the intrinsic contractile state of cardiac muscle (Sonnenblick, 1962), and it is now possible to examine the function of the heart in terms of myocardial muscle mechanics by considering instantaneous force, velocity, and shortening. Recent investigations have utilized these concepts to obtain an understanding of the hypertrophied and failing heart as abnormal cardiac muscle, with secondary emphasis on the function of the heart as a pump. Determination of the contractile state of hypertrophied and failing heart muscle, under controlled conditions, was most readily accomplished by study of experimental animal models of ventricular hypertrophy and congestive heart failure. The purpose of the current discussion is to present some of the data and conclusions derived from recent studies of animals with experimentally produced ventricular hypertrophy and congestive heart failure (Spann *et al.*, 1967a,b).

The basic experimental plan in these investigations was to examine the contractile performance of intact right ventricles and isolated muscles of three groups of cats: (1) normal controls, (2) cats with right ventricular hypertrophy but without congestive failure; and (3) cats which, despite the development of right ventricular hypertrophy, developed heart failure. Right ventricular hypertrophy with and without overt heart failure was produced in the cat by chronic constriction of the pulmonary artery (Spann *et al.*, 1967c).

Development of Ventricular Hypertrophy

Severe ventricular hypertrophy promptly followed the obstruction of the ventricular outflow tract (Fig. 1). Right ventricular weight averaged 0.94 ± 0.04 (SEM) gm/kg body weight after only two days of constriction of the pulmonary artery, a value almost two times the right ventricular weight in normal cats which averaged 0.55 ± 0.02. Within 1 month the right ventricular weight had tripled (Fig. 1). When examined under the electron

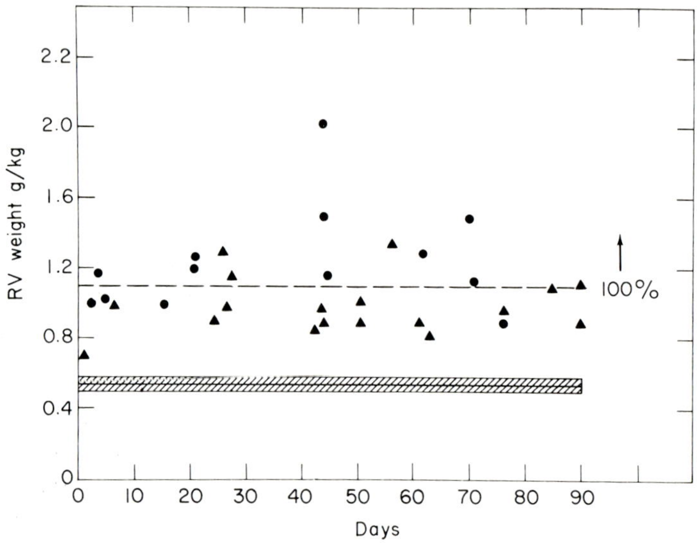

FIG. 1. Relation between right ventricular weight and the time at which the pulmonary artery was constricted. Average normal right ventricular weight and standard error are represented by cross-hatched area; average right ventricular weight was 0.55 ± 0.02 gm/kg body weight. Circles represent animals in which the remaining lumen of the pulmonary artery after constriction was 10% or less. Triangles represent animals in which the remaining pulmonary artery lumen after constriction was greater than 10% and usually 20%. The abscissa represents days after the pulmonary artery was constricted.

microscope, this hypertrophied heart muscle appears relatively normal with the usual relationships between contractile and noncontractile elements. This increase in ventricular weight was not due to a relative increase in tissue water since the wet weight to dry weight ratio was the same in the normal and hypertrophied groups. Myocardial protein concentration per unit dry weight of ventricular tissue also remained constant, indicating that there was no appreciable increase in the nonprotein elements of the myocardium. It has also been shown that the myocardial RNA synthesis is increased within

24 hrs. after an excessive work load is imposed on the left ventricle (Nair *et al.*, 1968). Thus, it is quite clear that when the heart is faced with an abnormal load there is a very rapid increase in contractile element mass. The changes in connective tissue elements of the hypertrophied heart are discussed in the chapter by Spann *et al.*, page 141.

Contractile State of Hypertrophied and Failing Heart Muscle Studied in the Papillary Muscle and Intact Ventricle

The hemodynamic status of each cat in the three groups was determined by right heart and aortic catheterization while the animal was lightly anesthetized. In some of the animals from each group, the right ventricular papillary muscles were then studied in a myograph in oxygenated Krebs solution (Sonnenblick, 1962). This system allowed measurement of force, muscle length, and the first derivatives of these variables under controlled conditions and comparison of data from the three groups of cats (Spann *et al.*, 1966). Length–tension relations, the isometric contraction, force–velocity relations, and responses to inotropic interventions were determined. In other animals from each group, the cardiac catheterization was done, then the chest was opened and contractile mechanics of the intact right ventricle were determined during isovolumic contractions prior to removal of the papillary muscle for study in the myograph. In this manner ventricular pump function, as reflected by circulatory dynamics, could be determined and then a quantitative description of both ventricular contractile state and isolated muscle performance could be obtained in each animal.

Length–Tension Relationships

In the papillary muscle the length of the muscle at the apex of the active length-tension curve was defined as L_{max}; changes in muscle length were expressed as percentages of L_{max}. Tensions were calculated as force per unit cross-sectional area of each muscle. In both the hypertrophy and failure groups the active developed tension was less than normal at all muscle lengths along the length–tension curve (Fig. 2). Maximum active tension in the muscles from cats with hypertrophy averaged 5.3 ± 0.6 gm/mm^2 compared with the normal value of 6.2 ± 0.7 gm/mm^2, whereas the maximum isometric tension for the muscles from cats with congestive heart failure was markedly reduced, averaging 2.4 ± 0.4 gm/mm^2. In the studies of the intact heart a segment of the length–tension curve was determined for each ventricle in the following manner. After determination of spontaneously occurring right ventricular maximum systolic wall tension during an isometric contraction, dextran was infused into the normal animals to increase resting ventricular

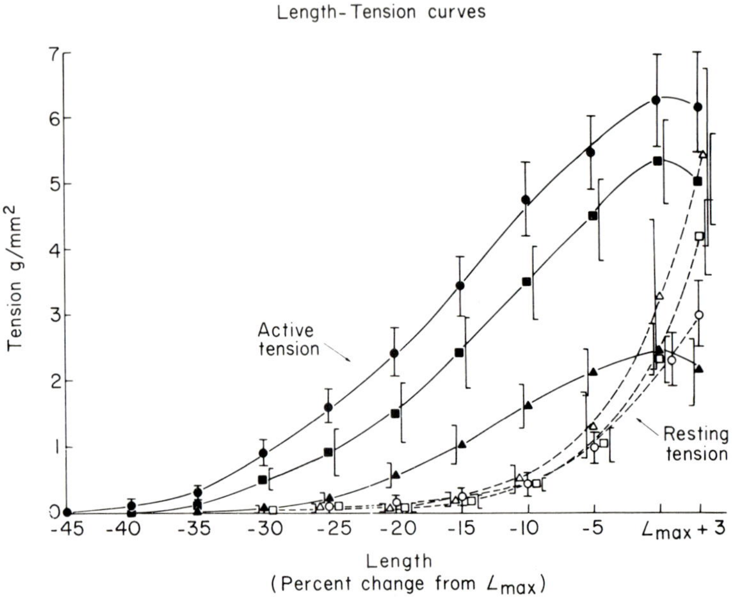

FIG. 2. Relation between muscle length and tension of the papillary muscles from 14 normal (circles), 10 hypertrophied (squares), and 11 failing (triangles) right ventricles. Open symbols represent resting tension; solid symbols, actively developed tension. Each value is the average of the group; vertical lines with cross bars equal ± 1 S.E.M. Tension is corrected for cross-sectional area (gm/mm^2). Data from Spann *et al.*, 1967a.

circumference, while the animals with ventricular hypertrophy and heart failure were bled to decrease diastolic ventricular circumference. The isovolumic contractions were then repeated, and maximum systolic wall tension was determined at the new resting lengths. When ventricular length–tension (Frank-Starling curves) were obtained by these manipulations of end-diastolic volume in the intact right ventricle, the hypertrophied and failing ventricles, like the hypertrophied and failing papillary muscles, were found to be operating along the ascending limb of a depressed length-active tension curve, rather than along the descending limb of a normal curve. When comparisons were made at similar end-diastolic ventricular circumferences, active ventricular wall tension was only one half normal in both the hypertrophied and the failing heart. The hypertrophied and failing ventricles, although operating on depressed length active tension curves, were able to maintain relatively normal peak isovolumic ventricular wall tension by means of an increased end-diastolic volume at the expense of increased end-diastolic ventricular pressure.

Interestingly, in the hypertrophied or failing cardiac muscle there does not appear to be a decrease in diastolic compliance per unit of muscle mass. There were no significant differences among the average resting length–tension curves in any of the three groups of papillary muscles, as shown by the dotted lines in Fig. 2. Also, in the intact ventricles, the diastolic tension was normal at all points along the resting length–tension curve, indicating no decrease in diastolic compliance in the hypertrophied and failing intact ventricles.

In the papillary muscle, the time course of the development of isometric tension was analyzed in terms of the maximum rate of tension development and the time from stimulation to the development of peak tension. The rate of tension development in an isometrically contracting muscle is an expression of the intensity of the active state in cardiac muscle, while the time from stimulation to development of peak tension is related directly to the duration of active state in cardiac muscle (Sonnenblick, 1967). In the isolated muscle from both hypertrophied and failing hearts the rate of tension development was markedly depressed while the time to peak tension was normal (Fig. 3). The depression of rate of rise of tension reflects a decrease in an intrinsic speed of the contractile element since the series elastic component of the hypertrophied and failing heart has recently been shown to be normal (Parmley *et al.*, 1968). The normal time to peak tension demonstrates that the duration of active state is unchanged in hypertrophy and

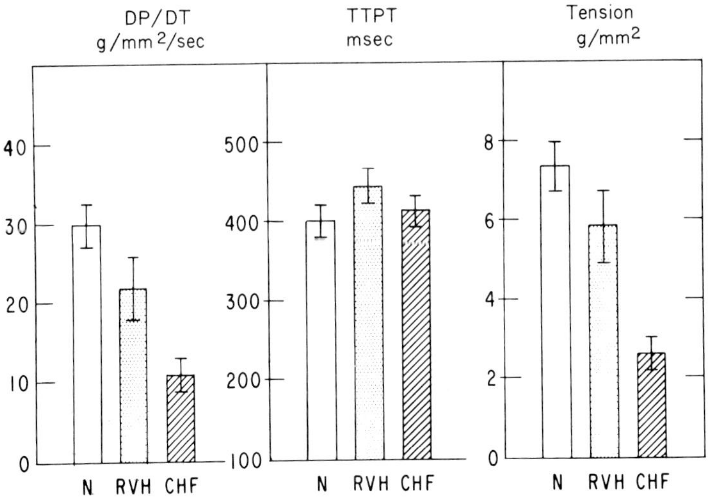

FIG. 3. Left, maximum rate of isometric force development shown for the three groups of muscles in gm/mm²/sec. All muscles were studied at the apex of their length–tension curves. Center, time from peak stimulation to the peak of developed isometric tension in msec. Right, maximum isometric tension in gm/mm². All muscles were studied at the apex of their length–tension curves. Each bar represents the average value and the vertical lines with cross-hatching equal ± 1 S.E.M.

heart failure and that the depression of force does not result from an abnormal abbreviation of the duration of the force generating processes between actin and myosin. This latter finding is in agreement with recent clinical evidence that the pre-ejection phase of the intact failing human ventricle is prolonged with a shortening of the duration of the ejection phase with unaltered duration of total electromechanical systole (Weissler *et al.*, 1969).

Force–Velocity Relationships

The force–velocity relationship allows the most precise characterization of the intrinsic contractile state of cardiac muscle and can best be studied in the isolated muscle; these relationships were examined in papillary muscles from the three groups of animals. Initial muscle length were set by a small preload which was constant for each force-velocity curve, and the effects on the velocity of shortening of progressively increasing afterload were then determined. Velocity of shortening was corrected for muscle length and was expressed in muscle lengths per second, whereas the force was expressed in gm/mm^2. The velocity of shortening at the smallest load (0.5 gm/mm^2) was used to approximate the maximum velocity of shortening (V_{max}) to avoid errors that might result from extrapolation of the curve to zero load. At each load, the velocity of shortening was less in muscles from both those cats with hypertrophy and those with failure, and the entire force velocity curve was shifted downward and to the left (Fig. 4). The maximum velocity of shortening

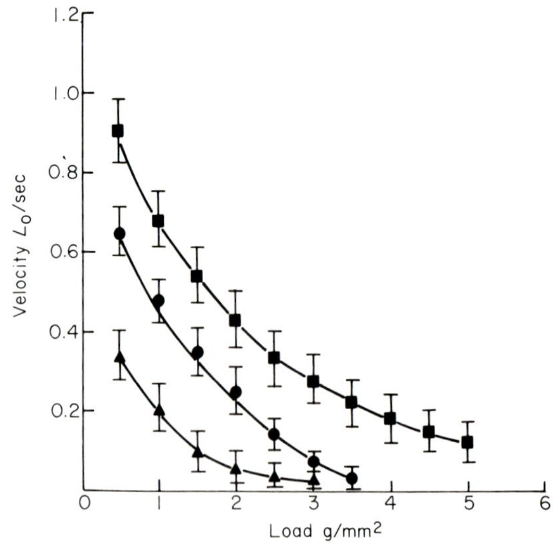

Fig. 4. The force–velocity relations of the three groups of cat papillary muscles. Average values with ± S.E.M. are given for each point. Velocity has been correct to ML/sec (L_0/sec). ■, Normal (15); ●, RVH (11); and ▲, CHF (11). Data from Spann *et al.*, 1967a.

at the load of 0.5 gm/mm^2 averaged 0.90 ± 0.08 ML/sec in normal muscles and was significantly lower, averaging 0.65 ± 0.60 ML/sec in muscles from cats with hypertrophy. V_{max} was significantly lower in the muscles from cats with failure than in the muscles from normal cats or those with hypertrophy and averaged 0.34 ± 0.06 ML/sec. Thus, in cardiac muscle isolated from the hypertrophied and failing heart there is a very severe depression of the contractile state which is reflected by a downward shift of the force velocity curve with substantial reductions in the maximum intrinsic speed of contraction. These findings provide further evidence for a depression of the intensity of the active state in muscles from the failing and hypertrophied heart. It also should be emphasized that the abnormalities of contractility demonstrated in the isolated preparation are intrinsic properties of the cardiac muscle of the hypertrophied and failing heart. They are not dependent on altered humoral or environmental factors since they are present *in vitro* in a situation in which the chemical and physical conditions are controlled in an identical manner for all groups of muscles studied.

It is possible to determine the maximum contractile element velocity of shortening and the entire force velocity relationship in the intact ventricle during an isometric contraction (Levine and Britman, 1964; Fry *et al.*, 1964; Ross *et al.*, 1966). As tension is developed during an isometric contraction, the contractile element shortens and there is an equivalent elongation of the series elastic element. The velocity of lengthening of the series elastic and the velocity of shortening of the contractile element are equivalent in an isometric contraction. Thus, contractile element velocity may be represented by the rate of extension of the series elastic. Since Parmley *et al.* (1968) recently have shown that there is no change in the series elastic properties in right ventricular hypertrophy or heart failure in the cat, the same constants for the series elastic can be used in calculations for the normal, failing, and hypertrophied hearts. The whole force–velocity curve was shifted downward and to the left in both the hypertrophied and the failing ventricles, a finding exactly like that seen in the isolated papillary muscle. The maximum velocity of contractile element shortening (V_{max}) in the intact ventricle was depressed to 60% of the normal value in both the hypertrophied and the failing hearts.

The Effects of Positive Inotropic Interventions

The effects of sustained post extrasystolic potentiation produced by paired electrical stimulation on the maximum active tension of the normal, hypertrophied, and failing muscles are shown in Fig. 5. The increments in tension produced by paired electrical stimulation was significantly reduced from the normal value of 3.8 ± 0.3 gm/mm^2 to 2.2 ± 0.4 gm/mm^2 in the muscles from the failing group and to 2.8 ± 0.6 gm/mm^2 in the muscles from the cats in the hypertrophied group. The average maximum tensions achieved were

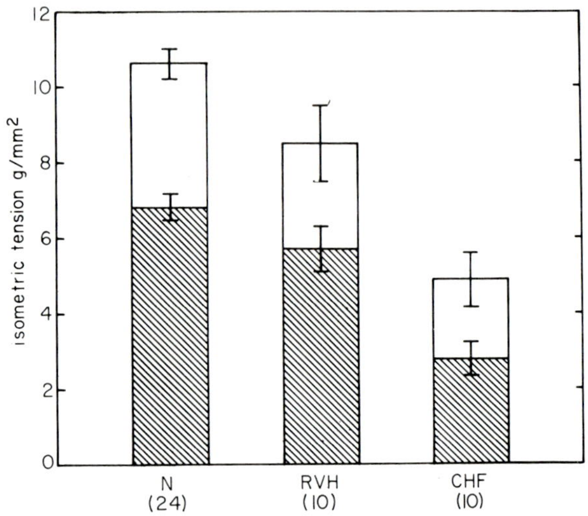

FIG. 5. Effects of sustained postextrasystolic potentiation produced by paired electrical stimulation on the maximum isometric force contraction at L_{max} in the three groups of muscles. The cross-hatched area represents control force with single electrical stimulation; the clear area above represents the augmentation with sustained paired electrical stimulation. Numbers in parentheses = number of animals. Vertical lines with cross bars equal $\pm$ 1 S.E.M. (From Spann *et al.*, 1967a.)

significantly reduced in muscles from both hypertrophied and failing hearts, averaging 8.5 ± 1.0 gm/mm^2 and 4.9 ± 0.7 gm/mm^2 respectively compared to the value of 10.6 ± 0.4 gm/mm^2 observed in normal muscles ($p < 0.05$). Thus, the depression of contractile state of hypertrophied and failing heart muscle could not be completely corrected by paired electrical stimulation. Similarly, there was a decrease in the positive inotropic response of hypertrophied and failing muscle to a progressive increase in the frequency of contraction from 6 to 48 stimuli per minute (Fig. 6). In each muscle there was a progressive elevation in both the rate of tension rise and the developed tension with a decrease in the time from stimulation to peak tension when frequency of contraction was increased. However, the increments in the rate of rise of tension and total tension in response to increases in frequency were reduced in the hypertrophied and failing muscles. For example, the increase in the rate of rise of tension per unit increment in frequency per minute averaged 0.43 gm/mm^2/sec, 0.13 gm/mm^2/sec and 0.07 gm/mm^2/sec in the normal, hypertrophied, and failing groups, respectively. The third positive inotropic intervention was the addition of strophanthidin to the muscles while they were contracting isometrically at the apex of the length–tension curve. Following strophanthidin, the maximum tension achieved by the muscles from cats in the congestive failure group averaged 4.6 ± 0.7 gm/mm^2, a value significantly less than the normal value of 8.4 ± 0.5 gm/mm^2.

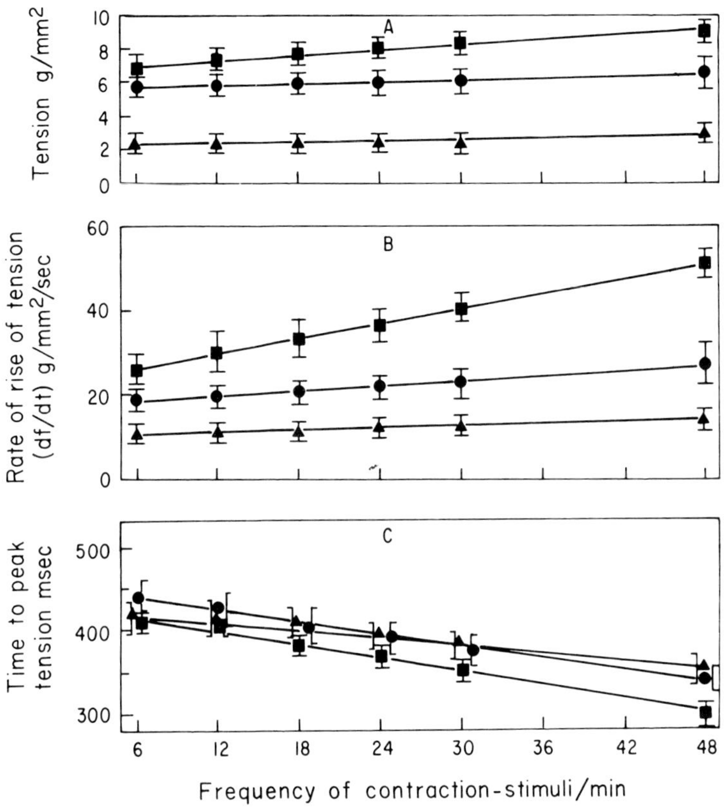

FIG. 6. Force–frequency relations in the three groups of muscles. Average maximum isometric tension (upper), rate of tension development (middle), and time from stimulation to peak tension (lower) are shown as functions of the frequency of contraction. ■, 8 Normal; ●, 9 RVH; ▲ 10 CHF. Vertical lines with cross bars equal ± 1 S.E.M. (From Spann *et al.*, 1967a.)

Thus, in addition to the depression of the functional level of the contractile state, papillary muscles obtained from animals with right ventricular hypertrophy and heart failure also have depressions of responses to positive inotropic interventions. Furthermore, although the absolute levels of force and rate of force development in the muscles from hypertrophied and failing hearts were augmented by these procedures, in the failing muscles they did not even reach the basal level observed in the normal muscles. It would appear that the contractile state is reduced even with inotropic potentiation and that the intrinsic defect of contractility in cardiac hypertrophy and heart failure can only be partially corrected by these positive inotropic interventions. However, in severe heart failure, even a small increase in contractile state can be of vital importance. As shown in Fig. 7, when the active length–tension

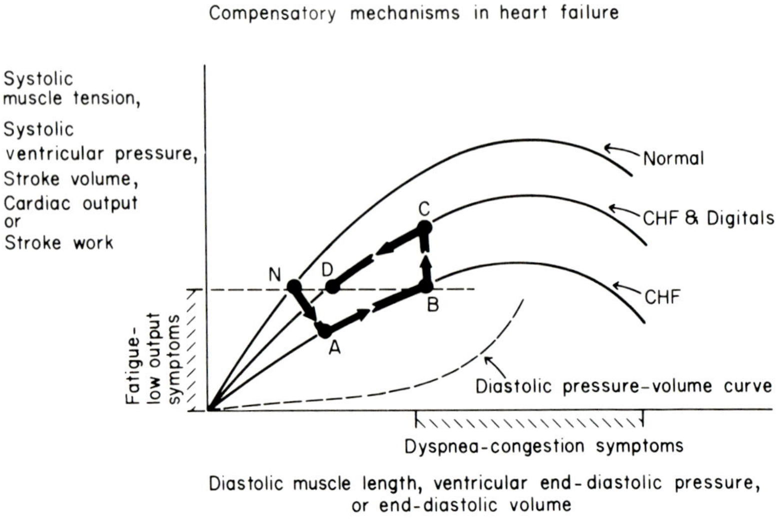

FIG. 7. Diagrammatic representation of the use of the Frank-Starling mechanism as a compensation for congestive heart failure. The three curves represent length–tension or ventricular-function curves in normal, congestive heart failure, and heart failure after treatment with digitalis. Points N–D represent in sequence: a depression of contractility, Frank-Starling compensation, increase in contractility with digitalis, and the reduction in the use of the Frank-Starling compensation which digitalis allows. Of note is the fact that points N, B, and D all lie on the same line in the vertical axis and thus all represent the same stroke volume, but each is on a different end-diastolic pressure on the horizontal axis. The levels at which symptoms of congestion, such as dyspnea, and symptoms of low cardiac output, such as fatigue, occur are represented by the cross-hatched areas. The dashed curve represents a diastolic pressure–volume curve relating end-diastolic pressure on the ordinate to end-diastolic volume or muscle length on the abscissa (from Spann *et al.*, 1970). (N to A) Initial reduction of contractility due to CHF; (A to B) use of Frank-Starling compensation to maintain cardiac output; (B to C), increase in contractility when digitalis is administered; (C to D) digitalis allowed reduction in the use of Frank-Starling compensation.

or Frank-Starling curve is severely depressed from point N to points A and B, and that individual is treated with digitalis, the positive inotropic action of the glycoside increases the contractile force obtained at any end-diastolic volume and shifts the ventricle to point C on the middle function curve. On this improved curve, the required systolic tension or stroke volume can be achieved with a lower resting tension or end-diastolic volume, at point D. This reduction in end-diastolic volume may be of considerable importance in reducing pulmonary venous hypertension, the symptoms of pulmonary congestion, and peripheral venous congestion while maintaining cardiac output.

Comparison of Cardiac Muscle Contractile State and Ventricular Pump Function in Hypertrophy and Failure

The cardiac output and other hemodynamic values, reflecting the status of the heart as a pump in the intact closed chest animal, were compared with the quantitative values for contractile performance of heart muscle in the intact ventricle and isolated papillary muscle. While contractile state of the isolated cardiac muscle and intact ventricle uniformly was depressed both in right ventricular hypertrophy and in heart failure, the circulatory functions of the heart were not depressed uniformly. In the studies of isolated papillary muscle, the values for right ventricular end-diastolic pressure, systemic arterial pressure, cardiac output and arterio-mixed venous oxygen difference were normal in all eleven animals in the hypertrophy group, despite the subsequently documented severe depression of the contractile state of isolated ventricular muscle. In studies of the intact ventricle, the average cardiac output of the closed chest animal was normal in the ventricular hypertrophy cats that were subsequently found to have severe depressions of tension development and velocity of contraction. In these hypertrophy animals with normal cardiac outputs, the maximum ventricular wall tension at similar end-diastolic circumferences was reduced to values averaging one-half of normal and the maximum velocity of contractile element shortening averaged only one-third of the normal value.

How then is circulatory function maintained with this degree of cardiac muscle dysfunction? It would appear that when the ventricle is chronically stressed by an abnormal pressure load, its initial response is to increase the total muscle mass. This increase in muscle mass, operating in conjunction with the Frank-Starling mechanisms and increased sympathetic stimulation, maintains overall circulatory compensation despite depression of the intrinsic contractile state of each unit of myocardium. These compensatory mechanisms, however, produce problems. Prior to the fall in resting cardiac output, the distressing abnormalities associated with the syndrome of congestive heart failure can be considered as side effects of the compensatory mechanisms as they attempt to maintain cardiac output. Thus, the compensatory mechanisms, in themselves, produce undesirable secondary effects that limit the degree which they can be utilized (Spann *et al.*, 1970). For example, an increase in myocardial mass by hypertrophy provides a basic compensatory mechanism for the heart when its work load is increased. Although the intrinsic contractile state of each unit of myocardium is depressed, the total mass of myocardium is increased, thus returning the total contractile performance of the heart toward normal. Pain of cardiac ischemia, when the oxygen requirements of the hypertrophied myocardium exceed the ability of the coronary arteries to provide oxygen, is the undesirable and limiting side effect of severe ventricular hypertrophy.

The Frank-Starling compensation through an increase in ventricular end-diastolic volume causes an increase in systolic tension and stroke volume, thereby tending to prevent the fall in cardiac output which would otherwise occur with the depression of myocardial contractile state which is represented in Fig. 7 as the movement from point N to A. Actually, many of the classic symptoms and physical findings in the syndrome of congestive heart failure are due to the body's utilization of the Frank-Starling mechanism by salt and water retention. By moving up and to the right to point B on the depressed length–tension curve, myocardial active tension and cardiac output are maintained at the expense of increases in resting muscle length and ventricular end-diastolic volume. It is apparent from the dotted curve representing the passive length–tension curve in Fig. 7 that such an increase in end-diastolic volume causes an elevation of the intraventricular pressure, the mean left atrial pressure, the pulmonary venous pressure, and the consequent development of pulmonary congestion and dyspnea or pulmonary edema. Thus, the compensatory mechanism has associated deleterious side effects, which are expressed as "symptoms," even while the overall compensation of the heart maintains cardiac output, at least during rest. These symptoms, in turn, limit the extent to which this mechanism of compensation can be used. Thus, as these limits are approached, these side effects are the signs and symptoms of compensated heart failure. A reduction in cardiac output is a relatively late manifestation of the hypertrophied and failing heart; when the compensatory mechanisms are no longer sufficient to overcome the intrinsic depression of contractile state, cardiac output falls and organ perfusion and function are impaired.

Possible Relation of the Impaired Contractile State to Alterations in the Sympathetic Nervous System

When an excessive burden or stress is placed on the heart, sympathetic activity increases in order to help maintain cardiocirculatory function near a normal level (Chidsey *et al.*, 1962; 1965). As this process continues a severe depletion (Chidsey *et al.*, 1963; Spann, *et al.*, 1965) of cardiac norepinephrine stores takes place due to defects in synthesis (Pool *et al.*, 1967) uptake and binding (Spann *et al.*, 1965) of catecholamines by the cardiac sympathetic nerves. In the current studies marked depressions of the cardiac norepinephrine concentrations were observed in the right and left ventricle in both

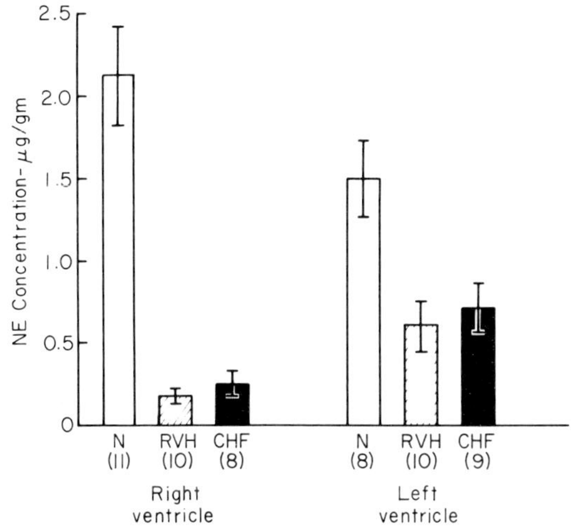

FIG. 8. The average norepinephrine concentration of the right and left ventricles of cats in the normal, RVH and CHF groups. Vertical lines with cross bars equals ± 1 S.E.M. Numbers in parentheses = number of animals in each group (from Spann *et al.*, 1967a.

right ventricular hypertrophy and heart failure. The extent of the norepinephrine depression was comparable in ventricular hypertrophy and failure (Fig. 8). Of particular interest is the depression of left ventricular norepinephrine concentration in animals with right ventricular hypertrophy. Since, in the hypertrophy group, there was no circulatory failure, this represents an alteration in a constituent of the nonstressed, nonhypertrophied, contralateral ventricle of an animal with severe stress placed on the opposite ventricle. No explanation is available currently for either this finding or the finding of the similar alterations in the collagen concentration in the nonstressed, nonhypertrophied contralateral ventricle (Buccino *et al.*, 1969) as discussed in the chapter by Spann, page 141 of this book).

What is the effect of this profound depletion of cardiac norepinephrine on the contractile performance of the heart? Is cardiac norepinephrine depletion a basic cause of the intrinsic weakness of hypertrophied and failing heart muscle? To assess the possibility that the cardiac norepinephrine depletion, *per se*, was responsible for the intrinsic depression of contractile performance in the failing heart muscle, the contractile state of cardiac muscle removed from hearts which were depleted of norepinephrine by a mechanism other than heart failure was examined. In 12 cats, cardiac norepinephrine depletion was produced by chronic cardiac denervation and the contractile function of papillary muscles isolated from these hearts were studied in the same manner

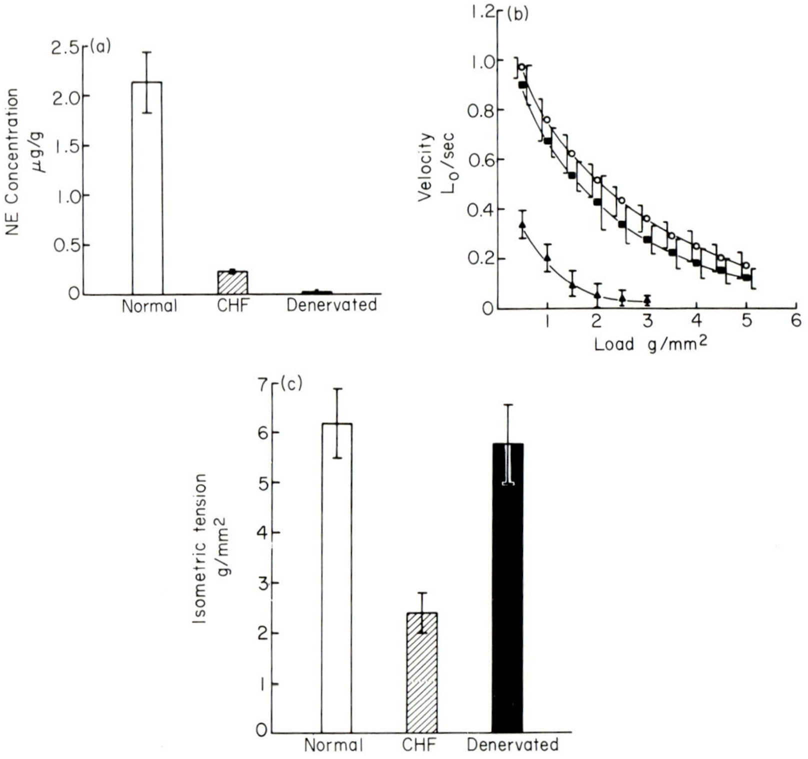

FIG. 9. (a) The average right ventricular norepinephrine concentration in normal cats (N), cats with chronic heart failure due to pulmonary artery constriction (CHF), and cats with surgically produced total cardiac denervation but no heart failure (D). (b) The average force–velocity relationship in right ventricular papillary muscles isolated from N, CHF, and D cats. Velocity is expressed on the ordinate as muscle lengths (L_o)/sec and total load is expressed on the abscissa as gm/mm^2. ■, 15 Normal; ○, 12 denervated; ▲ 11 CHF. (c) The average maximum active tension developed at the apex of the length–tension curve in isolated right ventricular papillary muscles from the N, CHF, and D groups, is expressed as gm/mm^2. All vertical bars equal $\pm$ S.E.M. and each number in parentheses represents the number of animals in that group (from "Pre- and Postoperative Management of the Cardiopulmonary Patient" Grune and Stratton, 1970, p. 207).

as in the muscles from the failing hearts (Spann *et al.*, 1966). The cardiac norepinephrine concentrations of the cardiac denervated animals were reduced to levels of 0.006 ± 0.003 μg/gm, a value even lower than the values in the heart failure group [Fig. 9(a)]. However, the contractile function of cardiac muscle from the norepinephrine depleted, denervated heart was not depressed as shown by the force–velocity curve [Fig. 9(b)] and by the maximum isometric tension developed [Fig. 9(c)]. It can be concluded that cardiac stores of norepinephrine are not fundamental for maintaining the basic contractile state of the myocardium and that the cardiac norepinephrine depletion which occurs in ventricular hypertrophy and congestive heart failure is not the primary cause of the intrinsic depression of cardiac contractility in hypertrophied or failing heart muscle. What then are the effects of this cardiac norepinephrine depletion?

In the intact heart Covell *et al.* (1966) demonstrated that this norepinephrine depletion interferes with the transmission of sympathetic impulses to the heart. In dogs with severe cardiac norepinephrine depletion and right heart failure due to tricuspid insufficiency and pulmonary stenosis, the chronotropic and inotropic responses to graded stimulation of the sympathetic nerves were markedly reduced in animals with heart failure. Furthermore, these investigators showed that the myocardium of the dog with heart failure responded to exogenously administered norepinephrine. It was concluded that the quantity of neurotransmitter released per nerve impulse is reduced markedly in experimental heart failure with cardiac norepinephrine depletion. Thus, it would appear that even an abnormal increase in the impulse traffic along the cardiac sympathetic nerves would not augment the contractile state of the failing myocardium to a substantial degree. Of further interest, the norepinephrine depleted cardiac muscle of the hypertrophied and failing heart is supersensitive to the effects of exogenous catecholamine (Spann *et al.*, 1967a). The positive inotropic effects of L-norepinephrine were determined in papillary muscles from eight normal cats and from six cats with cardiac norepinephrine depletion due to right ventricular hypertrophy and heart failure. The increments in tension in response to norepinephrine were greater in papillary muscles from the hypertrophied and failing hearts, and the dose response curve was shifted upward in these muscles (Fig. 10). At a concentration of 10^{-7} M L-norepinephrine, the increment in isometric force averaged 1.47 ± 0.23 gm/mm^2 in muscles from cats with right ventricular hypertrophy and heart failure, a value significantly greater than that observed in the normal muscles, 0.84 ± 0.20 gm/mm^2 ($p < 0.05$). Since the circulating arterial norepinephrine concentration is increased in heart failure (Chidsey *et al.*, 1962) and the failing heart is not only responsive but even supersensitive to its positive inotropic actions, the circulating catecholamine represents an important compensatory mechanism for the hypertrophied and failing heart. This conclusion has been borne out by the clinical experience with the β-adrenergic receptor blocking agent, propranolol; overt congestive and circulatory failure may appear or increase when this agent is given to patients with advanced cardiac disease and a critical dependence on sympathetic activity (Stephen, 1966).

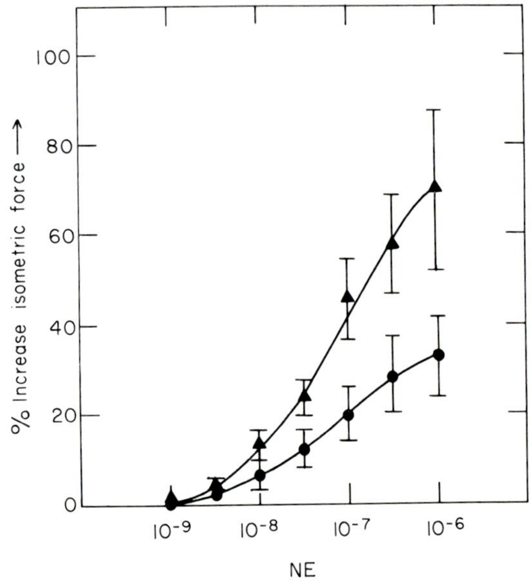

FIG. 10. Effects of exogenous norepinephrine on isometric tension of papillary muscles of cats in the RVH and CHF groups. L-norepinephrine was added to the muscle bath at 5-min intervals in increasing concentrations starting at $10^{-10}M$, while isometric tension achieved at each concentration was recorded. The percent increase in isometric force is shown on the ordinate and the concentration of added norepinephrine (NE) on the abscissa. ●, Normal muscles from normal hearts; ▲, muscles from the norepinephrine depleted hearts of animals in the RVH and CHF groups. Vertical lines with cross bars equal ± S.E.M.

Conclusions

The major conclusion developed in the research reviewed in this chapter is that *the fundamental abnormality in congestive heart failure is a depression of myocardial contractility*. Except in massive acute cardiac damage, heart failure is not a sudden event but is part of a continuum initiated either by an excessive cardiac work load or direct myocardial injury, and which progresses from depressed myocardial performance into ventricular hypertrophy and compensation, with or without congestive symptoms, and on to final overt failure of the circulation. When the ventricle is chronically stressed by an increased work load or is directly damaged by coronary or myocardial disease, it responds by increasing the total muscle mass. This ventricular hypertrophy, operating in conjunction with the Frank-Starling mechanisms and increased sympathetic stimulation, maintains overall circulatory compensation despite depression of the intrinsic contractile state of each unit of myocardium; however, each compensatory mechanism has a built-in set of limitations that, when exceeded, produce signs and symptoms. As the intrinsic contractile state of each unit of myocardium is further depressed, circulatory compensation can no longer be maintained, despite maximum utilization of the compensatory mechanisms. Overt heart failure then occurs with a fall in cardiac output at rest and organ function is compromised due to inadequate blood flow. Thus, overt congestive heart failure represents the final expression of deteriorating cardiac function. *Compensated congestive heart failure* may be defined as the condition in which cardiac muscle function is deprcssed and the heart and circulation utilize compensatory mechanisms, often with resultant symptoms, to prevent a fall in cardiac output to less than systemic requirements at rest. *Overt congestive heart failure* can be defined as the pathological state in which a severe abnormality of cardiac function results in an inability of the heart to pump blood at a rate commensurate with the systemic requirements.

References

Buccino, R. A., Harris, E., Spann, J. F., Jr., and Sonnenblick, E. H. (1969). *Amer. J. Physiol.* **216,** 425.

Chidsey, C. A., Harrison, D. C., and Braunwald, E. (1962). *N. Eng. J. Med.* **267,** 650.

Chidsey, C. A., Braunwald, E., Morrow, A. G., and Mason, D. T. (1963). *N. Eng. J. Med.* **269,** 653.

Chidsey, C. A., Braunwald, E., and Morrow, A. G. (1965). *Amer. J. Med.* **39,** 442.

Covell, J. W., Chidsey, C. A., and Braunwald, E. (1966). *Circ. Res.* **19,** 51.

Fry, D. L., Griggs, D. M., Jr., and Greenfield, J. C., Jr. (1964). *Circ. Res.* **14,** 73.

Hill, A. V. (1938). *Proc. Roy. Soc. (London) Ser. B* **126,** 136.

Levine, H. J., and Britman, N. A. (1964). *J. Clin. Invest.* **43,** 1383.

Nair, K. G., Cutilletta, A. F., Zak, R., Koide, T., and Rabinowitz, M. (1968). *Circ. Res.* **23,** 451.

Parmley, W. W., Spann, J. F., Jr., Taylor, R. R., and Sonnenblick, E. H. (1968). *Proc. Soc. Exp. Biol. Med.* **127,** 606.

Pool, P. E., Covell, J. W., Levitt, M., Gibb, J., and Braunwald, E. (1967). *Circ. Res.* **20,** 349.

Ross, J., Jr., Covell, J. W., Sonnenblick, E. H., and Braunwald, E. (1966). *Circ. Res.* **18,** 149.

Sonnenblick, E. H. (1962). *Fed. Proc. Fed. Amer. Soc. Exp. Biol.* **21,** 972.

Sonnenblick, E. H. (1967). *J. Gen. Physiol.* **50,** 661.

Spann, J. F., Jr., Chidsey, C. A., Pool, P. E., Braunwald, E. (1965). *Circ. Res.* **17,** 312.

Spann, J. F., Jr., Sonnenblick, E. H., Cooper, T., Chidsey, C. A., William, V. L., and Braunwald, E. (1966). *Circ. Res.* **19,** 317.

Spann, J. F., Jr., Buccino, R. A., Sonnenblick, E. H., and Braunwald, E. (1967a). *Circ. Res.* **21,** 341.

Spann, J. F. Jr., Eckberg, D. L., Covell, J. W., Sonnenblick, E. H., Ross, J., Jr., and Braunwald, E. (1967b). *Circulation* **36,** Suppl. 2, 241.

Spann, J. F., Jr., Buccino, R. A., and Sonnenblick, E. H. (1967c). *Proc. Soc. Exp. Biol. Med.* **125,** 522.

Spann, J. F., Jr., Mason, D. T., and Zelis, R. F. (1970). *Mod. Concepts Cardiov. Dis.* **39,** 79.

Stephen, A. (1966). *Amer. J. Cardiol.* **18,** 463.

Weissler, A. M., Harris, W. S., and Schoenfeld, C. D. (1969). *Amer. J. Cardiol.* **23,** 577.

Part VI
Energetics of the Hypertrophied Heart

DETERMINANTS OF MYOCARDIAL ENERGY UTILIZATION

Henry Neal Coleman

Introduction

It is generally accepted that aerobic metabolism is the principal metabolic pathway for myocardial energy production. Therefore, measurement of myocardial oxygen consumption ($M\dot{V}O_2$) reflects the sum of energy-utilizing reactions of myocardial contraction.

The determinants of $M\dot{V}O_2$ have been the subject of many investigations during the past 50 years. Initial studies were concerned primarily with the effects of hemodynamic factors such as pressure, flow (Evans and Matsuoka, 1915), or their derivatives (Sarnoff *et al.*, 1958), however, Fenn (1923). and subsequently Hill (1938) demonstrated that the rate of energy utilization in skeletal muscle was controlled by the mechanical conditions during contraction, focusing attention on the relation of the mechanics of myocardial contraction to $M\dot{V}O_2$. Thereafter, recent studies have considered the relationship between $M\dot{V}O_2$ to multiple factors including tension development in the ventricular wall (McDonald *et al.*, 1966), alterations in the velocity of contraction (Krasnow *et al.*, 1964; Sonnenblick *et al.*, 1965), and calculated contractile element work (Britman and Levine, 1964). However, these studies were performed in the intact heart where it is difficult to make correlations because of the complex architecture of the ventricle and the problem in isolating single variables. The study of isolated papillary muscle with its linear arrangement of fibers, a simplified geometry, and mechanical controls allows direct measurement of myocardial mechanics. With the development of a polarographic oxygen electrode method for determining $M\dot{V}O_2$ of cat papillary muscle (Lee, 1953) and the subsequent elucidation of the mechanics of myocardial contraction (Abbott and Mommaerts, 1959; Sonnenblick, 1962), it is now feasible to systematically investigate the relationship between myocardial mechanics and $M\dot{V}O_2$. The purpose of this chapter is to review the results of recent investigations of the determinants of $M\dot{V}O_2$ as studied in isolated cat papillary muscle.

Methods

Measurement of Mechanical Activity

Papillary muscles were excised rapidly from the right ventricle of cats anesthetized with intraperitoneal sodium pentobarbital (30 mg/kg) and transferred to a Petri dish containing oxygenated Krebs–Ringers solution. Ties of noncapillary 4–0 silk were placed on each end of the muscle, which was then mounted from the bottom of the central tubular muscle chamber of a lucite bath as shown in Fig. 1. Details of this bath and apparatus have been previously presented (Coleman, 1967). The muscle was fixed at its base to the rod entering the bottom of the bath through a mercury seal, and the upper end of the muscle attached to a Schilling isotonic transducer (Schilling, 1960) mounted on a Palmer adjustable screw stand. The use of a lever permitted examination of afterloaded contractions where (1) preload or initial tension was the determinant of initial fiber length, (2) afterload was the amount of tension that the muscle must develop before shortening could occur, and (3) total load, equaling preload plus afterload, was the load at which both the extent and velocity of shortening were determined. Isometric

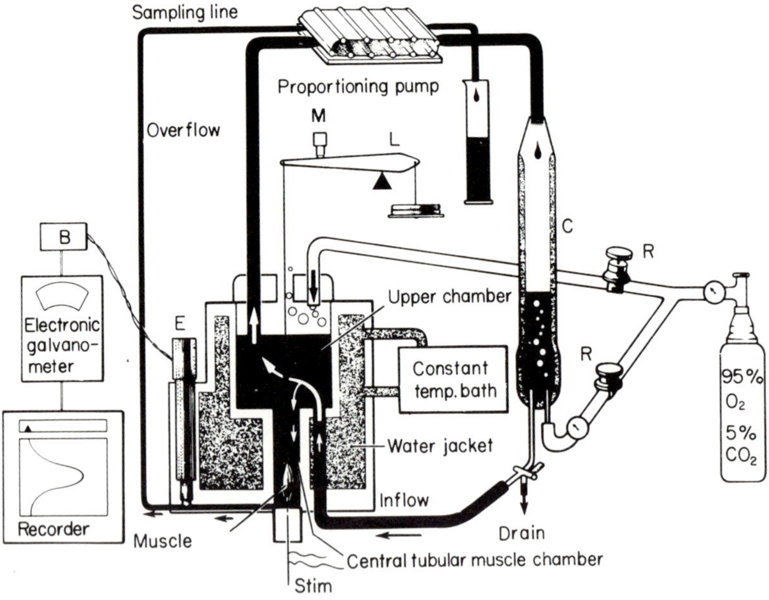

FIG. 1. Schematic illustration of the experimental apparatus. B represents electrode controls for position and polarizing voltage; C, condenser column; E, electrode; M, lever stop; L, lever; and R, pressure regulator. (Reproduced with permission of Circulation Research.)

tension was determined from above the bath by attaching a Statham force transducer (model G-1-1000) to the lever with a noncompliant segment of jeweler's chain.

A Grass S4E stimulator coupled with a Tektronix waveform generator was utilized to provide supramaximal square wave stimulus (3–6 V) for 2.5 msec, at a frequency of 30/min for all experiments. The temperature of the condenser column, muscle bath, and electrode was maintained at 29°C with a Haake constant-temperature pump. All tracings were recorded on a multichannel oscillographic recorder. The velocity of muscle shortening, expressed in mm/sec, was determined from the tangent to the shortening trace at each load, whereas the rate of force development, expressed in gm/sec, was obtained in a similar fashion from the isometric twitch. The tangent was located at the point of peak velocity on each trace with the use of an R.C. differentiator (time constant equals 1 msec).

The performance of the muscle was evaluated in terms of a mechanical model in which a contractile element (CE), capable of generating force and shortening, is arranged in series with two elastic components (SEC). Values for internal contractile element work (CEW) in gm•mm were obtained by integration of the load extension curves of the series elastic component (Parmley and Sonnenblick, 1967) as a function of load for each preload. In addition, work performed on the extension of the equipment, principally the sutures holding the muscle, was determined by integration of the load extension curve of the equipment as a function of load. This external work, in combination with the work performed in extending the SEC, comprises the total work performed during tension development in isometric contractions. Total CEW for afterloaded contractions is the sum of the tension development work (termed "internal" CEW) and the external work (load × distance shortened), the former including the above-mentioned correction for equipment distensibility.

Measurement of Oxygen Consumption

The bath and apparatus were perfused with a modified Krebs–Ringers solution (Na^+ 152, K^+ 3.6, Cl^- 135, HCO_3^- 25, Mg^{2+} 1.2, $H_2PO_4^-$ 1.3, SO_4^- 1.2 and Ca^{2+} 5.0 mEq/liter, glucose 5.6 mmoles/liter), which had a pH of 7.4 when bubbled with 95% O_2–5% CO_2. The solution was circulated at 6.7 cc/min from a reservoir (not shown), by a Technicon model I proportioning pump to a column where it was equilibrated with 95% O_2–5% CO_2 before passing by gravity through the inflow line to the upper part of the muscle bath. The fluid in the upper chamber in excess of that circulated past the muscle was removed and returned to the reservoir through the overflow line, while the atmosphere above the solution was saturated with a continuous flow of 95% O_2 and 5% CO_2. The solution was circulated through a central tubular muscle chamber and withdrawn (rates ranging from 3.5 to 4.0 cc/hr in individual experiments) into a capillary containing an oxygen electrode. This capillary had a diameter of 0.8 mm and length of 39 mm, dimensions adequate to insure uniform diffusion of oxygen across the capillary at the electrode site (Carlson *et al.*, 1950).

Oxygen tension was polarographically measured using Clark-type (Clark *et al.*, 1953) oxygen electrodes.* The current from the electrode, proportional to the oxygen tension, was amplified by a Kintel electronic galvanometer and recorded on a Brown–Honeywell 12-in. chart recorder. Each electrode was tested for linear response by evaluating the current produced in oxygen concentrations of 100%, 90%, 20.9% (room air), and 0% (nitrogen). Thereafter, the electrode was calibrated in place during each experiment by changing the gas equilibrating the solution from 95% O_2–5% CO_2 to 90% O_2–5% N_2. Gas mixtures were analyzed either with a Haldane apparatus using the method of Peters and Van Slyke (1932) or by gas chromatography.

The oxygen consumption of the papillary muscle ($M\dot{V}O_2$) was calculated by use of solubility of O_2 at 29°C, the calibration curve, and the deflection in the O_2 record produced by each intervention at a constant flow.

Results

Effects of Afterload on Myocardial Mechanics and $M\dot{V}O_2$

The development of tension has long been recognized as an important determinant of energy utilization of both skeletal muscle (Fenn, 1923; Hill, 1938) and the intact heart (Rhode, 1912; Sarnoff *et al.*, 1958). In Fig. 2 the effects of progressive increments in afterload (tension) at a constant preload (initial muscle length) on myocardial mechanics and $M\dot{V}O_2$ is depicted. With progressive increments in afterload, both the velocity of shortening [Panel (a)], and the extent of shortening [open circles, panel (b)], decrease. External work, the product of afterload and displacement, shown as closed circles in panel B, is zero at zero load, increases with progressive increments in afterload to reach a maximal value of 50% of isometric load, and declines thereafter to zero at isometric contraction. As shown in panel (c), $M\dot{V}O_2$ increases along with increments in afterload up to ~50% of isometric force. Thereafter, further additions of afterload are associated with only small increments in $M\dot{V}O_2$. Thus, $M\dot{V}O_2$ cannot be correlated directly with tension development alone.

* Constructed by Mrs. Zena Taylor McCallum.

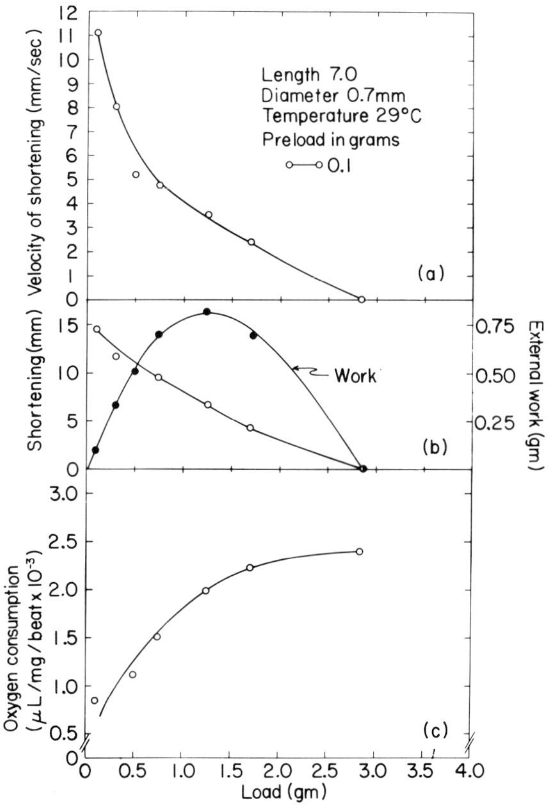

FIG. 2. Effect of increasing afterload at a constant preload on myocardial mechanics and $M\dot{V}O_2$. Ordinates are velocity of shortening (upper panel) shortening and external work (middle panel), and oxygen consumption (lower panel). Abscissa is total load. (Reproduced with permission of *Amer. J. Physiol.*)

In order to evaluate the contribution of shortening and external work to $M\dot{V}O_2$, 13 experiments were performed comparing $M\dot{V}O_2$ of isometric contraction to the $M\dot{V}O_2$ of afterloaded contractions in which shortening and external work occurred at the same level of tension development. In each experiment, preload was held constant and measurements of mechanical performance and $M\dot{V}O_2$ were made at various points on a force–velocity curve by progressive additions of afterload (range of preload in all experiments from 0.50 to 0.75 gm). Subsequently, initial tension was decreased in order to allow measurement of $M\dot{V}O_2$ for isometric contractions in which tension development was equal to that attained during the afterloaded isotonic contractions. The order of procedure was reversed in some experi-

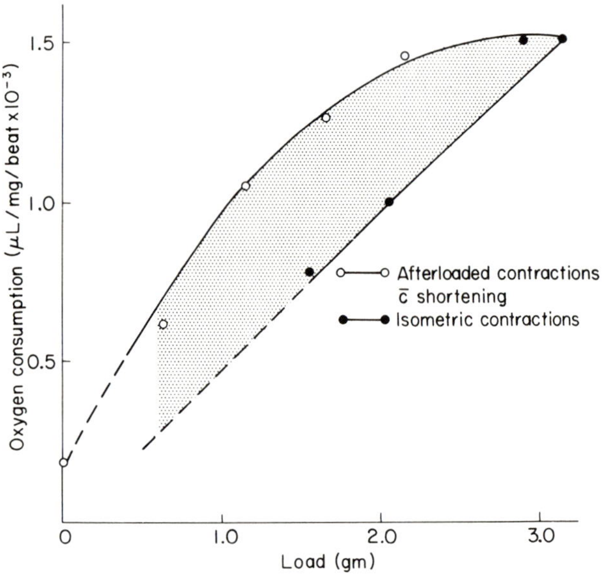

FIG. 3. Comparison of the $M\dot{V}O_2$ of isometric contractions (filled circles) to the $M\dot{V}O_2$ of afterload isotonic contractions at equal levels of tension development (open circles). The dotted area is change in $M\dot{V}O_2$ associated with onset of shortening and external work in afterloaded contractions. The point on the ordinate at $0.23 \pm 0.05\ \mu$L/mg/beat $\times 10^{-3}$ represents an average intercept as determined in five experiments (see text). (Reproduced with permission of *Amer. J. Physiol.*)

ments, and values for $M\dot{V}O_2$ of isometric contractions were obtained prior to those of afterloaded contractions. The results of one such experiment are depicted in Fig. 3. It is apparent from a comparison of the $M\dot{V}O_2$ of isometric contractions with the $M\dot{V}O_2$ of afterloaded contractions that the performance of fiber-shortening work was associated with an additional oxygen consumption over and above that associated with tension development alone (the stippled area in Fig. 3). In five experiments in which measurements were obtained at one-half isometric load, this additional oxygen consumption attributable to shortening and external work accounted for an average of $48\% \pm 9$ SEM of the total $M\dot{V}O_2$.

In Fig. 4, the relationship between the increment in MVO_2 above that associated with tension development in an isometric contraction and external work performed during afterloaded contraction at that level of tension is shown for the group of 13 experiments. These variables are linearly related and are described by the least-squares regression equation $y = (0.02 \pm 0.06) + (0.57 \pm .08) \times$. Statistical evaluation revealed the slope of the line is significant from zero ($p < 0.01$) with a coefficient of correlation of 0.82.

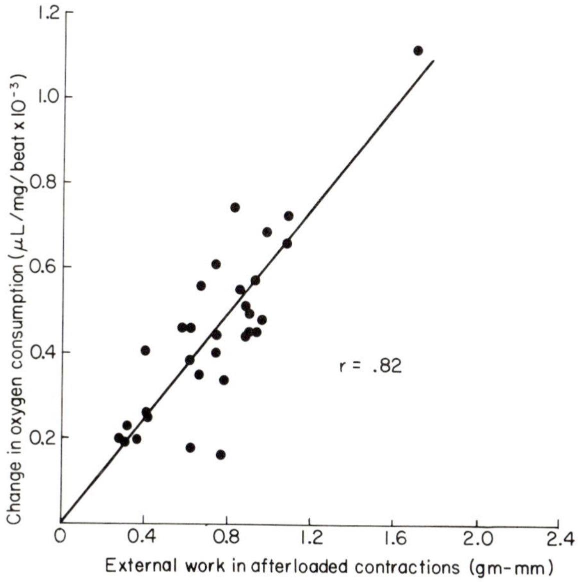

FIG. 4. Relationship between the change in M$\dot{V}O_2$, when isometric and afterloaded contractions were compared at constant levels of tension development, and the external work performed in the after loaded contractions (13 experiments). Relationship is described by the least-squares regression equation $y = (0.02 \pm 0.06) + (0.57 \pm 0.08) \times, r = 0.82$. (Reproduced with permission of *Amer. J. Physiol.*)

EFFECT OF ALTERATIONS IN INITIAL MUSCLE LENGTH

The effect of altering initial muscle length on M$\dot{V}O_2$ was determined by initiating contraction against the same total load from two different preloads. This effectively redistributes the load with afterload decreasing at the longer muscle length for each level of total load. The results from a typical experiment of this type are graphically presented in Fig. 5. Panels (a) and (b) of this figure illustrate the increments in the initial velocity of shortening with an increase in preload from a control level of 0.1–0.5 gm. Figure 5 (c) illustrates the effect on M$\dot{V}O_2$ of initiating contraction from two different preloads against a constant total load. At each load, initiation of contraction from the greater muscle length resulted in increments in shortening and thus external work. These changes in mechanical behavior were associated with an increased M$\dot{V}O_2$. Similar results were found in 18 additional experiments in which preloads ranged from 0.1 to 1.0 gm (Coleman, 1968).

CONTRACTILE ELEMENT WORK AND M$\dot{V}O_2$

In the development of tension the contractile elements shorten as the series elastic components are stretched and work of the contractile element (CEW) can be calculated (Britman and Levine, 1964; Sonnenblick, 1964). Contractile

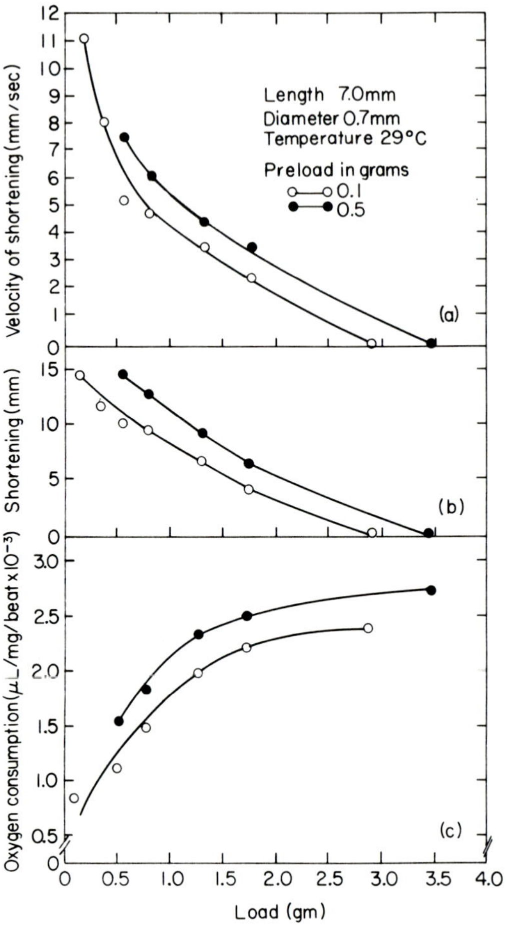

FIG. 5. Effect of increasing reload at a constant total load on myocardial mechanics and $M\dot{V}O_2$. (a) Ordinates are velocity of shortening; (b) shortening; (c) oxygen consumption. Abscissa demonstrates total load. (Reproduced with permission of American Journal of Physiology.)

element work was calculated for the 13 experiments in which afterloaded and isometric contractions were compared at the same level of tension development. The results from a typical experiment are shown in Fig. 6(a). In the upper panel of Fig. 6, values determined for contractile element work (CEW) during tension development (series elastic + equipment extension work) are plotted as closed circles. The external work performed during shortening in afterloaded contractions is represented by the stippled area between the open and closed circles, whereas total CEW for afterloaded contractions is portrayed as open circles. These values for CEW were determined for the experiment depicted in Fig. 3 in order to evaluate the relationship between CEW and $M\dot{V}O_2$ over a wide range of loads. Evaluation of the CEW for afterloaded contractions reveals that this function reaches a maximal value at 60% of isometric load and declines thereafter to the point at which isometric contraction occurs. Contrasted with this, $M\dot{V}O_2$ increased with addition of afterload and reached a maximal value at isometric contraction [Figs. 3 and 6(b)], indicating a lack of correlation between $M\dot{V}O_2$ and total calculated CEW over a considerable range of loads. This absence of direct

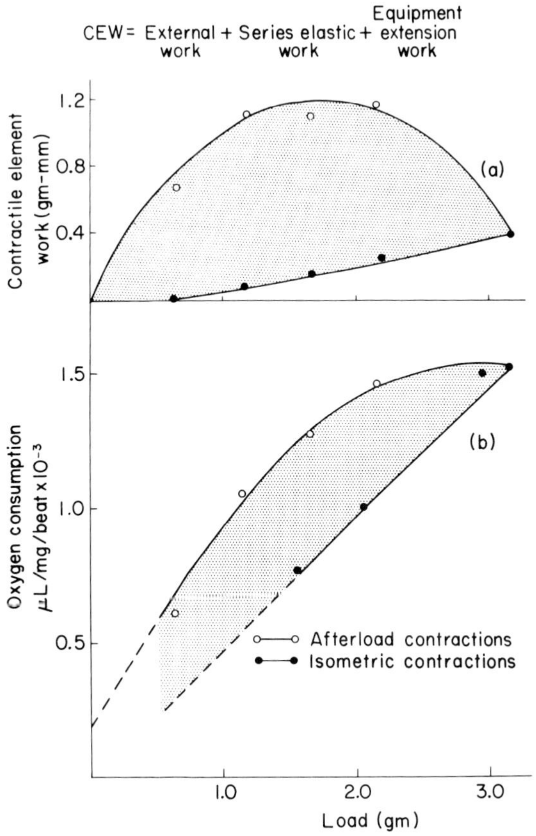

FIG. 6. Panel (a) Relationship between contractile element work (CEW) and load. Filled circles are calculated internal CEW (comprised of series elastic work + equipment extension work). The dotted area illustrates external work. Total CEW for afterloaded contractions is displayed as open circles. (b) Relationship between $M\dot{V}O_2$ (shown in Fig. 2) and total CEW in panel (a) for afterloaded contractions.

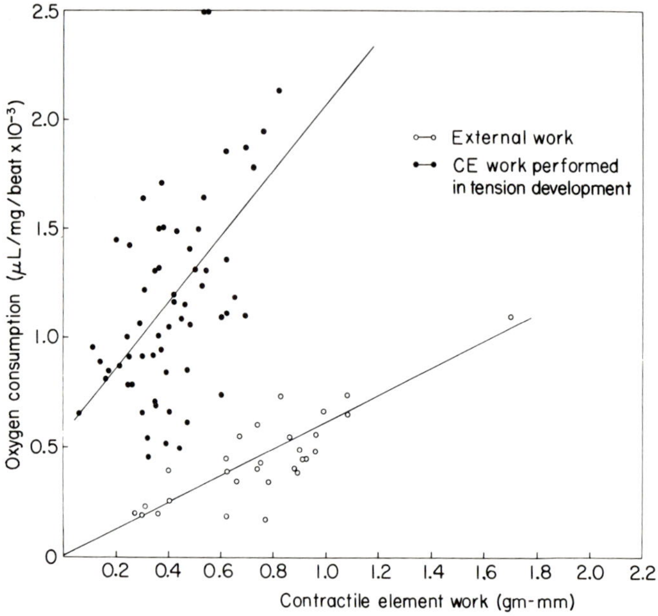

FIG. 7. Comparison of the relative $M\dot{V}O_2$ of external work to internal CEW. Relationship between external work and $M\dot{V}O_2$ associated with external work (open circles) is described by the regression equation $y = (0.02 \pm 0.06) + (0.57 \pm 0.08)x$. The relation betweem $M\dot{V}O_2$ of isometric contractions and calculated "internal" CEW during tension development (filled circles) is described by the regression equation $y = (0.63 \pm 0.14) + (1.34 \pm 0.31)x$. The difference between the slopes of the two lines is significant ($p < 0.05$). (Reproduced with permission of *Amer. J. Physiol.*)

correlation between CEW and $M\dot{V}O_2$ of afterloaded contractions [Fig. 6(b)] is consistent with the hypothesis that the work performed on stretching the series elastic component is much more costly in terms of $M\dot{V}O_2$ than is the work performed in shortening the muscle. In Fig. 7 this difference in the relative amount of energy utilization for the two types of contractile element is presented for the group of 13 experiments in which isometric and isotonic contractions were compared. Values for "internal CEW" and $M\dot{V}O_2$ obtained in six additional experiments in which isometric contractions were evaluated are also depicted. The relationship between $M\dot{V}O_2$ and CEW associated with isometric tension development, represented as filled circles, is described by the least squares regression equation $y = (0.63 \pm 0.14) + (1.34 \pm 0.31) \times$. For purposes of comparison, the relationship between external work and the $M\dot{V}O_2$ associated with external work is shown (open circles) for the 13 experiments in which both afterloaded and isometric contractions were compared (previously depicted in Fig. 4). The difference between these two regression equations is significant ($p < 0.05$) when analyzed by Students'

T test. These data suggest that the performance of external work is associated with a substantially smaller unit energy cost than is the performance of internal contractile element work during tension development.

M$\dot{V}O_2$ Associated with Activation

As outlined above, the experiments protocol required that afterloaded contractions be performed, at preloads ranging from 0.5 to 0.75 gm. However, this requirement prevents accurate extrapolation of the M$\dot{V}O_2$ curve to the intercept on the ordinate and thus limits definition of the energy utilization associated with activation (and perhaps shortening independent of load) (Hill, 1938). In order to obtain a more precise extrapolation of M$\dot{V}O_2$ to zero load, values for M$\dot{V}O_2$ were determined for contractions with a preload of only 50 or 100 mg on the lever and then with a preload plus afterload of 50 mg in each of five experiments. The extrapolation of these points resulted in an average intercept on the ordinate of 0.23 ± 0.05 SEM μL/mg beat $\times 10^{-3}$ M$\dot{V}O_2$.

Effect of Alterations in Contractile State on M$\dot{V}O_2$

The effects of digitalis glycosides on myocardial contractility and M$\dot{V}O_2$ have been of particular interest to investigators. Although it has been demonstrated that cardiac glycosides augment the force of contraction of both the failing (Bloomfield *et al.*, 1948) and nonfailing myocardium (Braunwald *et al.*, 1961), the effects of glycosides on M$\dot{V}O_2$ remains a matter of controversy. Accordingly, the effects of acetylstrophanthidin on force–velocity relations and M$\dot{V}O_2$ were determined in 13 papillary muscle preparations. The results from a representative experiment are depicted in Fig. 8. In panel (a) it is evident that the administration of acetylstrophanthidin (0.15 γ/cc) shifted the force–velocity relationship to the right with augmentation of both the maximum velocity of shortening (V_{max}) and the maximum force of isometric contraction. Thus, values for both the extent and velocity of shortening at comparable loads [panels (a) and (b)] were increased after the addition of acetylstrophanthidin to the perfusate. Further, panel (c) shows that changes in force–velocity relations, produced by augmentation of the inotropic state with the glycoside, are associated with an increased M$\dot{V}O_2$ over the entire range of loads which were evaluated. Similar results were obtained in 10 additional experiments for concentrations of acetylstrophanthidin between 0.015 and 0.20 γ/cc. In two experiments a concentration of 0.010 γ/cc produced no alterations in myocardial mechanical behavior or M$\dot{V}O_2$.

That such changes in M$\dot{V}O_2$ are not unique properties of digitalis-induced augmentation of the contractile state can be seen in Fig. 9, where the contractile state has been augmented by increasing the calcium ion concentration of the perfusate from 2.5 to 7.5 mEq/liter. As shown in panel (a),

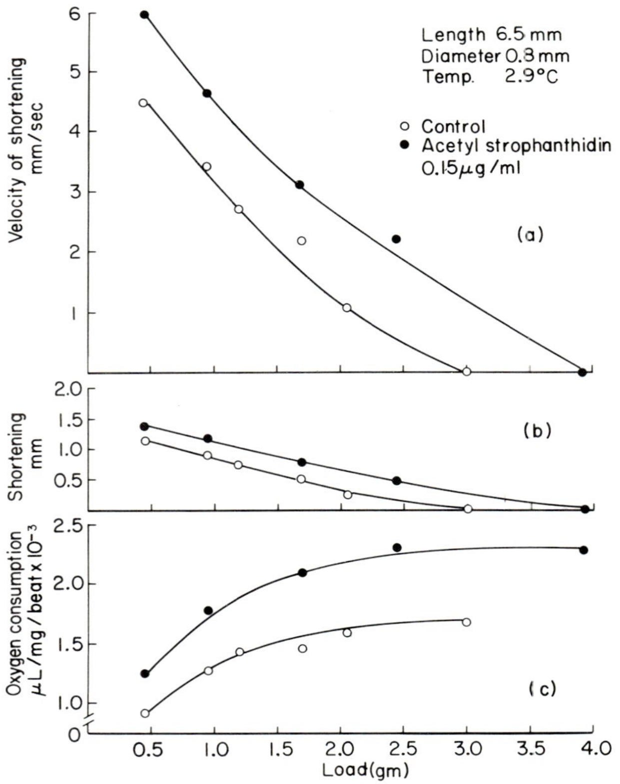

FIG. 8. Effect of acetylstrophanthidin, 0.15/cc on force–velocity relations and $M\dot{V}O_2$. The ordinates represent (a) velocity of shortening; (b) shortening, and (c) oxygen consumption. The abscissa represents total load. (Reproduced with permission of *Circ. Res.*)

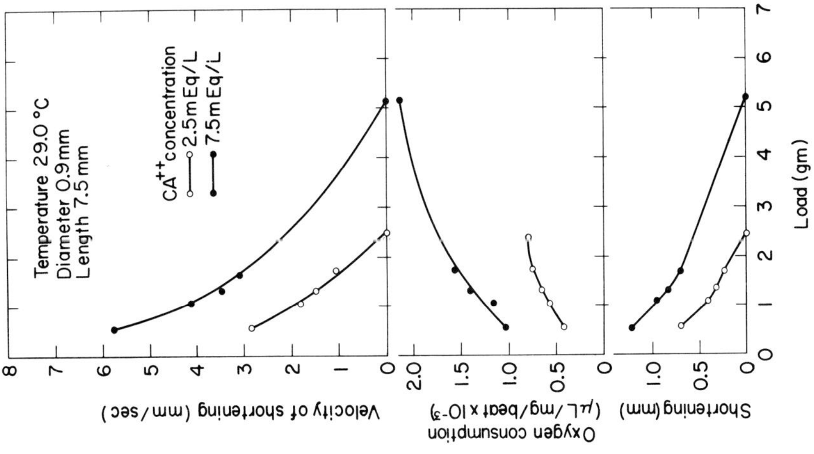

FIG. 9. Effect of calcium ion concentration on force–velocity relations and $M\dot{V}O_2$. Ordinates illustrate (a) velocity of shortening; (b) oxygen consumption; and (c) shortening. Abscissa, load.

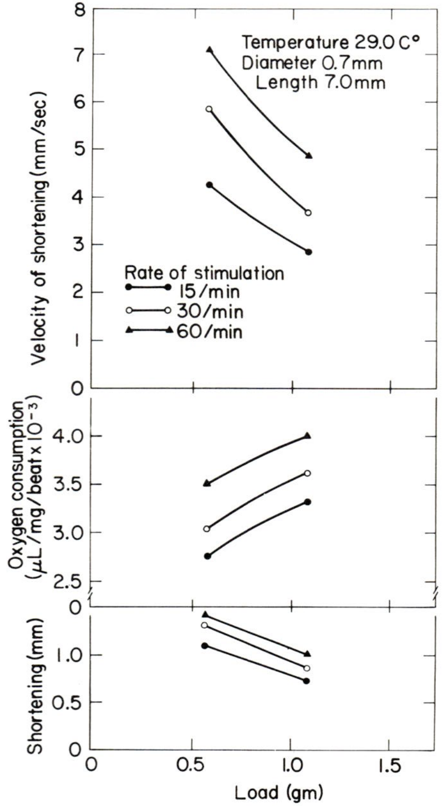

FIG. 10. Effect of alterations in rate of stimulation on force–velocity relations and $M\dot{V}O_2$. Ordinates illustrate (a) velocity of shortening; (b) oxygen consumption per beat; and (c) shortening. Abscissa, load.

the force–velocity relation is shifted to the right with increments in both force of isometric contraction and the intrinsic velocity of shortening (V_{max}). In addition the extent of shortening and thus external work was increased [panel (c)]. These changes in myocardial mechanical behavior are associated with a sizeable increment in $M\dot{V}O_2$, as evident in panel (b). Similar results were obtained in six additional experiments for changes in Ca^{3+} concentrations from 3.75 to 6.25, 5.0 to 7.5, and 2.5 to 5.0 mEq/liter.

In Fig. 10, the effects of changes in the rate of stimulation on myocardial mechanics and $M\dot{V}O_2$ are presented. Increments in the rate of stimulation from 15 to 30 to 60 per minute resulted in increments in both the velocity of shortening at a given load [panel (a)] and extent of shortening and external work [panel (c)]. As shown in panel (b), these changes in myocardial mechanical behavior following augmentation of the contractile state by increasing the rate of stimulation are also associated with an increase in the $M\dot{V}O_2$ per contraction.

When the contractile state was augmented by the addition of norepinephrine 5×10^{-8} *M* to the perfusate; the force–velocity curve was shifted to the right with augmentation of both intrinsic velocity and peak isometric tension. In addition, the extent of shortening and thus external work were increased following norepinephrine. As has been illustrated for the previous inotropic interventions, these changes in the mechanics of myocardial contraction were associated with increased $M\dot{V}O_2$.

Since, in the experiments cited above, augmentation of the contractile state resulted in increments in the velocity of shortening for a given load, in the extent of shortening and thus the work performed in V_{max} and in $M\dot{V}O_2$, it was not possible to determine the individual effects of these mechanical variables on $M\dot{V}O_2$. In order to eliminate the effect of external work and evaluate the effect of alterations in velocity of contraction and thus contractile state on $M\dot{V}O_2$, additional experiments were performed to evaluate isometric contractions prior to and following augmentation of the contractile state with acetylstrophanthidin (six experiments) and norepinephrine (nine experiments). In each experiment, initial tension was decreased following acetylstrophanthidin and/or norepinephrine in order to achieve comparable levels of tension development for both the control and augmented contractile state. In this manner, external work was eliminated, tension was maintained constant, and the contractile state was characterized by a single mechanical parameter, the intrinsic velocity of contraction. The results from a typical experiment of this type are depicted in Fig. 12. At each of three levels of isometric tension, augmentation of the contractile state with acetylstrophanthidin was associated with an increased $M\dot{V}O_2$. Thus, this experiment describes a qualitative relationship between contractile state and $M\dot{V}O_2$.

In order to define the quantitative aspects of the relationship between contractile state and $M\dot{V}O_2$ additional isometric experiments were performed in which norepinephrine was utilized to augment the contractile state. At each level of isometric tension, norepinephrine induced augmentation of the contractile state was associated with increased $M\dot{V}O_2$, thus quantifying the changes in $M\dot{V}O_2$. The alterations in contractile state were measured from force–velocity curves obtained at a preload of 0.2 gm for both the control and augmented contractile states. In order to eliminate possible errors in extrapolation of force–velocity curves to define V_{max}, the change in contractile state was taken as the change in velocity of shortening with only the preload of 0.2 gm from each force–velocity curve. In Fig. 12 the relationship between change in isometric $M\dot{V}O_2$ at a constant tension and change

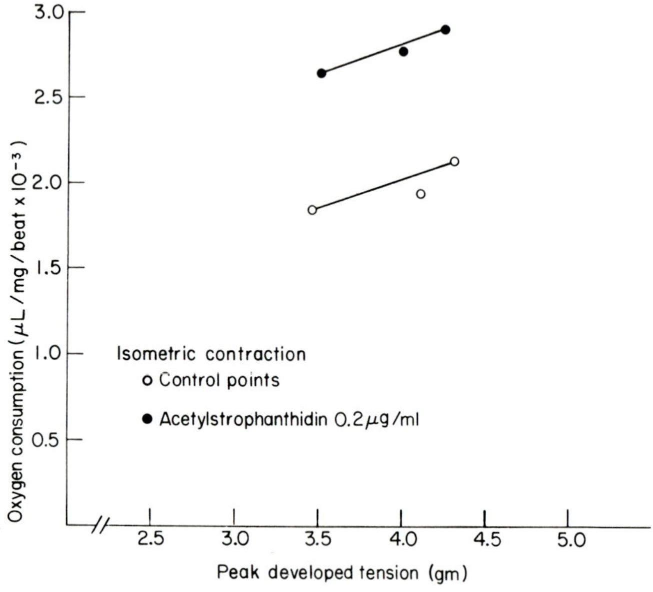

FIG. 11. Effect of acetylstrophanthidin, 0.20/cc on $M\dot{V}O_2$ os isometric contractions at constant levels of developed tension. Ordinate; oxygen consumption. Abscissa; peak developed tension. (Reproduced with permission of *Circ. Res.*)

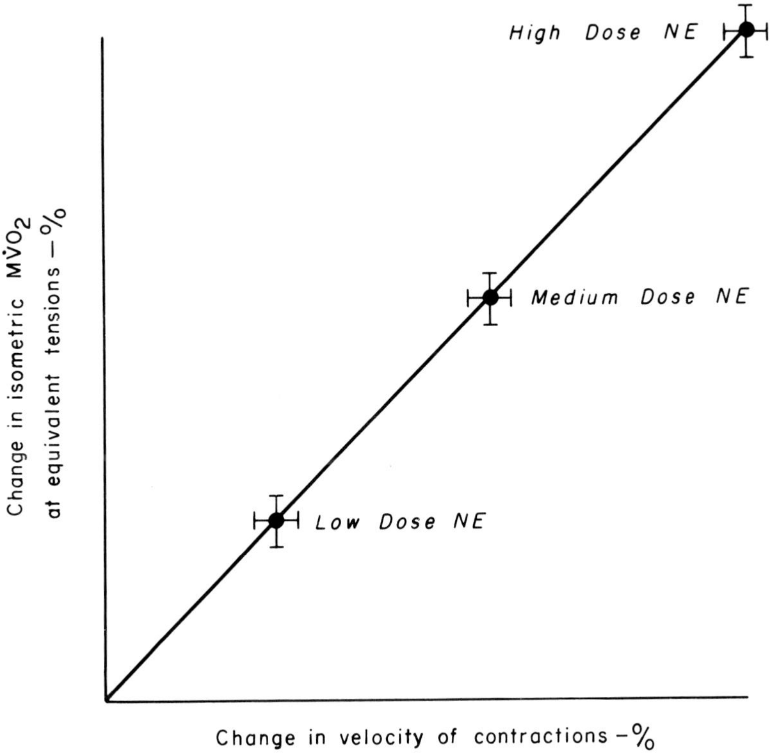

FIG. 12. Sketch of relationship between changes in $M\dot{V}O_2$ of contractions at a constant tension and alterations in contractile state following norepinephrine (nine experiments). Ordinate, change in $M\dot{V}O_2$ of isometric contraction; abscissa, change in velocity of contraction. This relationship is described by the least-squares linear regression $y = (8.96 \pm 3.22) + (8.12 \pm 0.19) \times$.

in contractile state following various concentrations of NE is depicted for a group of nine experiments. This relationship is described by the least-squares linear regression equation $y = (8.96 \pm 3.22) + (0.81 \pm 0.19) \times$. The slope of the regression line is significantly different from zero ($p < 0.001$).

Basal Oxygen Consumption

The $M\dot{V}O_2$ of quiescent muscle was determined in 18 muscles in one phase of these studies and averaged 2.58 ± 0.16 SE uL/mg dry tissue/hr. In order to evaluate the possible effects on $M\dot{V}O_2$ of muscle thickness, the muscles were divided into two groups on the basis of diameter, 0.4–0.7 mm for eight muscles and 0.8–1.0 mm for 10 muscles. $M\dot{V}O_2$ averaged 2.66 ± 0.20 and 2.53 ± 0.24 μL/mg dry tissue/hr in these two groups, values that do not differ significantly. Further, it was observed that the muscles selected for study did not demonstrate an increase in basal $M\dot{V}O_2$ when stretched by increments in preload from 0.1 to 1.0 gm, while muscles having diameters greater than 1.1 mm consistently demonstrated increased $M\dot{V}O_2$ when stretched by addition of preload. The addition of norepinephrine 10^{-7} *M* to 15 muscles did not change basal $M\dot{V}O_2$. Basal $M\dot{V}O_2$ following acetylstrophanthidin 0.20 γ/cc was increased (2.97 ± 0.33 μL/mg/hr for 9 muscles) when compared with control value cited above. However, the difference in resting $M\dot{V}O_2$ between the two groups was not significant.

Discussion

The development of tension, recognized as an important factor influencing energy utilization of the heart by Rhode in 1912, has subsequently been characterized as a major determinant of the heart's oxygen consumption (Sarnoff *et al.*, 1958; McDonald, 1966). The importance of tension, also recognized in the initial investigations into the factors determining oxygen consumption of isolated heart muscle (Lee, 1953; Whalen, 1960), was re-emphasized by McDonald (1966) in a systematic evaluation of the relationship between alterations in developed tension and $M\dot{V}O_2$ of isolated cat papillary muscles. Similar results were found in the present data which describe a linear relationship between $M\dot{V}O_2$ and isometric tension development. However, although both the present data and that presented by McDonald demonstrate that increments in developed tension brought about by increasing afterload result in substantial changes in $M\dot{V}O_2$, the relationship between developed tension and $M\dot{V}O_2$ is not linear for afterloaded contractions.

In addition to myocardial tension development, the results of these experiments demonstrate that $M\dot{V}O_2$ is determined by external shortening against a load. This effect of external work has been shown by comparing the $M\dot{V}O_2$ of isotonic and isometric contractions at equal levels of tension development. Thus, the $M\dot{V}O_2$ of afterloaded contractions was associated with that resulting from the development of tension plus an additional energy utilization directly proportional to the external work performed by the muscle. Additional evidence for external work as a determinant of myocardial energy utilization has been found in the initial measurements of myocardial heat production where a load dependent heat was described in isotonic contractions (Gibbs *et al.*, 1967). The present data describe the role of external work as a determinant of myocardial energy utilization over and above that $M\dot{V}O_2$ associated with tension development and are analogous to the effect of external work on the energetics of skeletal muscle, as described by Fenn (1923).

In experiments on skeletal muscle performed by Fenn, the heat production associated with the maximal amount of external work was increased an average of 39% (range 23–50%) above the heat produced by a tetanic contraction developing a similar level of tension. The present data indicate that, in heart muscle at one half of isometric load, the point at which maximal external work is performed at a given initial muscle length (Fig. 1), 48% of the total $M\dot{V}O_2$ is associated with external work. Thus, in addition to qualitative similarities established between the effects of external work on the energetics of cardiac and skeletal muscle, these data indicate a general quantitative similarity for the Fenn effect on the energetics of the two types of muscle.

In addition to the effect of external work, it has been shown in skeletal muscle that the onset of shortening per se results in an increased heat production which was proportional to the extent of shortening and was independent of load, and thus work (Hill, 1938). However, this "heat of shortening," described only when heat production was determined during the initial phases of contraction, has not been demonstrated when either creatine phosphate utilization (Mommaerts *et al.*, 1962; Carlson *et al.*, 1963), heat production (Carlson *et al.*, 1963), or reduction of mitochondrial NAD (Jobsis and Duffield, 1967) was measured over an entire contraction. These divergent findings led Davies *et al.* (1967) to suggest that the "heat of shortening" was due to changes in entropy of the chemical processes within the muscle and did not represent degraded free energy. In the present study, the $M\dot{V}O_2$ in excess of that associated with tension development when shortening occurred in afterloaded contractions was proportional to the external work performed. The fact that the intercept of the regression equation describing this relationship (Fig. 4) was not significantly different from zero suggests that shortening per se did not have a detectable effect on $M\dot{V}O_2$ in these experiments. Although this view is consonant with the results of Carlson *et al.* (1963) and Davies *et al.* (1967), in skeletal muscle, delineation of the precise effect of shortening per se on myocardial energy utilization is not possible from these experiments. Of recent note are measurements of heat production in cardiac muscle (Gibbs *et al.*, 1967) which again suggest the true existence of energy use attributable to the effect of shortening.

From the model of Hill (1938) in which contractile activity with a passive elastic component SEC, tension development can be considered in terms of the work performed by the CE in stretching the SEC, plus the work performed against equipment compliance. This form of work has been considered as "internal" contractile element work. On the other hand, the work the CE does in moving a load comprises the external work. From the analysis of the present data, it is evident that $M\dot{V}O_2$ is linearly related to both external work (Fig. 4) and internal work (Fig. 6). It is also clear from the present experiments that the performance of internal work by series elastic extension during tension development has approximately twice the unit energy cost of performing external fiber shortening work. These data, quantifying the difference between energetic cost of tension development and external work are in agreement with the observations of Evans and Matsuoka (1915) who noted that work performed by the intact heart against an increasing pressure load resulted in a much higher $M\dot{V}O_2$ than work performed by increasing the stroke volume. Thus, at a constant contractility the factors determining $M\dot{V}O_2$ might be represented by the equation

$$M\dot{V}O_2\ \mu L/mg/beat \times 10^{-3} = 0.57 \text{ external work gm}\cdot\text{mm} + 1.30 \text{ tension development work gm}\cdot\text{mm} \quad (1)$$

The values of 0.57 and 1.30 $\mu L/mg/beat \times 10^{-3}$ $M\dot{V}O_2$ per gm • mm of work represent the slope of each of the least squares regression equations of the data presented in Fig. 6. The inequality of the unit energy cost between the two types of CEW (internal vs. external work) provides limitations to the usefulness of total CEW as a unifying determinant of $M\dot{V}O_2$ (Britman and Levine, 1964). In addition the sum of the relative energy costs of the two types of work produces the observed nonlinear relation between $M\dot{V}O_2$ and total CEW when a force–velocity curve is inscribed.

As noted above, alterations in initial muscle length result in a redistribution of load with afterload decreasing at the greater preload for each level of total load. Since the intrinsic velocity of contraction is not altered by changes in initial muscle length, the $M\dot{V}O_2$ of afterloaded contractions at any given muscle length is determined by the sum of the energy costs of the two types of work performed. Thus, the Frank-Starling principle affects myocardial energy utilization through alterations in the level of tension developed and external work performed.

The " internal " CEW values in these experiments were obtained from the SE load-extension curves recently determined by Parmley and Sonnenblick (1967), where SE extensibility was found to be 5–6% of muscle length for isometric contractions. Although utilization of these latest SEC extension curves which were somewhat different for different initial tensions resulted in a lack of correlation between $M\dot{V}O_2$ and total CEW of afterloaded contraction, a similar lack of correlation was observed when internal CEW was calculated by the initial formula proposed by Sonnenblick on the basis of SEC extension of 8–10%, where CEW equals external work + Afterload/3.2

(Sonnenblick, 1964). Thus, regardless of the method utilized to calculate CEW, this function does not correlate with $M\dot{V}O_2$ of isolated papillary muscle when both internal and external work are performed.

Although the present study indicates that, in afterloaded contractions, calculated CEW cannot be considered the primary, sole determinant of $M\dot{V}O_2$, it should be emphasized that the present data do not exclude CEW as one determinant of $M\dot{V}O_2$. In fact, this concept may have increased credibility when it is observed that external work has now been demonstrated to affect $M\dot{V}O_2$. Validation of the exact relationship between $M\dot{V}O_2$ and CEW must await delineation of the manner in which $M\dot{V}O_2$ is affected by alterations in tension maintenance, a factor recently reemphasized by Jöbis and Duffrield (1967) to affect the energy utilization of skeletal muscle. This factor may have contributed significantly to the increased $M\dot{V}O_2$ seen during tension development, since internal CEW is a function of peak developed tension and independent of the finite period of time that tension is maintained. It was not possible, however, to determine the relative effects of internal CEW and tension maintenance on the $M\dot{V}O_2$ associated with tension development in these experiments.

That an additional term should be considered in this mathematical representation describing the process utilizing energy during contraction is suggested by studies performed in skeletal muscle (Hill, 1938), in which analysis of the energy utilized included a term for activation processes. Although the processes included in the activation term for skeletal muscle are different from those of cardiac muscle because of the inability to tetanize the latter, recent investigations (Pool and Sonnenblick, 1967) in heart muscle of creatine phosphate utilization have described an energy utilization associated with activation which is distinct from the creatine phosphate hydrolysis associated with tension development or work performance. Preliminary indication of the existence of a consumption of oxygen which may be related to activation events as electrical depolarization (Klocke *et al.*, 1966) and binding of calcium by the sarcoplasmic reticulum (Hasselback, 1964) was found by determining the $M\dot{V}O_2$ for contractions with a preload of 50 mg and extrapolating these values to zero tension, i.e., the intercept on the ordinate. The validity of assigning the determined $M\dot{V}O_2$ value of 0.23 μL/mg/beat $\times 10^{-3}$ to these activation events assumes that unloaded shortening *per se* utilizes no energy.

The observation that the intercept of the regression equation describing the relationship between internal CEW and $M\dot{V}O_2$ of isometric contractions (filled circles, Fig. 6) occurred at 0.63 μL/mg/beat $\times 10^{-3}$ is further indication that activation processes resulted in an energy utilization in the present experiments. The $M\dot{V}O_2$ values of 0.23 ± 0.05 μL/mg/beat $\times 10^{-3}$ for very lightly loaded isotonic contractions and 0.63 ± 0.14 μL/mg/beat $\times 10^{-3}$ for isometric contractions are dissimilar ($p < 0.05$), an observation that may again suggest a role for tension maintenance in determining $M\dot{V}O_2$.

Separation of a factor for activation which, in the present data is included in the second term of Eq. (3), would result in the mathematical formulation of the present data as

$$M\dot{V}O_2 = K_1 \text{ external work} + K_2 \text{ tension} + O_2 \text{ cost of activation} \qquad (2)$$

In addition to the factors outlined in Eq. (2) as determinants of $M\dot{V}O_2$ for a given contractile state, recent studies in the intact heart (Krasnow *et al.*, 1964; Graham *et al.*, 1968) have demonstrated that alterations in the velocity of contraction were associated with substantial changes in $M\dot{V}O_2$ of similar direction. Similar increases in $M\dot{V}O_2$ were found in the present data where augmentation of the contractile state was achieved with acetylstrophanthidin, norepinephrine, increments in rate of stimulation, and an increase in calcium ion concentration. Analysis of the mechanics of myocardial contraction in these afterloaded contractions revealed that agumentation of the contractile state was associated with increments in V_{max}, the velocity of shortening, and the extent of shortening and external work in muscles developing a constant level of tension. These alterations in mechanical behavior were associated with increased $M\dot{V}O_2$ in each instance. However, in these studies as well as other investigations of the effects of inotropic agents on $M\dot{V}O_2$ (Krasnow *et al.*, 1964; Sonnenblick *et al.*, 1965; Covell *et al.*, 1966) both the velocity of contraction and the extent of shortening and external work were increased by the intervention, thus precluding individual consideration of the effects of these parameters on $M\dot{V}O_2$.

On the other hand, when comparison of the effects of acetylstrophanthidin and norepinephrine on $M\dot{V}O_2$ of isometric contractions at equal levels of developed tension was undertaken, external contractile element shortening and thus external work were eliminated. The small remaining contractile element shortening is produced by the extension of the series elastic component by the contractile element and, although the stiffness of the series elastic is somewhat decreased by the changes in initial length (Sonnenblick, 1964; Parmley and Sonnenblick, 1967), contractile element shortening for contractions at a given developed force can be assumed to be of similar magnitude. Thus, the increments in $M\dot{V}O_2$ in Figs. 11 and 12 following glycoside and norepinephrine administration can be associated with augmentation of the contractile state independent of changes in tension development, external work, and contractile element shortening.

While the data presented only indicated a qualitative relationship between contractile state and $M\dot{V}O_2$ following acetylstrophanthidin, the experiments with norepinephrine characterize a linear relationship between these two variables when tension was maintained constant in isometric contractions (Fig. 14). From these data, as well as the recent report by Graham *et al.* (1968), it is apparent that the contractile state is, in addition to tension, a major determinant of $M\dot{V}O_2$. Further, the present data and the data of Covell *et al.* (1966) would suggest that in earlier studies in which hemodynamic parameters were controlled, a lack of consideration of the alterations in myocardial mechanical behavior following digitalis glycosides could account for the observed lack of change in $M\dot{V}O_2$ after glycosides. Indeed, a consideration of the relationship between norepinephrine induced alterations in contractile state and $M\dot{V}O_2$ offers a possible explanation for the increased $M\dot{V}O_2$ which has heretofore been attributed to an " oxygen wasting " effect of norepinephrine.

It should be noted that the present delineation of the relative energy utilization of the CEW work factors must be superimposed on a given contractile state. The constants K_1 and K_2 accounting for the overall $M\dot{V}O_2$ are valid only for a given contractile state. The manner in which these constants and/or the oxygen cost of activation may change with alterations of the contractile state remains a subject for further investigation.

The determination of resting oxygen consumption has assumed increasing importance since various investigators (Cranefield and Greenspan, 1960) have utilized the relation of resting oxygen consumption to changes in muscle diameter as a method of investigating the problem of diffusion limitations for isolated papillary muscle. The muscle diameters in this investigation at which increments in length resulted in increased resting oxygen uptake are somewhat larger than those previously reported (Cranefield and Greenspan, 1960; Lee, 1953), a finding which may have resulted from differences in the technique of determining oxygen consumption. Although the data presented here on resting oxygen consumption do not provide a solution to the problem of the critical diameter for adequate diffusion, the lack of difference in resting oxygen consumption between muscles grouped from smaller (0.4–0.7 mm) versus larger diameters (0.8–1.0 mm) would suggest that below 1.0 mm, muscle diameter is not a significant factor in determining resting oxygen consumption.

In summary, the present data demonstrate that myocardial energy utilization is determined by the mechanics of myocardial contraction. At a constant contractility, $M\dot{V}O_2$ for afterloaded contractions could be described by the equation: $M\dot{V}O_2$ μL/mg/beat $\times 10^{-3} = 0.57$ external work gm•mm + 1.30 internal work gm•mm. The unit $M\dot{V}O_2$ cost of performing " internal " contractile element work during tension development was found to be twice the $M\dot{V}O_2$ consumed in performing external work. Thus, total CEW of afterloaded contractions was not a simple linear correlate of $M\dot{V}O_2$. Moreover, at a constant tension, the data describe a linear relationship between $M\dot{V}O_2$ and contractile state, as characterized by velocity of contraction.

References

Abbott, B. C., and Mommaerts, W. F. H. M. (1959). *J. Gen. Physiol.* **42,** 533.

Bloomfield, R. A., Rapoport, B., Milnor, J. P., Long, W. K., Mebane, J. G., and Ellis, L. B. (1948). *J. Clin. Invest.* **27,** 588.

Braunwald, E., Bloodwell, R. D., Goldberg, L. I., and Morrow, A. G. (1961). *J. Clin. Invest.* **40,** 52.

Britman, N. A., and Levine, H. J. (1964). *J. Clin. Invest.* **43,** 1397.

Carlson, F. D., Brink, F., Jr., and Brink, D. (1950). *Rev. Sci. Instrum.* **21,** 923.

Carlson, F. D., Brink, F., Jr., Brink, D., Hardy, D. J., and Wilkie, D. R. (1963). *J. Gen. Physiol.* **46,** 851.

Clark, L. C., Jr., Wolf, R., Granger, D., and Taylor, Z. (1953). *J. Appl. Physiol.* **6,** 189.

Coleman, H. N. (1967). *Circ. Res.* **21,** 487.

Coleman, H. N. (1968). *Amer. J. Physiol.* **214,** 100.

Coleman, H. N., Sonnenblick, E. H., and Braunwald, E. (1969). *Amer. J. Physiol.* **271,** 291.

Coleman, H. N., Sonnenblick, E. H., and Braunwald, E. (1971). *Amer. J. Physiol.* Submitted for publication.

Covell, J. W., Braunwald, E., Ross, J., Jr., and Sonnenblick, E. (1966). *J. Clin. Invest.* **45,** 1535.

Cranefield, P. F., and Greenspan, K. (1960). *J. Gen. Physiol.* **44,** 235.

Davies, R. E., Kushmerick, M. J., and Larson, R. E. (1967). *Nature (London)* **214,** 148.

Evans, C. L. and Matsuoka, Y. (1915). *J. Physiol. (London)* **49,** 378.

Fenn, W. O. (1923). *J. Physiol. (London)* **58,** 175.

Gibbs, C. L., Mommaerts, W. F. H. M., and Ricchiuti, N. (1967). *J. Physiol. (London)* **191,** 25.

Graham, T. P., Jr., Covell, J. W., Sonnenblick, E. H., Ross, J., Jr., and Braunwald, E. (1968). *J. Clin. Invest.* **47,** 375.

Hasselback, W. (1964). "Progress in Biophysics and Molecular Biology," Vol. 14, pp. 167–217. McMillan, New York.

Hill, A. V. (1938). *Proc. Roy. Soc. Ser. B* **126,** 136.

Jobsis, F., and Duffield, J. (1967). *Science* **156,** 1388.

Klocke, F. J., Braunwald, E., and Ross, J., Jr. (1966). *Circ. Res.* **18,** 357.

Krasnow, N., Rolett, E. L., Yurchak, P. M., Hood, W. B., Jr., and Gorlin, R. (1964). *Amer. J. Med.* **37,** 514.

Lee, K. S. (1953). *J. Pharmacol. Exp. Ther.* **109,** 304.

McDonald, R. H., Jr. (1966). *Amer. J. Physiol.* **210,** 351.

McDonald, R. H., Jr., Taylor, R. R., and Cingolani, M. E. (1966). *Amer. J. Physiol.* **211,** 667.

Mommaerts, W. F. H. M., Seraydarian, K., and Marechal, G. (1962). *Biochim. Biophys. Acta* **57,** 1.

Parmley, W. W., and Sonnenblick, E. H. (1967). *Circ. Res.* **20,** 112.

Peters, J. P., and Van Slyke, D. D. (1932). "Quantitative Clinical Chemistry," Vol. 2, p. 84. Williams and Wilkins, Baltimore.

Pool, P. E., and Sonnenblick, E. H. (1967). *J. Gen. Physiol.* **50,** 951.

Rhode, E. (1912). *Arch. Exp. Pathol. Pharmakol.* **68,** 406.

Sarnoff, S. L., Braunwald, E., Welch, C., Case, R. B., Stainsby, W. N., and Macruz, R. (1958). *Amer. J. Physiol.* **192,** 148.

Schilling, M. O. (1960). *Rev. Sci. Instrum.* **31,** 1215.

Sonnenblick, E. H. (1962). *Amer. J. Physiol.* **202,** 931.

Sonnenblick, E. H. (1964) *Amer. J. Physiol.* **207,** 1330.
Sonnenblick, E. H. Ross, J., Jr., Covell, J. W., Kaiser, G. A., and Braunwald, E. (1965). *Amer. J. Physiol.* **209,** 919.
Whalen, W. H. (1960). *J. Physiol.* (*London*) **157,** 672.

STUDIES ON MITOCHONDRIA FROM NORMAL, HYPERTROPHIED, AND FAILING MYOCARDIUM

Arnold Schwartz

Introduction

Since the initial observations and description of minute cytoplasmic organelles by Altmann in 1894, the recognition of the importance of mitochondria has received the attention of numerous investigators (Bresnick and Schwartz, 1968). For many years only one specific function of mitochondria was recognized: the generation of adenosine triphosphate from energy-laden substrates (Lehninger, 1964). Since it is well recognized that in normally functioning, adult mammalian cardiac muscle, the primary source of ATP is the mitochondrion, these organelles have received a good deal of attention with respect to function in pathological situations. The processes of contraction, relaxation and active transport all require energy donated from ATP (Bresnick and Schwartz, 1968). Consequently, any one of these energy-utilizing aspects of heart muscle would require adequately functioning mitochondria in order to maintain a normal stable myocardium. The relationship between mitochondria and the various energy-utilizing systems in the cardiac muscle cell is schematically pictured in Fig. 1. Note that the processes of contraction and relaxation require calcium, but that both systems are under the influence of separate enzymatic systems which require ATP. The Na^+, K^+-ATPase enzyme system is thought to be located in the cell membrane, and also requires ATP for adequate function.

Within recent years, it has become apparent from numerous investigations that mitochondria can carry out a number of very important energy-linked processes. These include ion transport and the production of reduced coenzymes, both required for growth and differentiation (Lehninger, 1964; Bresnick and Schwartz, 1968). Figure 2 (a, b) presents a generalized modern picture of the complexity of the mitochondrion with its associated reactions. It is of particular interest that all animal and plant mitochondria have now been

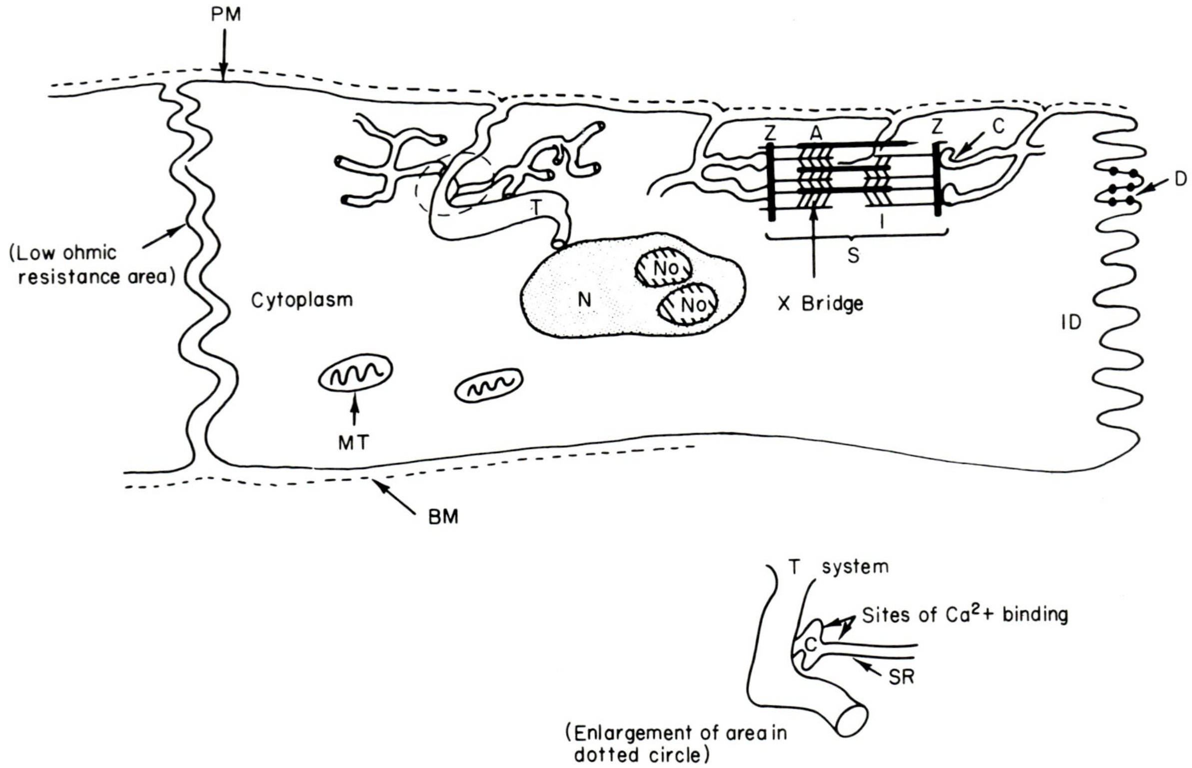

FIG. 1. Diagrammatic sketch of cardiac muscle cell. PM, plasma membrane; BM, basement membrane; T, T-system; C, cisterna of SR; MT, mitochondrion; S, sarcomere of myofibril; I, I band of sarcomere (actin); A, A band of sarcomere (myosin) (X, cross bridges between A and I); N, nucleus; No, nucleolus; ID, intercalated disc; D, desmosome; SR, sarcoplasmic

shown to contain a specific DNA, which is quite different from nuclear DNA. In addition, mitochondria also contains specific species of transfer RNA and aminoacyl-transfer RNA synthetases which presumably catalyze the selective attachment of amino acids to RNA in protein synthesis (Nass, 1969; Wagner, 1969). Tables I and II summarize some of the interesting properties of DNA and protein in mitochondria. It is apparent that mitochondrial DNA can be synthesized and replicated within the organelle. Furthermore, mitochondria are capable of synthesizing RNA. They also contain ribosomes and ribosomal RNA's which differ from cytoplasmic nucleic acids. It has also been shown that these organelles can, in fact, incorporate amino acids into protein and, in particular, into the inner membrane of the organelle. The incorporating system is different from the cytoplasmic protein synthetic system in that the former is specifically sensitive to several antibacterial antibiotics (Nass, 1969). Mitochondrial RNA polymerase can be inhibited by actinomycin-D and, consequently, is probably DNA-dependent. From a wide variety of experiments by numerous investigators, one can assume that mitochondrial DNA (mDNA) is genetically active. However, it is improbable that mDNA can code for the synthesis of the entire mitochondrion. The DNA molecule, which is circular, has a molecular weight of approximately 9 to 10×10^6, which is equivalent of approximately 15,000 base pairs. Mitochondrial DNA can, therefore, code for about 5000 amino acids or 30 polypeptide chains of molecular weight 20,000. It is generally agreed, therefore, that mitochondrial DNA probably codes for at least *part* of the inner membrane system. Note from Fig. 2 that this membrane system contains the entire apparatus for oxidative phosphorylation. The outer membrane of mitochondria probably is synthesized in the cytoplasm and is under the control of nuclear genes. Accordingly, it has been suggested that, in terms of evolution, mitochondria might have arisen from microorganisms. It has been suggested that mitochondrial DNA could code for the synthesis of perhaps cytochromes a, b, and c_1 (Slater *et al.*, 1968). It is apparent, therefore, that mitochondrial DNA accounts for "cytoplasmic heredity," and can be considered as part of a second genetic system of the cell. Investigations in our own laboratory have suggested a role for polyamines, particularly histones, in the control of mitochondrial activity. The interesting possibility of an interaction of these substances with mitochondrial nucleic acids is presently being studied (Johnson *et al.*, 1969; Johnson and Schwartz, 1969; Schwartz *et al.*, 1966). Specific histones derived from cardiac muscle have been shown to effect an energy-linked movement of potassium from heart mitochondria into the cytoplasm of the cell (Safer and Schwartz, 1967). Figure 3 indicates the effects of histones on potassium transport and the possibility that these basic proteins participate in the respiratory control of heart mitochondria. Basic proteins have also been found to specifically affect isolated contractile

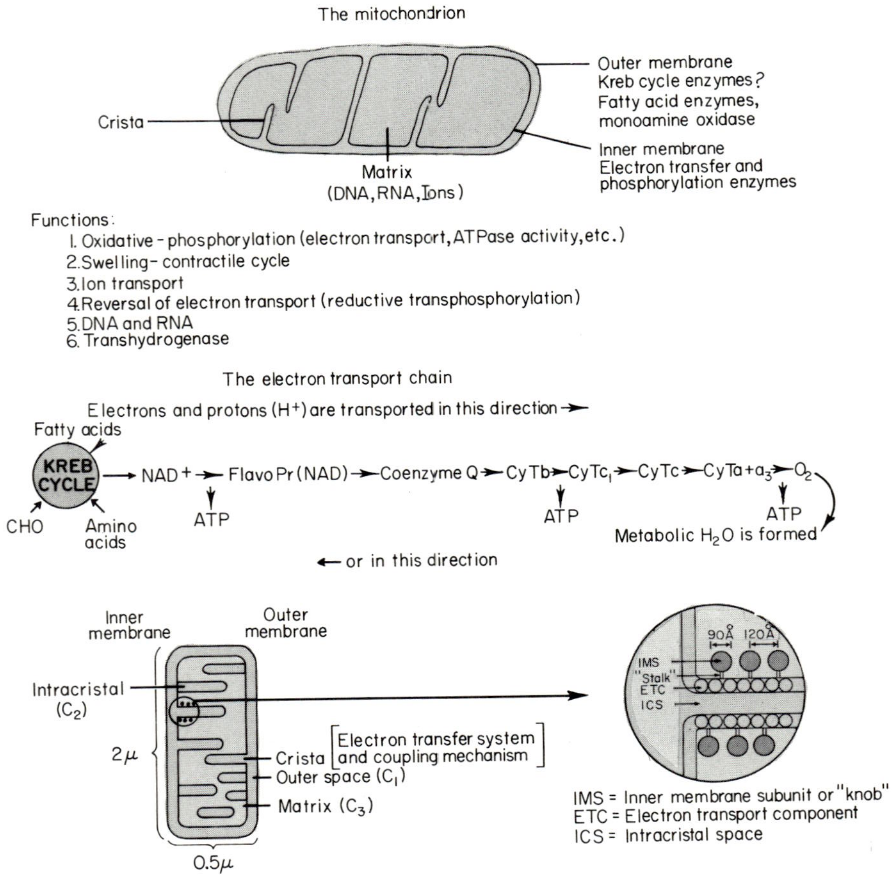

FIG. 2(a). The mitochondrion.

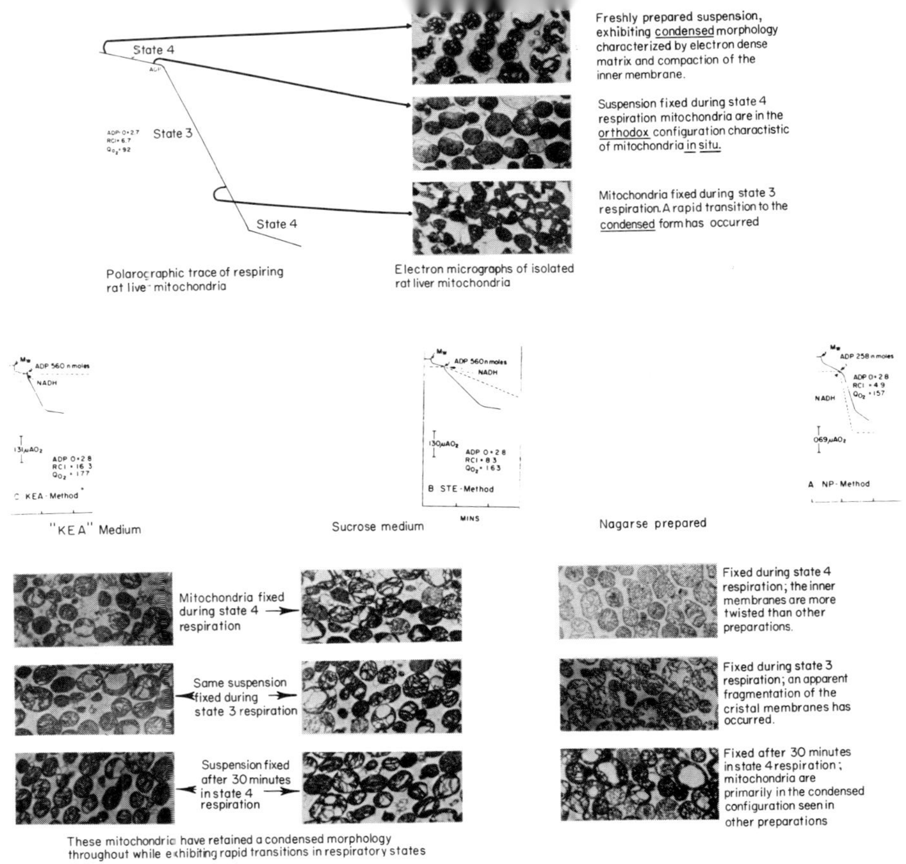

FIG. 2(b). Ultrastructural changes in mitochondria associated with biochemical states.

TABLE I

CONTENT OF DNA AND PROTEIN IN MITOCHONDRIA[a]

Cell type	DNA related to mitochondrial protein (μg/mg)	Protein per single mitochondrion (gm × 10^{-13})	DNA per single mitochondrion (gm × 10^{-16})[a]
	Adult tissues		
Beef heart	0.24	1.1	0.26
Rat liver	0.65, 0.8	2.0	0.9–1.6
	0.46, 0.51		
Hamster liver	0.58		
Mouse liver	0.55		
Chicken liver	0.5		0.7
	Eggs (nondividing)		
Frog oocytes	0.52		
Sea urchin			0.23
	Rapidly growing cells		
L cells (mouse fibroblasts)	1.1, 1.0–1.2[b]	0.80	0.88
Mouse embryo	1.3		
Mouse placenta	0.9		
Rat embryo	1.8		
Rat placenta	1.7		
Hamster embryo	1.3		
Hamster placenta	1.1		
	Tumors		
Ascites tumor (mouse)	2.5		
Hepatoma (rat)	5.3		
Walker-carcinoma (rat)	4.7, 8.2		
Jensen-sarcoma (rat)	4.7, 5.4		
Sarcoma (mouse drug-induced)	4.7		
Sarcoma (hamster, polyoma virus-induced)	4.7		
	Eukaryotic microorganisms		
Yeast	0.7–1.0, 1.1–4.3	0.85	0.6–3.7
Tetrahymena[b]			3.7
Neurospora	0.7		
	Higher plants		
Mung bean[b]	0.8	6.2	5.0
Turnip[b]			5.0

[a] A molecular weight of 60 × 10^6 daltons corresponds to 1.0 × 10^{-16} gm of DNA. Taken from Nass (1969).

[b] Mitochondrial DNA was isolated on cesium chloride gradients rather than extracted by acid hydrolysis.

TABLE II

CHEMICAL AND ELECTRON MICROSCOPICAL ESTIMATE OF CIRCULAR AND LINEAR DNA MOLECULES ISOLATED FROM MITOCHONDRIA IN THREE BANDS ON CESIUM CHLORIDE–ETHIDIUM BROMIDE GRADIENTS (DNA I, LOWER BAND; DNA Im, INTERMEDIATE BAND; DNA II, UPPER BAND)[a]

Mitochondria		DNA I Circular monomers, dimers (covalently closed)		DNA Im Circular monomers, dimers interlocked dimers, oligomers		DNA II Nicked circles, some oligomers, linear DNA	
Source	Deoxy-ribo-nuclease[a]	DNA/protein (μg/mg)	Monomers: dimers (%)	DNA/protein (μg/mg)	Monomers: dimers (%)	DNA/protein (μg/mg)	Circles: linear (%)
L cells	—	0.44	94:6[b]	0.08	24:76[c]	3.9	1:100
L cells	+	0.56	95:5	0.12	21:79[c]	0.50	70:30
			48% of total)		(10% of total)		(42% of total)
HeLa cells	—		90:10[d]		40:60		
Normal leukocytes	—		99:1				
Leukemic leukocytes,							
Case 1	—		68:32[c]				
			(15 to 50% of total)				
Case 2	—		89:11[c]				
Sea urchin whole							
eggs	—		95:5		33:67		

[a] If treatment of mitochondria with deoxyribonuclease is omitted, variable amounts of nuclear DNA are present as linear DNA. Taken from Nass (1969).

[b] 80–90% of dimers consist of open double-size circles; the others, of two joined monomers.

[c] Figures include interlocked dimers and 1–3% interlocked oligomers.

[d] Dimers consist of two joined monomers.

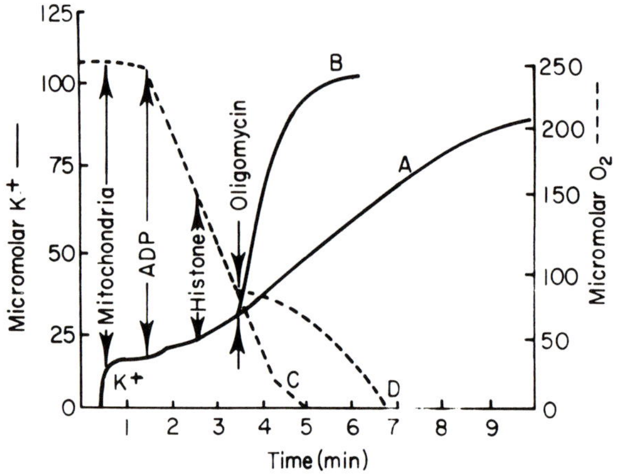

FIG. 3. Inhibition of the effects of histone by ADP. For curves A and B, the medium consisted of 0.25 *M* sucrose, 10 m*M* trischloride (pH 7.4), 5 m*M* trisphosphate, 1 m*M* tris-glutamate, and 17 mg mitochondrial protein in a final volume of 10.0 ml. The additions for curve A were 500 μM tris-ADP and 250 μg β-7 histone. The additions for curve B were 500 μM tris-ADP, 250 μg β-7 histone, and 25 μg oligomycin. Curves A and B denote the efflux of K^+ from the mitochondria. For curves C and D, the medium was the same as for curves A and B except that the final volume was 2.0 ml and 4.3 mg of mitochondrial proteins were added. The additions for curve C were 500 μM tris-ADP and 50 μg β-7 histone. The additions for curve D were 500 μM tris-ADP, 50 μg β7 histone, and 10 μg oligomycin. Curves C and D represent the uptake of O_2 by the mitochondria.

preparations from cardiac muscle (Schwartz *et al.*, 1965). It is possible, therefore, that specific basic proteins or polyamines, present in the cardiac muscle cell, are released at specific times, perhaps during stressful periods, and control intramitochondrial nucleic acid metabolism as well as cardiac muscle function. Studies in other laboratories have suggested an interaction of the nuclear genetic system with that of the mitochondrial genetic system, so that perhaps in situations which require the growth and development of heart muscle, such as in hypertrophy, the mitochondria may participate to an important degree in the process. The role of the mitochondrial genetic system in diseases is at present being seriously considered by numerous investigators (Nass, 1969). Emphasis is being placed in this introductory section on the presence of active and specific nucleic acid metabolism in mitochondria because this may be of importance in considering the role of mitochondria in hypertrophy and heart failure.

This chapter will discuss experiments carried out in this laboratory and in other laboratories concerning the importance of mitochondria in the normal and diseased cardiac muscle cell.

Methods

The procedures for isolation and assay of respiratory control, oxygen consumption, potassium transport and nucleic acid metabolism in mitochondria have been completely discussed in previous papers (see reference section). The methodology employed for the induction of congestive hypertrophy and congestive heart failure in the guinea pig has also been discussed in detail (Schwartz and Lee, 1962). The cardiomyopathic Syrian hamsters were obtained from Dr. E. Bajusz of Cambridge, Massachusetts. The human heart preparations were obtained from recipient patients during transplantation procedure at the Methodist Hospital, Brown-Fondren Cardiovascular Research and Training Center, and at St. Luke's Hospital, Houston, Texas, through the courtesy of Dr. Michael E. De Bakey and Dr. Denton A. Cooley. Nonfailing human heart tissue was obtained from experiments carried out using the Portable Preservation Chamber, through the courtesy of Drs. Michael E. De Bakey and E. B. Diethrich.

Results

Heart Mitochondria in Failure

In a series of experiments involving failing guinea pig heart, produced by a partial coarctation of the proximal portion of the ascending aorta, specific defects in mitochondrial oxidative phosphorylation were found. This is shown in Table III. Furthermore, defects in anaerobic glycolysis were also observed (Fig. 4). It should be emphasized that these animals were all in severe congestive heart failure. The hearts were markedly hypertrophied (as well as dilated), and the animals exhibited all signs and symptoms of congestive heart failure, rather similar to that observed in the human. These findings were also repeated in heart–lung preparations, failed by pressure loading (Procita *et al.*, 1965). The experiments alluded to above were all carried out using the classic manometric procedure. This method employs a highly fortified medium, and requires rather prolonged incubation conditions. It is possible, therefore, that during the incubation, mitochondria may be damaged. Certainly, it is rather difficult to ascertain adequate respiratory control using this procedure.

TABLE IIIa

HEART AND BODY WEIGHT RATIOS (HW/BW) OF CONTROL AND CHF GUINEA PIGS

Type	No. of animals	Body weight (gm)	Heart weight (gm)	HW/BW × 10^3
Control	30	738 ± 12.6	2.06 ± 0.017	2.73
CHF	12	708 ± 39.9	3.10 ± 0.030	4.38

TABLE IIIb

P:O RATIOS AND OXYGEN CONSUMPTION OF MITOCHONDRIA FROM CONTROL AND CHF GUINEA PIG HEARTS[a]

Type	Substrate	No. of experiments	P:O	Q_{O_2} (μ atoms O_2/mg. protein/hr.)
Control	Glutamate	20	3.13 ± 0.05	9.53 ± 0.05
CHF	Glutamate	20	1.78 ± 0.05	6.86 ± 0.40
Control	Succinate	10	1.97 ± 0.06	8.60 ± 2.7
CHF	Succinate	11	1.12 + 0.23	4.52 ± 0.70

[a] The main compartment of each flask contained the following: $MgCl_2$, 8 m*M*; KCl, 50 m*M*; ATP (disodium salt, Sigma), 2.5 m*M*; cytochrome C (from beef heart, Sigma), 0.017 m*M*; DPN (Sigma), 0.5 m*M*; malic acid, 0.52 m*M*, NaF, 12 m*M*, substrate, 13 m*M*; glucose, 56 m*M*, and hexokinase (Sigma, type III), 20 units; K-phosphate buffer, pH 7.4, 20 m*M*. 0.25 *M* sucrose containing 0.001 *M* EDTA, at pH 7.4 to make a total flask volume of 3.0 ml. The temperature was 37.5 C; reaction time was 20 min; each determination was run in triplicate. Each flask received approximately the same amount of mitochondrial protein (an average of 5 mg per flask) in each experiment. The gas phase was air.

Consequently, a number of laboratories have suggested that the results originally reported could, in fact, be due to artifacts resulting from the assay procedure. Accordingly, Sobel *et al.* (1967) repeated our experiments using the same animal, but employed a more sensitive and more modern assay procedure, namely a polarographic method that does not involve the use of a highly fortified media as well as prolonged incubation at higher temperatures. These investigators found no alteration in oxidative phosphorylation of animals purportedly in the same degree of congestive failure that we employed. However, it is well known that when the manometric procedure is employed

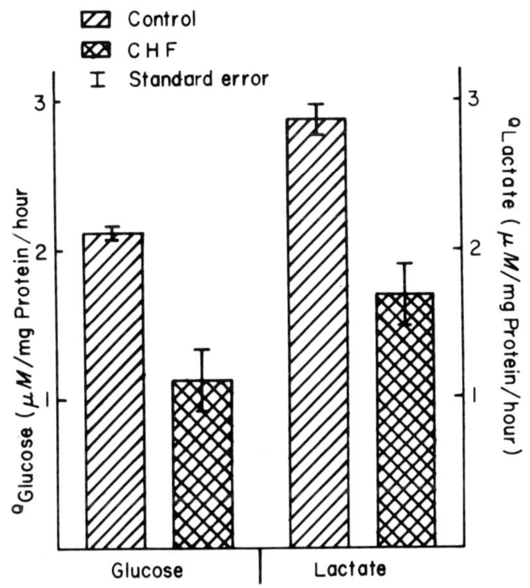

FIG. 4. Anaerobic glycolysis of control and CHF guinea pig homogenates.

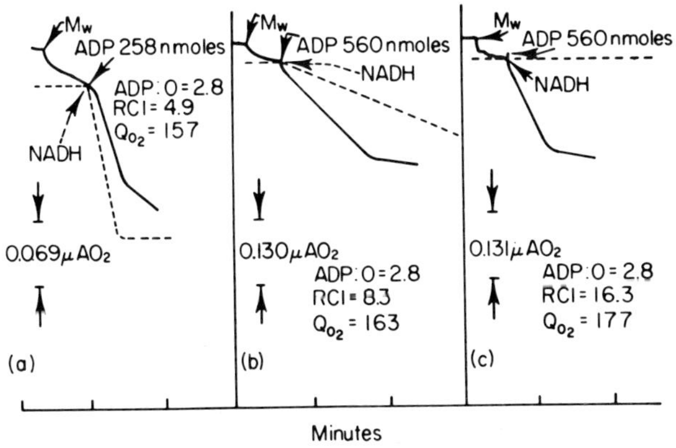

FIG. 5. Oxygen electrode tracings of rat heart mitochondria isolated in medium containing Nagarse (A), sucrose, tris, 10 m*M* EDTA (B) and KCl-EDTA-albumin (C). The polytron was used in C and a glass homogenizer in A and B. RCl = respiratory control index; QO_2 = oxygen consumption in nanoatoms O_2/min/mg mitochondrial protein. Glutamate is the substrate. Dotted lines indicate the rate of oxidation of NADH added at the same point at which ADP was added but in different experiments and in the absence of substrate and ADP and in the presence of inorganic phosphate. Assay temperature was 25°C. M_w = washed mitochondria; nmoles = nanomoles. Similar results were obtained with guinea pig heart mitochondria.

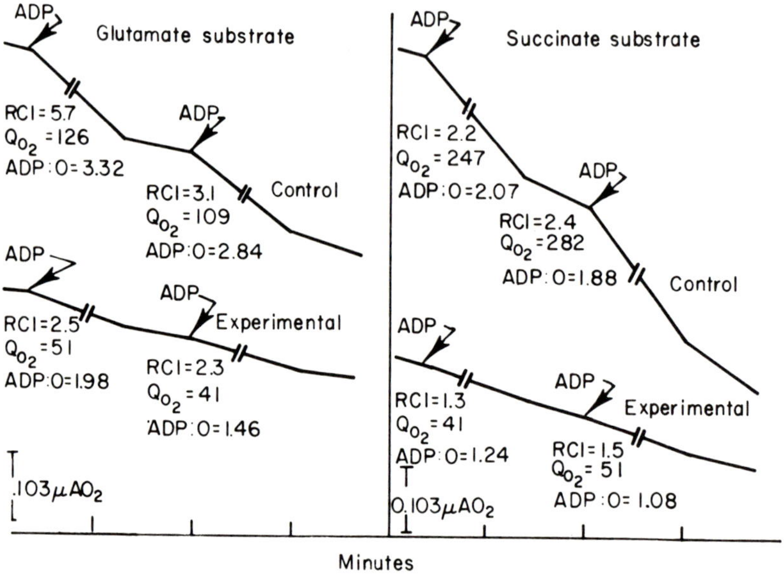

FIG. 6. Representative oxygen electrode tracings of mitochondria from a normal guinea pig heart and one in congestive heart failure. The mitochondria were isolated in 0.25 *M* sucrose, 10 m*M* tris, 1 m*M* EDTA. Glutamate or succinate was used as the substrate (5 m*M*-final concentration); assays were carried out in the sucrose-tris medium at 30°C. ADP, 550 nanomoles, was added where indicated. RCl = respiratory control index; QO_2 = oxygen consumption in nanoatoms O_2/min/mg mitochondrial protein.

properly, and mitochondria isolated with intact membranes, little or no damage to mitochondria, even under prolonged incubation conditions, should occur. Consequently, we repeated our original experiments employing a number of different isolation and assay procedures, as well as both the manometric and oxygen-electrode methods. Figure 5 indicates the three particular procedures employed (Lindenmayer *et al.*, 1968). It should be noted that the proteinase procedure (used by Sobel *et al.*, 1967), which is frequently employed for the isolation of cardiac mitochondria, is inadequate because it produces damage to the outer membrane. An appropriate procedure was devised for isolation of intact mitochondria, which could remain viable for prolonged periods of time, at various temperatures and under various incubation conditions. Guinea pigs in severe heart failure, similar to those previously employed (Schwartz and Lee, 1962), exhibited heart mitochondria which also showed an aberration in oxidative phosphorylation similar to

TABLE IV

QUANTITATIVE EVALUATION OF OXIDATIVE PHOSPHORYLATION IN GUINEA PIGS BY USE OF DIFFERENT ISOLATION MEDIA[a]

	Control			Experimental		
Medium	RCI	ADP:O	QO_2	RCI	ADP:O	QO_2
STE	5.0 ± 0.6	2.9 ± 0.1	141 ± 19	2.0 ± 0.3	2.2 ± 0.1	50 ± 5
KE	15.6 ± 1.3	3.1 ± 0.3	105 ± 9	4.9 ± 1.6	2.7 ± 0.1	67 ± 5
KEA	18.5	2.9	205	5.6	2.8	96
CE	5.9	3.0	154	3.7	3.0	131
NP	6.3	3.0	127	4.8	2.6	57

[a] Control refers to normal cardiac mitochondria. Experimental refers to mitochondria isolated from guinea pig hearts in congestive failure. The mitochondria were assayed at 30°C with glutamate as substrate. Values are means ($\pm$SE) of 5 experiments (STE) or 4 experiments (KE) or the average of 2 experiments (KEA, CE, NP). STE = 0.25 *M* sucrose, 10 m*M* tris, 1 m*M* EDTA; KE = 0.18 *M* KCl, 10 m*M*, EDTA; KEA = 0.18 *M* KCl, 10 m*M* EDTA, 0.5% albumin; CE = 0.18 *M* choline Cl, 10 m*M* EDTA; NP = Nagarse-containing medium. RCI = respiratory control index; QO_2 = nanoatoms O_2/min/mg mitochondrial protein. An experiment at room temperature (about 23°C) in KE medium gave results similar to the above.

those described (Fig. 6). Furthermore, even under conditions which yielded mitochondria with extremely high respiratory control, the defect was still observable (Table IV). Acute hypoxia could not be the cause of the defect, since experiments were carried out using both guinea pigs and rats wherein the heart was failed (acutely) by installation of nitrogen. Mitochondria, which were normally functioning, could still be isolated. These experiments indicate quite clearly that defective mitochondria can be isolated from animals in severe congestive heart failure. However, it is probable that the defect is either due to or associated with the failing process rather than the cause of the muscle failure. We have come to this conclusion by the use of an intriguing new model for the study of experimental heart failure.

THE ROLE OF MITOCHONDRIA IN HYPERTROPHY AND FAILURE IN THE CARDIOMYOPATHIC SYRIAN HAMSTER

The Syrian hamster, strain BIO 14.6, shows 100% incidence of a primary cardiomyopathy. This is obviously a genetically transmitted or conditioned degenerative process that always terminates in congestive heart failure. The

TABLE V

OXIDATIVE PHOSPHORYLATION AND Ca^{2+} UPTAKE OF HAMSTER HEART MITOCHONDRIA

Substrate	RCI		ADP:O		QO_2		Ca^{2+} Uptake	
	C	E	C	E	C	E	C	E
Glutamate	8.5± 0.8	4.3± 0.4	2.92± 0.07	3.04± 0.25	0.125± 0.012	0.092± 0.018		
Succinate	2.5± 0.5	2.4± 0.2	2.06± 0.16	1.91± 0.19	0.118± 0.017	0.093± 0.010	419± 17	348± 17

The mitochondria were isolated and assayed as described in Materials and Methods. Each value is the mean of 6 experiments (glutamate), 5 experiments (succinate), and 4 experiments (Ca^{2+} uptake) with the standard error of the mean. C is control hamster heart mitochondria; E is mitochondria from Syrian hamster hearts in congestive failure. RCI, respiratory control index; QO_2, oxygen consumption is μatoms/mg protein/min; Ca^{2+} uptake, nanomoles/mg protein/30 min; temp., 37°C.

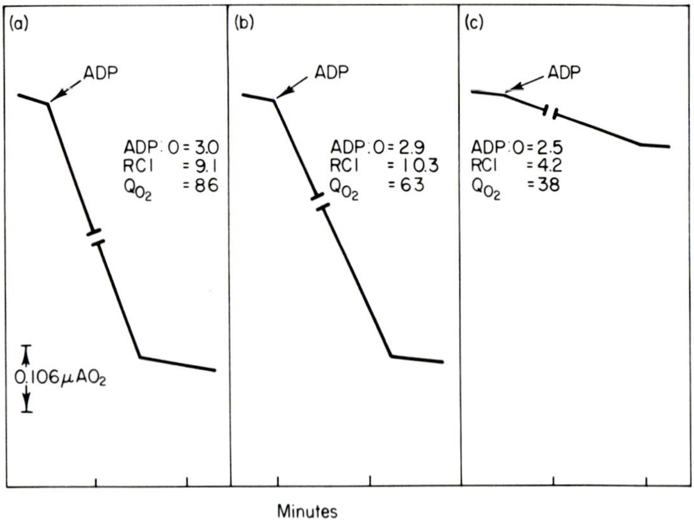

FIG. 7. Cardiomyopathic Syrian hamster. (a) Control; (b) early failure stage; (c) late failure stage (several).

animal offers a rather unique opportunity to study the sequence of events leading to cardiac insufficiency and to assay both the biochemistry and the morphology associated with the process of hypertrophy and failure (Bajusz *et al.*, 1969). In hamsters exhibiting severe congestive heart failure, quite

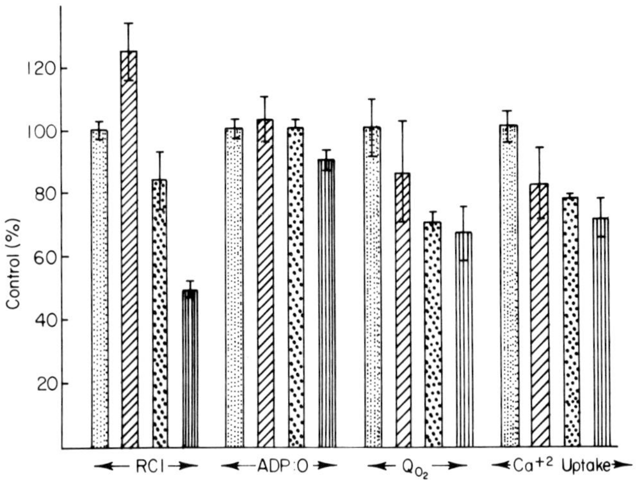

FIG. 8. Cardiomyopathic Syrian hamster. Bars filled with small dots represent the control group; cross-hatched, early failure stage; large dots, late failure stage (moderate); and vertically striped, late failure stage (severe).

similar to that found in the guinea pig and in the human, again a mitochondrial defect, similar to that described above, was found (Schwartz *et al.*, 1968). Associated with the aberration, a defect in calcium transport was also found. Table V summarizes the changes observed. We have recently undertaken a series of experiments employing much younger Syrian hamsters

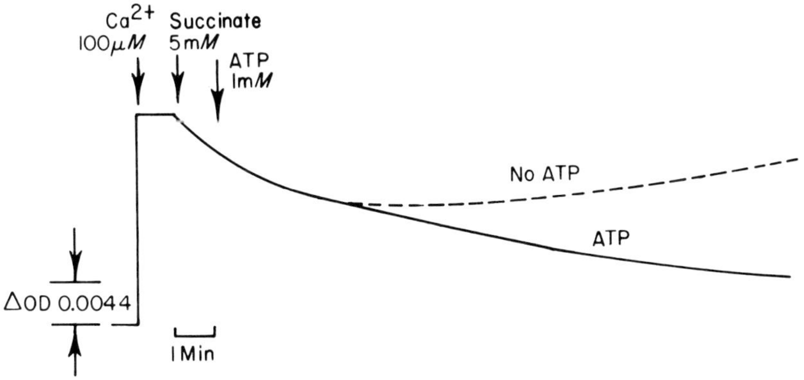

FIG. 9. Ca^{2+} uptake by rabbit cardiac mitochondria measured by dual-beam spectrophotometry. The reaction mixture consisted of 100 m*M* KCl, 10 m*M* $MgCl_2$, 20 m*M* tris-maleate buffer (pH 6.8), 4 m*M* inorganic phosphate, 0.3 m*M* murexide and 1 mg/ml mitochondrial protein. Ca^{2+}, succinate, and ATP were added as indicated by the arrows. The dotted line is the reaction in absence of ATP; the solid line in presence of ATP. The reaction was carried out at room temperature (about 23°C).

exhibiting cardiac hypertrophy, but not demonstrable peripheral congestive heart failure. We have found that the mitochondrial defect is associated with the *severity* of the failing process. In fact, in the early stage of failure, there is little or no change in mitochondrial oxidative phosphorylation, although calcium transport does appear to be diminished. Moreover, in the very early stage of hypertrophy, without demonstrable heart failure, there is a significant, but small, *increase* in respiratory control (Figs. 7 and 8) (Lindenmayer *et al.*, 1970). Notice, however, that even though respiratory control is normal or above normal, calcium transport is still diminished. Therefore, it seems possible that ion transport, particularly calcium, may be an early defect in the hypertrophied and failing process. Assuming that mitochondrial calcium transport is involved in cardiac muscle relaxation, as has been suggested by

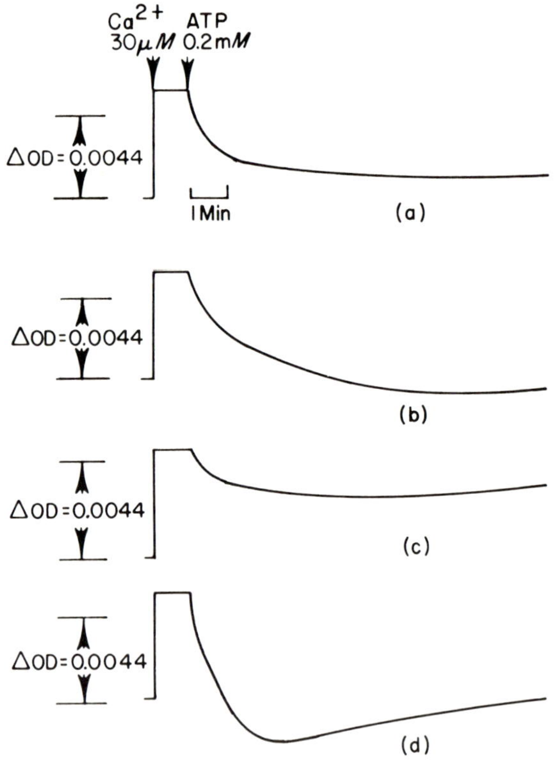

FIG. 10. Human heart. Dual-wave length spectrophotometric recordings [different protein concentrations (mg/ml)]. Ca^{2+} binding by human cardiac relaxing system measured by dual-beam spectrophotometry. Each experiment was carried out with a preparation obtained from a different heart. Membrane protein concentrations in mg/ml, respectively, = a, 1.0; b, 1.3; c, 0.5; d, 1.0. (See Harigaya and Schwartz, 1969.)

Chance (1965), some years ago, and by our own very recent data employing a very sensitive dual-beam spectrophotometric recording system (Fig. 9), the importance of the present findings may be twofold. (1) Calcium is accumulated and released by mitochondria by an energy-dependent process. Our recent results suggest that the partial mechanism for relaxation, perhaps calcium accumulation, may be impaired. Furthermore, the reactions required for contraction, that is calcium release, may also be altered. Since our kinetic measurements indicate the rapidity of both uptake and release of calcium by normal mitochondria, and since mitochondria are in abundance in the cardiac muscle cell, this finding may have relevance to the failing process. (2) It is well known that calcium can uncouple oxidative phosphorylation (Lehninger, 1949). If the system primarily responsible for relaxation in cardiac muscle failure, namely the sarcoplasmic reticulum is defective, mitochondria might be exposed to higher calcium concentrations, which could lead to impairment of oxidative phosphorylation causing a further increase in the severity of cardiac failure.

Studies in Human Heart

Fresh human tissue was obtained at the time of transplantation as indicated in the Methods section. Mitochondria derived from sections which were in severe failure, as ascertained by the pathologist, always exhibited an aberration similar to those observed in the experimental situation. However, mitochondria isolated from normal areas of the hearts were found to be normal with respect to oxygen consumption and respiratory control, as well as calcium transport. In four cases, we examined mitochondria derived from nonfailing hypertrophied human heart tissue (idiopathic subaortic stenosis). In all cases, the mitochondria exhibited extremely high "super normal" respiratory control indices and very high oxygen consumption rates. These results are consistent with the findings in the nonfailing cardiomyopathic Syrian hamster, as described above.

It may be of interest to the audience, that the only demonstrable and reproducible biochemical defect thus far found in the failing hearts was in the so-called relaxing system. A slower rate of uptake and release was always found (Fig. 10).

Addendum

In chronically overloaded and hypertrophied myocardium, which occurred in advance of *overt* circulatory failure in dogs, Wollenberger and his colleagues found both ultrastructural and enzymatic evidence of a mitochondrial defect (Wollenberger *et al.*, 1963).

Isoproterenol-Induced Cardiac Hypertrophy

It is now established that certain catecholamines, particularly isoproterenol, not only produce a striking growth of salivary glands (which include both hyperplasis and hypertrophy), but also induces hypertrophy of heart muscle (Zbinden and Moe, 1969; Schwartz and Matsui, 1967). Low doses of isoproterenol (5 mg or less/kg) usually produce a demonstrable heart hypertrophy without visual signs of necrosis. Higher doses, however (usually around 50–80 mg/kg), produce very definite areas of myocardial necrosis. Accordingly, this drug is useful for studying not only the process of cardiac hypertrophy, but also to evaluate potential antianginal drugs.

Employing high doses of isoproterenol, we have found, associated with the marked hypertrophy and necrosis of the heart, a significant diminution of respiratory control in mitochondria (Stanton and Schwartz, 1967).

Lower doses of isoproterenol (5 mg/kg or lower administered for a few days to rats) produces a definite increase in heart weight, protein synthesis and nucleic acid concentrations (based on mg/gm weight) (Stanton *et al.*, 1969).

Using still lower doses of isoproterenol and even prior to the hypertrophic event, we have recently found significant changes in the RNA pattern of both the nuclear and cytoplasmic fractions of heart muscle. This is exhibited in Figs. 11–13. Further studies are presently being carried out. Tentatively, it is attractive to assume that isoproterenol causes its dramatic results by a derepression of the genome.

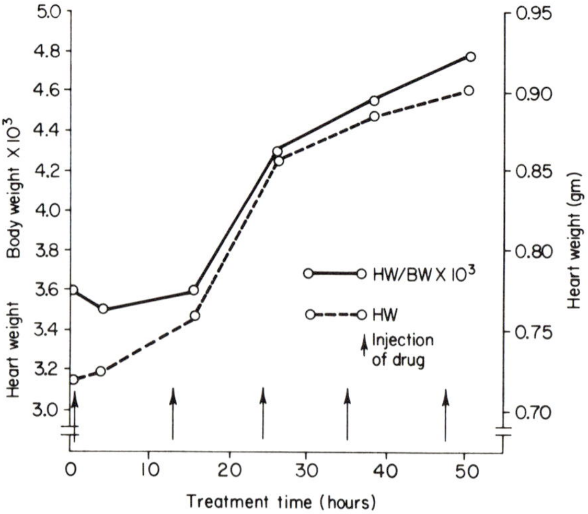

Fig. 11.

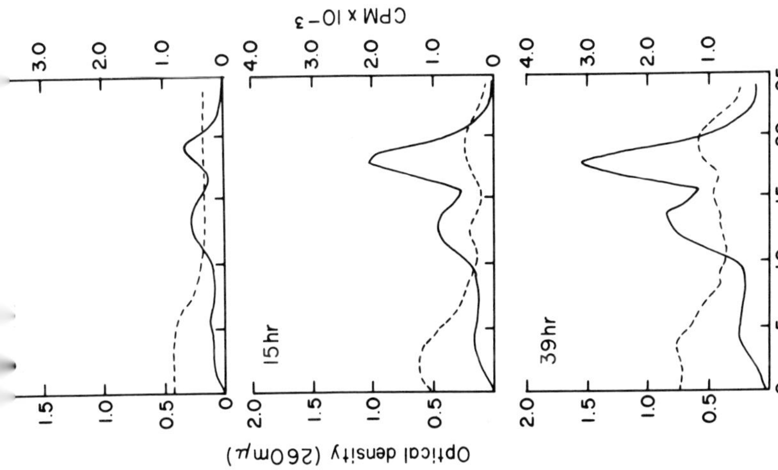

FIG. 12. "Nuclear" RNA.

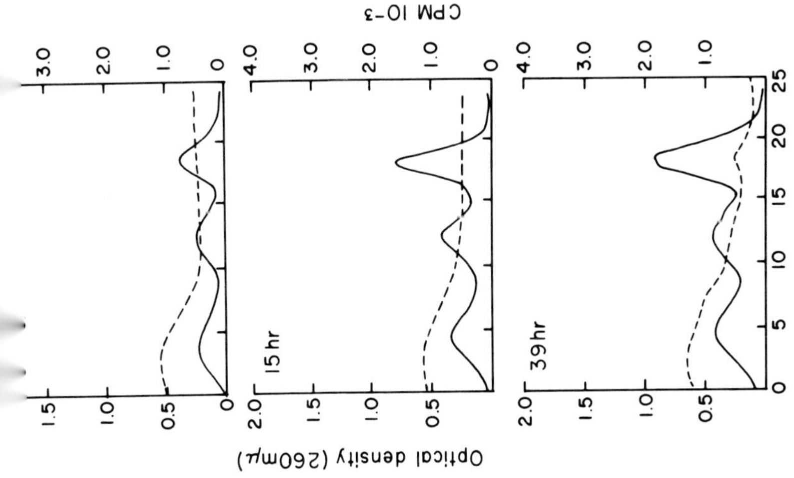

FIG. 13. Cytoplasmic RNA.

Possible Preventative Aspects

We have recently been carrying out a series of preliminary experiments designed to determine appropriate conditions for the maintenance of energy producing mechanisms in human and animal heart. We have now carried out studies on five normal human hearts, removed from young individuals who were in accidents involving cerebral tissue. The heart and lungs were removed intact and placed in a Portable Preservation Chamber, which is designed to perfuse the hearts normally with blood, and the lungs with mix-

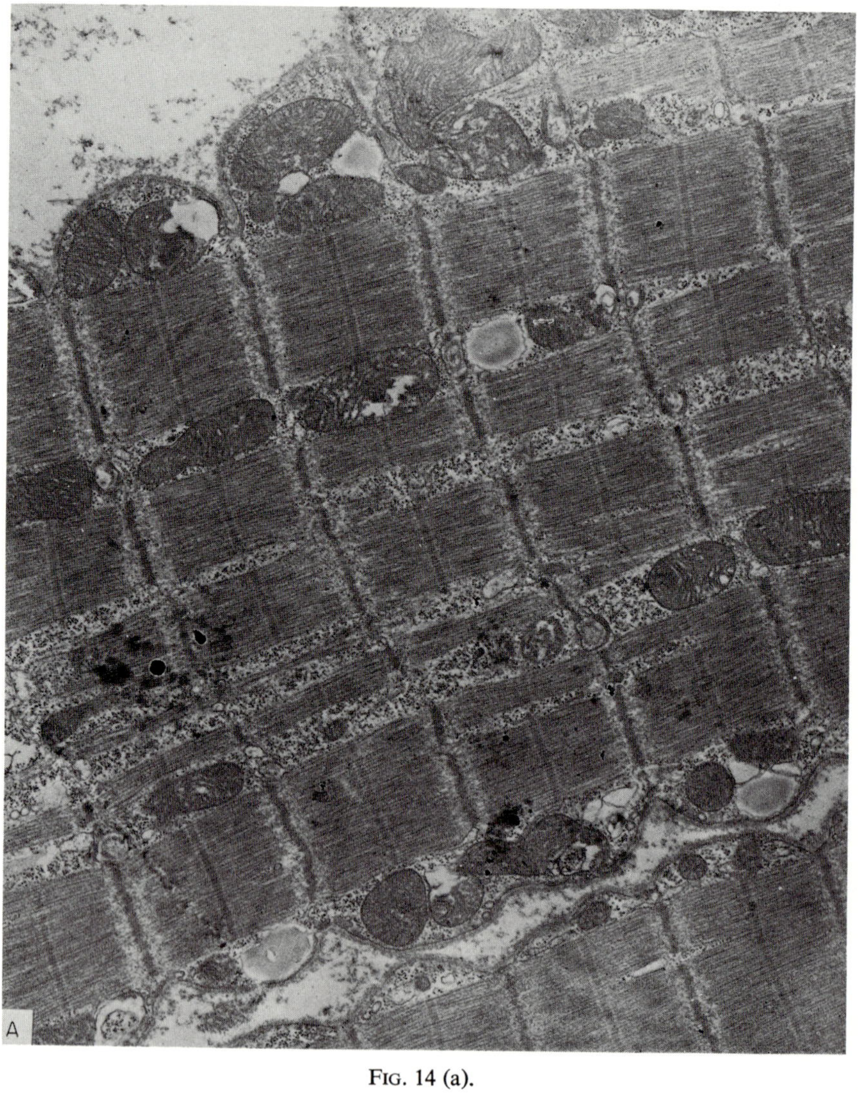

Fig. 14 (a).

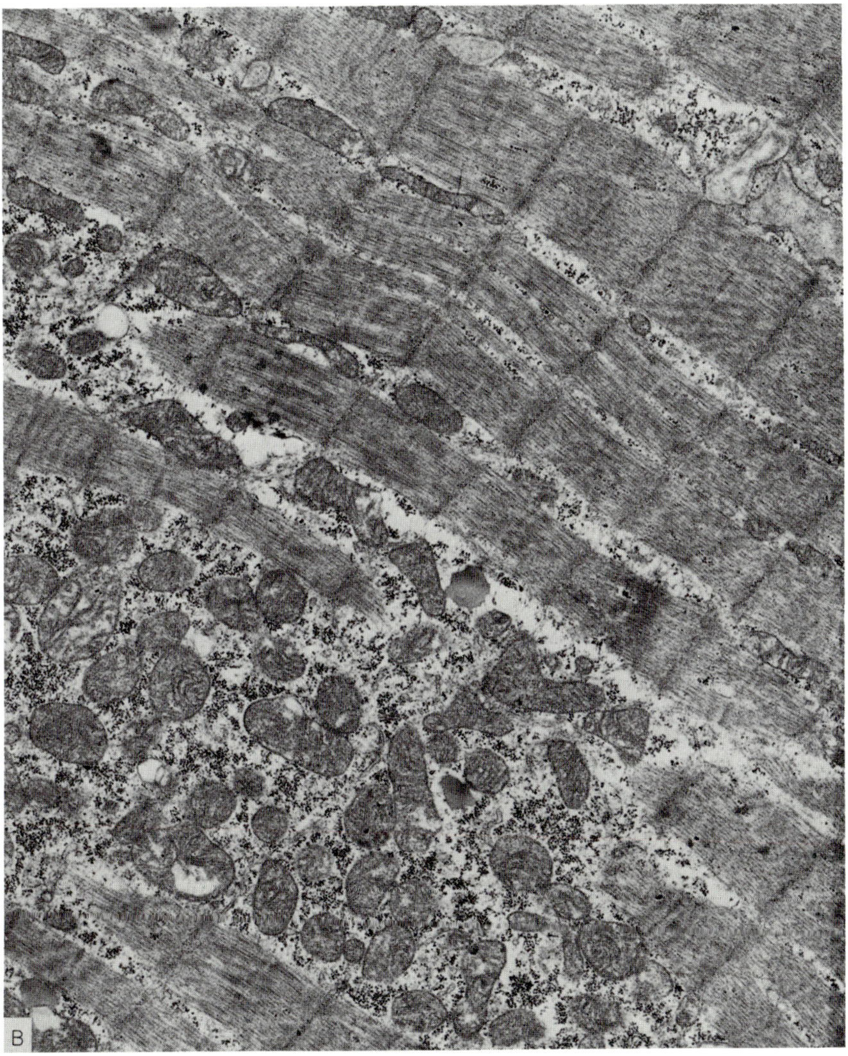

FIG. 14 (b).

tures of gases. The hearts were generally allowed to function for up to 36–48 hr, with physiological measurements being taken from time to time. In addition, periodically, small amounts of insulin and potassium were added to the perfusing fluid with the hope of maintaining appropriate membrane "permeability." At the termination of the experiment, the entire heart was processed for mitochondria. The resulting organelles exhibited extremely high respiratory control ratios, and very adequate oxygen consumption. More strikingly, however, these mitochondria maintained their function *in vitro* for up to one week. We have never observed this phenomenon in either human hearts, unperfused or hearts from a variety of animal species. We are now duplicating these experiments, omitting insulin and using dog hearts and have found, in preliminary experiments, that mitochondria do not exhibit these remarkable preservation characteristics. Electron micrographs of sections of the intact preserved human heart are included with this manuscript (Fig. 14); sample oxygraph tracings of animal and human mitochondria are also shown [Figs. 15(a), (b), and (c)]. We are presently employing a multi-parameter ion transport device which directly records, on one mitochondrial

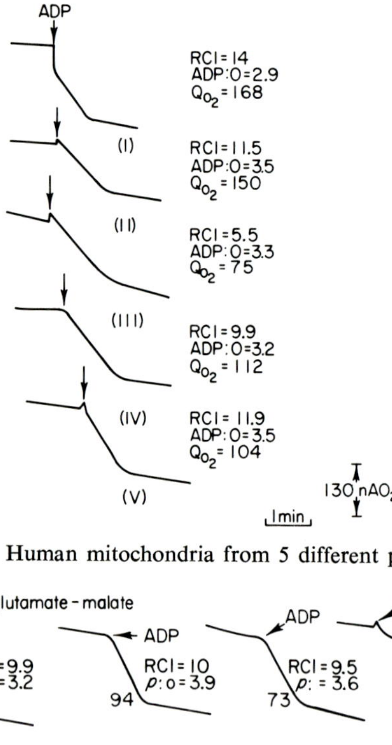

FIG. 15 (a). Human mitochondria from 5 different preparations.

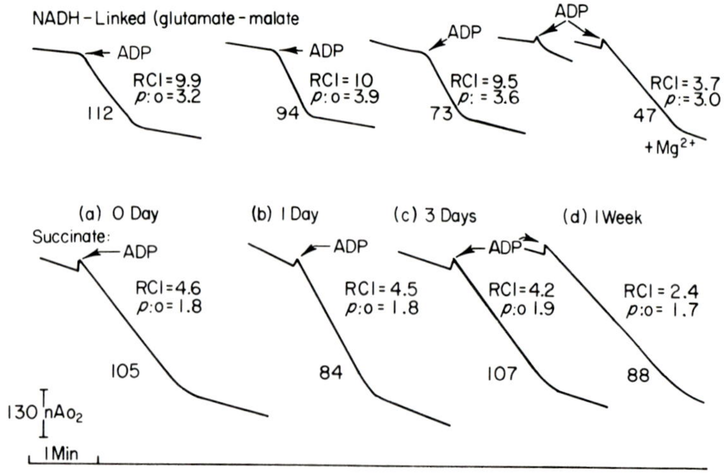

FIG. 15 (b). Human mitochondria (stored at 0°C). Note that addition of $MgCl_2$ restored function after prolonged storage.

sample, the following variables: light scattering ("swelling and contraction"), oxygen consumption, pyridine nucleotide, oxidation and reduction, potassium, sodium and hydrogen transport. Sample tracings of such events as influenced

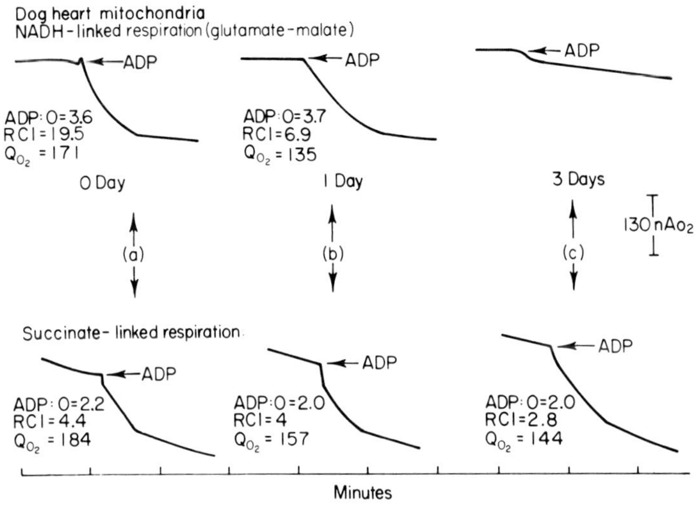

FIG. 15 (c). Dog mitochondria (stored at 0°C).

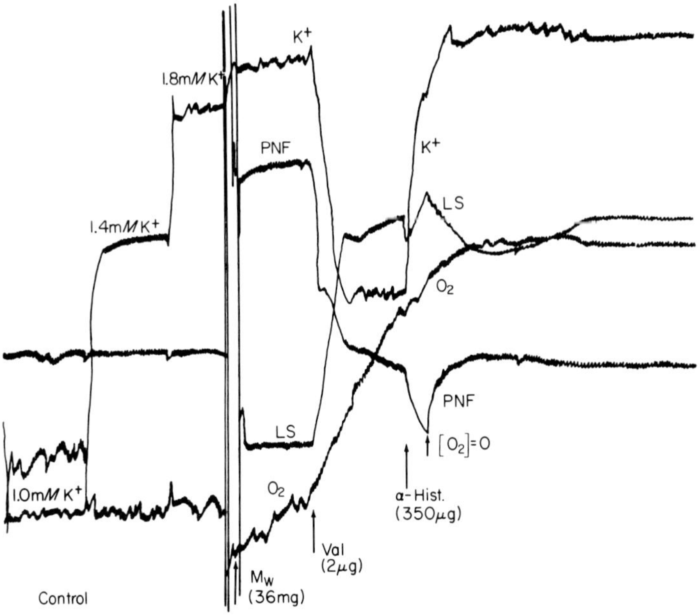

FIG. 16 (a). Use of the multiparameter ion transport device first introduced by Dr. B. C. Pressman (U. of Miami). (Appreciation is extended to Dr. Pressman for his generous advice and instruction.)

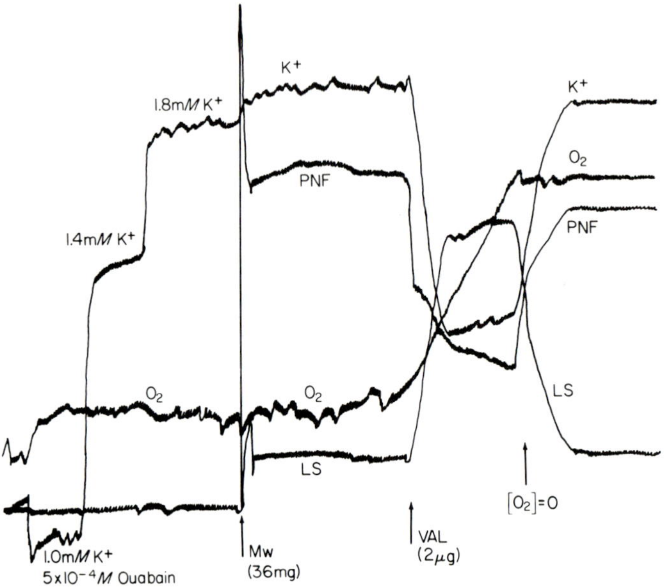

FIG. 16(a), (b). Use of the multiparameter ion transport device. Valinomycin, ouabain, and histone effects on mitochondria. (PNF) Pyridine nucleotide fluorescence; (LS) light scattering; and (Mw) washed mitochondria.

by an antibiotic and histone are shown in Figs. 16(a) and (b). Note that a cardiac glycoside has no effect.

Discussion

The specific biochemical and pathophysiological mechanisms which induce hypertrophy and subsequent failure are clearly unknown. In the present contribution, we have indicated that the severity of the failing process appears to be accompanied by a mitochondrial defect. However, prior to severe heart failure, mitochondria appeared to be functioning normally with respect to energy production but not with respect to calcium transport. Since our preliminary findings would suggest that the calcium uptake and release system, usually termed "sarcoplasmic reticulum" in skeletal muscle, may be an important factor in congestive heart failure, alterations in intracellular calcium metabolism may be an important future consideration in looking for etiological aspects of the diseased heart. The fact that in some stages of the process of hypertrophy, mitochondria appeared to be functioning "super-normally," at least with respect to the production of ATP, is consistent with the original hypothesis of Meerson (1962) and Meerson *et al.* (1964), who have defined three significant developmental stages in the hypertrophied and failing heart:

1. Transient breakdown stage which is characterized by contractile insufficiency, together with a deficiency of certain enzymes, presumably located in mitochondria.

2. Protracted stage of relatively stable hyperfunction which is characterized by the absence of cardiac insufficiency, by hypertrophy and by adequate or "superadequate" oxidative phosphorylation.

3. Protracted stage of progressing cardiosclerosis and gradual exhaustion of the hypertrophied heart which is characterized by disturbances in protein synthesis and sustained hypoxia.

Stage 3 would be characterized, we feel, by an aberration of mitochondrial function or functions. The second stage defined by Meerson might be characterized by increased protein synthetic activity, and possibly by either an increased number of size of mitochondria, or by an increase in respiratory control of mitochondria, the latter perhaps produced by an alteration of the inner membrane system. We and other investigators have shown a rather complex relationship between the functional state of mitochondria and the ultrastructure of the inner membrane system [Fig. 2(b)]. Can mitochondria grow? As discussed extensively in the introduction, the entire apparatus for protein synthesis is indeed present in mitochondria. Protein synthesis has, in fact, been shown to occur in mitochondria. There are a number of interesting recent studies which indirectly bear on this possible phenomenon. Gollnick and King (1969) have found that mitochondria were more numerous and appeared to be larger with more densely packed cristae in skeletal muscle derived from rats which were exercised exhaustively. These investigators suggested that the metabolic capacity of rat skeletal tissue can be enhanced by training. Prior to this work, Holloszy (1967) found that mitochondria derived from skeletal muscle of rats subjected to a strenuous program of treadmill running, exhibited a higher level of respiratory control and more tightly coupled oxidative phosphorylation than control tissues. This adaptation could partially account for the increase in aerobic work capacity that occurred with regularly performed, prolonged exercise. Furthermore, the following enzymes were increased approximately twofold in the hind limb muscles of exercised rats: succinate dehydrogenase, reduced DPN–cytochrome c reductase, succinate oxidase, and cytochrome oxidase. Furthermore, the *concentration* of cytochrome c was also increased twofold, suggesting that the rise in respiratory enzyme activity was, in fact, a result of the actual increase in enzyme protein production. In fact, the total protein content of the mitochondrial fraction increased approximately 60%. These results would be consistent with the capacity for mitochondria to synthesize mitochondrial proteins when required. It is entirely possible that the growing heart, either in health or disease, could also be characterized by an increased mitochondrial protein synthesis. The mechanism for the derepression of the mitochondrial genome is, of course, unknown, but it is attractive to speculate on the possibility of hormonal control (thyroxine, growth hormone, etc.). Similar results from those reported above were also found in mitochondria derived from heart muscle of rats subjected to exercise. The hearts were also hypertrophied by this process (Arcos *et al.*, 1968). These investigators presented both biochemical and ultastructural evidence of an increase in the number of mitochondria in the hypertrophied, but non-failing cardiac muscle.

It is of interest also to mention that other compensatory changes occur in enzymes not associated with mitochondria in experimental cardiac hypertrophy. For example, Valadares *et al.* (1969) found that 6 days after aortic coarctation in rats, myocardial glucose-6-phosphate dehydrogenase was increased 200% over the control values expressed either per gram wet weight or per organ itself. Administration of cycloheximide resulted in a significant inhibition of the increase in cardiac glucose-6-phosphate dehydrogenase after constriction. These authors concluded that "it is conceivable that the augmentation in the activity of this enzyme may be related to the increases in RNA and protein synthesis observed during development of cardiac hypertrophy." It is natural that during the hypertrophic process, both RNA and protein synthesis should be increased. This, of course, has been found by a number of investigators. Consequently, an important enzyme in this process should also be increased, namely glucose-6-phosphate dehydrogenase. However, for increased protein synthesis and RNA synthesis to occur, energy is also needed in the form of ATP. Increased protein synthesis in mitochondria and increased respiratory control of these organelles could conceivably supply the increased demand for energy.

References

Arcos, J. C., Sohal, R. S., Sun, S. C., Argus, M. F., and Burch, G. E. (1968). *Exp. Mol. Pathol.* **8,** 49.

Bajusz, E., Baker, J. R., Nixon, C. W., and Homburger, F. (1969). *Ann. N.Y. Acad. Sci.* **156,** 105.

Bresnick, E., and Schwartz, A. (1968). *In* "Functional Dynamics in Cell," pp. 97–163. Academic Press, New York.

Chance, B. (1965). *J. Biol. Chem.* **240,** 2729.

Gollnick, P. D., and King, D. W. (1969). *Amer. J. Physiol.* **216,** 1502.

Holloszy, J. O. (1967). *J. Biol. Chem.* **242,** 2278.

Johnson, C. L., and Schwartz, A. (1969). *J. Pharmacol. Exp. Ther.* **167,** 365.

Johnson, C. L., Oro, J., and Schwartz, A. (1969). *Arch. Biochem. Biophys.* **131,** 310.

Lehninger, A. L. (1949). *J. Biol. Chem.* **178,** 625.

Lehninger, A. L. (1964). "The Mitochondrion." Benjamin, New York.

Lindenmayer, G. E., Sordahl, L. A., and Schwartz, A. (1968). *Circ. Res.* **23,** 439.
Lindenmayer, G. E., Harigaya, S., Bajusz, E., and Schwartz, A. (1970). *Mol. Cell. Cardiol.* **1,** 249–259 (1970).
Meerson, F. Z. (1962). *Circ. Res.* **10,** 250.
Meerson, F. Z., Zaletayeva, T. A., Lagutchev, S. S. and Pshennikova, M. G. (1964). *Exp. Cell Res.* **36,** 568.
Nass, M. M. K. (1969). *Science* **165,** 25.
Procita, L., Schwartz, A. and Lee, K. S. (1965). *Circ. Res.* **16,** 391.
Safer, B., and Schwartz, A. (1967). *Circ. Res.* **21,** 25.
Schwartz, A., and Lee, K. S. (1962). *Circ. Res.* **10,** 321.
Schwartz, A., and Matsui, H. (1967). *In* "Secretory Mechanisms of Salivary Glands," (Leon, H. Schneyer and Charlotte A. Schneyer, eds.). Academic Press, New York.
Schwartz, A., Laseter, A. H. and Ferguson, G. G. (1965). *Circ. Res.* **17,** 555.
Schwartz, A., Johnson, C. L., and Safer, B. (1966). *Life Sci.* **5,** 2143.
Schwartz, A., Lindenmayer, G. E., and Harigaya, S. (1968). *Trans. N.Y. Acad. Sci.* **30,** 951.
Slater, E. C., Tager, J. M., Papa, S. Quagliariello, E., eds. (1968). "Round Table Discussion on Biochemical Aspects of the Biogenesis of Mitochondria." Published in *Bari* by Adriatica Editrice.
Sobel, B. E., Spann, J. F., Pool, P. E., Sonnenblick, E. H., and Braunwald, E. (1967). *Circ. Res.* **21,** 355.
Stanton, H. C. and Schwartz A., (1967). *J. Pharmacol. Exp. Ther.* 157, 649.
Stanton, H. C., Brenner, G., and Mayfield, E. D. (1969). *Amer. Heart J.* **77,** 72.
Valadares, J. R. E., Singhal, R. L., Parulekar, M. R., and Beznak, M. (1969). *Can. J. Physiol. Pharmacol.* **47,** 388.
Wagner, R. P. (1969). *Science* **163,** 1026.
Wollenberger, A. Kleitke, B., and Raabe, G. (1963). *Exp. Mol. Pathol.* **2,** 251.
Zbinden, G., and Moe, R. A. (1969). *Ann. N.Y. Acad. Sci.* **156,** 294.

ENERGY STORES AND ENERGY UTILIZATION IN THE MYOCARDIUM IN HYPERTROPHY AND HEART FAILURE

Peter E. Pool

It is commonly agreed that heart failure may be defined as failure of the heart to meet the demands of the circulation. Since we know that the state of myocardial hypertrophy and heart failure is associated with a depression of the mechanical function of the myocardium, we must also seek to explain the underlying cause of this deficient mechanical function. Ultimately, a biochemical lesion must be sought; the purpose of this presentation is to briefly review those investigations which have involved energy stores and energy utilization in the hypertrophied and failing myocardium in an attempt to determine whether or not a biochemical defect in these processes could be a causal factor in the development of heart failure in the hypertrophied heart.

In order to adequately delineate the alterations in energy metabolism which take place during hypertrophy (and with the onset of heart failure), it would be necessary to study these processes in the presence of the various types of experimental heart failure such as pressure overload and flow overload and at various stages of heart failure. Although a complete delineation of this spectrum is not available at the present time, it is possible from currently available information to determine whether or not certain aspects of energy metabolism are causally involved in the genesis of heart failure. It is interesting that a defect in energy metabolism is not commonly implicated in the process of hypertrophy, since heart failure is thought by many to be a continuation of the process of hypertrophy. At some point, however, it seems obvious that whether it is composed of normal muscle or of muscle qualitatively inferior to that normally present in the myocardium, the hypertrophied myocardium must be inadequate to provide for the increased demands of the circulation. At this point, some process must have failed, or at least ceased to expand so that heart failure ensued.

The process of energy production has been discussed at some length in this volume. Basically, this process involves the uptake of substrates from the coronary capillary blood in the form of carbohydrates, fats, and proteins, and their oxidation to three- and four-carbon fragments which enter the Krebs cycle. During oxidation in the Krebs cycle, electrons are passed to oxygen via coenzymes and cytochromes, and this flow of electrons is coupled with the phosphorylation of ADP. Defects in these processes are no longer felt to be causally involved in the onset of congestive heart failure (Chidsey *et al.*, 1966; Sobel *et al.*, 1967; Lindenmayer *et al.*, 1968). Very severe heart failure, however, has occasionally been associated with abnormalities in the process of oxidative phosphorylation, e.g., Lindenmayer *et al.*, (1968).

The results of the process of energy production are the cellular stores of ATP which represent the immediate source of energy for cellular work. ATP is in equilibrium with a larger store of energy in the form of creatine phosphate, the result of the transfer of a high-energy phosphate bond from ATP to creatine in a reaction catalyzed by creatine phosphokinase. However, creatine phosphate is not capable of directly supplying energy necessary for muscle contraction.

Early studies of myocardial energy stores in heart failure indicated that a deficiency of these stores could be responsible for the heart-failure state. Some of these conclusions were derived from studies of acute experimental heart failure produced by hypoxia or ischemia, and it was reasoned by analogy that in the hypertrophied heart there might exist a state of relative hypoxia leading to a depressed store of energy insufficient for the maintenance of normal contractile force.

In some other studies, chronic severe hypertrophy and heart failure have been associated with diminished high-energy phosphate stores, e.g., Fleckenstein *et al.* (1959); Minton *et al.* (1960). However, it was not possible in any of these studies to determine whether or not these diminished stores had a causal role in the heart-failure state. In order to delineate this problem, Chidsey *et al.* (1966) examined high-energy phosphate stores in samples of myocardium taken from 14 patients with heart failure in whom replacement of the mitral or aortic valve, or both, was performed. In all of these patients, rheumatic heart disease was responsible for the valvular deformity and all were on maintenance doses of digoxin. The types of valvular lesion included aortic stenosis, aortic insufficiency, mitral stenosis, mitral insufficiency, and a combination of these.

Biopsy material was derived from left ventricular papillary muscles which were removed during the routine course of operation. For comparison, biopsies were also taken at the time of operation from eight patients without previous history of heart failure who were undergoing repair of septal defects or pulmonic stenosis. These biopsies were obtained from the right ventricle, and in all cases right ventricular hypertrophy was present.

Creatine phosphate concentrations assessed in the biopsies obtained from patients with heart failure and those with hypertrophy alone were similar averaging 3.9 ± 0.5 and 4.0 ± 0.9 μmoles/gm, respectively. ATP concentrations were also similar averaging 3.6 ± 0.6 μmoles/gm in biopsies from patients patients without heart failure, and 3.2 ± 0.5 μmoles/gm in those from patients with heart failure.

Whereas in some ways the availability of human tissue provided an optimum opportunity to examine the effects of heart failure under conditions in which the results would be most relevant to human biology, there were several limitations to this type of study. All patients were on cardiopulmonary bypass at the time of biopsy, although the period of bypass was brief. In addition, it was necessary to compare biopsies obtained from the contralateral ventricles of patients with and without heart failure.

In other studies, in which experimental chronic heart failure was induced in dogs and guinea pigs, this state was found to be associated with modest depressions of myocardial CP stores (Fox *et al.*, 1965; Feinstein, 1962). It has been shown that the mechanical function of guinea pig hearts subjected to acute asphyxia could recover at a time when high-energy phosphate stores were still depressed (Feinstein, 1962). It has also been shown that acute hypoxic and ischemic heart failure may be produced in dogs at a time when no reductions of high-energy phosphate compounds have occurred (Pool *et al.*, 1966; Covell *et al.*, 1967).

These data all indicated that reductions in myocardial energy stores were probably not involved in the onset of heart failure. To test this hypothesis, experiments were designed in which heart failure was produced and in which the effects on the myocardium could be carefully documented both from observations *in vivo* and from the mechanical behavior of samples of myocardium isolated *in vitro*. Myocardial energy stores could then be correlated with the mechanical performance of the myocardium itself, rather than with its effects on the peripheral circulation.

In this investigation, right ventricular hypertrophy or right ventricular hypertrophy with heart failure was produced in cats by a graded constriction of the pulmonary artery 3 weeks to 3 months prior to the time of study (Pool *et al.*, 1967). Just prior to sacrifice, all animals were anesthetized, their chests were opened, and biopsies of the right ventricle were obtained using a rapid freezing technique to preserve high-energy phosphates.

The energy stores found in these samples are shown in Fig. 1. In specimens of right ventricle obtained from cats with heart failure, concentrations of ATP and inorganic phosphate did not differ significantly from those found in right ventricular tissue obtained from normal animals or animals with right ventricular hypertrophy. On the other hand, concentrations of both total creatine and creatine phosphate were significantly reduced. Total creatine

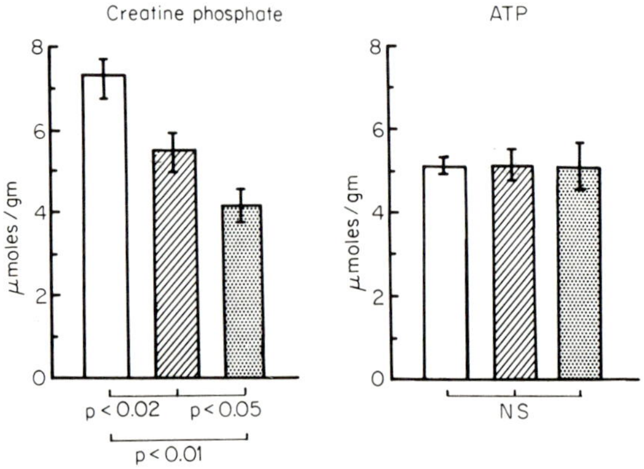

FIG. 1. *In vivo* right ventricular high-energy phosphate stores in normal cats and in cats with right ventricular hypertrophy (RVH) and congestive heart failure (CHF). Open bar represents control group (17); striped bar, RVH (10); dotted bar, CHF (8).

averaged 15.5 ± 0.6, 12.5 ± 0.9, and 9.7 ± 0.6 μmoles/gm, respectively in the normal, hypertrophied, and failing groups, whereas creatine phosphate averaged 7.2 ± 0.5, 5.4 ± 0.5, and 4.2 ± 0.4 μmoles/gm in these three groups. Since both total creatine and creatine phosphate were proportionately reduced in the hypertrophied and failing groups, the fraction of total creatine present as creatine phosphate was similar, averaging 46 %, 43 %, and 43 %, respectively, in the three groups.

Since the hemodynamic stress on the *in situ* heart may have been different in the three conditions studied and because of alterations in circulatory dynamics which may have been produced by the thoracotomy, energy stores were also investigated in papillary muscles isolated from these hearts, all of which were contracting under similar conditions *in vitro*.

The changes produced in the myocardium by the induction of ventricular overload leading to heart failure were evident in the mechanical performance of the papillary muscles isolated from these hearts. Peak isometric tension development at the top of the length-active tension curve in muscles from normal animals averaged 5.2 gm/mm^2, whereas the tension in muscles from animals with heart failure averaged 1.1 gm/mm^2. After contracting for 30 min at the top of their length-active tension curves at a frequency of 12/min, muscles from all three groups were rapidly frozen and their high-energy phosphate stores determined in order to evaluate the relationship of these stores to the mechanical performance of the muscles.

In all three groups of muscles, ATP and creatine phosphate concentrations were found to be similar. This indicated that muscles derived from the animals with heart failure had the ability to increase their high-energy phosphate stores when isolated *in vitro* and exposed to lesser rates of work performance than the *in vitro* condition. In addition, it indicated that the depressed mechanical performance of muscles derived from animals with hypertrophy and heart failure could not be attributed to depressions in total high-energy phosphate stores. Of course, the possibility remains that the depletion of a discrete compartment of high-energy phosphate stores could have occurred in the animals with heart failure and that this specific depletion might not have been detected in the presence of a large store of high-energy phosphate compounds from other compartments within the myocardium.

Because the failing myocardium had a slightly depressed creatine phosphate store that could be replenished in part following isolation of muscle samples *in vitro*, the possibility existed that there was an imbalance between energy production and energy demand in heart failure. This imbalance could have resulted from several possible derangements.

One of these possibilities would be that energy production was not adequate to meet the demands of energy utilization. Studies cited above have shown that energy production in the presence of heart failure remains at normal levels at least until very severe heart failure occurs. Thus, this possibility seemed unlikely. On the other hand, increased energy utilization could also appear as an imbalance between energy production and energy utilization. This could result from the failing heart performing more work per minute than the normal heart. This possibility also seemed unlikely because the myocardium in heart failure is capable of less tension development than the normal myocardium. Nonetheless, *in vivo*, the failing myocardium works at a relatively higher position on its length-active tension curve than does the normal heart, and thus the normal heart seldom works to full capacity while the failing heart works close to full capacity. This difference, in addition to derangements in circulatory status that might lead to inadequate oxygenation of the hypertrophied and failing heart, could lead to the disparities noted above.

A major possibility that remained, however, was that energy utilization in the heart failure state could be an inefficient process so that greater amounts of energy would be required to perform a given amount of work. This could occur if the contractile proteins were an inefficient transducer. Although abnormalities of energy utilization attributable to abnormalities of the contractile proteins have been considered for some time (Olson, 1964), only indirect measurements of the process of energy utilization have been available.

In order to approach this problem directly and to answer the question of whether or not an inefficient process of energy conversion might be involved in the heart failure state, we directly measured the utilization of ATP and creatine phosphate in the right ventricular papillary muscle of the cat under conditions in which no energy production could occur. This was accomplished by inhibiting ATP synthesis by blockade of both oxidative phosphorylation and anaerobic glycolysis, and by subsequently determining the utilization of energy stores at rest and during activity. Since energy production was inhibited, it was possible to determine efficiency in terms of the amount of energy utilized to perform a given amount of work. Muscles were stimulated to contract, and both the amount of work performed and the diminution of high-energy phosphate stores which resulted were measured (Pool *et al.*, 1969).

In these studies right ventricular hypertrophy and right ventricular hypertrophy with failure was produced by graded stenosis of the pulmonary artery in cats. These animals were sacrificed between 3 weeks and 1 month postoperative, considerably earlier than for the animals in the previous study.

Right ventricular papillary muscles were isolated in Krebs solution *in vitro* and isometric tension was determined at the top of the length-active tension curve. Depressions in maximum tension development were noted in those muscles from animals with heart failure and were similar in extent to those found in the previous study (Pool *et al.*, 1967). Initially, basal energy utilization, the energy utilization of the muscle at rest, was determined in normal muscles and in those from animals with heart failure. This was accomplished by freezing groups of muscles either at the point when energy production had been arrested completely (following treatment with iodoacetic acid and nitrogen) or at subsequent periods of 3, 7, or 10 min. High-energy phosphate stores were assessed in these muscles, and the diminution of these stores with time was used to calculate the basal rate of energy utilization as shown in Fig. 2.

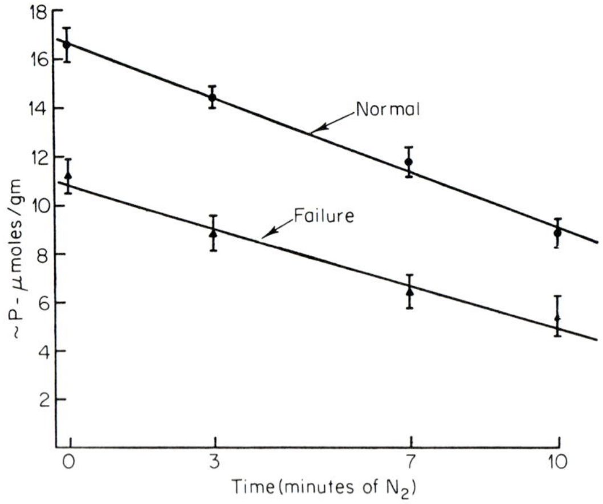

FIG. 2. Resting energy utilization in *in vivo* right ventricular papillary muscles from normal cats and from cats with heart failure as determined by regression analysis. $\sim P =$ sum of creatine phosphate and ATP; $T =$ minutes of nitrogenation. Normal: $\sim P = (16.7 \pm 0.5)–(0.77 \pm 0.07)T$; failure: $\sim P = (10.9 \pm 0.5)–(0.60 \pm 0.09)T$.

When energy production had been inhibited, energy stores in the papillary muscles from animals with heart failure were lower than those from normal animals. These differences could be attributed to the fact that the animals in heart failure were acutely stressed, and in addition, muscles from these animals had undergone treatment with iodoacetic acid, which inhibits glycolysis. These results would be expected if the failing myocardium depended to a greater extent than the normal heart upon glycolytic production of ATP.

In muscles from animals with heart failure, the basal rates of energy utilization, indicated by the progressive fall in energy stores with time, were similar in muscles from normal animals and in those from animals with heart failure. In the normal animals this basal rate of energy utilization was 0.77 ± 0.07 μmoles/gm/min, whereas that in the muscles from animals with heart failure was 0.60 ± 0.09 μmoles/gm/min.

Similar results were obtained in muscles stimulated to contract and perform work. The mechanical function of muscles from cats with heart failure was severely depressed (Table I). Those muscles from animals with heart failure

TABLE I

COMPARATIVE AVERAGE VALUES FOR MUSCLES FROM NORMAL CATS WITH HEART FAILURE

	63 Normal muscles	42 Failure muscles	(Failure/normal) X 100
~P (μmoles/gm)	3.15	0.23	7
No. of contractions	34.4	21.9	64
Contractile element work performed (gm · cm/gm)	312	41	13

produced only 41 gm · cm/gm of work while contracting an average of 21.9 times; however, the normal muscles produced 312 gm · cm/gm of work while contracting an average of 34.4 times. Thus the total work performance of the muscles from animals with heart failure was only 13% as great as that from normal animals and the number of contractions only 64% as many.

It was interesting, however, that the muscles from animals with heart failure, in addition to having depressed mechanical performance, also used substantially less energy than the normal muscles, 0.23 μmoles/gm as compared to 3.15 μmoles/gm of high-energy phosphate compounds. This meant that muscles from animals with heart failure used only 7% as much energy as those from normal animals, and the overall efficiency with which chemical energy was transformed into mechanical work under these conditions was not decreased. These results indicate that the failing heart is able to transform chemical energy into ventricular tension with at least as great efficiency as the normal heart. However, these results do not rule out the possibility that there may be an inefficiency in the conversion of ventricular wall tension to useful external work. Thus, from the available data, there is little evidence to suggest that disturbances in energy metabolism can be implicated as causal factors in the onset of congestive heart failure in the hypertrophied heart. The hypertrophied and failing myocardium has slightly decreased concentrations of creatine phosphate *in vivo*, which may be attributed in part to depressions in total creatine stores. Concentrations of ATP are not significantly changed, but these decreases in creatine phosphate concentrations may reflect some imbalance between energy production and energy demand. However, the fact that similar energy stores are found in papillary muscles from both normal animals and animals with heart failure at a time when their mechanical performance is vastly different indicates that one cannot attribute the depression in myocardial mechanical performance to a deficiency of energy stores. In addition, other studies, such as those of Feinstein (1962), have shown that when myocardial energy stores are depressed by hypoxia, normal mechanical behavior may be restored following reoxygenation of the animal at a time when energy stores remain severely depressed. These findings also make it unlikely that even moderate depressions of energy stores *in vivo* can be responsible for the heart failure state.

The efficiency of energy utilization in the myocardium was also investigated, and it was determined that although the failing myocardium develops considerably less tension than the normal myocardium, it also utilizes considerably less energy in developing this tension; thus, the efficiency of the conversion of chemical energy to mechanical work in the myocardium in heart failure is not decreased.

Acknowledgments

Supported in part by Public Health Service Grant HE 12010 and Research Career Development Award 1-KE-HE 23005 from the National Heart and Lung Institute.

References

Chidsey, C. A., Weinbach, E. C., Pool, P. E., and Morrow, A. G. (1966). *J. Clin. Invest.* **45,** 40.

Covell, J. W., Pool, P. E., and Braunwald, E. (1967). *Proc. Soc. Exp. Biol. Med.* **124,** 126.

Feinstein, M. B. (1962). *Circ. Res.* **10,** 333.

Fleckenstein, A., Janke, J., and Gerlach, E. (1959). *Klin. Wochenschr.* **37,** 451.

Fox, A. C., Wikler, N. S., and Reed, G. E. (1965). *J. Clin. Invest.* **44,** 202.

Lindenmayer, G. E., Sordahl, L. A., and Schwartz, A. (1968). *Circ. Res.* **23,** 439.

Minton, P. R., Zoll, P. M., and Norman, L. R. (1960). *Circ. Res.* **8,** 924.

Olson, R. E. (1964). *Circ. Res. Suppl.* **2,** 109.
Pool, P. E., Covell, J. W., Chidsey, C. A., and Braunwald, E. (1966). *Circ. Res.* **19,** 221.
Pool, P. E., Spann, J. F., Buccino, R. A., Sonnenblick, E. H., and Braunwald, E. (1967). *Circ. Res.* **21,** 365.
Pool, P. E., Chandler, B. M., Spann, J. F., Sonnenblick, E. H., and Braunwald, E. (1969). *Circ. Res.* **24,** 313.
Sobel, B. E., Spann, J. F., Pool, P. E., Sonnenblick, E. H., and Braunwald, E. (1967). *Circ. Res.* **21,** 355.

SOME BIOCHEMICAL ASPECTS OF EXCITATION–CONTRACTION–RELAXATION COUPLING IN NORMAL AND FAILING HEART MUSCLE

Arnold Schwartz

There are two major membrane systems which are undoubtedly involved in the process of contraction and relaxation of cardiac muscle. These are the Na^+,K^+-ATPase enzyme system and the so-called relaxing system. The former may be located in the cell membrane, but might also be found in the *T*-system as well as in the sarcoplasmic reticulum. The latter, at least in skeletal muscle, is found in the sarcoplasmic reticulum, but in cardiac muscle is less well defined.

The present chapter discusses some recent findings concerning these two important membrane systems. Our preliminary experiments employing failing human tissues and cardiomyopathic Syrian hamsters (BIO 14.6), indicate a possible defect in the relaxing system. Furthermore, a series of studies carried out in this laboratory strongly suggest that the Na^+,K^+-ATPase is the pharmacological receptor for cardiac glycosides.

Methods

The procedures for the isolation of the Na^+,K^+-ATPase in a relatively purified form, and the isolation of the relaxing system vesicles (abbreviated in this paper CRS, cardiac relaxing system) have been discussed in detail in published communications (Matsui and Schwartz, 1966a; Harigaya and Schwartz, 1969; Schwartz *et al.*, 1969). The assays for these systems have also been described but we wish to emphasize the importance of rapid kinetic measurements of the relaxing system, using an Aminco-Chance dual-beam spectrophotometer and the use of a linked enzyme system for recording the activity of the Na^+, K^+-ATPase. These are delineated in Figs. 1 and 2.

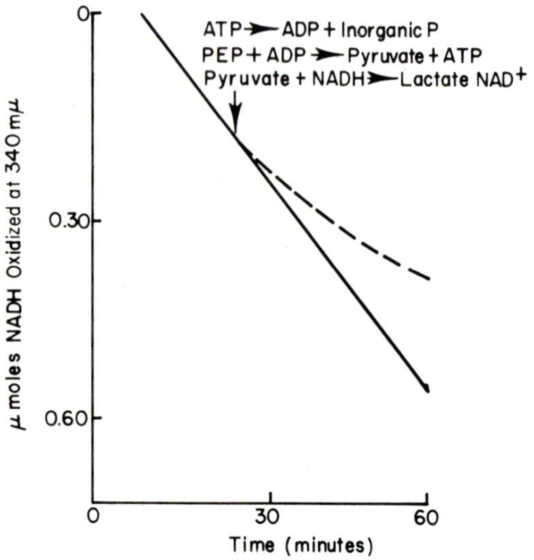

FIG. 1. Continuous recording spectrophotometric assay for Na^+ K^+-ATPase activity. At the arrow, 10^{-6} M ouabain was added to one cuvette, and water to the control. The dotted line (---) describes the course of the reaction in the presence of ouabain. Temperature: 37°C. (Reprinted from Schwartz *et. al.*, 1969)

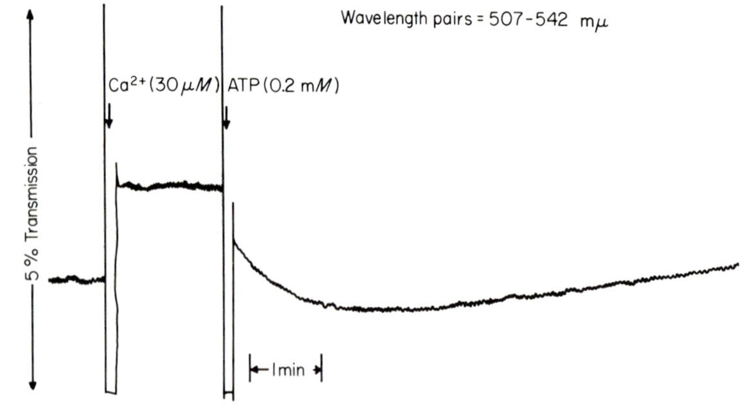

FIG. 2. Measurement of calcium binding by means of a dual-beam spectrophotometer (see Harigaya and Schwartz 1969 for details). The downward trace indicates calcium binding by the vesicles; the upward slope shows release of bound calcium.

Results

Na^+, K^+-ATPase Enzyme System

This enzyme system derived from cardiac muscle is quite similar to the Na^+, K^+-ATPases isolated from all other tissues. Figure 3 indicates the type of activity obtained and the effects of a cardiac glycoside, ouabain.
It is of interest that a number of inhibitors and ions act in a manner which is at least superficially similar to cardiac glycosides. Among these is calcium (Fig. 4), and tributyl tin, an inhibitor of oxidative phosphorylation (Fig. 5a).

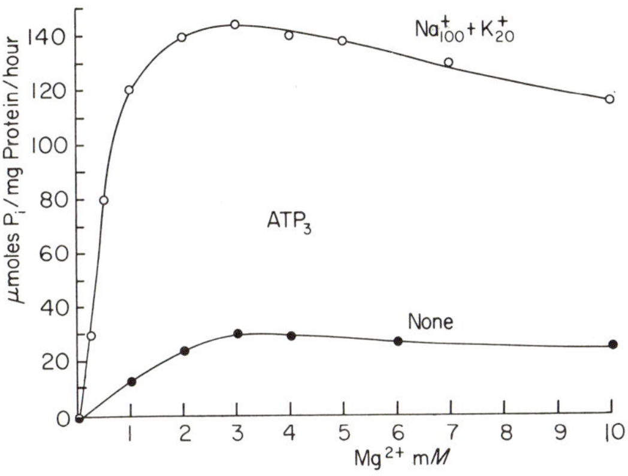

FIG. 3. The effect of Mg^{2+}, Na^+ and K^+ on parotid gland ATPase activity. The incubation medium contained 30 m*M* tris pH 7.0, 3 m*M* tris-ATP, and the various ions as indicated. The numerals appearing as subscripts in this and subsequent figures represent the concentration of the ions used in m*M* per liter. After a 5 min equilibration period at 38°C, in the presence of ATP, the enzyme suspension was added and the incubation was continued for 30 min. (Reprinted from Schwartz, Laseter, and Kraintz, 1963)

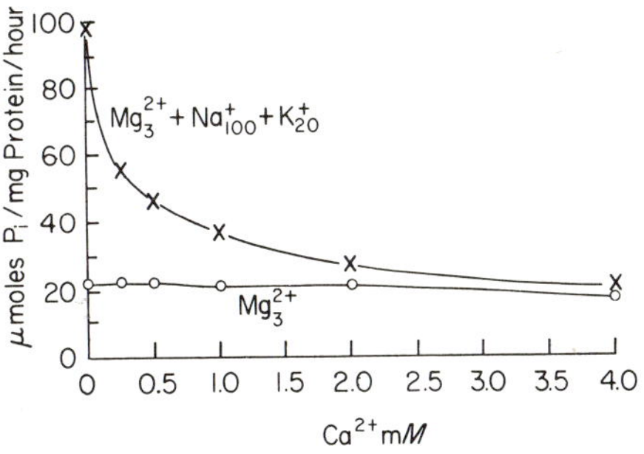

FIG. 4. The effect of calcium on the parotid ATPase activity in the presence and absence of Na^+ plus K^+. (Reprinted from Schwartz, Laseter, and Kraintz, 1963)

Another important characteristic is the fact that the inhibitory effects of cardiac glycosides are specifically reversed or overcome by increasing concentrations of potassium (Fig. 5).

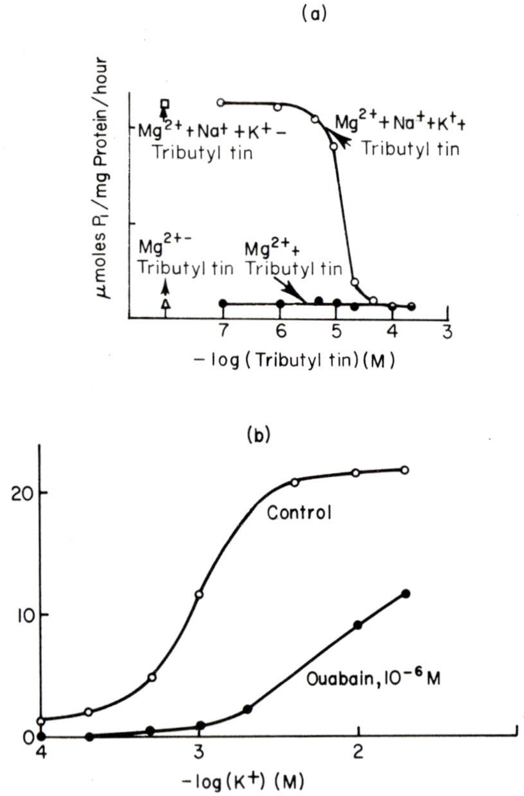

FIG. 5. (a) Effect of tri-*n*-butyltin on the ATPase activity. 40 m*M* tri-*n*-butyl tin in ethanol was diluted with water to the desired concentration. 1% or less concentration of ethanol did not affect ATPase activity. (b) Effect of K^+ concentration on the Na^+,K^+-dependent ATPase activity in the presence or absence of 10^{-6} *M* ouabain. Concentrations of $MgCl_2$ and NaCl were 5 m*M* and 100 m*M*, respectively. The basic Mg^{2+}-dependent activity was subtracted from the activity in the presence of Na^+ and K^+. (Reprinted from Matsui and Schwartz, 1966.)

A kinetic analysis of the inhibitory action of potassium reveals noncompetitive kinetics (Fig. 6a).

It is obvious then that cardiac glycosides affect the Na^+, K^+-ATPase in a rather complex manner requiring both Na^+ and K^+ ions, and in a specific ratio (Matsui and Schwartz, 1966b). Furthermore it has recently become apparent that the action of cardiac glycosides is both temperature- and time-dependent, at least in glycoside-sensitive species (Schwartz *et al.*, 1969). The half-maximal inhibitory concentrations of ouabain at various temperatures and times are exhibited in Table I.

Using a highly active labeled cardiac glycoside, it was possible to show a specific binding of the drug to the enzyme (Matsui and Schwartz, 1967, 1968; Schwartz *et al.*, 1968). The data indicated in Fig. 8 and Table II show the type of binding and characteristics of same, as well as those substances which support binding.

Furthermore only cardiotonic glycosides specifically bind to Na^+, K^+-ATPase preparations (Fig. 9).

TABLE I

OUABAIN CONCENTRATION REQUIRED FOR I_{50} OF Na^+, K^+-ATPASE, AS A FUNCTION OF INCUBATION TIME AND TEMPERATURE[a]

Time (min)	I_{50} Concentration of ouabain at μM		
	22°C	37°C	45°C
Beef heart			
2	—	0.5	0.25
10	1	0.35	0.1
20	0.75	0.25	0.07
30	0.35	0.06	0.025
Dog heart			
2	—	5	2.5
10	3.5	0.75	0.45
20	1	0.25	0.08

[a] Results represent a compilation of statistically significant data.

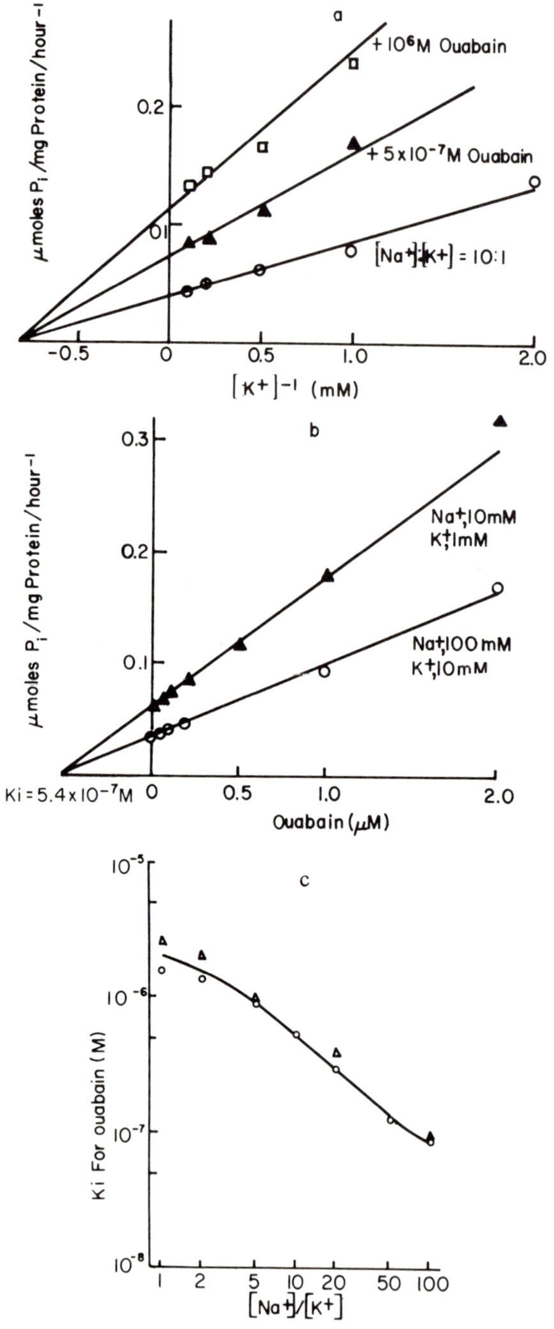

FIG. 6a–c. (a) Lineweaver-Burk a
sis of ouabain inhibition at a con
Na^+/K^+ ratio. Na^+,K^+-ATPase ac
was determined at various K^+ co
trations with a constant Na^+/K^+
of 10 in the presence and absen
5×10^{-7} *M* and 10^{-6} *M* ouabain
was plotted against $1/K^+$ (= 1
× 10). (b) Dixon plot of ouabain i
tion at a constant Na^+/K^+ rati
Relationship between Ki for ou
and Na^+/K^+ ratio. Ki obtained
plotted against Na^+/K^+ ratios on
logarithmic scale. O, △ represent d
ent enzyme preparations. [Parts (
reprinted from Matsui and Schv
1966].

Sulfydryl reagents also specifically affect the Na^+, K^+-ATPase, in a manner similar to cardiac glycosides (Fig. 7a and b).

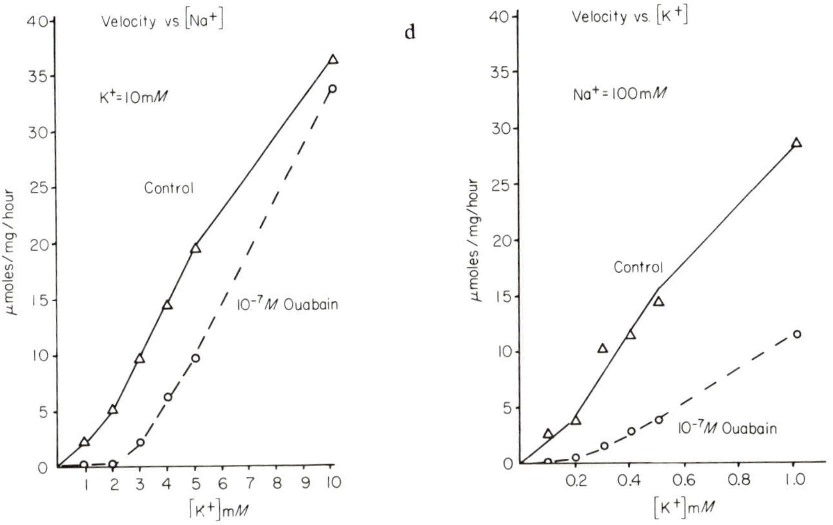

FIG. 6d. Na^+, K^+–ATPase activity vs. monovalent cation concentration: effect of ouabain. The enzyme (0.075 mg) was preincubated at 37° for 5 min in the presence of 5 m*M* $MgCl_2$, 50 m*M* tris–Cl, pH 7.4, NaCl, KCl, and ouabain as indicated. The reaction was started by the addition of tris–ATP (final conc. = 2.5 m*M*) and terminated after 15 min by ice cold TCA.

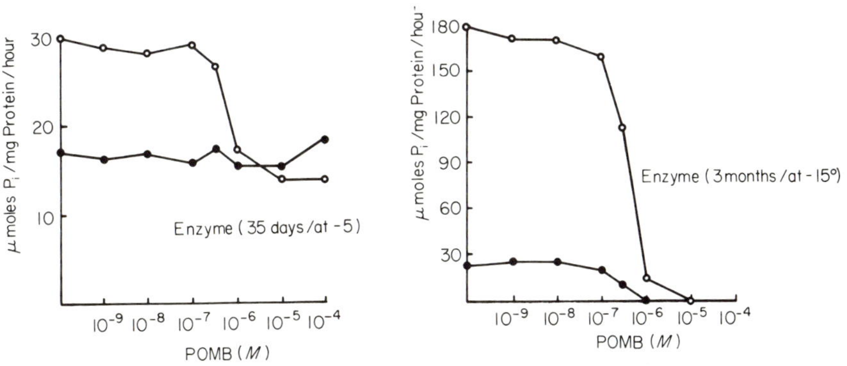

FIG. 7. From Schwartz and Laseter, 1964.

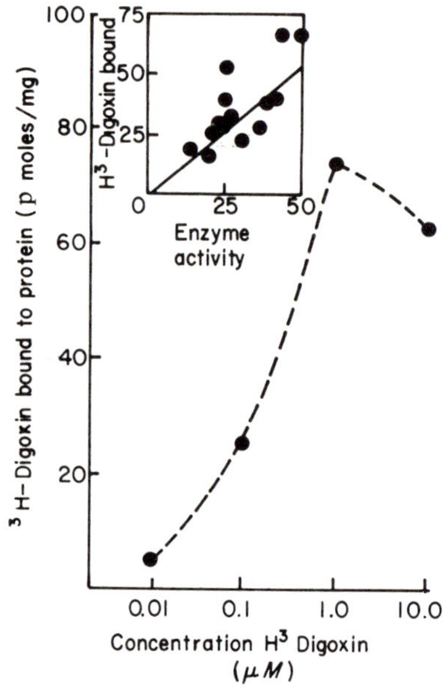

FIG. 8. Concentration and specific binding of ^{3}H-digoxin to a Na^+,K^+-adenosine triphosphatase. The enzyme was prepared from fresh calf heart and used within 1 week after isolation. The binding was carried out in tubes containing 50 m*M* tris • HCl (*pH* 7.4), 2 m*M* tris adenosine triphosphate, 5 m*M* $MgCl_2$, 100 m*M* NaCl, 1 m*M* EDTA, H^3-digoxin at indicated concentrations, with and without 10^{-4} *M* unlabeled ouabain; the tubes were shaken in a water bath at 37°C for 3 min. The binding reaction is complete in about 1 min. The inset represents specific binding of 10^{-6} *M* ^{3}H-digoxin as a function of specific activity of various preparations measured as the amount of inorganic phosphate released per milligram of protein per hour in a system identical to the binding experiment, except that KCl (10 m*M*) was added. ^{3}H-digoxin binding is expressed as picomoles per milligram of protein. The hydrolysis of adenosine triphosphate under these conditions is completely inhibited by 10^{-4} *M* ouabain. These results are typical of many experiments. (Reprinted from Schwartz, Matsui, and Laughter, 1968.)

Heretofore, it was thought that the Na^+,K^+-ATPase consisted of two separate reactions.

$$E + ATP \xrightleftharpoons{Na^+} E - P + ADP$$

$$E - P \xrightarrow{K^+} E + P_i$$

However the binding and other experiments indicate the additional complexity of this enzyme system. In addition we have now recently shown that in the presence of low concentrations of ouabain, nucleotide-free preparations will incorporate, to a very great extent, inorganic phosphate (Lindenmayer *et al.*, 1968) (Table III).

TABLE II

BINDING OF DIGOXIN TO Na^+, K^+–ATPase[a]

Addition	^{3}H-Digoxin bound to protein (pmole/mg)	
	Without Na^+	100 mM with Na^+
None	0	0
ATP	0	10.3
Mg^{2+} + ATP	14.5	37.3
ADP	0.5	0.7
Mg^{2+} + ADP	4.8	11.1
Mg^{2+} + CTP	14.3	26.1
(5 mM) Mg^{2+}	11.5	0
(5 mM) Mn^{2+}	31.7	16.3
(0.05 mM) Ca^{2+}	2.0	0
(0.5 mM) Ca^{2+}	2.7	0
(5 mM) Ca^{2+}	4.0	0.5
(20 mM) Ca^{2+}	9.0	2.9
(5 mM) Sr^{2+}	5.3	16.1
(4 mM) P_i	0.7	0
P_i + Mg^{2+}	42.8	1.4
Tris-arsenate (As)	0	0
As + Mg^{2+}	38.8	1.9
Tris-SO_4^{2-} (SO_4)	5.4	0
SO_4 + Mg^{2+}	5.6	0
Tris-acetate + Mg^{2+}	13.9	0

[a] Reprinted from Schwartz, Matsui, and Laughter, 1968.

TABLE III

LABELING WITH $^{32}P_i$ OF ATPASE SYSTEM[a]

Type	Carrier-free (cpm/mg protein) 1.5 × 10^6 cpm	Carrier added (cpm/mg protein)	
		3 × 10^6 cpm $^{32}P_i$/3 μM P_i	4 × 10^4 cpm $^{32}P_i$/30 μM P_i
3 mM Mg^{2+}	—	1455 (1.46)	—
3 mM Mg^{2+} and 0.1 mM ouabain	—	8800	—
3 mM Mg^{2+} and 20 mM K^+	485	0	0

[a] Numbers in parentheses represent amount of inorganic phosphate incorporated in pmoles. Values are typical of several experiments.

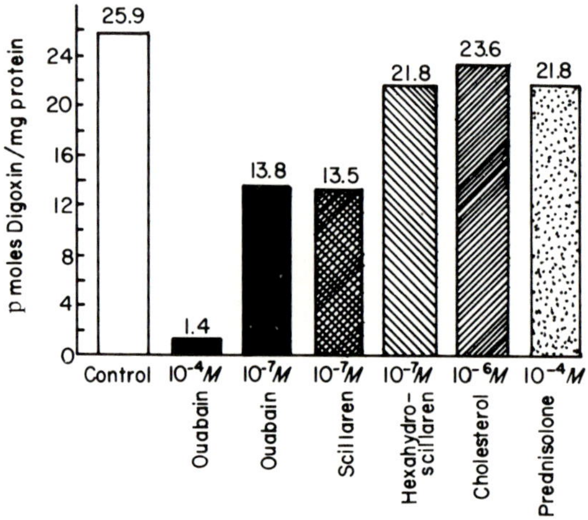

FIG. 9. Dilution of ^{3}H-digoxin binding by cardiac glycosides and steroids. Cardiac glycoside and noncardiac steroid was added in the reaction mixture containing ^{3}H-digoxin in the concentrations shown in the figure. Specific activity of the enzyme was 12.7 μM P_i per mg protein per *h*. (Reprinted from Matsui and Schwartz, 1968.)

We have now specifically shown that magnesium ions are required for the incorporation of inorganic phosphate in the presence of cardiac glycoside but that potassium specifically inhibits the reaction (Fig. 10a). The chemical nature of the phospho-enzyme is identical to the compound formed upon incubation with labeled ATP. Hence the substance could not be acyl phosphate as suggested by numerous authors, and the mechanism of the Na^+, K^+-ATPase should now be reconsidered. This has also been very recently concluded by Albers and his co-workers (Siegel *et al.*, 1969). In view of the information described, the conclusion we have reached is that cardiac glycosides act by allosterically affecting an important lipoprotein involved in the movements of Na^+ and K^+. A plausible scheme is presented in Fig. 10b. In order to directly demonstrate that cardiac glycosides could possibly affect this enzyme, *in vivo*, a number of experiments were carried out; one of which is described below. A supported isolated dog heart preparation was set up, and several indices of contraction were measured. This is pictured in Fig. 11.

At the peak of inotropic effect as well as at minimal positive inotropic effect, the heart was flushed with ice cold saline solution and three membrane systems were isolated; mitochondria, relaxing system, and Na^+,K^+-ATPase. Only the Na^+,K^+-ATPase was significantly inhibited by the drug (Figs. 12 and 13).

Cardiac glycosides in a wide range of concentrations under varying conditions do not affect the cardiac relaxing system (Fig. 12).

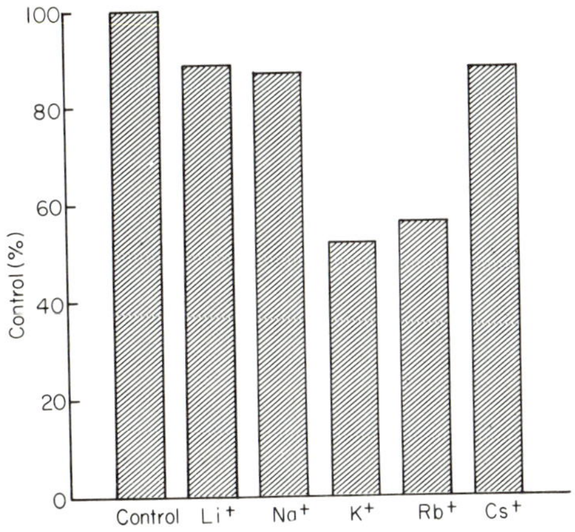

Fig 10(a). Ordinate represents incorporation of ^{32}Pi into Na^+, K^+-ATPase in presence of $MgCl_2$ and ouabain (percent). The effect of various cations on incorporation is shown in abscissa.

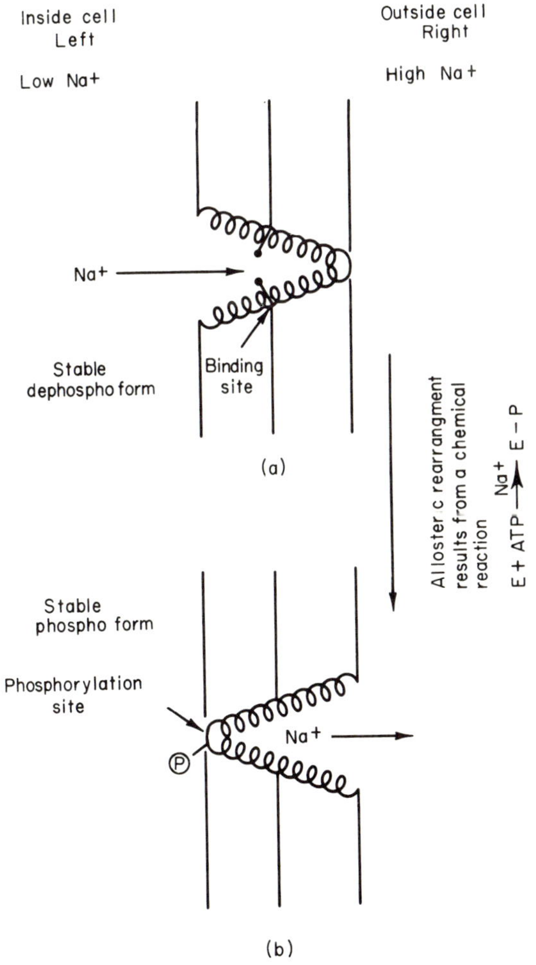

FIG. 10(b). Allosteric pump concept. (From Bresnick and Schwartz, 1968, redrawn from the concept of Jardetzky.)

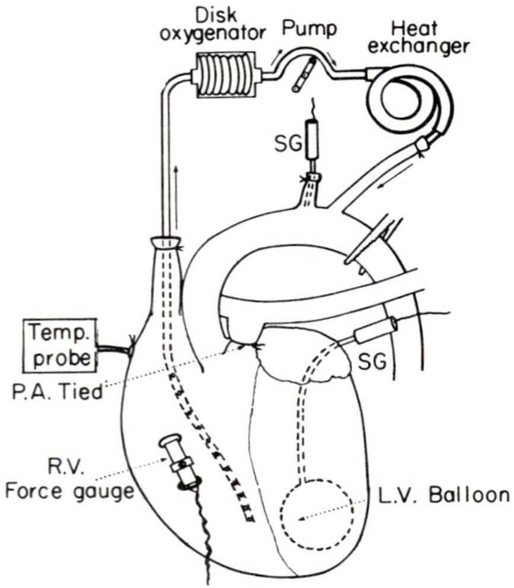

(a)

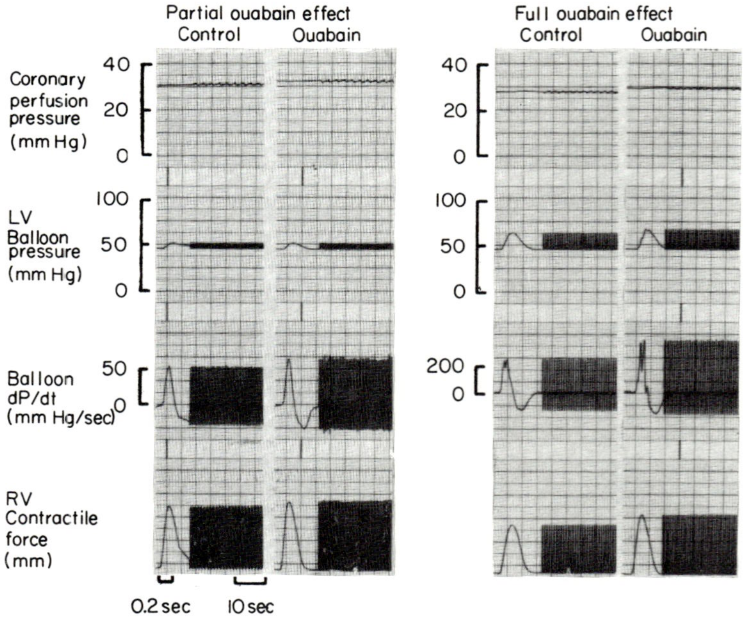

(b)

FIG. 11(a). Schematic diagram of *in situ* dog heart perfusion. S.G., strain-gauge pressure transducer; P.A., pulmonary artery. Ouabain, 10^{-2} *M*, was added to the disc oxygenator to produce a final concentration of 10^{-6} *M*. Total system volume = 1200 ml. Positive inotropic effects of ouabain were recorded from right ventricular force gauge and from left, ventricular balloon (*dP/dt*). (b) Representative records from partial and full ouabain perfusions and their respective controls taken immediately before addition of ouabain (10^{-6} *M* final concentration) to the perfusing fluid. Partial and full ouabain records taken after 6 min and 20 min of drug perfusion, respectively. Coronary perfusion pressure monitored with a pressure transducer from a cannula in the aortic arch. Changes in coronary perfusion pressure are not significant. Balloon *dP/dt* increased 23% and 53% in the partial and full ouabain perfusions, respectively, and right ventricular contractile force increased 16% in the partial ouabain, and 24% in the full ouabain perfusion in these hearts. Heart rates (electrically paced): partial ouabain, 114; full ouabain, 75. In other experiments, results were not affected by heart rates. (Reprinted from Besch *et al.*, 1970.)

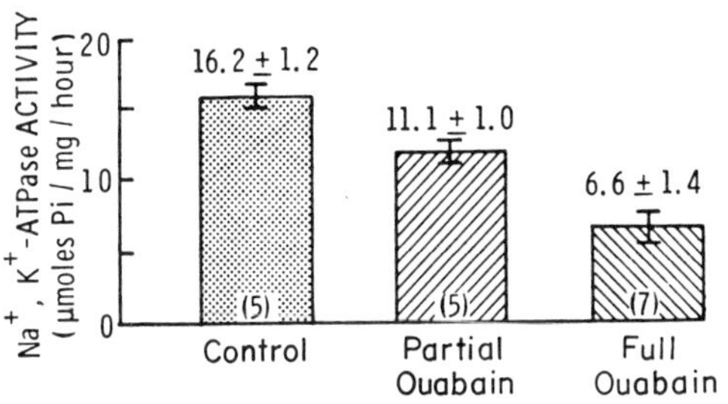

FIG. 12(a). Na^+,K^+-ATPase activity of the enzyme system isolated from control perfused and from partial and full ouabain-perfused canine myocardium. Enzyme activities were measured spectrophotometrically using a linked lactate dehydrogenase-pyruvate kinase system, in the presence of (final concentrations): NaCl, 100 m*M*; KCl, 10 m*M*; $MgCl_2$, 5 m*M*; tris-ATP, 5.0 m*M*; tris-Cl buffer (pH 7.4), 25 m*M*; 25 to 50 μg of protein; and, in the cuvettes measuring Mg^{2+} activity, 5×10^{-4} *M* ouabain. Reaction temperature, 37°C. The Na^+,K^+-ATPase activity of partial ouabain-perfused hearts was significantly lower than control ($P < 0.02$) and of full ouabain-perfused hearts, also significantly lower than control ($P < 0.001$). Values are mean ± S.E. Numbers in parentheses are numbers of experiments.

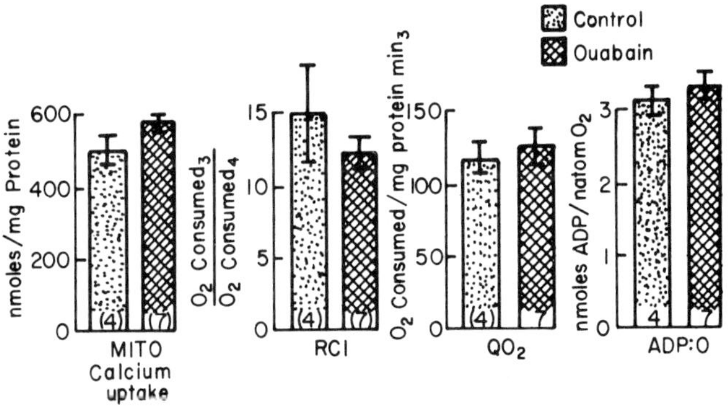

(b) Calcium uptake and oxidative phosphorylation measurements of mitochondria isolated from control perfused and ouabain-perfused canine myocardium. For calcium uptake, the standard assay conditions were (final concentration): Trissuccinate, 5 m*M*; KCl, 100 m*M*; $MgCl_2$, 10 m*M*; inorganic phosphate, 4 m*M*; disodium ATP, 2 m*M*; Trismaleate buffer (pH 6.8), 10 m*M*; EDTA, 0.1 m*M*; protein, 0.1 mg, in a final volume of 1 ml; temperature, 37°C; incubation time, 30 min. RCI = respiratory control index, the ratio of oxygen consumed per minute in state 3 to oxygen consumed per minute in state 4; Q_{O_2} = oxygen consumed per milligram of protein per minute in state 3; ADP/O (P/O) = nanomoles of ADP used per nanoatom of oxygen (state 3). For oxidative phosphorylation measurements, the standard assay conditions were (final concentrations): Trissuccinate or trisglutamate, 5 m*M*; sucrose, 0.25 *M*; inorganic phosphate, 5 m*M*; tris-Cl (pH 7.4), 10 m*M*; protein, 1 to 2 mg/ml; temperature, 30°C. ADP (approximately 500 nmole) was added to produce state 3 respiratory bursts. No significant differences in calcium uptake or oxidative phosphorylation were found between control and experimental preparations. Values from partial and full ouabain experiments are pooled for presentation. Values are mean ± S.E. Numbers in parentheses are numbers of experiments. (Reprinted from Besch *et al.*, 1970.)

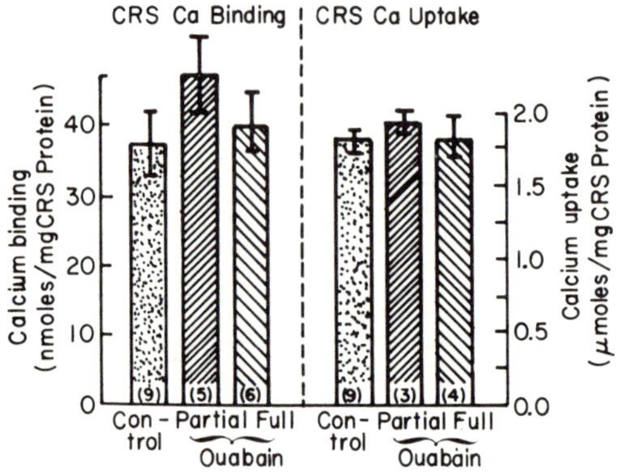

FIG. 13. Maximum ATP-dependent calcium binding and uptake by cardiac relaxing system (CRS) obtained from control and partial and full ouabain-perfused canine myocardium. The standard assay conditions were (final concentration): KCL, 100 m*M*; $MgCl_2$, 10 m*M*; disodium ATP, 2 m*M*; trismaleate buffer (pH 6.8), 20 m*M*; and 0.2 mg of protein (binding) or 0.05 mg of protein and 5 m*M* sodium oxalate (uptake) in a final volume of 1 ml. Binding: Temperature, 25°C; time, 5 min. Uptake: temperature, 37°C; time, 30 min. No significant differences were found for binding or uptake between control and experimental preparations. Numbers in parentheses are numbers of experiments.

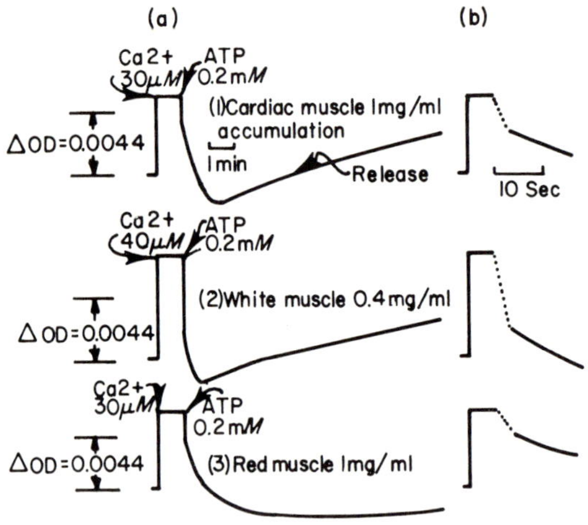

FIG. 14. Rate of Ca^{2+} binding by relaxing preparations from various muscles of rabbit, measured by dual-beam spectrophotometry. Reaction mixture consisted of 100 m*M* KCl, 10 m*M* $MgCl_2$, 20 m*M* trismaleate buffer (pH 6.8), 0.3 m*M* murexide, 0.4–1 mg/ml membrane protein, 30–40 μ*M* Ca^{2+} and 0.2 m*M* ATP. Incubation at room temperature (about 23°C). A and B are the same, except for different time scales. The ordinate in this figure represents changes in transmitted light expressed in units of optical density (OD). (Reprinted from Harigaya and Schwartz, 1969.)

Rapid Kinetic Studies of The Cardiac Relaxing System

Employing a new isolation procedure for the cardiac muscle relaxing system which involves the use of a Polytron blending apparatus and a Na^+ bicarbonate-azide solution, we have obtained fairly stable, very highly active preparations which rapidly remove calcium from solution, *in vitro*. Figure 14 compares cardiac muscle to white and red skeletal muscle.

The rate constant, initial rate and half maximal rate for calcium *binding* by membrane vesicles for various muscles is shown in Table IV.

Notice that the rates of uptake and release are decidedly different when compared to a similar system isolated from human failing cardiac muscle (Table V).

The Ca^{2+} binding rate was calculated from the measurement at the 10 sec period. All hearts were obtained at the time of implant surgery and all were in varying stages of failure. This is a consistent finding which appears to be similar to that found by Chidsey (personal communication, 1969) employing a failing calf preparation.

TABLE IV

Rate of Ca^{2+} Binding by Membrane Vesicles from Various Muscles

Preparation	Rate constant (M^{-1} sec^{-1})	Initial rate (nM of Ca^{2+} mg^{-1} min^{-1})	Half-maximal time (sec)
Cardiac muscle	2375	256	10
White muscle	3450	1440	<3
Red muscle	1270	182	20

TABLE V

Ca^{2+} Binding Rate of Membrane Vesicles from Failing Human Cardiac Muscle

Human heart	Ca^{2+} binding rate (nM mg^{-1} min^{-1})	Half-maximal time (sec)	Maximal Ca^{2+} binding (nM mg^{-1})
1	36.4	20	24.2
2	34.8	70	35.2
3	34.3	33	25.6
4	69.6[a]	32	42.3

[a] The value calculated at the 3-sec period is 112.0 (nM mg^{-1} min^{-1}), which is significantly lower than the values obtained for animal preparations from heart (Harigaya and Schwartz, 1969).

Discussion

The evidence presented in this paper indicates quite strongly the importance of two membrane systems, Na^+,K^+-ATPase and the relaxing system. Unfortunately, there have been no definitive morphological or ultrastructural studies concerning the localization of these systems. It is often assumed that the pump enzyme is located in the cell membrane while the calcium sequestering system is located in the sarcoplasmic reticulum (SR). However, at least in the human muscle, there is a paucity of SR and there have been, again, no clear studies showing specific localization of the Na^+,K^+-ATPase. It would be of importance to devise clearcut experiments which will solve this important problem. Despite this, however, our biochemical studies suggest that the Na^+,K^+-ATPase is the pharmcological receptor for cardiac glycosides and that the cardiac relaxing system of muscle may, in fact, be involved in the failing heart. The latter has been shown both in failing human heart and in a cardiomyopathic strain of Syrian hamster (BIO 14.6) (Fig. 15).

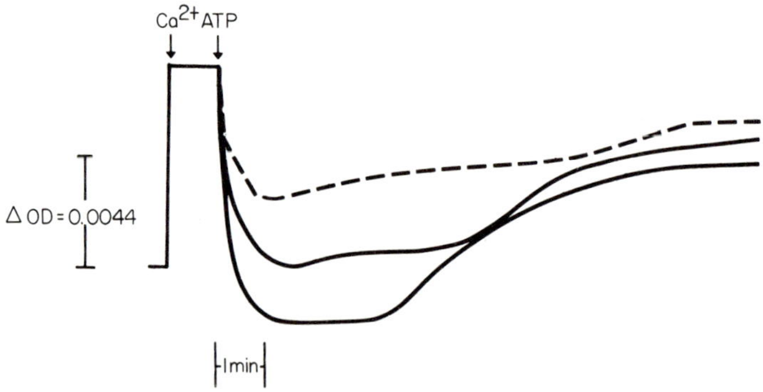

FIG. 15. Calcium binding of isolated cardiac relaxing system from normal and failing cardiomyopathic Syrian hamster (BIO 14.6). Calcium binding by CRS in presence of ATP regenerating system. The dotted lines represent CRS from cardiomyopathic hamsters in congestive heart failure (about 270 days/age) strain BIO 14.6; solid lines normal CRS. The reaction mixture consisted of 100 m*M* KCl, 10 m*M* $MgCl_2$, 20 m*M* trismaleate buffer (pH 6.8), 0.3 m*M* murexide, 0.6 mg CRS protein, 2 m*M* PEP and 0.05 mg/ml pyruvate kinase.

REFERENCES

Besch, H. R., Jr., Allen J. C., Glick, G., and Schwartz, A. (1970). *J. Pharmacol. Exp. Ther.* **171**, 1.

Bresnick, E., and Schwartz, A. (1968) "Functional Dynamics of the Cell." Academic Press, New York.

Harigaya, S., and Schwartz, A. (1969). *Circ. Res.* **25**, 781.

Lindenmayer, G. E., Laughter, A. H., and Schwartz, A. (1968). *Arch. Biochim. Biophys.* **127,** 187.
Matsui, H., and Schwartz, A. (1966a). *Biochim. Biophys. Acta* **128,** 382.
Matsui, H., and Schwartz, A. (1966b). *Biochim. Biophys. Res. Commun.* **25,** 147.
Matsui, H., and Schwartz, A. (1967). *Proc. Fed. Amer. Soc. Exp. Biol.* **26,** 398.
Matsui, H., and Schwartz, A. (1968). *Biochim. Biophys. Acta* **151,** 655.
Schwartz, A , and Laseter, A. H. (1964). *Biochem. Pharmacol.* **13,** 337.
Schwartz, A., Laseter, A. H., and Kraintz, L., *J. Cell. Comp. Physiol.* (1963).**62**, 193.
Schwartz, A., Matsui, H., and Laughter, A. (1968). *Science* **159,** 323.
Schwartz, A., Allen, J. C., and Harigaya, S. (1969). *J. Pharmacol. Exp. Ther.* **168,** 31.
Siegel, G. J., Koval, G. J., and Albers, R. W. (1969). *J. Biol. Chem.* **244,** 3264

EVIDENCE FOR INCREASED GLYCOLYTIC METABOLISM IN CARDIAC HYPERTROPHY AND CONGESTIVE HEART FAILURE

Sanford P. Bishop and Ruth A. Altschuld

In an attempt to understand the metabolic abnormalities in myocardial hypertrophy and congestive heart failure (CHF), most investigators have directed their attention to the major source of energy production in the heart, the mitochondria and oxidative metabolism. Studies of heart mitochondria isolated from various animal species with hypertrophied and failing myocardia have given conflicting results. Function of the isolated mitochondria is reported to be either normal (Plaut and Gertler, 1959; Chidsey *et al.*, 1966; Sobel *et al.*, 1967; Stoner *et al.*, 1968), or depressed (Argus *et al.*, 1964; Wollenberger *et al.*, 1963; Schwartz and Lee, 1962; Lindemayer *et al.*, 1968). An additional factor which must be considered in the bioenergetics of the hypertrophied myocardium is the increased demand placed upon the energy producing resources of the heart by alterations in hemodynamic and mechanical factors. When oxidative metabolism is taxed to its limit, or if inhibitory factors are operating, it is reasonable to assume that reserve sources of energy production will be utilized. The role of glycolytic metabolism in meeting this increased energy demand has received little study.

In myocardial hypertrophy there is an increase in the cross-sectional diameter of the myocardial cell (Karsner *et al.*, 1925) while the capillary to fiber ratio remains constant (Wearn, 1940). It has been suggested that this increased diffusion distance from the capillary lumen to the center of the hypertrophied cell may result in a decreased oxygen availability in the center of the cell (Wearn, 1940). Since direct methods of determining the intracellular distribution of oxygen are not available, we looked for indirect means of detecting reduced availability of oxygen. The association of the isozymes of lactate dehydrogenase (LDH) with aerobic and anaerobic metabolism (Cahn *et al.*, 1962; Markert, 1963; Dawson *et al.*, 1964) and the shifts in isozyme distribution which have been shown to occur with altered environmental oxygen availability (Johansson, 1966; Lindy and Rajasalmi, 1966; Thorling and

Jensen, 1966) suggested a possible tool for evaluating myocardial intracellular oxygen availability.

Lactate dehydrogenase exists as two genetically determined subunits which have been designated as heart (H-LDH) and muscle (M-LDH) types corresponding to their respective preponderance in these tissues (Appella and Markert, 1961). These subunits combine in groups of four with pure heart and muscle forms and intermediate hybrids resulting in a total of five isozymes (Fig. 1). The theory that LDH isozymes are associated with the metabolic activity of the tissue is based on several observations. Tissues which are highly dependent on aerobic metabolism such as heart and brain have a preponderance of those LDH isozymes composed primarily of the heart-type subunit (Vessell *et al.*, 1962; Dawson *et al.*, 1964). Tissues such as white skeletal muscle and uterine smooth muscle which function well under anaerobic conditions, contain the electrophoretically slower moving LDH isozymes which are composed primarily of muscle-type subunit (Vessell *et al.*, 1962; Dawson *et al.*, 1964). It has been demonstrated *in vitro* that levels of pyruvate in the incubation medium which allow the reaction to proceed to lactic acid in the presence of M-LDH are inhibitory to the heart-type of LDH (Cahn *et al.*, 1962; Kaplan, 1966). This *in vitro* inhibition suggests that the heart-type subunit favors the entrance of pyruvate into the citric acid cycle to be

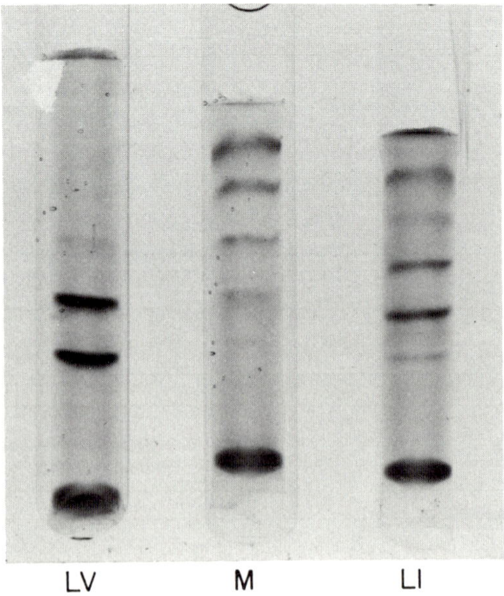

FIG. 1. Disc electrophoresis polyacrilamide gels of homogenates of myocardium (LV), skeletal muscle (M), and liver (Li) from a normal dog. The large-pore gel at the origin has been broken off. The dark band at the bottom (anode) end of the gel is a tracking dye. LDH-3 is very weak in myocardium, LDH-1 weak in skeletal muscle, whereas all five bands are present in liver.

oxidized by aerobic metabolism. Furthermore, decreasing oxygen availability in cultured liver cells (Johansson, 1966), chick embryos (Lindy and Rajasalmi, 1966), or in rabbit renal cortex (Thorling and Jensen, 1966) has been shown to produce a redistribution of LDH isozymes toward those isozymes containing M-LDH. These findings indicate that cells are capable of adapting their LDH isozyme content in response to environmental variations in oxygen availability. Based on this information, we theorized that if there is relative tissue hypoxia and metabolic adaptation with myocardial hypertrophy and failure, there should be an isozyme shift toward those isozymes favoring anaerobic metabolism. In addition, we would expect to see increased lactate production in tissues operating under decreased aerobiasis.

Experimental Animals

Three groups of dogs were investigated. The first group contained 8 dogs which were naturally infested with the canine heartworm *Dirofilaria immitis*. Animals in this group had signs of cardiopulmonary insufficiency from 2 months to over 2 years. The diagnosis was confirmed by the demonstration of typically dilated pulmonary arteries by cineangiocardiogram, a right ventricular hypertrophy pattern on the electrocardiogram (Detweiler and Patterson, 1965), elevated mean pulmonary artery and right ventricular systolic and end-diastolic pressure (Fig. 2), presence of *D. immitis* microfilaria in the peripheral blood, presence of adult parasites in the right ventricle and pulmonary artery at necropsy, and microscopic demonstration of obstructing vascular lesions in the pulmonary arteries and arterioles (Adcock, 1961).

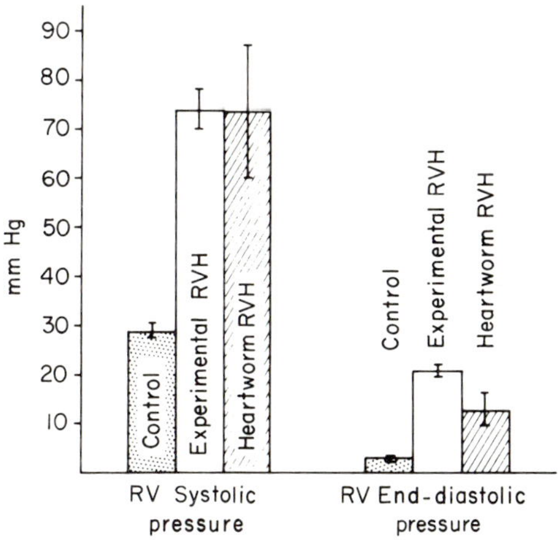

FIG. 2 Right ventricular (RV) pressures in experimental and naturally acquired right ventricular hypertrophy (RVH) and congestive heart failure. Bars represent mean values for each group ± S.E.M. (From Bishop and Altschuld, 1970.)

In the second group, progressive pulmonary arterial stenosis was produced in 11 dogs by means of a rubber Jacobson cuff surgically implanted around the main pulmonary artery (Bishop and Cole, 1969b). With the animal under methoxyflurane anesthesia, the pulmonary artery was progressively narrowed at biweekly intervals by percutaneous injection of fluid into a connecting bulb located subcutaneously. Right ventricular pressure was monitored during this procedure using a 15 gauge polyethylene catheter attached to a Statham P23AA transducer and displayed on a direct writing oscillograph. The right ventricle progressively increased in size as determined by a qualitative increase in heart size and wall thickness on thoracic radiographs and cineangiocardiograms, the appearance of a right ventricular hypertrophy pattern on the electrocardiogram (Detweiler and Patterson, 1965), and increased right ventricular mass determined at necropsy (Fig. 3). The experiment was terminated 55–80 days following surgery when the dogs were in advanced congestive heart failure as determined by the presence of the following signs: venous distention, palpable liver enlargement, ascites, an observed decrease in exercise tolerance, and an elevation of right ventricular end-diastolic pressure above 7 mm Hg.

The third control group contained nine unoperated normal animals and four dogs which had undergone a sham thoracotomy and pulmonary artery dissection 6–10 weeks previously. No differences in hemodynamic or metabolic data among unoperated and sham-operated animals were found and therefore they are considered as one group.

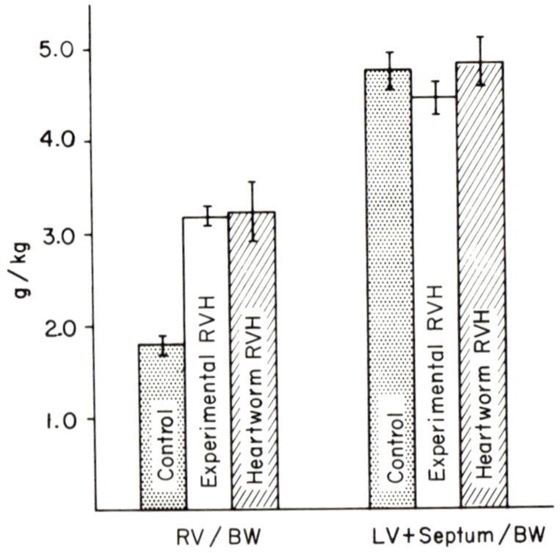

FIG. 3. Ventricular weight to body weight ratios in experimental and naturally acquired right ventricular hypertrophy (RVH) and congestive heart failure. RV/BW = right ventricular free-wall weight/body weight; LV + septum/BW = left ventricle plus septum weight/body weight.

The increase in right ventricular free-wall weight of dogs with both experimental and naturally occurring right ventricular hypertrophy (RVH) is compared with the control animals in Fig. 3. The mean value for the experimental animals is similar to that for dogs with naturally acquired RVH, although there is more variability in the latter group. Combined left ventricle and septum to body weight ratios were not altered. Right ventricular systolic and end-diastolic pressures are presented in Fig. 2; mean values are similar for both groups with RVH with more variability in the group infested with heartworms.

Determination of Lactate Dehydrogenase (LDH) Isozymes

Immediately after death of the animals by electrocution, approximately 3 gm of a full thickness sample of right and left ventricular free-wall were freed of epicardium, endocardium, visible blood vessels, connective tissue, and adipose tissue. A 10% homogenate was prepared with 0.154 *M* KCl using 15 strokes of a motor-driven teflon pestle in a Potter-Elvehjem glass homogenizer. The 10% homogenate was centrifuged at 10,000 × g for 1 hr and the supernatant used for total LDH enzyme activity and electrophoretic separation of the isozymes. To increase stability of the enzyme (Zondag, 1963), 10 mg/ml neutralized reduced glutathione was added to the supernatant. Protein was determined by the biuret method and total lactate dehydrogenase activity by the method of Wroblewski and LaDue (1955). The reaction was started by the addition of pyruvate (3.3×10^{-4} *M* final concentration) to the cuvette at 30°C and the oxidation of NADH followed at 340 mμ with either a Cary 15 or Beckman DU spectrophotometer with Gilford recorder.

Electrophoresis was performed at 4°C using a discontinuous polyacrilamide gel system according to a modified method of Davis (1964) with a constant voltage supply power source (Canalco, Rockville, Maryland) at 3 mA. An amount of sample containing 20 Wroblewski-LaDue units of enzyme was placed in 0.2 ml of a large pore 2.5% polyacrilamide sample gel pH 6.8. This was polymerized on top of a column of 5% polyacrilamide running gel pH 8.9. A sample of liver was run concurrently to ensure that the slower moving heat sensitive isozymes were retained.

After the completion of the electrophoretic separation, usually 40–80 min, the gels were removed from the glass columns and stained according to the tetrazolium method of Goldberg and Cather (1963). The gels were scanned with a Densicord recording densitometer with integrator attachment (Photovolt Corporation, New York, N. Y.) using a 595 mμ filter. The percentage of each isozyme was determined directly from the integrator marks. The relative amounts of heart (H-LDH) and muscle-type (M-LDH) isozyme were calculated from the isozyme percentages using the ratio of H-LDH and M-LDH subunits present in each isozyme as previously described (Appella and Markert, 1961; Cahn *et al.*, 1962; Markert, 1963). Values reported are the mean of two or more gels for each sample.

Total LDH activity and LDH isozyme distribution in the left and right ventricles are shown in Table I. Although total LDH activity varied considerably from one animal to another, left and right ventricles contained similar amounts in any individual dog and there was no significant statistical difference between mean values for any group when compared by Student's t-test with the control group at the 5% level. The results were not different whether related to wet weight of tissue or to protein in the supernatant.

Distribution of LDH isozymes in control dog left and right ventricles was very similar (Table I and Fig. 4). LDH-1, the most rapidly migrating isozyme,

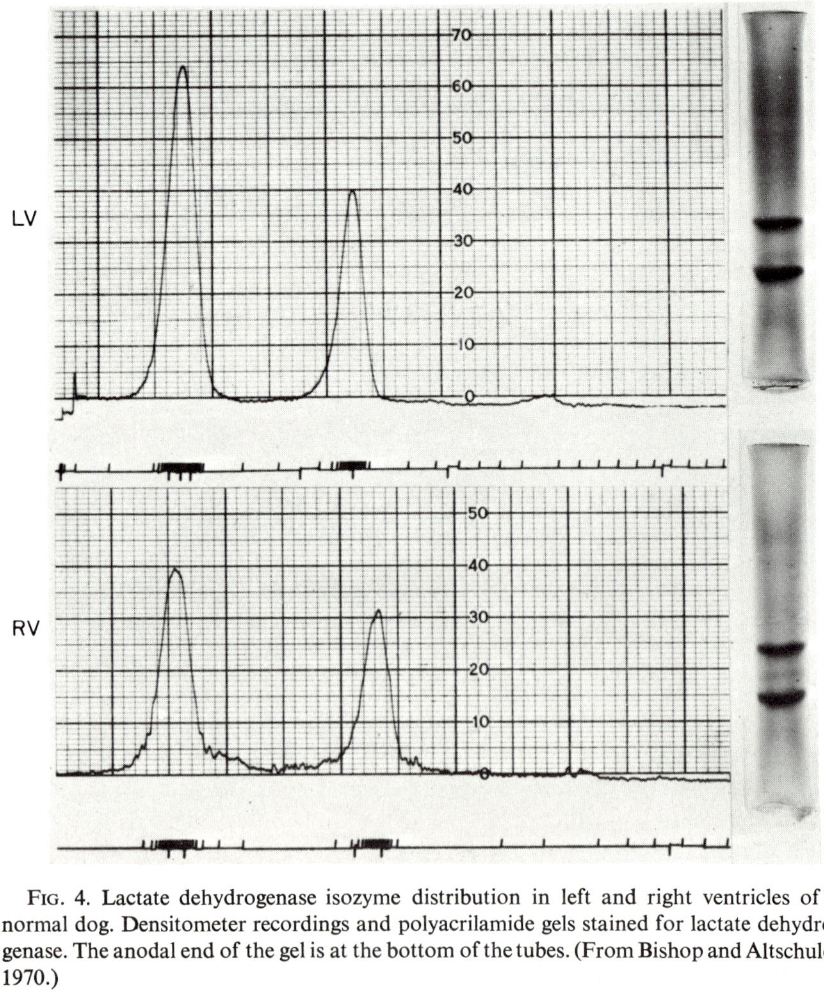

FIG. 4. Lactate dehydrogenase isozyme distribution in left and right ventricles of a normal dog. Densitometer recordings and polyacrilamide gels stained for lactate dehydrogenase. The anodal end of the gel is at the bottom of the tubes. (From Bishop and Altschuld, 1970.)

TABLE I

TOTAL LACTATE DEHYDROGENASE ACTIVITY AND ISOZYME DISTRIBUTION IN VENTRICLES OF DOGS WITH RIGHT VENTRICULAR HYPERTROPHY AND FAILURE[a,b]

Group	Right ventricle						Left ventricle					
	Units LDH/gm tissue	Isozyme (%)					Units LDH/gm tissue	Isozyme (%)				
	($\times 10^3$)	1	2	3	4	5	($\times 10^3$)	1	2	3	4	5
Control (14)												
	247	56.6	41.4	2.0	0	0	275	59.0	39.7	1.3	0	0
	± 24	± 1.9	± 1.8	± 0.6			± 25	± 1.9	± 1.8	± 0.4		
Experimental RVH and CHF (11)												
	268	32.4	58.3	9.3	0	0	289	48.2	49.1	2.7	0	0
	± 20	± 2.4	± 1.2	± 1.4			± 25	± 2.4	± 1.9	± 0.8		
	$P > 0.05$	< 0.001	< 0.001	< 0.001			> 0.05	< 0.01	< 0.01	> 0.05		
Dirofilariasis RVH and CHF (8)												
	220	34.6	53.5	11.9	< 1	0	257	44.6	47.8	7.6	< 1	0
	± 27	± 2.6	± 2.6	± 5.2			± 29	± 4.3	± 3.7	± 2.0		
	$P > 0.05$	< 0.001	< 0.001	< 0.001			> 0.05	< 0.001	< 0.05	< 0.01		

[a] Values are means $\pm$ SEM. Numbers in parentheses are number of animals in each group.
[b] From Bishop and Altschuld, 1970.

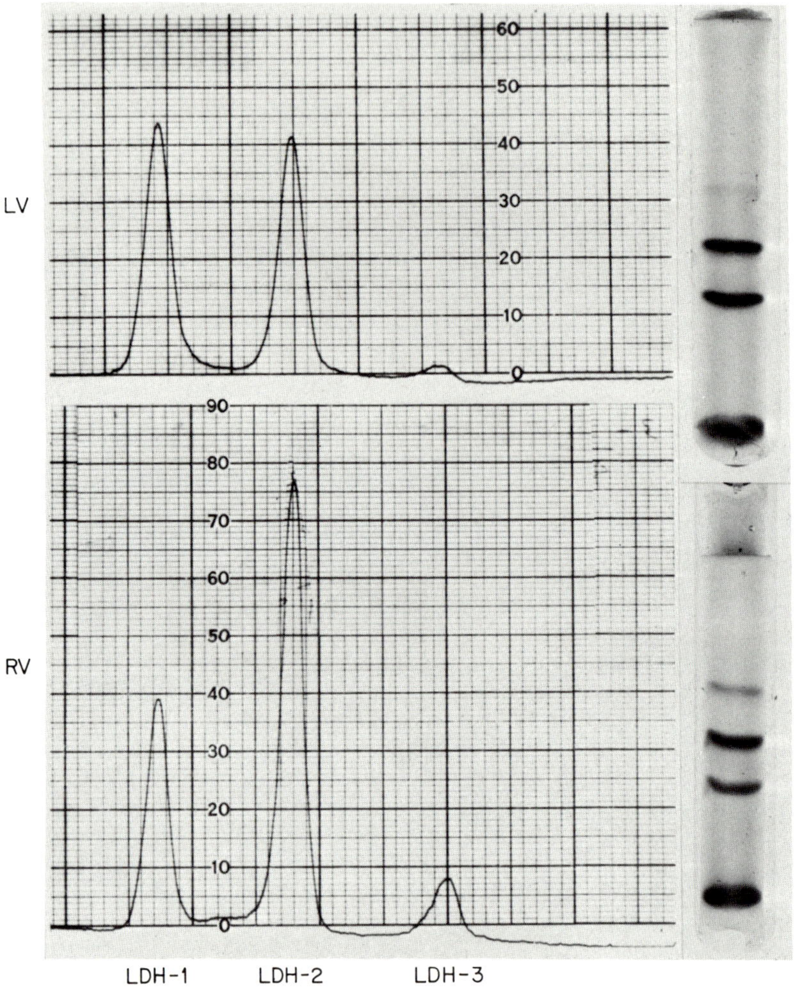

FIG. 5. Lactate dehydrogenase isozymes distribution in left and right ventricles of a dog with experimental RVH and CHF. In the right ventricle there is an appreciable increase in LDH-2 and 3, whereas the change is less apparent in the left ventricle. (From Bishop and Altschuld, 1970.)

exhibited the greatest enzyme activity, LDH-2 somewhat less, and LDH-3 was very weak. LDH-4 and 5 were not found in normal dog hearts. In both groups of dogs with RVH and CHF there was a relative decrease in LDH-1 activity and an increase in the activity of LDH-2 and 3 with the occasional appearance of LDH-4 in the right ventricle (Table I and Fig. 5). The LDH isozyme distribution in the left ventricle from dogs with RVH and CHF was more like the control dog left ventricle, but nevertheless had a significant isozyme shift toward those isozymes containing M-LDH.

The amount of M-LDH in the control dogs, when calculated as a percentage of total LDH activity had a mean of 11.4 ± 0.56 (S.E.M.)% and 10.6 ± 0.54% in the right and left ventricles, respectively (Fig. 6). In both experimental and naturally occurring RVH and CHF there was a significant increase to 19.2 ± 0.92% and 19.1 ± 1.14% M-LDH ($P < 0.001$), respectively, in the right ventricles. The left ventricles had a lesser increase to 13.6 ± 0.76 and 15.6 ± 1.43% M-LDH ($P < 0.01$).

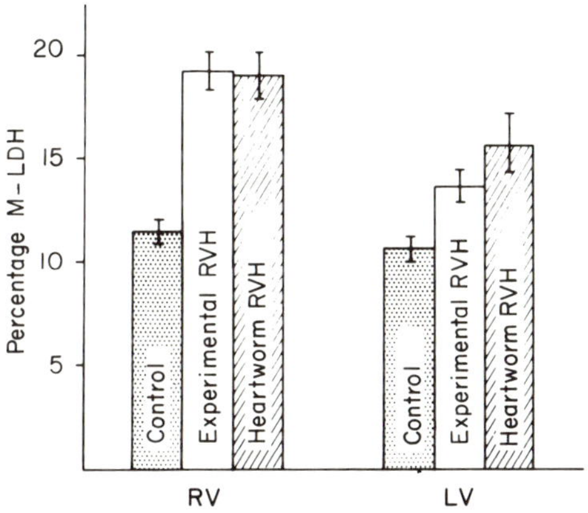

FIG. 6. Relative percentage of muscle type lactate dehydrogenase in right (RV) and left (LV) ventricles of control dogs and those with experimental and naturally acquired right ventricular hypertrophy (RVH) and congestive heart failure. (From Bishop and Altschuld, 1970.)

Determination of Glycolytic Activity

Glycolytic activity was measured by injecting 1.5 ml heart homogenate into stoppered bottles containing 6 ml modified LePage buffer (Potter, 1957) pH 7.6 which had been equilibrated at 37°C with 95% N_2, 5% CO_2. Final concentration of the incubation mixture was 3 m*M* K_2HPO_4, 50 m*M* nicotinamide, 8.3 m*M* $MgCl_2$, 0.25 m*M* NAD, 60 m*M* KCl, 4.2 m*M* ADP, 12.5 m*M* glucose, and 0.1 mg/ml type III yeast hexokinase (Sigma).

Samples were withdrawn at 0, 15, and 30 min of incubation and immediately deproteinized with an equal volume of chilled 0.6 *M* perchloric acid. Lactic acid was determined by the method of Scholz *et al.* (1959). Glucose concentration of the homogenates was determined by a glucose oxidase method (Glucostat, Worthington Biochemical Corp., Freehold, N.J.). Equal volumes of perchloric acid extract and 0.4 *M* triethanolamine buffer, pH 7.6, to which sufficient K_2CO_3 had been added to bring the final concentration to 0.55 *M* K_2CO_3 were combined, mixed and allowed to stand in the cold for 10 min. Aliquots of the clear supernatant fluid were used immediately for the determination of metabolic intermediates. Glucose-6-phosphate and fructose-6-phosphate were measured enzymatically according to the method of Hohorst (1963). Fructose-1,6-diphosphate and triose phosphates were determined by the method of Bücher and Hohorst (1963).

The production of lactic acid under anaerobic conditions by the right ventricular homogenates was significantly increased from a control group mean of 2.53 ± 0.58 m*M*/l to 4.05 ± 0.54 and 5.26 ± 0.90 m*M*/l in the experimental and heartworm RVH groups, respectively (Fig. 7). Although lactic

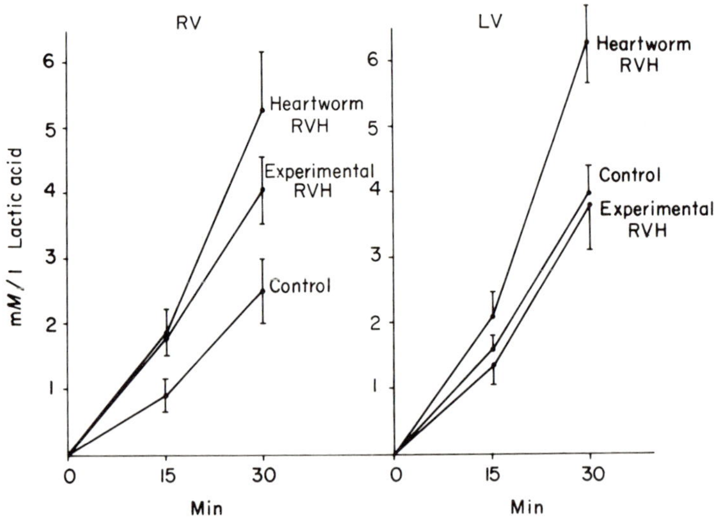

FIG. 7. Lactate production by anaerobically incubated left and right ventricular homogenates of control dogs and those with experimental and naturally acquired RVH and CHF. (From Bishop and Altschuld, 1970.)

acid production of left ventricular homogenates from dogs with experimental RVH and CHF was not different from that produced by control dog left ventricular homogenates, left ventricular homogenates from dogs with naturally acquired RVH and CHF produced 6.27 ± 0.68 m*M*/l lactic acid compared to 3.97 ± 0.39 m*M*/l for the controls. An unexplained but consistent finding was that left ventricular homogenates from control dogs produced more lactate than the corresponding right ventricular homogenates.

The utilization of glucose by left and right ventricular homogenates under anaerobic conditions is shown in Table II. Glucose utilization was slightly,

TABLE II

GLUCOSE UTILIZATION DURING 30 MIN ANAEROBIC INCUBATION OF HEART HOMOGENATES[a]

Group	Right ventricle mM/1	Left ventricle mM/1
Control	4.9 ± 0.57	6.5 ± 0.51
Experimental RVH	5.9 ± 0.55	5.6 ± 0.94
Heartworm RVH	7.1 ± 0.25[b]	8.5 ± 0.63[b]

[a] From Bishop and Altschuld, 1970.
[b] $P < 0.05$, when compared to control.

but not significantly, increased in the experimentally hypertrophied right ventricle. Utilization was significantly increased compared to controls in both ventricles of the dogs with the more chronic, naturally occurring RVH and CHF secondary to infestation with *D. immitis*.

The concentration of glycolytic intermediates produced by anaerobic incubation of homogenates is shown in Table III. In Fig. 8 the various glycolytic intermediates have been plotted as ratios of their concentrations in hypertrophied ventricular homogenates to that in control homogenates. The control

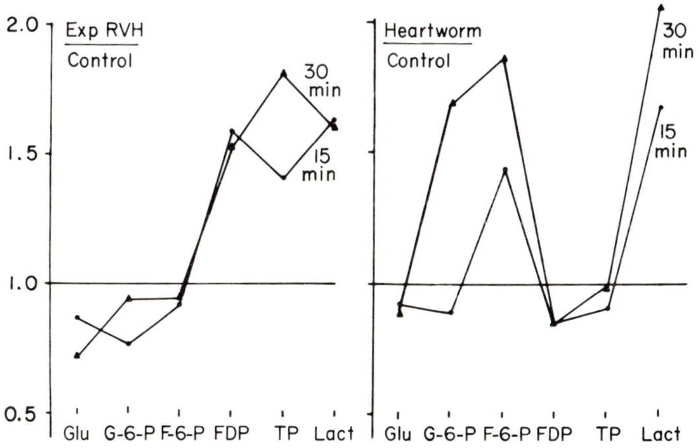

FIG. 8. Glycolytic intermediate metabolites of experimental (Exp RVH) and heartworm produced right ventricular hypertrophy and congestive heart failure. Values are plotted as ratios of their concentrations in the hypertrophied ventricular homogenates to that in the control homogenates. The control values are represented by the horizontal line with a value of 1.0. See text for discussion. Glu = glucose; G-6-P = glucose-6-phosphate; F-6-P = fructose-6-phosphate; FDP = fructose-1,6-diphosphate; TP = triose phosphates; Lact = lactate.

TABLE III

GLYCOLYTIC INTERMEDIATE METABOLITE CONCENTRATIONS DURING ANAEROBIC INCUBATION OF HEART HOMOGENATES[a,b]

Group	Glucose	G-6-P	F-6-P	FDP	TP	Lactate	Total triose mEq
A. Metabolite Concentrations following 15-min Incubation							
Left ventricle							
Control	17.87 (1.08)	2.61 (0.29)	0.66 (0.10)	0.40 (0.09)	0.47 (0.06)	1.55 (0.26)	23.56
Experimental RVH	18.58 (2.08)	2.82 (0.60)	0.72 (0.15)	0.39 (0.04)	0.38 (0.07)	1.36 (0.30)	24.25
Heartworm RVH	18.57 (2.02)	2.92 (0.90)	0.92 (0.26)	0.33 (0.08)	0.36 (0.07)	2.08 (0.44)	25.18
Right ventricle							
Control	19.66 (1.11)	2.43 (0.32)	0.62 (0.12)	0.39 (0.11)	0.39 (0.05)	0.93 (0.25)	24.42
Experimental RVH	17.08 (1.91)	1.86 (0.49)	0.69 (0.15)	0.63 (0.13)	0.54 (0.06)	1.79 (0.28)	22.58
Heartworm RVH	18.12 (1.42)	2.61 (0.76)	0.89 (0.22)	0.34 (0.12)	0.35 (0.06)	1.86 (0.36)	24.16

B. Metabolite Concentrations following 30-min Incubation

Left ventricle							
Control	12.18 (1.35)	3.74 (0.51)	0.98 (0.16)	0.68 (0.17)	0.77 (0.13)	3.97 (0.39)	22.33
Experimental RVH	14.69 (1.97)	4.63 (1.06)	1.07 (0.28)	0.53 (0.13)	0.49 (0.14)	3.76 (0.69)	25.16
Heartworm RVH	10.41 (1.25)	5.86 (1.36)	1.77 (0.41)	0.63 (0.18)	0.66 (0.09)	6.27 (0.69)	25.60
Right ventricle							
Control	15.48 (1.29)	3.20 (0.50)	0.93 (0.19)	0.76 (0.24)	0.63 (0.14)	2.53 (0.54)	23.52
Experimental RVH	14.52 (1.67)	3.00 (0.82)	0.87 (0.24)	1.15 (0.14)	1.14 (0.16)	4.05 (0.54)	24.72
Heartworm RVH	11.45 (0.72)	5.42 (1.25)	1.73 (0.40)	0.64 (0.24)	0.62 (0.18)	5.26 (0.90)	25.12

[a] Values are means ± 1 SEM in parentheses; G-6-P, glucose-6-phosphate; F-6-P, fructose-6-phosphate; FDP, fructose-1,6-diphosphate; TP, triose phosphates.

[b] mEq (Triose equivalents)/1 2% heart homogenate.

values are represented by the horizontal line with a value of 1.0. For animals with experimental RVH and CHF there is a definite crossover point between fructose-6-phosphate and fructose-1,6-diphosphate. According to the crossover theorem (Chance *et al.*, 1958), this suggests that there is an increased activity of phosphofructokinase, the enzyme required for this reaction to proceed in a forward direction. This could well represent the specific locus of increased activity in the glycolytic pathway in the hypertrophied myocardium. In the heart worm-infested group of dogs, however, no clear single site of increased enzyme activity is demonstrated by this method. The apparent decrease in phosphofructokinase activity suggested by the negative crossover between fructose-6-phosphate and fructose-1,6-diphosphate cannot be accepted as such, since there is an increased steady state of lactate production in these homogenates. Although any interpretation of these results in the heartworm group of dogs becomes pure speculation, it is possible that there are increased levels of activity in the later steps of the glycolytic pathway producing increased levels of ATP and thereby accelerating hexose monophosphate synthesis. The increased length of time during which the heartworm group of dogs had been exposed to conditions producing RVH and CHF may have been sufficient to cause changes in the glycolytic metabolic pathway which had not yet developed in the group with experimental hypertrophy.

Discussion

The finding of an increased proportion of muscle-type LDH isozyme in the hypertrophied ventricles lends support to the hypothesis that there is an adaptive metabolic change in the hypertrophied myocardial cell. The theories relating LDH isozymes to metabolic activity, however, are not entirely uncontested. It has been pointed out that pyruvate levels required to inhibit H-LDH *in vitro* are probably not attained *in vivo* (Vessell and Pool, 1966). Certain mammalian tissues utilizing anaerobic metabolism such as erythrocytes, platelets, and bovine lens fibers contain isozymes with predominantly the heart-type subunit (Vessel, 1965). In addition, certain fish are able to function with only one isozyme in both heart and skeletal muscle which appears to be homologous to LDH-5 of mammals (Markert, 1968). These discrepancies with the theory relating LDH isozyme function with a metabolic role have yet to be explained.

In addition to possible hypoxia due to increased diffusion distance in the hypertrophied myocardial cell, other factors must also be considered to explain the redistribution of LDH isozymes. Possible sources of the increased muscle-type LDH in hypertrophied myocardium include (1) contamination with tissues high in M-LDH; (2) systemic or local factors resulting in altered oxygen availability in the tissue; (3) new muscle cells or embryonic myocardium in the hypertrophied tissue; and (4) a hormonally related mechanism, perhaps associated with increased protein metabolism in the cell. The finding of increased amounts of M-LDH in the nonstressed and nonhypertrophied left ventricles of the dogs in this study and as previously reported by us (Bishop and Altschuld, 1969) is in contrast to the results of a similar study reported by Fox and Reed (1969). Our findings suggest that an increased work load on one ventricle results in alterations in the opposite ventricle as well. This phenomenon has also been noted with respect to decreased catecholamines (Chidsey *et al.*, 1964), decreased myofibrillar adenosine triphosphatase activity (Chandler *et al.*, 1967), increased hydroxyproline content (Buccino *et al.*, 1969), morphologically altered Z-bands (Bishop and Cole, 1969a), and increased cell length (Laks *et al.*, 1969) in nonstressed left ventricles from animals with right ventricular hypertrophy.

To minimize contamination with connective tissue, myocardial samples were carefully trimmed of fat, endocardium, epicardium, and large blood vessels. The participation of connective tissue elements in myocardial hypertrophy has not been clearly defined. A recent report indicated that hydroxyproline content is elevated in both ventricles of cats with experimental RVH (Buccino *et al.*, 1969), presumably the result of increased fibroblastic activity in the myocardium. Although the possibility that increased fibroblasts may be responsible for the increased proportion of M-LDH in hypertrophied hearts cannot be completely discounted, on the basis of histologic examination this appears unlikely. Only small amounts of increased connective tissue were found in hypertrophied right ventricles and there was no apparent correlation between those hearts with histologically evident increased connective tissue and LDH isozyme redistribution. The left ventricles did not have histologically demonstrable increased connective tissue.

Leukocytes contain predominantly the muscle-type of LDH isozyme (Fox and Reed, 1969) and therefore must be considered as possible contaminants. Histological examination of the myocardium did not reveal the presence of white blood cells, and LDH isozymes 4 and 5 which are the predominant ones in white blood cells, were not found in the electrophoresis gels of myocardial tissue.

Due to the difficulty in measuring cellular levels of oxygen in the working myocardium, there is no direct experimental evidence concerning the availability of oxygen at the cellular level in myocardial hypertrophy. Attempts to produce LDH isozyme redistribution by altering the oxygen and blood supply to the myocardium have yielded conflicting results. Experimental coronary artery stenosis to produce myocardial ischemia did not result in a shift in myocardial LDH isozymes in the absence of myocardial fibrosis (Fox and Reed, 1969). On the other hand, animals made hypoxic by exposure to simulated high altitudes did have an increase in myocardial

M-LDH in the absence of hypertrophy (Mager *et al.*, 1968). In addition, human myocardial tissue from patients with combined ischaemic heart disease and myocardial hypertrophy was found to have an increase in the amount of M-LDH. Either condition alone did not result in an alteration in the LDH isozyme pattern (Ballo and Messer, 1968). Although reported studies suggest a decreased level of oxygen is present in the subendocardial layers of the normal and stressed left ventricle (Kirk and Honig, 1964; Moss, 1966), no difference was found in LDH isozyme distribution in either left or right ventricular subendocardial or subepicardial myocardium of dogs with right ventricular hypertrophy (Fox and Reed, 1969).

Sobel *et al.* (1969) found an increased amount of M-LDH in the hypertrophied left ventricles of guinea pigs studied as early as two days after bands were placed on the ascending aorta. We have found an increased proportion of M-LDH in both ventricles of dogs which were killed with mild degrees of right ventricular hypertrophy and without evidence of congestive heart failure (unpublished observations). These findings suggest that a metabolic adaptive change takes place in the stressed myocardium during the early stages of hypertrophy. It should be noted that both of these models limit the cardiac output of the animal which may result in embarrassment of the coronary circulation. This would be especially true of the afterloaded ventricle with its increased requirement for blood flow and oxygen.

The possibility that new tissue which is added to the enlarging myocardium is biochemically similar to embryonic myocardium is quite attractive. Embryonic and young growing myocardial tissue, which is less susceptible to the effects of hypoxia than adult myocardium, contains greater amounts of M-LDH than adult myocardium (Dawson *et al.*, 1964). Available evidence would indicate that entirely new cells are not added to the heart during hypertrophy, at least during the early stages (Linzbach, 1960). It is possible, however, that those portions of the hypertrophying myocardial cell which are newly formed are metabolically similar to embryonic myocardial tissue and thereby contribute to the increased M-LDH in this tissue.

Kaplan (1966) has shown that various hormones may have a stimulatory effect on the isozymes of LDH. It is possible that the increased M-LDH found in hypertrophied myocardium is the result of hormonal action, perhaps through the stimulation of mRNA which is specific for M-LDH. Actinomycin will partially prevent the development of estradiol induced increased M-LDH in the rabbit uterus suggesting that newly synthesized mRNA is involved in the production of M-LDH (Kaplan, 1966).

The finding of an increased rate of lactate production and glucose uptake by anaerobically incubated homogenates of hypertrophied ventricles is additional evidence suggesting that hypertrophied myocardium utilizes anaerobic glycolytic metabolism to a greater degree than normal myocardium.

Although there is no general agreement, several studies have suggested that mitochondria isolated from hypertrophied failing myocardium have normal respiratory control and oxidative phosphorylation (Plaut and Gertler, 1959; Chidsey *et al.*, 1966; Sobel *et al.*, 1967; Stoner *et al.*, 1968) and that normal levels of ATP are present (Fox *et al.*, 1965; Chidsey *et al.*, 1966; Pool *et al.*, 1967). In the afterloaded heart, mitochondrial energy-producing mechanisms may nevertheless be inadequate to meet increased energy requirements. Depressed levels of creatine phosphate have been found in hypertrophied and failing myocardium (Fox *et al.*, 1965; Pool *et al.*, 1967) suggesting an imbalance between energy production and utilization. Our findings suggest that in the hypertrophied myocardium the oxidative mechanisms of energy production are augmented through utilization of the glycolytic pathway.

Few studies have been concerned with glycolytic metabolism in cardiac hypertrophy and congestive failure. Gudbjarnason *et al.* (1964) found increased activity of glyceraldehyde phosphate dehydrogenase in the myocardium of patients who died with congestive heart failure, lending further support for increased activity of the glycolytic pathway in this condition. In contrast to the present study, Schwartz and Lee (1962) found decreased anaerobic lactate production and glucose utilization in the cell-free supernatant of homogenized failing guinea pig ventricles. A possible explanation for this discrepancy resides in the fact that different systems were employed to measure anaerboic glycolysis. Schwartz and Lee incubated their homogenates with ATP and glucose, while ADP, glucose, and hexokinase were used in the present study. Only the reactions subsequent to the formation of glucose-6-phosphate are dependent on the activity of heart homogenate enzymes when ADP, glucose, and exogenous hexokinase are present. With this system as used in the present study, ADP is continuously regenerated, ATP concentrations are maintained at a low level, and inhibition of phosphofructokinase by high concentrations of ATP is avoided.

Glucose phosphorylation is not rate limiting in this system as shown by the fact that glucose-6-phosphate accumulates during incubation. Following fifteen minutes of incubation the glucose-6-phosphate concentration averaged 2.54 mM compared to 4.31 mM after 30 min of incubation. There were no significant differences between control and hypertrophied myocardium. The ATP necessary for phosphorylation of glucose is generated initially via the myokinase reaction (2 ADP $\leftrightarrow$ ATP + AMP) and subsequently from both myokinase activity and as a product of anaerobic glycolysis.

Further evidence supporting use of glucose, ADP, and hexokinase rather than glucose and ATP to measure anaerobic glycolysis has recently been presented (Altschuld *et al.*, 1969). Lactic acid production by heart homogenates incubated with glucose and hexokinase was greater than that obtained by incubating with an equal amount of glucose-6-phosphate. Moreover, lactic acid production from fructose-1,6-diphosphate was less than that from glucose and hexokinase or glucose-6-phosphate. The inclusion of an ATP consuming system (2-deoxyglucose plus hexokinase) greatly enhanced lactic acid production from glucose-6-phosphate and fructose-1,6-diphosphate. It would appear, therefore, that continual removal of ATP is necessary for a maximal rate of anaerobic glycolysis.

Wittels and Spann (1968) recently reported that in cardiac hypertrophy and congestive failure in the guinea pig there is defective oxidation of fatty acids associated with decreased levels of carnitine necessary for transport of fatty acids into mitochondria. They found that although fatty acid oxidation was decreased, glucose oxidation was not impaired in homogenates of hypertrophied failing guinea pig ventricles. They suggested, in agreement with the present study, that the failing heart may be forced to utilize pathways other than fatty acid oxidation for ATP production. Further experimental evidence is required to define the mechanisms involved in the LDH isozyme redistribution and increased capacity for *in vitro* glycolytic metabolism demonstrated in the hypertrophied dog heart.

Acknowledgments

Supported in part by grant GM 1052 and a program project grant (HE-09884) from the USPHS and a research grant from the Ohio Heart Association.

References

Adcock, J. L. (1961). *Amer. J. Vet. Res.* **22,** 655.

Altschuld, R. A., Weiss, A., Kruger, F. A., and Weissler, A. M. (1969). *J. Clin. Invest.* **48,** 1905.

Appella, E., and Markert, C. (1961). *Biochem. Biophys. Res. Commun.* **6,** 171.

Argus, M. F., Arcos, J. C., Sardesai, V. M., and Overby, J. L. (1964). *Proc. Soc. Exp. Biol. Med.* **117,** 380.

Ballo, I. M., and Messer, J. V. (1968). *Biochem. Biophys. Res. Commun.* **33,** 487.

Bishop, S. P., and Altschuld, R. A. (1970). *Amer. J. Physiol.* **218,** 153.

Bishop, S. P., and Cole, C. R. (1969a). *Lab. Invest.* **20,** 219.

Bishop, S. P., and Cole, C. R. (1969b). *J. Appl. Physiol.* **26,** 659.

Buccino, R. A., Harris, E., Spann, J. F., Jr., and Sonnenblick, E. H. (1969). *Amer. J. Physiol.* **216,** 425.

Bücher, T., and Hohorst, H. J. (1963). *In* "Methods of Enzymatic Analysis" (H. U. Bergmeyer, ed.), p. 246. Academic Press, New York.

Cahn, R. D., Kaplan, N. O., Levine, L., and Zwilling, E. (1962). *Science* **136,** 965.

Chance, B., Holmes, W., Higgins, J., and Connelly, C. M. (1958). *Nature* (*London*) **182,** 1190.

Chandler, B. M., Sonnenblick, E. H., Spann, J. F., Jr., and Pool, P. E. (1967). *Circ. Res.* **21,** 717.

Chidsey, C. A., Kaiser, G. A., Sonnenblick, E. H., Spann, J. F., and Braunwald, E. (1964). *J. Clin. Invest.* **43,** 2386.

Chidsey, C. A., Weinbach, E. C., Pool, P. E., and Morrow, A. G. (1966). *J. Clin. Invest.* **45,** 40.
Davis, B. J. (1964). *Ann. N.Y. Acad. Sci.* **121,** 404.
Dawson, D. M., Goodfriend, T. C., and Kaplan, N. D. (1964). *Science* **143,** 929.
Detweiler, D. K., and Patterson, D. F. (1965). *Ann. N.Y. Acad. Sci.* **127,** 481.
Fox, A. C., and Reed, G. E. (1969). *Amer. J. Physiol.* **216,** 1026.
Fox, A. C., Wikler, N. S., and Reed, G. E. (1965). *J. Clin. Invest.* **44,** 202.
Goldberg, E., and Cather, J. N. (1963). *J. Cell. Comp. Physiol.* **61,** 31.
Gudbjarnason, S., DeSchryver, C., Hunn, G., and Bing, R. J. (1964). *J. Lab. Clin. Med.* **65,** 796.
Hohorst, H. J. (1963). *In* "Methods of Enzymatic Analysis" (H. U. Bergmeyer, ed.), p. 134. Academic Press.
Johansson, G. (1966). *Exp. Cell Res.* **43,** 95.
Kaplan, N. O. (1966). *J. Cell. Comp. Physiol.* **66,** 1.
Karsner, H. T., Saphir, O., and Todd, T. W. (1925). *Amer. J. Pathol.* **1,** 351.
Kirk, E. S., and Honig, G. R. (1964). *Amer. J. Physiol.* **207,** 661.
Laks, M. M., Morady, F., and Swan, H. J. C. (1969). *Circ. Res.* **24,** 705.
Lindemayer, G. E., Sordahl, L. A., and Schwartz, A. (1968). *Circ. Res.* **23,** 439.
Lindy, S., and Rajasalmi, M. (1966). *Science* **153,** 1401.
Linzbach, A. J. (1960). *Amer. J. Cardiol.* **5,** 370.
Mager, M., Blatt, W. F., Natale, P. J., and Blatters, C. M. (1968). *Amer. J. Physiol.* **215,** 8.
Markert, C. L. (1963). *Science* **140,** 1439.
Markert, C. L. (1968). *Ann. N.Y. Acad. Sci.* **151,** 14.
Moss, A. J. (1966). *Circulation* **34,** Suppl. 3, 176.
Plaut, G. W. E., and Gertler, M. M. (1959). *Ann. N.Y. Acad. Sci.* **72,** 515.
Pool, P. E., Spann, J. F., Jr., Buccino, R. A., Sonnenblick, E. H., and Braunwald, E. (1967). *Circ. Res.* **21,** 365.
Potter, V. R. (1957). *In* "Manometric Techniques" (W. W. Unbreit, R. H. Burris, and J. F. Stauffer, eds.), p. 182. Burgess, Minneapolis, Minesota.
Scholz, R., Schmitz, H., Bücher, T., and Lampen, J. O. (1959). *Biochem. Z.* **331,** 71.
Schwartz, A., and Lee, K. S. (1962). *Circ. Res.* **10,** 321.
Sobel, B. E., Spann, J. F., Jr., Pool, P. E., Sonnenblick, E. H., and Braunwald, E. (1967). *Circ. Res.* **21,** 355.
Sobel, B. E., Henry, P. D., and Bloor, C. M. (1969). *Fed. Proc. Fed. Amer. Soc. Exp. Biol.* **28,** 451.
Stoner, C. D., Ressalat, M. M., and Sirak, H. D. (1968). *Circ. Res.* **23,** 87.
Thorling, E. B., and Jensen, K. (1966). *Acta Pathol. Microbiol. Scand.* **66,** 426.
Vessell, E. S. (1965). *Science* **150,** 1735.
Vessell, E. S., and Pool, P. E. (1966). *Proc. Nat. Acad. Sci. U.S.* **55,** 756.
Vessell, E. S., Osterland, K., Bearn, A. G., and Kunkel, H. G. (1962). *J. Clin. Invest.* **41,** 2012.
Wearn, J. T. (1940). *Harvey Lect.* **35,** 243.
Wittels, B., and Spann, J. F., Jr. (1968). *J. Clin. Invest.* **47,** 1787.
Wollenberger, A., Kleitke, B., and Raabe, G. (1963). *Exp. Mol. Pathol.* **2,** 251.
Wroblewski, F., and LaDue, J. S. (1955). *Proc. Soc. Exp. Biol. Med.* **90,** 210.
Zondag, H. A. (1963). *Science* **143,** 965.

Part VII
Electrical Correlates of the Hypertrophied Heart

INTRODUCTION TO "ADVANCED" ELECTROCARDIOGRAPHY IN CARDIAC HYPERTROPHY

A. C. L. Barnard

Introduction

The present chapter concerns electrocardiographic diagnosis, particularly diagnosis of hypertrophy, using methods still in the research stage. These methods offer the hope of more detailed diagnosis, at the expense of being more complicated than conventional electrocardiography. For want of a better term, the methods may be called "advanced." The use of the quotation marks denotes an awareness that this appellation must be earned rather than claimed.

Information Flow in Diagnosis

To gain a perspective on "advanced" electrocardiography, it is convenient first to generalize about the electrocardiographic diagnostic process. As indicated in Fig. 1, electrical measurements of some kind are made somewhere on the individual. The measurements then undergo processing by an external device and the results are displayed to the cardiologist. Internal processing of the information occurs in the cardiologist's mind, and finally a conclusion is enunciated.

Figure 1 is a generalized information flow diagram and in certain methods some of the stages may be absent. For instance, in conventional scalar electrocardiography there is essentially no external processing, the raw data being presented directly to the cardiologist. Frank-lead vectorcardiography provides an example of a method with simple external processing: The measured waveforms are combined by a resistor network before being seen by the cardiologist.

The most common measurement is of potential waveforms at points on

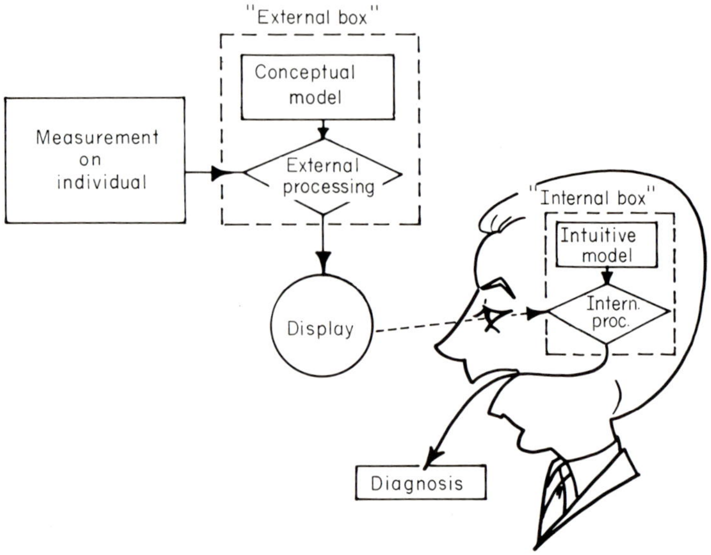

FIG. 1. Schematic diagram of information flow in the generalized diagnosis process.

the body surface, but other quantities, such as resistivity, and other locations, such as the epicardial surface, can be used. In particular situations, such unconventional measurements assume considerable importance.

Research workers hoping to develop new methods of electrocardiographic diagnosis focus their attention on the "external box" of Fig. 1. If we want a certain amount of diagnostic information to come out of the complete procedure, then the complexity of the internal and external boxes is complementary. If the external box is extremely simple or absent, raw data are presented to the cardiologist. The whole information-processing load is then thrown on him and his thought processes must be correspondingly complex. Making the external box more elaborate can leave the cardiologist with a simpler task.

In the present crisis of medical manpower, it is clearly desirable to investigate the possibility of taking the load off the cardiologist by making the external processing more elaborate. This could also afford side benefits, since some operations which are executed slowly and imprecisely in the human mind are performed rapidly and accurately by some machines, particularly computers. Thus, some methods which would be impossibly tedious when performed by the human mind become trivial when accomplished by computer, and the possibility of more accurate and extensive diagnosis arises. A word of caution should be inserted here, however. There is no guarantee that more elaborate methods will give better diagnosis than simple methods!

The responsibility is squarely on the research worker to show that elaboration is not done for its own sake, but is justified in some way, such as improved diagnosis.

The External Box

Conceptual Models in Diagnosis

Consider now the external box of Fig. 1 in more detail. In electrocardiography the external processing may involve a conceptual model of the heart as an electrical source and the thorax as an electrical conductor. Such a two-step model can be used to relate body surface potentials to myocardial excitation. The use of an external model is not mandatory, however, e.g., the measured data could be organized into a convenient display, such as an isopotential map, which could then be studied by a cardiologist. According to Schmitt (1961), we should then think of the cardiologist as using a "fuzzy and intuitive" mental model to relate surface events to those in the myocardium.

Table I shows the external processing methods used by four authors and indicates whether or not the methods involve a model.

TABLE I

External Processing Methods

Method	Model?	Presentation
Display isopotential maps	No	Boineau
Multipoles	Yes	Geselowitz
Multiple dipoles	Yes	Holt
Moving dipole sheet	Yes	Selvester (1970)

Forward and Inverse Modes of Model Usage

It is convenient to distinguish two modes in which a model may be used to relate events on the surface and in the myocardium. In either case we have a model source, with certain adjustable parameters, which is coupled with a thoracic model to give events on the thoracic surface.

The "forward" or "direct" mode is the simpler, since it proceeds logically from cause to effect. Various choices are made for the values of the source model parameters, and the surface effects are evaluated for each choice. These synthetic effects may be compared with those actually observed, to determine which source parameter values are most appropriate.

In the situation encountered clinically, it is more convenient to use the model in the "inverse" mode. In this procedure, the surface measurements themselves are used to calculate the most appropriate values of the source model parameters.

Outline of Projects

We can now put the work presented by Boineau, Selvester (1970), Geselowitz, and Holt in perspective. This is shown in Table II.

Discussion

The use of a model may be viewed as a data-reduction device. Less information is transmitted to the cardiologist than is present in the raw data. If the model is well chosen, the information lost is of low diagnostic value—that is, the model generates a meaningful abstract of the raw data. This is something that remains to be proved for the 12-dipole and the dipole–quadrupole approaches described by Holt and Geselowitz, respectively. On the other hand, if the isopotential mapping approach described by Dr. Boineau is used as a diagnostic method, essentially all the information is transmitted to the cardiologist, and he is left to make his own abstract.

At the present state of the art, it would be wise to continue work on all of these methods. However, if at some future time it could be shown that one of the machine-generated abstracts enables the cardiologist to make as good a diagnosis as the abstract he develops himself, then presumably this method could be adopted and the load on the cardiologist thereby reduced.

It is interesting to compare the multipole and multiple dipole approaches, since their advantages and disadvantages are opposite. To see this, divide either method into two stages.

1. Obtain the model parameters (dipole or multipole strengths) from the measured data.

2. Deduce the myocardial condition and behavior from the model parameters.

The multipole approach is very elegant in the first stage. An infinite series of orthogonal functions is available and can be used to represent the data to any desired degree of accuracy merely by taking more and more terms. On the other hand, when the multiple dipole model is used, the construction of the dipole set is somewhat arbitrary. The effects of changing it, for example, by adding another dipole in the hope of improving the representation of a certain myocardial segment, are not entirely predictable. The number of dipoles probably cannot be increased indiscriminately, because the problem may become ill-conditioned.

TABLE II

OUTLINE OF PROJECTS

	Measurement		Model		
Author	Quantity	Location	Source	Thorax	Mode
Boineau	Potential	Skin Epicardium Intramyocardium	—	—	—
Selvester (1970)	—	—	Moving dipole sheet	?	Forward
Geselowitz	Potential	Skin	Multipoles	Homogeneous realistic shape	Inverse
Holt	Potential	Skin	12-Dipole	Inhomogeneous realistic shape	Inverse

However, in the second stage the rankings are reversed. The multiple dipole model becomes much more convenient, since it is simple to interpret. The relationship between the dipole strength curve and the dimensions of the myocardial segment was hypothesized years ago by Selvester *et al.* (1965), and the hypothesis seems to be borne out by the work presented by Holt. Thus, for example, high dipole activity in the left ventricular free wall implies hypertrophy. In contrast, when the multipole approach is used the meaning of, for example, one of the quadrupole moments being abnormally negative is far from obvious.

Acknowledgment

Preparation of this manuscript was supported by UHPHS grant HE 11310.

References

Schmitt, O. H. (1961). *In* "Differentiation between Normal and Abnormal in Electrocardiography" (Ernst Simonson, ed.), Mosby, St. Louis, Missouri.

Selvester, R. H. (1970). Unpublished data.

Selvester, R. H., Collier, C. R., and Pearson, R. B. (1965). *Circulation* **31**, 45.

BASIS OF THE ELECTRICAL FIELD SURROUNDING THE HYPERTROPHIED RIGHT VENTRICLE

John P. Boineau and E. Neil Moore

Introduction

During excitation and recovery of the myocardium, an electrical field is produced which is distributed throughout the body. The characteristics of this field can be described by its intensity, its distribution, and its time course. Although it is well known that this field has characteristic variations that can be correlated with differences in shape, size, and state of the heart, the parameters that result in variation of the cardiac field are not well understood.

Linzbach (1960) has shown that in concentric hypertrophy the increased mass is primarily the result of an increase in cell volume (length and diameter). Others have speculated as to the effect of an increase in cell volume, as well as an increase in cell population, on the cardiac electrophysiology during excitation of the myocardium. The question is whether the increased potentials recorded from the body surface in RVH are a result of changes in the number of cells, or to the properties of individual cells, or to the more global effects of the total activation distribution and balance. Uhley (1961) has suggested that the transmembrane potentials of hypertrophied cardiac muscle are normal. If the transmembrane potentials are the same for normal and hypertrophied myocardium, what causes the difference in the field generated in the torso during activation?

The present studies were undertaken to determine quantitatively the parameters that result in an altered electrical field during ventricular activation of the hypertrophied myocardium.

Methods

Body Surface Potentials

Body surface potentials were recorded from normal dogs and dogs with spontaneous right ventricular hypertrophy (Fig. 1) through a McFee and Parungao, 1961) resistor network and also from 150 points over the torso surface. Both XYZ displays and equipotential contour maps were obtained in all subjects studied. The technique of producing equipotential maps has been described previously (Boineau *et al.*, 1966). These maps display the relationship between instantaneous potentials at all 150 locations. The maps are produced for each millisecond of QRS, and the time course of the electrical field is followed by inspection of a series of instantaneous potential distributions.

Ventricular Activation

Bipolar electrograms were recorded from the epicardial surface of the exposed dogs' hearts, and from intramural electrodes placed in the ventricular walls and septum. The local activation of various regions of the heart can be determined from the peaks of bipolar signals recorded from electrodes in these areas. Time alignment is accomplished by relating the individual peaks to a constantly recorded bipolar reference signal (Boineau *et al.*, 1968).

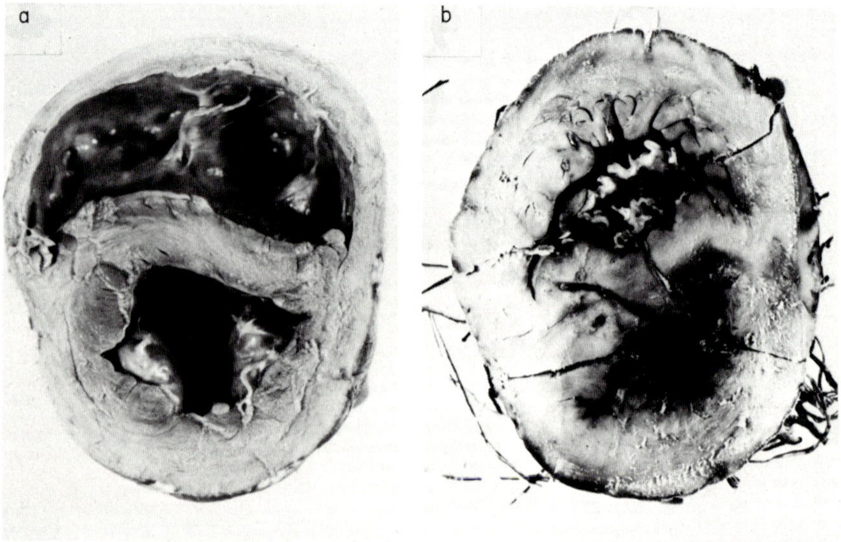

FIG. 1. Cross sections at midventricular level of a normal dog's heart (a) and a dog with RVH (b).

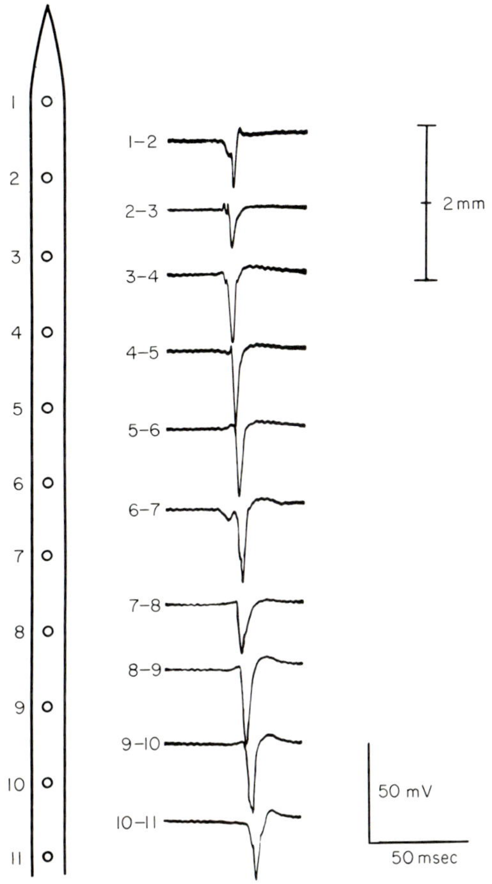

FIG. 2. Bipolar potentials recorded from an intramural multipoint electrode. The peaks of the bipolar tracings occur progressively later from point 1 near the endocardium to point 10 nearest the epicardium.

Figure 2 shows the bipolar potentials recorded from an electrode in a dog with right ventricular hypertrophy. The electrode terminals are 1 mm apart, and the potentials are recorded from between adjacent points. The peaks of the bipolar tracings occur progressively later from point 1 near the endocardium to point 10 nearest the epicardium. The intramural propagation velocity was 0.4 mm/msec, which is normal. Also, note that the potentials are smaller near the endocardium of the ventricle. The voltages were similar to those recorded from the normal left ventricle. Purkinje potentials were frequently recorded from endocardial areas of the right ventricle and there was no evidence of delay in endocardial excitation.

The relationship between ventricular thickness and the length (area) of the dipole layer is demonstrated in Fig. 3. A section through a normal right ventricle is shown above, and a section through a hypertrophied right ventricle, below. The dark lines represent the instantaneous activation front. The activation time in milliseconds is indicated in the bar graph below each section on the left, and time zero in relationship to the QRS complex recorded in lead II is shown below each section on the right. Note that the thicker ventricle permits a greater length (area) of the dipole layer. In the normal right ventricle (above), a wide dipole layer is present for only 5 msec, whereas in the hypertrophied right ventricle (below), a wider dipole layer exists for more than 10 msec. Assuming that the dipole moment per unit area of wavefront is the same in normal and hypertrophied muscle, the greater area of the wavefront in the thicker ventricle would result in a greater number of instantaneous generators, and this situation would persist for a longer period of QRS.

An indication of the relationship between generator activity and ventricular wall thickness is illustrated in Fig. 4. In this figure, peak bipolar potential is

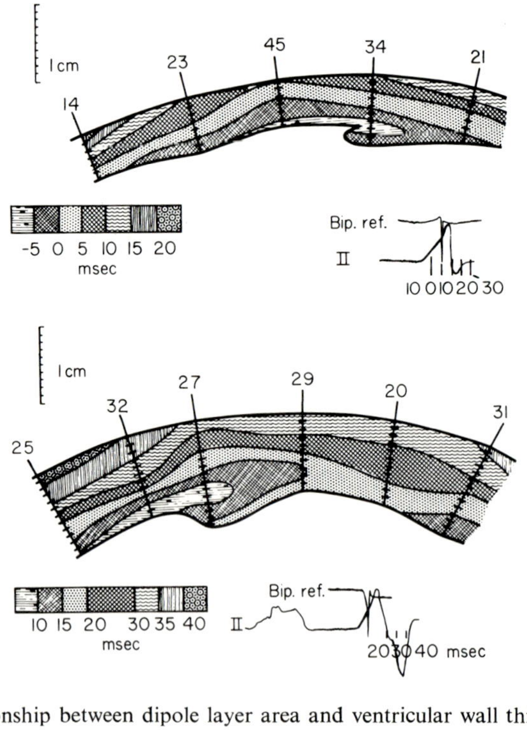

FIG. 3. Relationship between dipole layer area and ventricular wall thickness. Normal dog above. Dog with RVH below. The length of the activation front, the phase of ventricular activity in relationship to the total period of QRS are indicated.

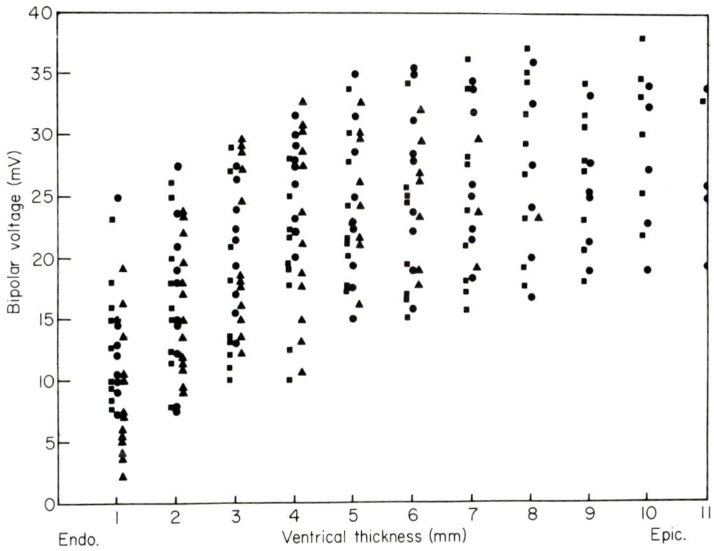

FIG. 4. Relationship between bipolar voltage and ventricular wall thickness. Peak bipolar potentials recorded from intramural electrodes at 1-mm increments from endocardium to epicardium. These potentials were recorded from ▲, the normal dog's right ventricle (NRV); ■, the normal left ventricle (NLV); and ●, from the right ventricle in dogs with right ventricular hypertrophy (RVH).

plotted against the intramural depth at which these potentials were recorded, in normal right ventricles (NRV), normal left ventricles (NLV), and in hypertrophied right ventricles (RVH). Although there is a wide distribution in peak voltage at each intramural level, there is an obvious trend of increasing peak potential from endocardium to epicardium. This trend is most obvious in the inner half of the ventricles and tends to level out in the outer half of the ventricles. There is considerable overlap in the results for normal right ventricle, normal left ventricle, and RVH. Partial separation occurs only at the point 1 mm beneath the endocardial surface. The data suggest that discontinuous, asynchronous activation of the irregular endocardium produces nonuniformity in the initial activation. With propagation of this activity into more compact myocardium, the wavefront becomes more uniform and synchronous. Therefore, some increase in generator intensity would be expected away from the endocardium.

The global aspect of activation is determined experimentally by constructing isochronous maps depicting the sequence and distribution of activation of the ventricles. In Fig. 5, the normal sequence of epicardial excitation of the dog is shown in the anterior and left lateral views. The activation time in milliseconds is indicated in the bar graph below, and the frontal and left

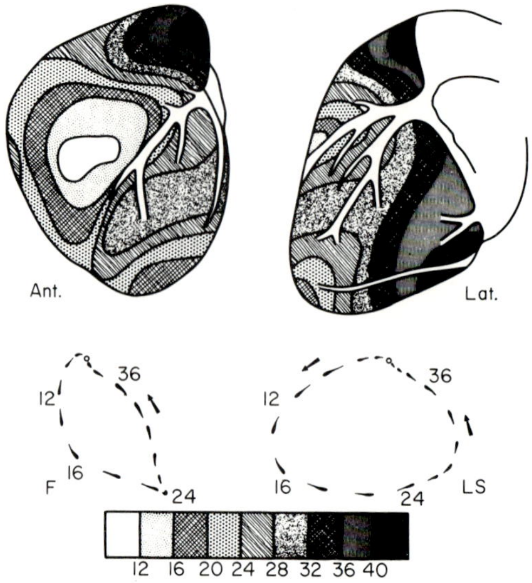

FIG. 5. The sequence of epicardial activation of the normal dog. Anterior and left lateral views are presented. Activation time in msec is indicated in the bar graph below and on the accompanying frontal (F) and left sagittal (LS) vectorcardiograms.

sagittal McFee vectorcardiograms are displayed for correlation with the activation data. Epicardial activity begins in the central right ventricle near the ventricular septum and spreads radially from this location. The earlier onset of epicardial activity in the right ventricle indicates an earlier completion of activity in this structure, whereas excitation persists in the left ventricle. The epicardial activity spreads in an anterior-to-posterior sequence. The intramural activation of a normal dog is shown in Fig. 6. Upon completion of activation moving through the thinner right ventricle, largely unopposed wavefronts are still present in the left ventricle. This balance of forces in favor of the left ventricle at 25 msec is shown here. Again, the McFee vectorcardiogram is presented for correlation with the activation data.

In Fig. 7, the sequence of epicardial activation of the anterior (ventral) and posterior (dorsal) surface of the heart in a dog with right ventricular hypertrophy is shown. The bar graph below indicates the activation time in milliseconds, and the frontal and left sagittal McFee vectorcardiograms are presented for correlation with the activation data. Note that in contrast to the normal dog, activation reaches the epicardium and terminates first in left ventricle. The intramural sequence of activation in this same dog is shown in Fig. 8. The thicker right ventricle permits a greater than normal area of the instantaneous dipole layer, and activation lasts longer. The electrical field produced by the large persistent wavefronts in the right ventricle is

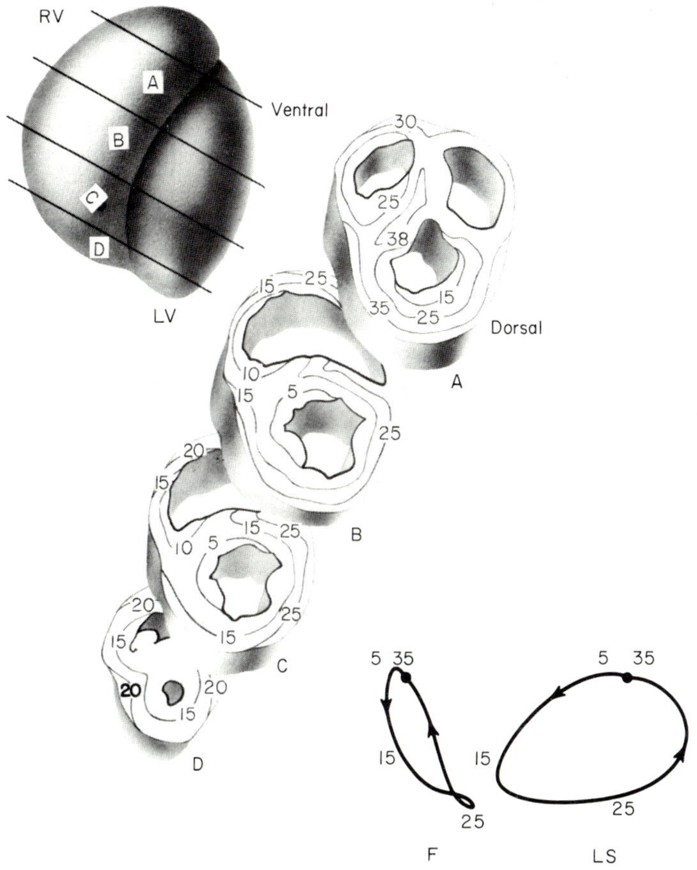

FIG. 6. Intramural ventricular activation in four sections of the normal dog's heart. F represents frontal; LS, left sagittal vectorcardiograms.

relatively unopposed by the effects of left ventricular generators, which terminate earlier.

The relationship between the instantaneous distribution of cardiac generators and the electrical field on the body surface during activation is shown in Fig. 9, in which (a) represents a normal dog, and (b) represents a dog with right ventricular hypertrophy. The equipotential distribution on the transparent torso surface is indicated. Maxima, or zones of highest positive potential are indicated by a plus sign, and minima or regions of highest negative potential are indicated by a minus sign. A transparent heart contained within the torso surface is shown, and the generator distribution during a specific instant of ventricular excitation is distributed within the walls of the transparent heart. These data were obtained from surface potentials and ventricular

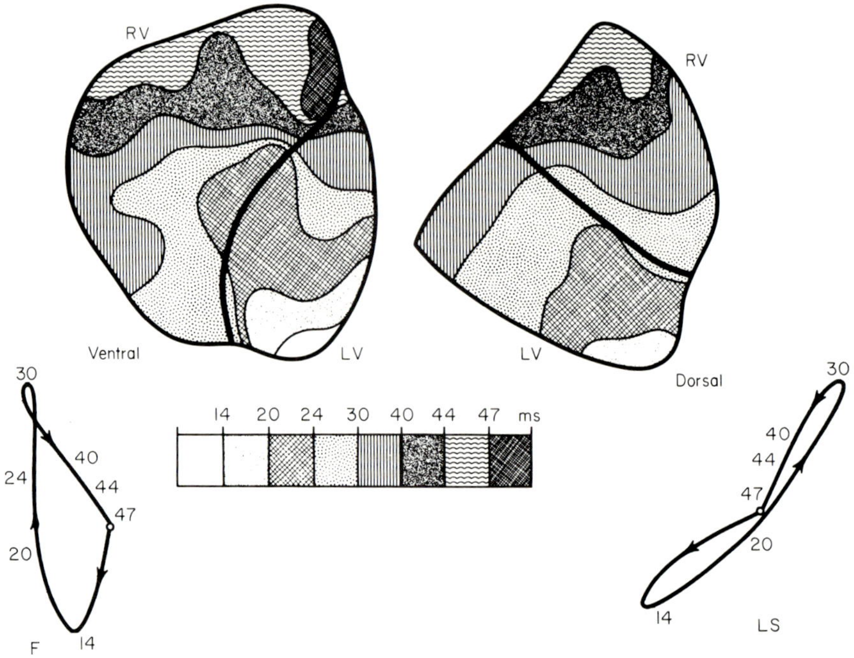

FIG. 7. The sequence of epicardial ventricular activation in a dog with right ventricular hypertrophy. Anterior (ventral) and posterior (dorsal) views are presented. The activation time in msec in indicated in the bar graph below and on the accompanying frontal (F) and left sagittal (LS) vectorcardiogram.

activation recorded from the same animals and time aligned. The surface of excitation is distributed over both ventricles, and its boundaries are determined by the natural discontinuities such as epicardium, endocardium, and valve areas. The torsos are viewed anteriorly and slightly to the dog's left in both cases. The anterior discontinuity in the generator surface represents the point at which the wavefront contacts the epicardium. The posterior boundary represents the point at which the wavefront contacts the endocardium or one of the other natural cardiac boundaries, such as the mitral and tricuspid valve areas. Activation moving toward the observer is indicated by positive charges, and activity moving away from the observer (posteriorly) is indicated by negative charges. Current flows toward the torso in areas overlying "outward" oriented generators (positive charges) and results in positive potentials on the torso in regions overlying these generators. Current flows inward from the torso in areas overlying "inward"-directed generators (negative charges) and results in negative surface potentials at these torso locations. Figures 9(a) and 9(b) represent similar instants at ~24 msec after the beginning of ventricular activation.

In the normal dog the wider surface area of LV generators, coupled with

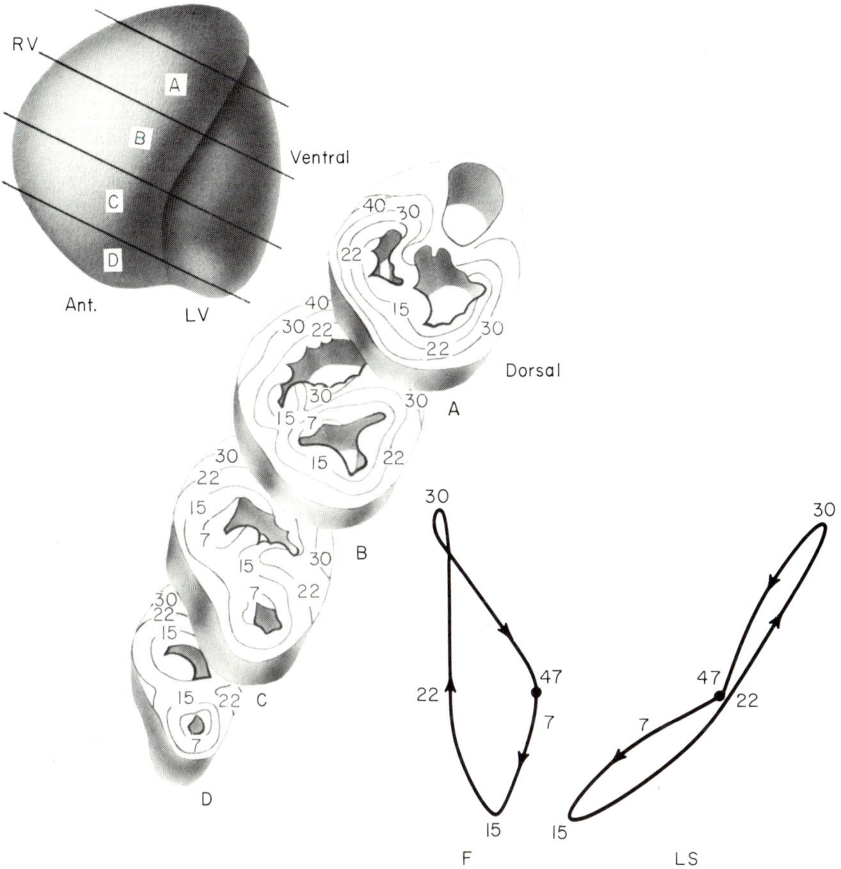

FIG. 8. Intramural ventricular activation in four sections of the dog's heart with right ventricular hypertrophy. This heart is the same as the one shown in Fig. 7.

the anterior "opening" in the activation front (primarily over the right ventricle, but also the anterior left ventricle), results in an anterior minimum. There is also a minimum on the right lateral chest, and an intermediate relative maximum or "saddle," so that the potential distribution is non-dipolar (Taccardi, 1963). The relative maximum results from the outward current from RV generators, which is superimposed on the predominantly negative field caused by LV activity at this instant. This distribution results from the earlier termination of activity in the thinner right ventricle, while broad wavefronts of activity still persist in the left ventricle.

In the dog with RV hypertrophy [Fig. 9(b)], activity terminates earlier in the left ventricle, and there is persistence of a wide surface of generators in the thicker right ventricle, resulting in a characteristically different potential distribution on the torso.

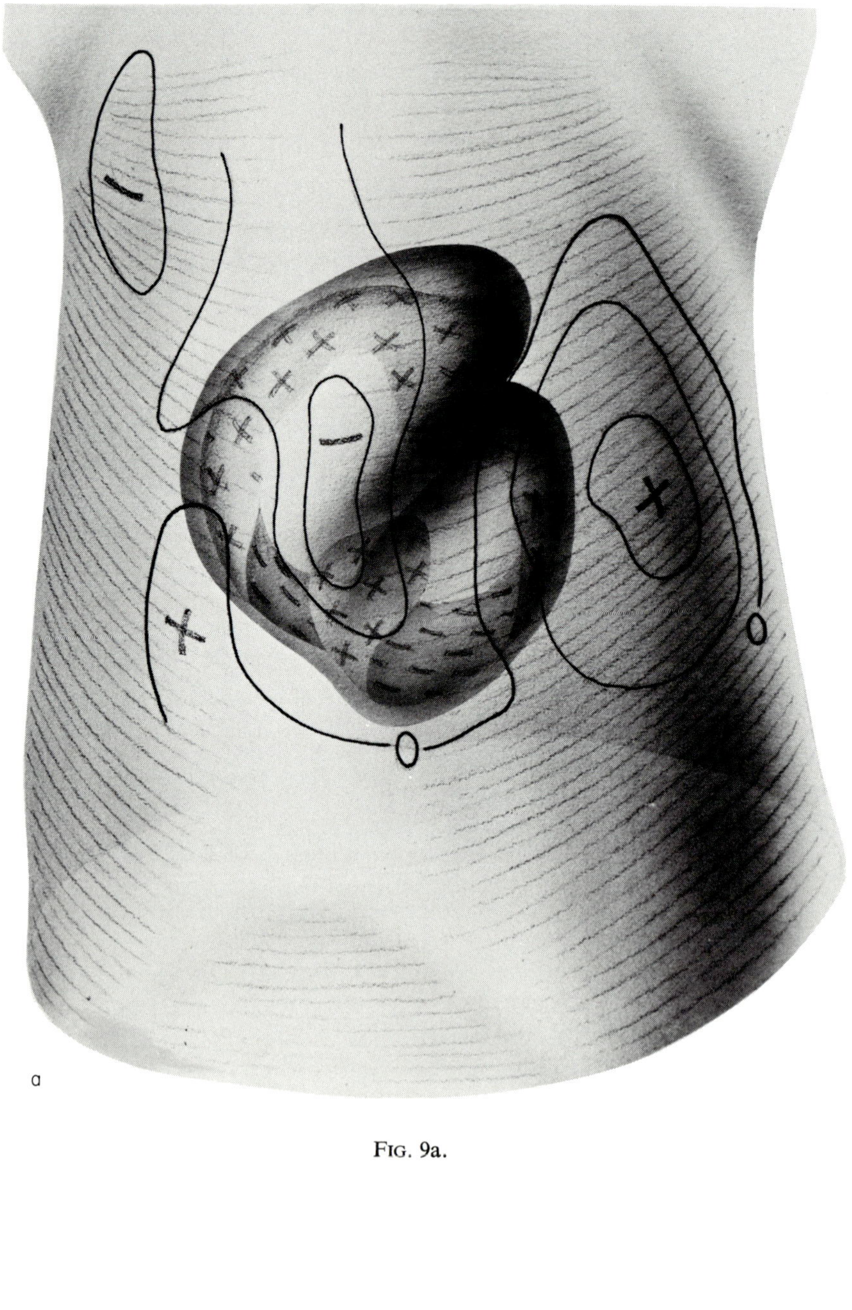

FIG. 9a.

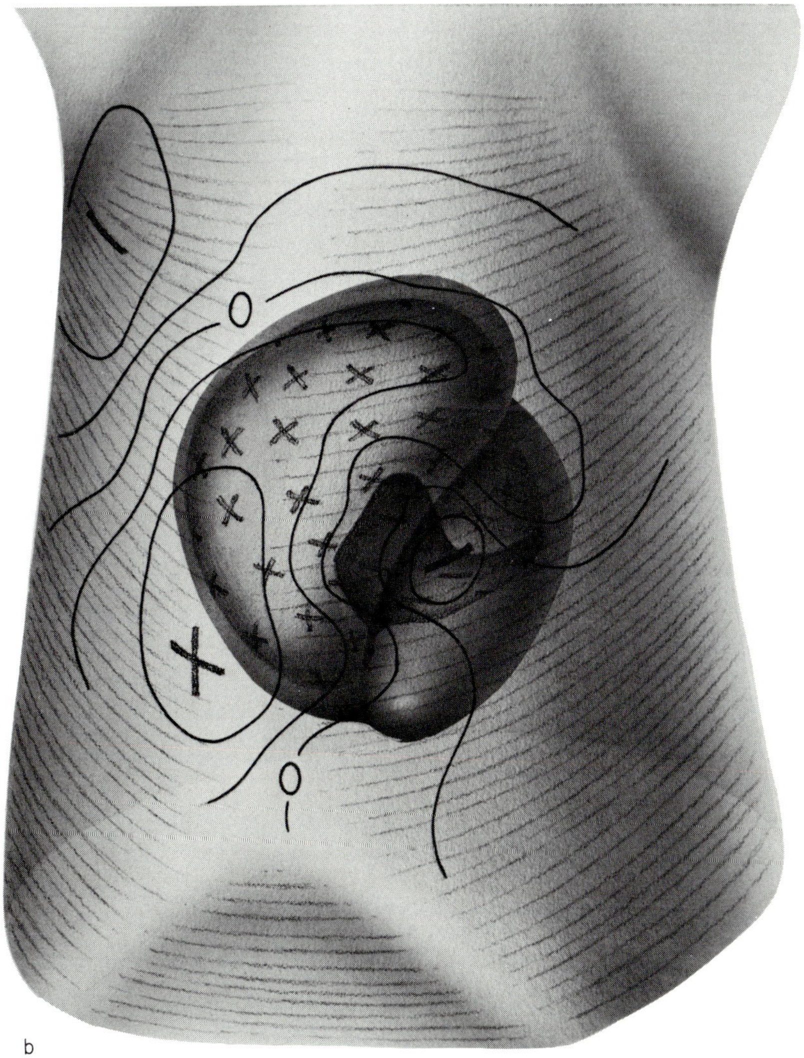

b

FIG. 9b. Relationship between electrical field (torso potentials) and cardiac generator distribution in a normal dog (a), and in a dog with RV hypertrophy (b). This figure is a representation of the generator distribution and surface potentials for the 24-msec instant after the beginning of ventricular excitation.

Although these latter illustrations are derived from physiological studies, the events can also be simulated with a mathematical model. The model is based on a numerical technique of Barr *et al.* (1966) and its physical characteristics are based on geometric and physiologic measurements made in one normal dog (Boineau *et al.*, 1967). Figure 10 illustrates the measurement of

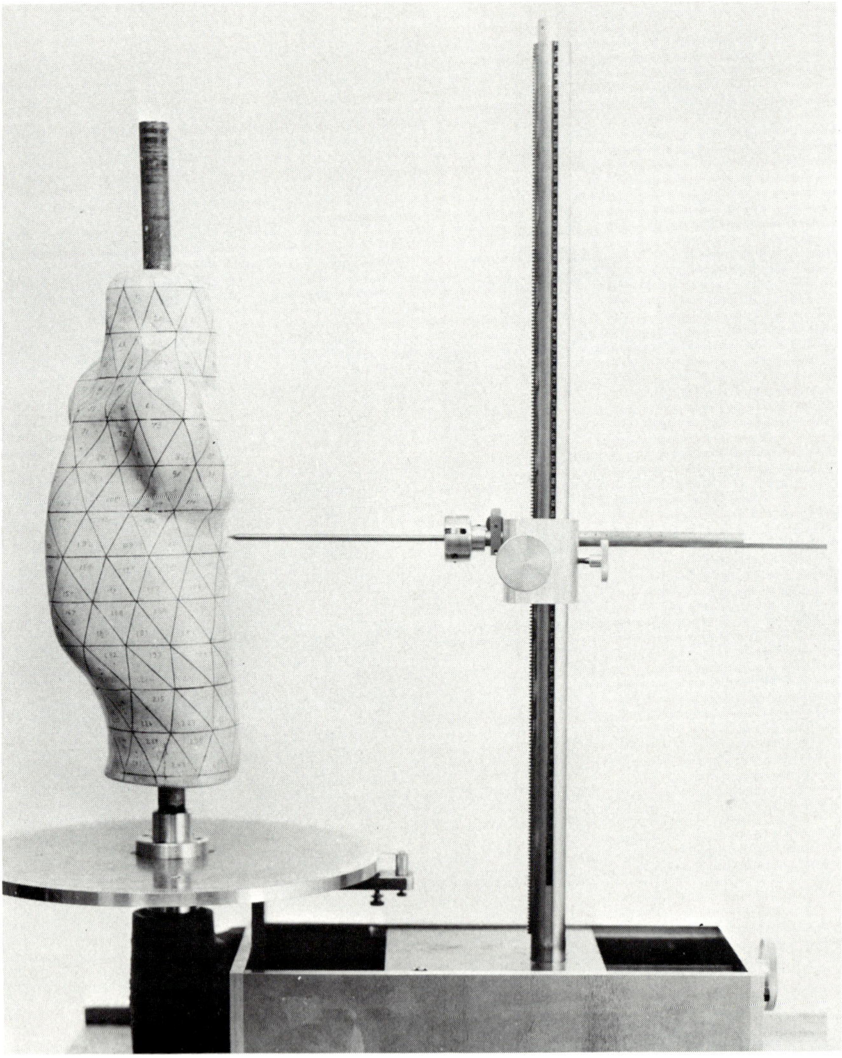

FIG. 10. The physical model of the torso, used in a mathematical-physical model of the electrocardiogram of the dog. Coordinates are determined for the torso model by the measuring apparatus on the right.

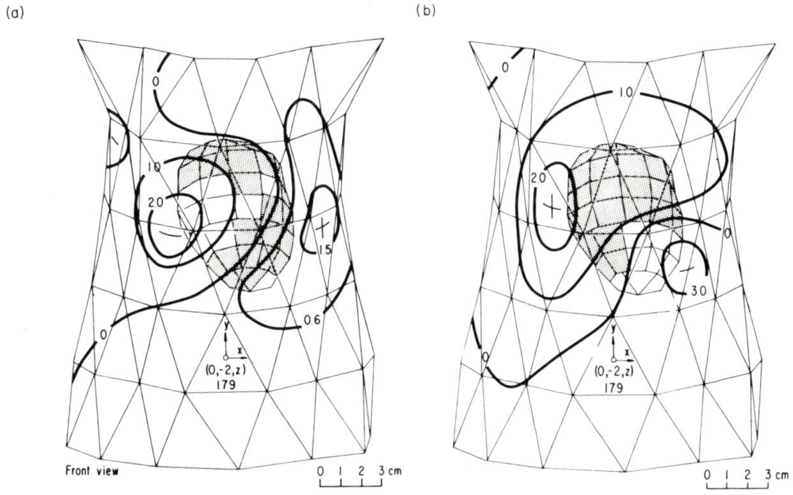

FIG. 11. Simulation of the body surface equipotential distribution for an instant in normal ventricular activation (a), and for an instant in activation of a dog with RV hypertrophy (b). A partial representation of the torso surrounding the heart is shown. The equipotentials are indicated on the torso. The stippled segments of the heart represent instantaneously active generators and the nonstippled cardiac segments represent generators which have recently "turned off," simulating epicardial breakthrough. Note the similarity of the equipotential distribution in these two examples to the distributions of potential in the normal and RV hypertrophy dog in Fig. 9.

the torso model constructed from this dog. The heart of this dog was similarly measured and was related to the torso using X rays and cineangiocardiograms. Cardiac generator activity in this model was simulated by dividing up the heart into 76 segments which could be turned on or off according to the sequence of activation recorded from the dog on which the model was based.

Figure 11 shows the torso potentials and generator activity at 24 msec in a normal dog (a), and in a dog with right ventricular hypertrophy (b). The stippled segments within the heart represent generators which are active. The unstippled segments of the model heart represents areas where activity has broken through to the epicardium and terminated. In Fig. 11(a), the simulated potentials resemble those recorded for this instant in time in the normal dog illustrated in Fig. 9(a), and in Fig. 11(b) the simulated equipotentials are quite similar to those recorded from a dog with spontaneous right ventricular hypertrophy in Fig. 9(b). The respective generator configurations are also similar. The effect of individual generators acting singularly and in groups can be studied by this technique. Since the simulated potentials closely resemble those recorded from the living subjects, and because the sequence of activation is based on physiological data obtained in a living dog, succinct conclusions as to the relationship between generators and the electrical field in hypertrophy can be reached.

Discussion

The data suggest that the increased intensity of the electrical field in ventricular hypertrophy is the result of the following:

(1) An increase in the dipole layer area which can be accommodated by a thicker ventricle. Since the surface of activity is not absolutely parallel with the endocardial and epicardial surfaces, but is somewhat oblique, its area must increase with increased ventricular thickness. The result is that more dipoles of the same density per unit area of the active surface are present at any instant in the wavefront.

(2) Slight increase in the generator EMF in the outer ventricular wall of the thicker right ventricle: The normal right ventricle is heavily trabeculated and in many areas quite thin (less than 4 mm). The potentials recorded from these thin areas are quite small in comparison to potentials in the outer half of the normal left ventricle, or a thickened right ventricle. This effect is not related to an increase in the dipole moment of single fibers, but is a physical effect resulting from greater homogeneity of the wavefront as it departs the endocardial boundary.

(3) The prolonged phase of RV activation results in an altered balance between right and left ventricular activity: The result is a larger area of RV activity, which persists longer and is decreasingly opposed by activity generated by LV generators.

These three factors contribute to the increased intensity of the electrical field of the hypertrophied right ventricle. There may be other factors, such as changes in tissue resistivity in RVH, which might also be important variables.

The distribution and time course of the electrical field and potentials on the body are largely determined by the distribution of wavefronts of intramural activity and the sequence of epicardial activation. These parameters can be simulated by a mathematical-physical model, which allows a more exact determination of the mechanism.

The questions of cell size and population in ventricular hypertrophy, the intensity of the *single cell* generator, and their relationship to the altered electrical field are irrelevant. The myocardium functions as an electrical matrix and the determinants of the external field on the body are unrelated, or are only indirectly related, to transmembrane potentials. The characteristics of the field can be related, however, to the features of the *global* activation front which is itself shaped and modified by variations in cardiac structure.

Acknowledgments

This work was supported in part by USPHS Grants HE-5732, HE-5716, HE-11307, HE-4885, and HE-10995; and Grants from the North Carolina Heart Association and the American Heart Association.

References

Barr, R. C., Pilkington, T. C., Boineau, J. P., and Spach, M. S. (1966). *IEEE Trans. Bio-Med. Eng.* **13,** 88.
Boineau, J. P., Spach, M. S., Pilkington, T. C., and Barr, R. C. (1966). *Circ. Res.* **19,** 489.
Boineau, J. P., Pilkington, T. C., Rogers,. L., and Spach, M. S. (1967). *Digest of the 7th Int. Conf. Med. Biol. Eng.*p. 412.
Boineau, J. P., Hill, J. D., Spach, M. S., and Moore, E. N. (1968). *Amer. Heart J.* 76, 605.
Linzbach, A. J. (1960). *Amer. J. Cardiol.*, **5,** 370.
McFee, R., and Parungao, A. (1961). *Amer. Heart J.* **62,** 93.
Taccardi, B. (1963). *Circ. Res.* **12,** 341.
Uhley, H. N. (1961). *Amer. J. Cardiol.* 7, 211.

BODY SURFACE POTENTIALS IN VENTRICULAR HYPERTROPHY—ANALYSIS USING A MULTIPLE DIPOLE MODEL OF THE HEART

John H. Holt, Jr., Anthony C. L. Barnard, and John O. Kramer, Jr.

Introduction

Durrer (1966) has remarked that in the early days of electrocardiography, reading electrocardiograms was like identifying a stamp: One looked up in a book the illustration resembling as closely as possible the record considered. One then copied the legend of the illustration, and the job was finished. Burton (1965), on the other hand, chose the analogy of bird-watching, noting the similarity between statements such as, "If it has an orange strip just above big black beady eyes, ... it is a Wilson's Warbler," and definitions of electrocardiographic conditions.

These statements by Durrer and Burton were, of course, designed to shock their audience, and are repeated for the same purpose here. However, there is a serious point underlying the statements: Electrocardiography as we know it today has developed largely on an empirical basis, not on the basis of sound theory. In making this statement we do not imply that conventional electrocardiographic methods are invalid. For example, empirical correlations between electrocardiographic findings and those at autopsy are a perfectly good way to establish the validity of a technique. Indeed, in the last analysis, they are the only method of validating a clinical technique. However, in the absence of a theoretical understanding, one is always left with the nagging doubt that some other system of electrocardiography might work better than that which happened to be adopted.

This is the question considered by the various research workers in the field of "advanced" electrocardiography. None of them doubt the usefulness of conventional electrocardiography. All of them doubt that it is the optimal system for deducing the myocardial condition from potential measurements made on the body surface.

The work to be reported here was the outcome of a basic study of the relationship between electrical activity in the heart and potentials observed on the body surface. The method involves a multiple dipole model of the heart as an electrical source, a realistically shaped electrically inhomogeneous model of the thorax, and potential measurements at many points on the thoracic surface.

Models of the Heart as an Electrical Source

It has been known since the time of Helmholtz that it is not possible to take potentials measured on the surface of a volume and deduce the source that gave rise to them. There are an infinite number of source configurations which, when located within the volume, would produce identical surface potentials. Thus, if we pose the basic question of electrocardiography as "given the surface potentials, determine the source," we are forced to conclude that electrocardiography is impossible.

Luckily, the situation is not so inauspicious. We have more information about the source, which we can use to discriminate against the infinite number of possible sources that are of no interest (including those not located in the myocardium) and pick out source configurations that do interest us. That is, we use our additional information to form conceptual models of the heart as an electrical source, and we interpret the surface potentials in terms of these models.

The complication of biological systems is almost limitless, and any model which is of practical interest must involve drastic simplifications. By choosing approximations at each stage in a conscious and rational manner, we can be aware of both the limitations of and the alternatives to the model we eventually adopt. The ventricular myocardium contains very large numbers of cells, but in modeling normal depolarization an enormous simplification immediately arises because the cells are not electrically isolated and cardiac muscle is a functional syncytium. Work with intramyocardial electrodes (Scher, 1962; Durrer, 1966; Boineau and Moore, this volume) has shown that at each instant in time during the depolarization period, the cells depolarizing at that instant are not distributed randomly through the myocardium. Rather, they form a simpler geometric arrangement indicated by the surfaces in Fig. 1(a), where it is shown that sources of current lie on one side of the surface and sinks on the other. Thus, the surface can be regarded as a current dipole layer, which moves through the ventricular myocardium as time progresses through the QRS interval.

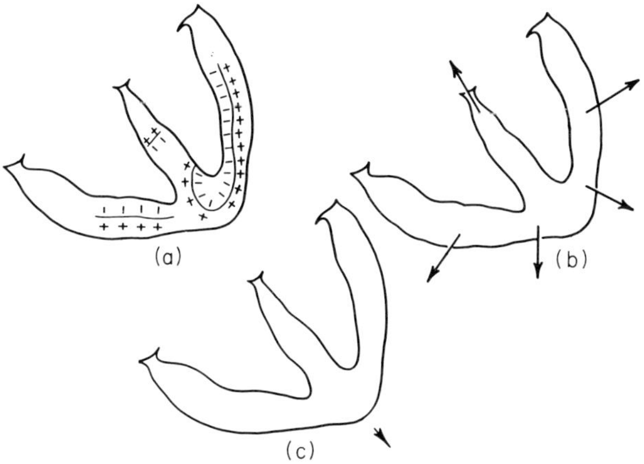

FIG. 1. Three possible models of the heart as an electrical source. (a) Most accurate; (c) least accurate. Multiple dipole model (b) is intermediate in accuracy.

The moving dipole layer is a possible model of the heart as an electrical source. It is studied, for example, by Selvester (1970). For our purposes, however, we must approximate further.

We can go to the extreme of simplification by approximating the dipole layer by a single dipole (the simplest possible battery), which is the resultant of all the elemental dipoles [Fig. 1(c)]. This "single dipole model" was used by Einthoven *et al.* (1913) and has dominated the development of electrocardiography. Its use is quite explicit in vectorcardiography, whose proponents claim that at any instant there are only three things to be known about the electrical heart, namely the three components of a single dipole.

We noted that any model is an approximation, and certainly the single dipole, indicated in Fig. 1(c), is only a crude approximation to the dipole layer in Fig. 1(a). Information has been discarded in making the transition from Fig. 1(a) to 1(c). To prove this, we need only note that it would be impossible to make the reverse transition: Given only the single resultant dipole we could not reconstruct the dipole layer. The vectorcardiographers are hopeful that the information discarded was not diagnostically useful, but this is far from obvious *a priori*. The only way to investigate this point is to test more accurate models, and see if they give better diagnoses than the single dipole model. This, in a nutshell, is the research program of any group working in "advanced electrocardiography." We might note, however, that the single dipole model makes very little sense from the point of view of modeling strategy. If we make the reasonable assumption that the objective of electrocardiography is to determine what occurs in different segments of the heart, then by choosing a single dipole model (in which the activity of the entire heart is lumped together), we automatically ensure that the model fails in this objective!

One way of looking at the information discarded in going from Fig. 1(a) to (c) is that the higher multipole moments of the source in Fig. 1(a) have been dropped. Thus, one approach to the problem is to include the next terms, the quadrupole terms, and see if any diagnostic improvement results. This is the course followed by Geselowitz and Briller, page 623.

Figure 1(b) shows an alternative approach. Instead of representing the dipole layer by one dipole, we use several dipoles. Obviously, the multiple dipole representation is more accurate than that with one dipole. Further, since each segment of myocardium is being represented by a dipole, if we can determine the behavior of this dipole in an individual, we can deduce the behavior of the particular myocardial segment in that individual.

Details of the Heart Model Used

When developing a conceptual model, it is necessary to decide what will be regarded as known, and therefore fixed in the model, and what will be regarded as unknown. The unknowns will form the variable parameters in the model. Deciding what is known may not appear arbitrary at first thought, but a little more reflection shows that it is, in fact, somewhat arbitrary. As a relevant example, let us consider that the instantaneous dipole layer of Fig. 1(a) is known from penetrating electrode work. Once we have decided on a segmentalization of the myocardium, both the directions and strengths of the dipoles in Fig. 1(b) are determined at that instant. However, these directions and strengths would only apply to the particular individual in whom the intramyocardial measurements were made.

If we move to another individual, what might we expect? The most general assumption would be that both the directions and strengths would be different and in principle a multiple dipole model could be used in this way. However, we assume (without having proved) that there would be practical difficulties in using the model in this way. We therefore adopt a further simplifying assumption: The direction of the dipole, that is, the direction of propagation of the depolarization wave in a particular segment, does not vary much from individual to individual. Then the dipole direction can be fixed, and only its strength left variable.

This is the manner in which we use the multiple dipole model. We conceptually divide the ventricular myocardium into 12 segments, locate a dipole in each, and choose the dipole directions on the basis of the intramyocardial measurements. This much is fixed on the model. The 12 dipole strengths are left as unknown functions of time, to be determined for each individual on the basis of surface potential measurements.

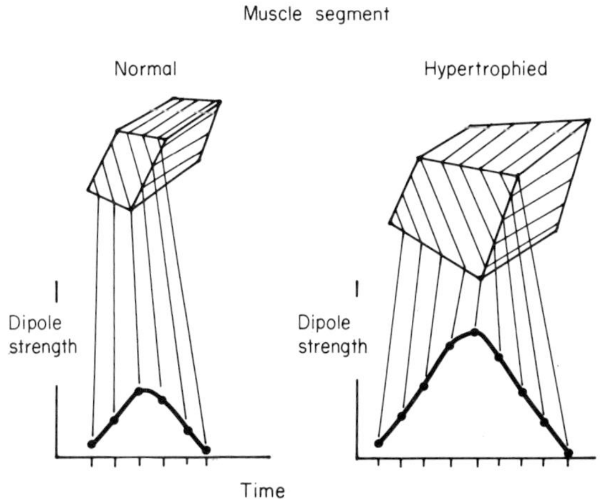

FIG. 2. A schematic representation of the postulated relationship between the volume of cardiac muscle and the time-varying dipole strength in normal and hypertrophy. The dipole time–strength integral is called dipole activity (DA).

Some features of the dipole strength–time curves can be anticipated as illustrated in Fig. 2. Before the depolarization wave has entered a segment, the corresponding dipole strength would be zero. As the wavefront enters the segment, the dipole strength rises and then declines again as the wavefront leaves. It was pointed out by Selvester *et al.* (1965) that the duration of the dipole strength–time pulse would be expected to be proportional to the thickness of the myocardial segment and that the dipole strength at any instant should be proportional to the area of the depolarization wavefront in the segment at that instant. If we assume that the speed of propagation of the depolarization wave is constant, it follows that the dipole strength–time integral is proportional to the mass of electrically active myocardium in the segment. This hypothesis is the basis of all interpretation of multiple dipole electrocardiograms presented in this chapter. The hypothesis implies that segmental hypertrophy manifests itself as an elevated strength–time integral (Fig. 2). For convenience, we give the strength–time integral the name "dipole activity" (DA).

Model of the Thorax

The model of the heart as an electrical source must be coupled with a model of the thorax as an electrical conductor before the relationship between source and observed potentials can be defined.

We use a thoracic model which is anatomically accurate [the anatomy being

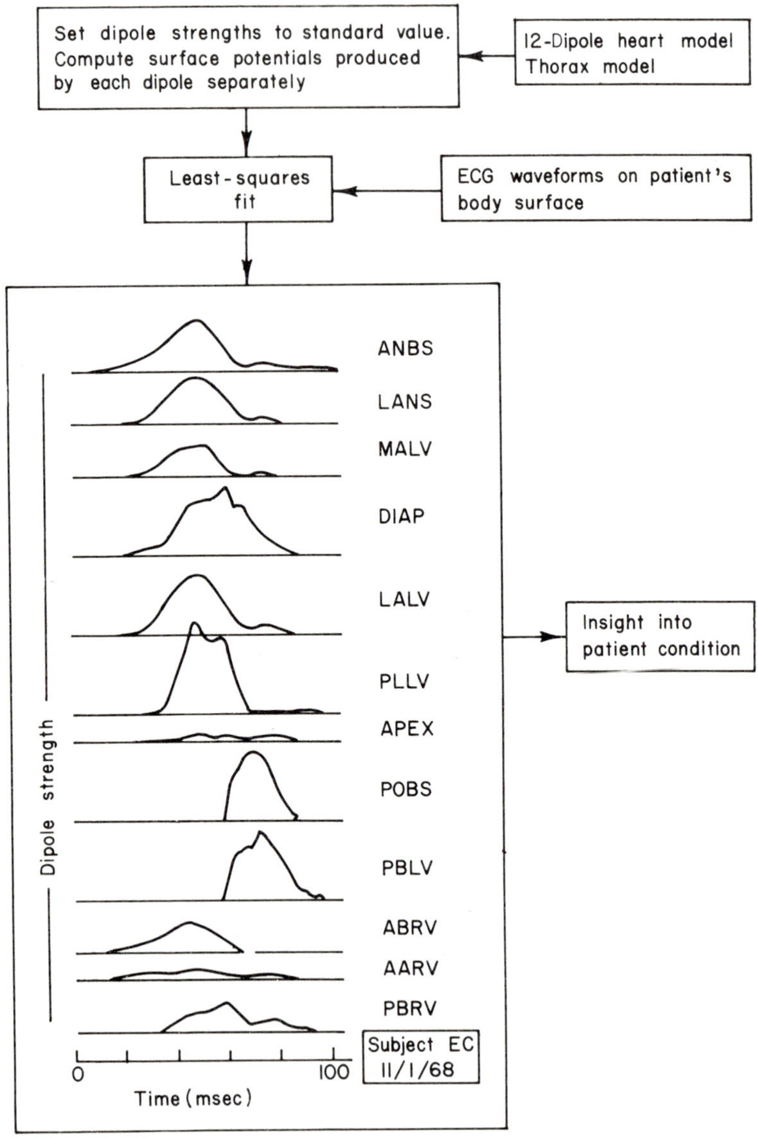

FIG. 3. A flow chart of the multiple dipole electrocardiographic method and the dipoles computed from a normal subject (see text for details). The dipole abbreviations are (ANBS), anterobasal septum; (LANS), low anterior septum; (MALV), midanterior left ventricle; (DIAP), diaphragmatic left ventricle; (LALV), lateral left ventricle; (PLLV), posterolateral left ventricle; (APEX), apex of septum; (POBS), posterobasal septum; (PBLV), posterobasal left ventricle; (ABRV), anterobasal right ventricle; (AARV), anteroapical right ventricle; and (PBRV), posterobasal right ventricle.

taken from a cross section anatomy text (Eycleshymer and Shoemaker, 1911] and which consists of several regions. The regions are internally homogeneous, but the electrical conductivity varies from region to region. Six regions are used: the two intracardiac blood masses, the two lungs, the remainder of the thorax (lumped into one region), and the surrounding air. This subdivision follows the guidance of Rush *et al* (1963), and the conductivities used were similar to those found by him.

Method

The method is outlined in Fig. 3. It is necessary first to determine the potentials produced on the surface by each myocardial segment separately, i.e., by each dipole with standard strength. If anatomical differences between individuals are ignored, these computations need only be performed once. The results can then be combined with instantaneous potential data from the body surface of an individual to determine the 12 dipole strengths that best fit the individual's body surface data at that instant. The procedure is similar to that of least-squares fitting and is repeated at intervals of either 1 or 2 msec through QRS. In this way, 12 dipole strength–time curves are built up. Since each instant is treated independently of all other instants, no constraints are imposed on the form of the dipole strength–time curves.

The 12-Dipole Electrocardiogram in Normal Subjects

Studies on about 75 normal subjects have been reported in the literature (Holt *et al.*, 1969a) and will be only briefly described here. The form of the dipole strength–time curves is often found to be a single pulse, which is as expected if the dipoles truly represent segmental activity (Fig. 3). Further, the sequence of onset of dipoles is consistent between normal individuals, and is in general agreement with the depolarization sequence determined by workers with direct intramyocardial measurements. When the segmental DA's are combined into activities for the septum, left ventricular (LV) free wall, and right ventricular (RV) free wall, the implied distribution of myocardial mass agrees fairly well with that determined by other workers in an autopsy series.

The 12-Dipole Electrocardiogram in LV Hypertrophy

Since this workshop concerns hypertrophy, these are the most relevant results. The main interest lies in the validity of the hypothesis that DA is proportional to segmental mass. If this is true, we then have a method for determining left or right ventricular muscle weight (LVMW or RVMW) using a completely noninvasive technique.

To examine this question in the LV, a series was selected from those individuals for whom 12-dipole electrocardiograms (MDECG's) were available and for whom LVMW's were known from LV biplane angiograms (Rackley *et al.*, 1964). The following groups of patients were excluded:

1. those with bundle-branch blocks, since the assumed depolarization directions would be inappropriate in such cases;

2. those with myocardial infarctions, since part of the tissue detected angiographically would not be electrically active (in a small series of such patients we have observed that the electrical mass is anomalously low soon after the occurrence of infarction, but recovers over a period of a few months);

3. those with Starr–Edwards valve prostheses at the time of the multiple dipole recording, since the short-circuiting effect of the metal cage is not included in the thoracic model;

4. those 25 years of age or less, since it has been established that young individuals tend to have high electrocardiographic voltages even when the heart is normal.

After these exclusions, the refined series contained 70 individuals, with a wide variety of cardiac diseases (including, for example, aortic stenosis, mitral stenosis, and ventricular septal defect).

Let us first consider the standard electrocardiograms of these patients. For many years, the Sokolow and Lyon (1949) criterion ($SV_1 + RV_{5,6} > 35$ mm) has been used as an indicator of left ventricular hypertrophy (LVH). In Fig. 4 this quantity is plotted against the LVMW determined from the biplane angiograms. The upper limit of LVMW in normal subjects, found by Kennedy *et al.* (1967), is indicated. It can be seen that the correlation is only fair, the coefficient of determination being $r^2 = 30\%$. Other criteria including the point-score method of Romhilt and Estes (1968) gave similar results. It may be argued that the Sokolow–Lyon criterion is only intended to detect LVH, not to quantify it. In this case it is relevant to note that the sensitivity of the criterion is 76% and the specificity 72% for this series of patients. A total of 26% of the individuals were misdiagnosed for the presence or absence of LVH.

In Fig. 5 the results obtained with the MDECG are shown. The dipole activity in the septum and left ventricular free wall (LVSDA) is plotted against the angiographic LVMW. It can be seen that the correlation is much better, the coefficient of determination being $r^2 = 90\%$. Apparently this noninvasive method enables us to estimate the LVMW with a standard error of 43 gm in this series of patients. If we use an upper limit of LVSDA in normal subjects, derived from a series of 58 individuals (Holt *et al.*, 1969a), we find the sensitivity and specificity of the method for diagnosis of LVH to be

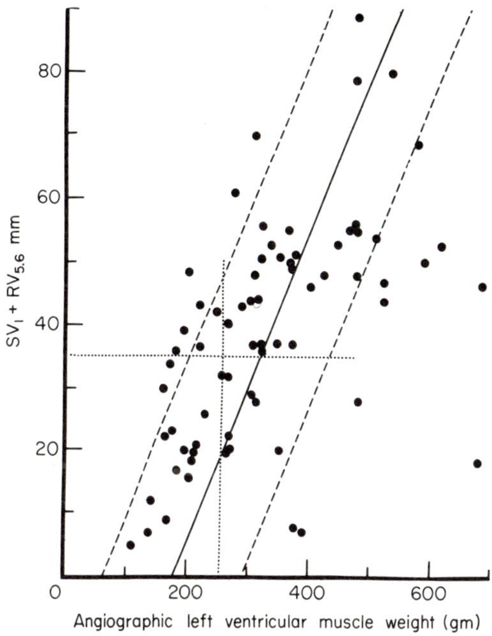

FIG. 4. The sum of the $SV_1 + RV_{5,6}$ from the electrocardiogram is plotted against angiographic left ventricular muscle weight (LVMW) from the same patients in Fig. 4. The short-dashed lines are the upper limits of normal used in the evaluation of diagnostic performance. The regression equation is $LVMW = 4.06(SV_1 + RV_{5,6}) + 177$. The long-dashed lines represent the standard error of the estimate (SEE). $n = 70$; $r^2 = 30\%$; SEE = 114 gm; sensitivity = 76%; and specificity = 72%.

98% and 81%, respectively. A total of 7% of the individuals were incorrectly diagnosed concerning the presence or absence of LVH. Similar results have been previously reported (Holt *et al.*, 1969b).

The 12-Dipole Electrocardiogram in RV Hypertrophy

As previously pointed out, not only are DA's computed for the LV and septum but also for the RV (RVDA's). In many of the LVH patients, the RVDA's as well as the LVDA's were elevated. This result is not unreasonable since many of these patients had chronic RV overload secondary to mitral valve disease or LV failure. Patients with clinical conditions resulting in only right ventricular hypertrophy (RVH) have increased RVDA's. As in pure LVH with increased LVDA, the RVDA in RVH is due to increased dipole strengths and durations. This presumably reflects increased RV wall thickness. In order to determine whether these results are correct, it is necessary to have

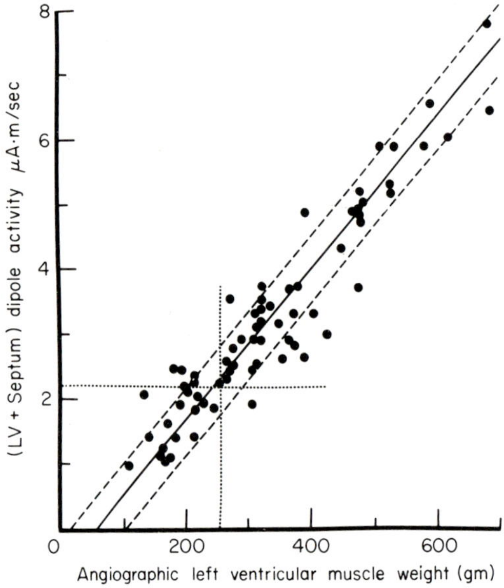

FIG. 5. The dipole activity in the left ventricle and septum (LVSDA) is plotted against angiographic left ventricular muscle weights (LVMW) for patients with various cardiac diseases. The short-dashed lines are the upper limits of normal used in the evaluation of diagnostic performance. The regression equation is LVMW = 85 • LVSDA + 59. The long-dashed lines represent the standard error of the estimate. $n = 70$; $r^2 = 90\%$; SEE = 43 gm; sensitivity = 98%; and specificity = 81%.

an independent method of gauging the RVMW. Unfortunately, no angiographic technique for measuring RVMW is available to us, and we do not have adequate autopsy data. The only independent data consistently available have been hemodynamic measurements.

We have used right ventricular systolic pressure (RVSP) as independent evidence of the RV condition. At best, RVSP indicates RVMW only in patients with conditions leading to RV pressure overload. In a series of 27 patients with such conditions, the correlation of determination between RVSP and RVDA was $r^2 = 86\%$. A sensitivity of 85% for RVH diagnosis by MDECG was obtained, and the specificity based upon the normal series was 94% (Holt *et al.*, 1969c). This diagnostic and quantitative ability was considerably better than that of conventional electrocardiography. Thus, we would conclude that the MDECG may be very useful in separating RV from LV electrical activity, an area in which conventional electrocardiography has been generally unsatisfactory. Although these results are encouraging, further studies currently in progress are clearly indicated.

Summary

Body surface potentials in patients with ventricular hypertrophy were evaluated using a method in which the electrical heart is regarded as a multiple dipole generator. The thoracic electrical inhomogeneities and geometry are considered in the model. The time-varying strengths of 12 dipoles (representing the depolarization of the ventricles) were calculated. In patients with left or right ventricular hypertrophy the respective dipole strengths and durations are increased over normal.

Acknowledgments

This work was aided by research funds from the Veterans Administration; Research Grants HE 11310-02, 2M01-FR00032-09, and Contract PH 43-67-1441 from the U. S. Public Health Service; Research Grant RD 2219-M from the Vocational Rehabilitation Administration; and a grant-in-aid from the Alabama Heart Association. The work reported here is the continuation of a project which began as a joint project between the University of Alabama School of Medicine and the IBM Houston Scientific Center. Many individuals at both locations made substantial contributions, but we would particularly like to mention the work of Dr. M. Stuart Lynn in laying foundations upon which the present results rest.

References

Burton, A. C. (1965). *In* "Physiology and Biophysics of the Circulation," pp. 115–120. Year Book Medical Publishers, Chicago, Illinois.

Durrer, D. (1966). *Trans. Stud. Coll. Physicians Philadelphia* **33,** 159.

Einthoven, W., Fahr, G., and de Waart, A. (1913). *Pfluegers Arch. Gesampte Physiol. Menschen Tiere* **150,** 275 [Translated by H. E. Hoff and P. Sekelj (1950), *Amer. Heart J.* **40,** 163.]

Eychleshymer, A. C., and Shoemaker, D. M. (1911). *In* "A Cross-Section Anatomy." D. Appleton, New York.

Holt, J. H., Jr., Barnard, A. C. L., Lynn, M. S., and Svendsen, P. (1969a). *Circulation* **40,** 687.

Holt, J. H., Jr., Barnard, A. C. L., and Lynn, M. S. (1969b). *Circulation* **40,** 697.

Holt, J. H., Jr., Barnard, A. C. L., Lynn, M. S., and Kramer, J. O., Jr. (1969c). *Circulation* **40,** 711.

Kennedy, J. W., Reichenbach, D. D., Baxley, W. A., and Dodge, H. T. (1967). *Amer. J. Cardiol.* **19,** 221.

Rackley, C. E., Dodge, H. T., Coble, Y. D., and Hay, R. E. (1964). *Circulation* **29,** 666.

Romhilt, D. W., and Estes, E. H., Jr. (1968). *Amer. Heart J.* **75,** 752.

Rush, S., Abildskov, J. A., and McFee, R. (1963). *Circ. Res.* **12,** 40.

Scher, A. M. (1962). *In* "Handbook of Physiology" (W. F. Hamilton and P. Dow, eds.), Vol. I, Sec. 2: Circulation, pp. 287–322. American Physiological Society, Washington, D.C.

Selvester, R. H. (1970). Unpublished data.

Selvester, R. H., Collier, C. R., and Pearson, R. B. (1965). *Circulation* **31,** 45.

Sokolow, M., and Lyon, T. P. (1949). *Amer. Heart J.* **37,** 161.

MULTIPOLE APPROACH TO ELECTROCARDIOGRAPHY

David B. Geselowitz and Stanley A. Briller

The electrocardiogram arises from electrical sources in the myocardium during depolarization and repolarization of the membranes of cardiac cells. In principle, knowledge of the distribution and strength of these sources throughout the myocardium at each instant of time in conjunction with knowledge of the electrical conductivity of the body tissues is sufficient for calculation of the surface electrocardiogram. This is called the "forward" problem.

By contrast, the "inverse" problem is the determination of cardiac electric sources from the surface electrocardiogram. It follows from the laws of electricity, however, that one cannot unambiguously calculate the internal sources from the surface potential distribution in the absence of detailed electrophysiological information about the heart and surrounding tissues (Helmholtz, 1853). In other words, the "inverse" problem does not have a unique solution.

Suppose a region such as the heart contains electrical sources, but that we are restricted to measurements *outside* this region. No matter how much detail the electric potential distribution is measured in, the only available information concerning the sources would be provided by their multipole components (Yeh *et al.*, 1958; Geselowitz, 1960; Brody *et al.*, 1961). These components are obtained by expanding the electrical potential in an infinite series with a point in the source region used as an origin. This infinite series is the multipole expansion (Stratton, 1941).

Consider, for example, current sources in an unbounded homogeneous conductor of conductivity, g. When the electric potential, V', outside the source region is expressed as a function of spherical coordinates (r, θ, ϕ), it must be of the form

$$V' = \frac{1}{4\pi g} \sum_{n=0}^{\infty} \sum_{m=0}^{n} (2 - \delta_{mo}) \frac{(n-m)!}{(n+m)!} \frac{1}{r^{n+1}} (a_{nm} \cos m\phi + b_{nm} \sin m\phi) P_n^m(\cos \theta) \tag{1}$$

where n and m are positive integers, δ_{mo} is the Kronecker delta (which is equal to unity for $m = 0$ and zero otherwise), P_n^m is an associated Legendre polynomial, and a_{nm} and b_{nm} are constants. This equation can be written more compactly if we define a set of complex functions ψ_{nm} such that

$$\psi_{nm} = (2 - \delta_{mo}) \frac{(n-m)!}{(n+m)!} r^n \exp(im\phi) P_n^m(\cos\theta) \tag{2}$$

Then

$$V' = \text{Re}\left\{ \sum_{n=0}^{\infty} \sum_{m=0}^{n} (a_{nm} + ib_{nm}) r^{-(2n+1)} \psi_{nm} \right\} \tag{3}$$

when Re denotes the real part of the complex number and $i = \sqrt{-1}$.

The information concerning the sources is contained in the set of multipole coefficients a_{nm} and b_{nm}. It is convenient to consider the cardiac sources as a distribution of current dipoles. In a very small region of the heart of volume dv the current dipole is $\mathbf{m}\, dv$, where $\mathbf{m}$ is then the current dipole moment per unit volume. Since $\mathbf{m}\, dv$ has the dimensions of current times length e.g., *ma–cm*, m has the dimensions of current per unit area.

The particular relation between the multipole coefficients and the source distribution $\mathbf{m}$, can be shown to be (Geselowitz, 1960, 1967)

$$a_{mn} + ib_{nm} = \int \mathbf{m} \cdot \nabla \psi_{nm}\, dv \tag{4}$$

where the integration is over the region containing sources.

In the case of electrocardiography, the sources are not in an unbounded conductor. Rather the potential distribution, V, is accessible on the surface of the torso, which is a bounded volume conductor. The multipole coefficients are related to V as follows (Geselowitz, 1960, 1967):

$$a_{nm} + ib_{nm} = \int gV \nabla \psi_{nm} \cdot d\mathbf{S} \tag{5}$$

where $d\mathbf{S}$ is an element of area on the body surface.

If the associated Legendre polynomials are written out, Eq. (1) becomes

$$\begin{aligned} V' = \frac{1}{4\pi g} \Bigg\{ & \frac{a_{00}}{r} + \frac{1}{r^2}(a_{10}\cos\theta + a_{11}\sin\theta\cos\phi + b_{11}\sin\theta\sin\phi) \\ & + \frac{1}{r^3}[a_{20}(\cos^2\theta - \tfrac{1}{2}\sin^2\theta) + (a_{21}\cos\phi + b_{21}\sin\phi)\cos\theta\sin\theta \\ & + \tfrac{1}{4}(a_{22}\cos 2\phi + b_{22}\sin 2\phi)\sin^2\theta] + \dots \Bigg\} \end{aligned} \tag{6}$$

The potential contributed by the first term in the multipole expansion, a_{00}, varies inversely with the distance from the source region. Since each dipole element contributes zero net current, the monopole term, which is the net current contributed by all the dipoles, is zero. This result follows formally from Eqs. (2) and (4), since $\nabla\psi_{00}$ is zero. The monopole is the zero-order term of the expansion because it is the term for which $n = 0$.

The second term, or first-order term of the multipole expansion, is the dipole. It is the first nonvanishing term, and its contribution to the potential varies inversely with the square of the distance from the origin. The dipole term has three components a_{10}, a_{11}, and b_{11} which may be identified in Eq. (6) as the z, x, and y components, respectively, of a vector. This vector, the dipole term of the multipole expansion, is the vector sum over all the elemental dipoles, since it follows from Eq. (4) that

$$\begin{aligned} a_{10} &= \int m_z \, dv \\ a_{11} &= \int m_x \, dv \qquad (7) \\ b_{11} &= \int m_y \, dv \end{aligned}$$

The second-order term in the multipole expansion is the quadrupole. Its contribution to the potential varies inversely with the cube of the distance. A quadrupole may be thought of as a pair of equal and opposite dipoles, just as a dipole may be regarded as a pair of equal and opposite sources (charges or currents). A quadrupole is described by five components a_{20}, a_{21}, b_{21}, a_{22}, b_{22}.

It is possible that at some instant of time the vector sum over all the dipole sources in the heart vanishes, i.e., the dipole sources in one region of the heart "cancel" the dipoles in another region. Is the ECG potential then zero? No—there may still be nonzero quadrupole (or higher-order) terms which will give rise to a potential.* And even if the dipole term is nonzero, there may be a significant quadrupole contribution to the surface electrocardiogram.

The heart vector or dipole, a concept introduced by Einthoven *et al.* (1913), is the dipole term in the multipole expansion. Therefore, higher-order terms may be considered refinements of the Einthoven model that provide a progressively more detailed description of electrical activity in the heart. It is of historical interest that Wilson suggested that Einthoven had the multipole

* An example of a source distribution that does *not* give rise to an electric field is a *uniform* dipole layer (Helmholtz double layer) forming a *closed* surface. In this case, all the multipole coefficients vanish.

expansion in mind when he proposed the heart vector model (Wilson *et al.*, 1946).

It was stated above that the available information concerning the sources is contained in the multipole components. If nothing further is known about the source region, then no more specific information about the sources can be obtained, although the information can be presented in alternative mathematical forms (Gabor and Nelson, 1954). In fact, considerable knowledge is available about the heart and its milieu. We have a good idea of the heart's location, tissue conductivities, and the pattern of spread of excitation. Questions of current interest are how to utilize this information to describe the sources in more physiological detail, and what are the theoretical and practical limitations governing the amount of detail that can be obtained.

An approach to the problem was stated by Fischmann and Barber (1963) who proposed an "aimed lead" that would respond strongly to activity in a particular region of the heart muscle, and very weakly to activity elsewhere. They proceeded to investigate a six-dipole model of the heart, in which each dipole represented activity in a local region. The dipole locations and orientations were chosen on the basis of heart geometry and electrophysiology, thus incorporating in the analysis specific data about the source region.

With the advent of the digital computer and with increased knowledge of the spread of excitation obtained from myocardial plunge electrodes, interest in solving the forward problem in some detail has grown.

Selvester *et al.*, (1965) have studied a 20-dipole model of electrical activity in which the dipoles are fixed in position and orientation on the basis of anatomical considerations, and are made to vary in time on the basis of data obtained in plunge electrode studies. They have shown that this model accounts reasonably well for the normal and abnormal vectorcardiogram.

Thus, it is very tempting to venture to go backwards and calculate the dipole moments from the surface ECG. This general analytic technique in electrocardiography, called the multiple dipole model, is not essentially different from that suggested by Fischmann and Barber. The essential features include lumping distributed activity in a number of discrete dipoles and selecting dipole locations on the basis of heart geometry. In variations of the technique, the dipole orientations may or may not be fixed, and the torso may or may not be considered a homogeneous conductor (Bellman *et al.*, 1964; Barnard *et al.*, 1967; Horan and Flowers, 1967; Rogers and Pilkington, 1966; Barr and Pilkington, 1969; Plonsey, 1966).

Will this approach to the inverse problem work? Detailed studies have been reported by T. C. Pilkington and his students (Rogers and Pilkington, 1966; Barr and Pilkington, 1969), with somewhat pessimistic results. The difficulty can be illustrated as follows. If one chooses 20 dipoles, computes the potential on the body surface, and then uses this information in turn to calculate the 20 dipole moments, these moments can be retrieved exactly. But suppose some noise is added to the system—or suppose the dipole positions and orientations are shifted somewhat. What happens to the inverse solution? The answer is that even with unrealistically small amounts of noise, the solutions may change dramatically. In other words, the solution of the inverse problem may be a set of 20 dipole moments very much different from the original set, yet one which leads to the same potential distribution on the surface within the limits of the inevitably present added noise. An explicit theoretical relationship between multipole dipole solutions of this type and the distribution of current sources remains to be developed.

As the number of dipoles used to represent the heart is decreased, the ambiguity in calculating the dipole moments in the presence of noise diminishes (Barr and Pilkington, 1969). On the other hand, an error is introduced by lumping activity in larger regions of muscle into fewer dipole sources.

The multiple dipole model is being studied in other laboratories to determine whether it can be made a useful diagnostic tool (Holt *et al.*, this volume). We are currently investigating an aimed lead which has its theoretical basis in the multipole expansion and which incorporates information concerning heart geometry and electrophysiology. The derivation assumes the heart wall to be a spherical shell in which activity is radially propagated. The origin of the multipole expansion is at the center of the shell and the polar axis is rotated until it passes through the region of interest. The resulting lead is a linear combination of dipole, quadrupole, and higher-order terms (Geselowitz and Arthur, 1968; Arthur, 1968). Selectivity for the local region of interest increases as additional terms are added, and is limited by the number of multipole terms that can be measured from surface electrocardiograms.

Another transformation under investigation provides the location in the torso of the heart's electrical center (Arthur, 1968; Geselowitz, 1968). The electrical center is defined as the location at which the dipole alone best accounts for the electrocardiographic potential. The electrical center will vary during the cardiac cycle, and combined with the dipole (vectorcardiogram), it will give information to represent the heart as a moving dipole.

One of our students, R. M. Arthur, has recently completed a dissertation (Arthur, 1968) applying the multipole concept to the human electrocardiogram, and is preparing his results for publication. His data indicate that significant quadrupole components are present in the human electrocardiogram, that in one normal subject the dipole plus quadrupole components account very well for surface electrocardiograms, and that a clinically practical lead system for obtaining the dipole and quadrupole utilizing 17 body surface electrodes is feasible. For this subject, the moving electrical center was in the region of the atria during the inscription of the P wave, and in the region of the ventricles during QRS and T.

Development of aimed leads may provide a useful tool for diagnosing many cardiac abnormalities, including left, right, and biventricular hypertrophy. However, in order to achieve optimum utilization of aimed leads, it is essential that sufficient data be available concerning electrical excitation and recovery in the various diseased states of the heart. Hypertrophy is one of many clinical states for which such information is meagre at this time.

Acknowledgment

This work was supported by United States Public Health Service Grant HE-08805.

References

Arthur, R. M. (1968). Ph.D. Dissertation, University of Pennsylvania, Philadelphia.

Barnard, A. C. L., Lynn, M. S., Holt, J. M., and Sheffield, L. T. (1967). *Biophys. J.* **7,** 925.

Barr, R. C., and Pilkington, T. C. (1969). *IEEE Trans. Bio-med. Eng.* **16,** 205.

Bellman, R., Collier, C., Kagiwada, H., Kalaba, R., and Selvester, R. (1964). *Commun. ACM* **7,** 666.

Brody, D. A., Bradshaw, J. C., and Evans, J. W. (1961). *IRE Trans. Bio-Med. Electron.* **8,** 139.

Einthoven, W., Fahr, G., and de Waart, A. (1913). *Pfluegers Arch. gesampte Physiol. menschen Tiere* **150,** 275. (Translated in *Amer. Heart J.* **40,** 163, 1950.)

Fischmann, E. J., and Barber, M. R. (1963). *Amer. Heart J.* **65,** 628.

Gabor, D., and Nelson, C. V. (1954). *J. Appl. Phys.* **25,** 413.

Geselowitz, D. B. (1960). *Proc. IRE,* **48,** 75.

Geselowitz, D. B. (1967). *Biophys. J.* **7,** 1.

Geselowitz, D. B. (1968). *IEEE Trans. Bio.-Med. Eng.* **15,** 303.

Geselowitz, D. B., and Arthur, R. M. (1968). *Biophys. J. Soc. Abstr.* **8,** 47.

Helmholtz, H. (1853). Poggendorff's Ann. **89,** 211 and 353.

Horan, L., and Flowers, N. (1967). *Med. Res. Eng.* **6,** 28.

Plonsey, R. (1966). *Biophys. J.* **6,** 153.

Rogers, C. L., and Pilkington, T. C. (1966). *IEEE Trans. Bio-Med. Eng.* **15,** 312.

Selvester, R. H., Collier, C. R., and Pearson, R. B. (1965). *Circulation* **31,** 45.

Stratton, J. A. (1941). "Electromagnetic Theory," pp. 175–183. McGraw-Hill, New York.

Wilson, F. N., Johnston, F. D., Rosenbaum, F. F., and Barker, P. S. (1946). *Amer. Heart J.* **32,** 277.

Yeh, G. C. K., Martinek, J., and deBeaumont, H. (1958). *Bull. Math. Biophys.* **20,** 203.

SUBJECT INDEX

I

J

K

L

M

N

O

P

T